Dear Reader

Kathy Moore

I am pleased to present you with my most recent book in this Special First Edition...

"THE ENCYCLOPEDIA OF HYPNOTHERAPY" which represents a lifetime of interest and research in this important realm of hypnosis.

May you find this of value to yourself.

Hypnotically yours,

Ormond McGill

A Letter to You From Ormond McGill, PhD
The Dean Of American Hypnosis

"Something for everyone. Simple philosophy, profound wisdom, hundreds of inductions, scripts, & techniques that make life work & hypnotherapy what it is- powerful, transformational & exciting!"

  —Jillian LaVelle, CHt, Fellow
  Author
  Founder, International Association of Counselors & Therapists®

"After a lifetime of experience, the Dean of Hypnosis, Ormond McGill has written THE definitive book on the power of persuasion & hypnotizing yourself or another. If you are a therapist this is the one book you should have on your shelf."

  —Richard Neves, PhD
  Author, Trainer
  President, American Board of Hypnotherapy®

"I was influenced by Ormond McGill when I was beginning to practice hypnosis and I'm still influenced by him today, this book isn't just the work of a lifetime, it's the work of two or three lifetimes."

  —Richard Sutphen, CHt
  "We Were Born Again To Be Together"
  Founder, Valley of the Sun Publishing

"In this monumental work, Ormond shares the nuts and bolts of the profession; completely new and innovative ideas as well as the old timer's techniques. He shows the novice and seasoned professional how to do hypnosis easily and effortlessly. Our gratitude is beyond words for all that Ormond McGill has given to the art and science of hypnotism."

  —Anne Spencer-Beacham, PhD
  "The Complete Hypnotherapist's Kit: A Marketing Manual"
  Founder, International Medical & Dental Hypnotherapy Association®

"A masterpiece! This brilliant, clear, down-to-earth book is a must for anyone interested in harnessing the power of the mind."

  —Shelley Stockwell-Nicholas, PhD, Fellow
  "Hypnosis: How To Put A Smile On Your Face & $$$ In Your Pocket"
  Founder, International Hypnosis Federation®

"A renaissance man who has his hand on the pulse of humanity. I've read everything he's ever written and studied with him and am so impressed by his deep wisdom and respect for his clients. Ormond McGill is an Institution. "
—Maurice Kouguell, PhD, Diplomate/Fellow
"DAPTH©: Accessing the Unconscious in Hypnosis & Counseling"

"Brings the genius of McGill to all of us; from the lay person to the professional. I've put this book right next to my dictionary."
—Nica Lee, CEO, Orderly Systems

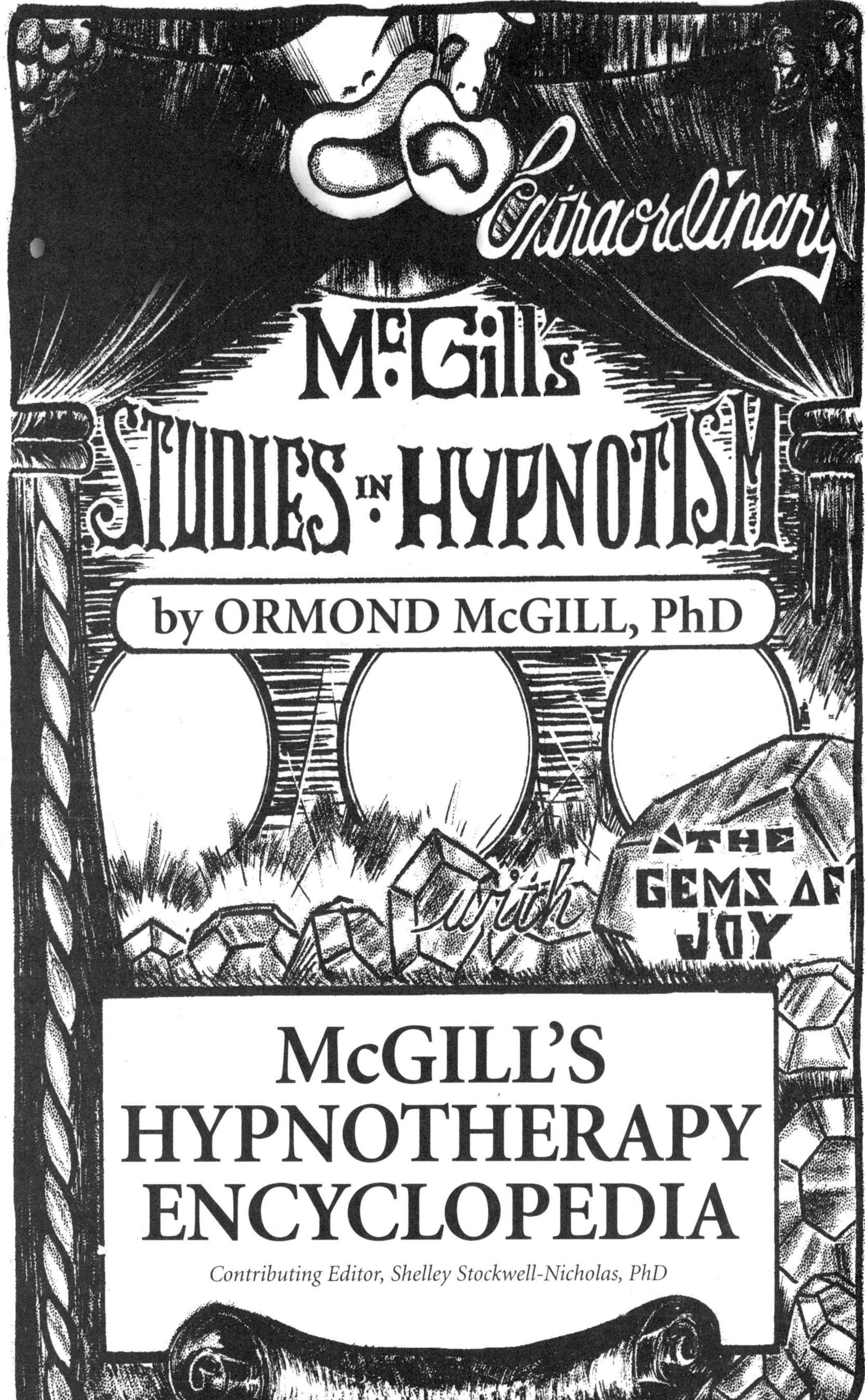

McGILL'S HYPNOTHERAPY ENCYCLOPEDIA

Contributing Editor, Shelley Stockwell-Nicholas, PhD

Illustration by Ormond McGill

ISBN Number: 0-912559-74-8
Library of Congress Number: 2003100604

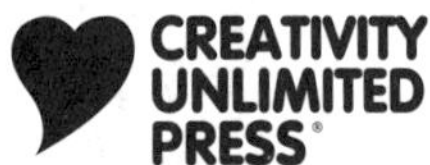

Creativity Unlimited Press®
30819 Casilina Drive, Rancho Palos Verdes, CA 90275, USA
www.internationalhypnosisfederation.com
(310) 541-4844

DISCLOSURE
Hypnotherapy is a legal health-care and help-care profession & not a licensed healing arts profession. Practitioners worldwide practice this proud profession in private and public. It is wildly popular because of its profound positive results. This book educates the reader on ways to use hypnosis and hypnotherapy for mind, body, social and spiritual wellness to cope with life, mood states, out-of-control behavior and illness and teaches how to help others do the same.

Based on personal observations, experience, case studies and research, the authors and publisher of this work expressly disclaim responsibility for any adverse effects arising from the use or application of the information contained in this book and the authors and publisher expressly claim responsibility for all good effects arising from the use or application of the information contained in this book.

Published in the USA

Credits

Contributing Editor: Shelley Stockwell-Nicholas
Photos and Cover Design: Jon Nicholas and Wendy Wilsing
Graphic Arts: Wendy Wilsing
Illustrations: Ormond McGill, Shelley Stockwell-Nicholas,
and Clark Dunbar (© RF RubberBall Productions)
Model: Kathy Kay

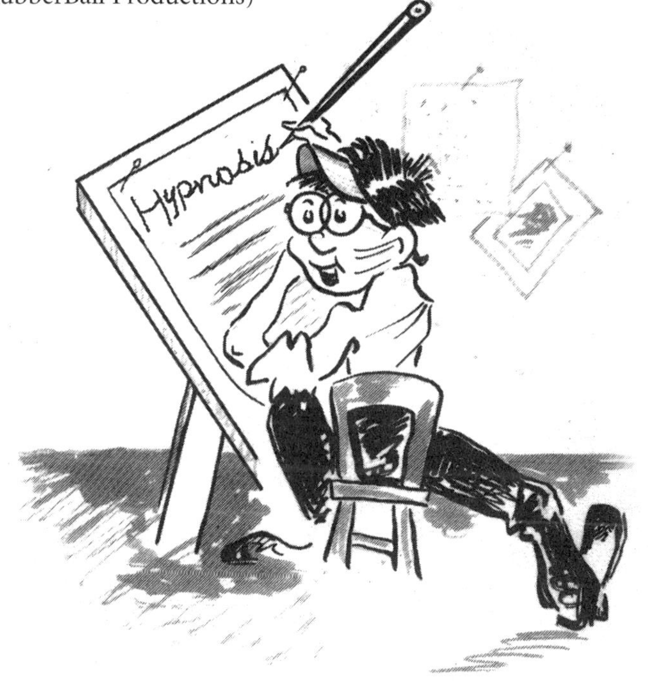

Illustration by Ormond McGill

Elder Contributors: Bernheim, Braid, Charcot, Coue`, de Puysegur, DeWaldosa, Erickson, Einstein, Elman, Esdaile, The Essenes, Jung, James, Liebeault, Mesmer, Munro, Perls, Tebbits, von Reichenbach and Vogel.

Moderns who contributed to this book: Charlene Ackerman, Norbert Bakas, Dwight Bale, Carl Joseph Berg, Peter Blum, Randal Churchill, Dewie Devers, Paul Durban, Michael Ellner, Diana L. England, Edith Fiore, Joe Hammer, Phillip Holder, William Horton, Roy Hunter, Gerald Kein, Dewey Kerr, Al Krasner, Jillian LaVelle, Alex Lessin, Serena Luminere, Irvin Mordes, Winifred Morice, Del Hunter Morrill, Marleen Mulder, Richard Neves, David John Oates, Robert Otto, Stephanie Rothman, Tom Silver, Anne Spencer (-Beacham), Barbara Stansberry, Shelley Stockwell (-Nicholas), Ernest Telkemeyer, Jeffrey Thompson, Niccolous Thompson, Sharon E. Toole, Jerry Valley, Anna Vitali, Gaye Wilson and Joseph Worrell for generously sharing your ideas and copyrighted work.

Heartfelt gratitude to Chuck Mignosa, Liz Fortini, Susan Gilmore, Nica Lee, Jon Nicholas, Wendy Wilsing & Stephanie Woolley for your loving help in producing this work and to each of Ormond McGill's treasured friends in the hypnosis field.

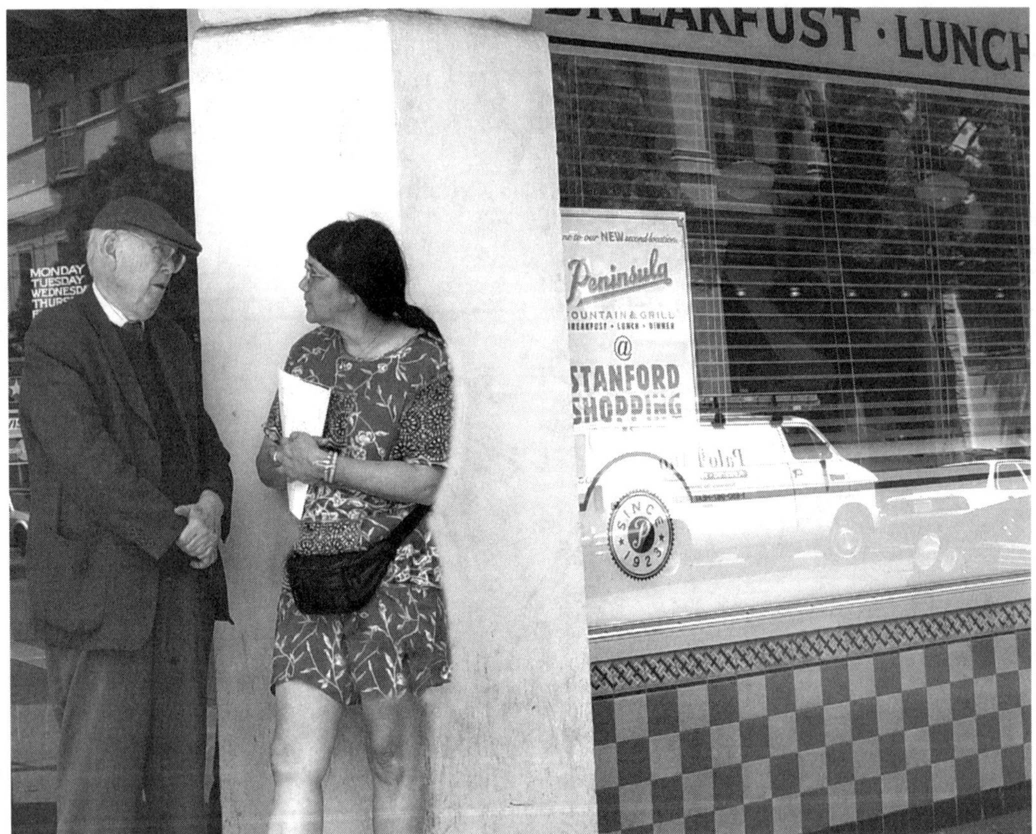

Photo by Jon Nicholas

Ormond and Shelley at the Creamery, Palo Alto, CA.

Forward

By Editor Shelley Stockwell-Nicholas, PhD

Welcome to the most original, comprehensive, step-by-step book of hypnotherapy ever written. If you are a neophyte or professional you will be enthralled by this adventure into the mysteries and use of mind. It's loaded with every conceivable hypnosis approach from classic Mesmerism to the newest cutting edge techniques. Many have never been written about before. You'll easily hypnotize yourself or others to joyously change the world one person at a time.

Those who meet the venerable author of this masterpiece, Ormond McGill, PhD are stunned by his wealth of knowledge, profound wisdom, velvet voice and the turquoise blue sparkle from his eyes. Over ninety-years-young, he knows more about hypnosis than any other living soul and generously shares his lifelong experience as a Teacher, Hypnotherapist and Performer. His 40 books are classics in the field and popular bestsellers in Europe, Asia and the United States.

In editing this one-of-a-kind book, I found myself saying again and again, "Ormond is a genius!" When I mentioned this to him he said, "I'm an expert on mocha chip milkshakes from the Creamery and butterflies." Ormond is a delightful and humble gem.

I have had the privilege of working and teaching with Dr. McGill for many years. When you read this masterpiece, you'll feel as if Ormond McGill is your own personal mentor and coach as well. I have carefully edited his wise words with the hope that they bring you to the greatest level of your own genius.

Thank you Ormond, for devoting so much of your life to bring us this amazing, one-of-a-kind experience of the hypnotherapy craft: I, and your readers, sit humbly at your feet.

Hypnotically Yours,

Shelley Stockwell-Nicholas

Shelley Stockwell-Nicholas

Dedication

This book is dedicated to the loving memory of Dave Elman, Master Instructor of Hypnotherapy. His wisdom is infused into the very pages of this work.

"When the activity of mind is under control, it becomes like pure crystal, reflecting equally without distortion, the perception, the perceiver and the perceived. It is through such mind that consciousness is known. Such a mind is a MASTERMIND."
 —Patanjali, 128 B.C.

Table of Contents

A PERSONAL LETTER FROM ORMOND McGILL
FOREWORD by Editor Shelley Stockwell-Nicholas ix
DEDICATION xi
CONTENTS xii
INTRODUCTION xix
PREFACE xxv

PART ONE: HYPNOTHERAPY BASICS
1. What Is Hypnosis? 1
2. Additional Thoughts 5
3. The Power Of Belief 7
4. Healing Waters 9
5. Were You Hypnotized? 11
6. The Question Of Will Power 15
7. Five Hypnotic Mind Myths 17
8. Hypnotic Hodge-Podge 19
9. Basic Structure Of A Session 23
10. The Consultation 29
11. Pre-Hypnosis Hypnosis 33
12. Direct Mental Marriage Hypnosis 35
13. Thoughts To Play With 37
14. Answers For Clients 39
15. Professional Wisdom & Protocols 45
16. Stockwell's Legal Requirements 47

PART TWO: INDUCING HYPNOSIS
17. Inductions 65
18. Hypnotic Sleep 75
19. Producing Somnambulism 79
20. Elman's Hypnotic Coma 83
21. The Art of Waking Hypnosis 87
22. From Waking To Trance 91
23. Establishing The Hypnotic Mood 93
24. Waking Hypnotic Inductions & Convincers 95
25. Rapid Induction To Profound Trance 103
26. More Rapid Inductions 105
27. The Relaxation Method 109
28. William James Let's Pretend 113
29. I Can, I Can't Rapid Inductions 117
30. Let's Pretend Some More 121
31. Acting Out Hypnosis For The "I Can't Be Hypnotized" 125
32. Ideomotor Induction 129
33. Sandy Beach Induction 131
34. Serenity (Symbiotical) Resonance Sound 133
35. Magnetic Mind Toning 137
36. The Holistic Method 141

37.   Quotation Induction 143
38.   Elman's Rapid Induction 147
39.   You Are The Star Hypnotherapy...153
40.   Bale's Outside/Inside Induction 157
41.   England's Rag Doll Induction 159
42.   Hypnotizing Children 163
43.   Candy Induction 171
44.   Blum's Singing Bowl Induction...173
45.   Transpersonal Induction 175
46.   Hypnodance 177
47.   Otto's Vertigo Induction 179
48.   Whirling Dervish Induction 181
49.   Instant Gamma Hypnosis 185
50.   Oriental Hypnotherapy Inductions 189
51.   Oriental Cobra Method..193

PART THREE: SUGGESTION FORMULAS SCRIPTS

52.   Fundamentals Of Successful Suggestions..199
53.   Self-Hypnosis 207
54.   The Power Of Suggestion 211
55.   Post-Hypnotic Suggestions 213
56.   Mental Set Hypnosis & The Sense Of Time..217
57.   Kein On The Law Of Compounding 221
58.   Self-Hypnosis For The Mature Adult 223
59.   Self Improvement Suggestions 225
60.   Suggestions With Deep Meaning 227
61.   Color Me Rich, Slim & Vital 229
62.   Sunshine Self-Esteem Suggestions 233
63.   Stop Smoking Today 235
64.   Sphere Of Energy To Stop Smoking 239
65.   Stockwell's Quit Smoking Approach 241
66.   Super Learning & Sports Performance..247
67.   Suggestions For Will & Memory...251
68.   Sleep Learning 253
69.   Stockwell's Poetry Hypnosis 255
70.   Energy, Confidence & Stamina 259
71.   Snuggle Down And Be Comfortable 261
72.   Tension, Stress And Depression 263
73.   Holder's Stress Management..265
74.   Einstein's Happiness Script 269
75.   The Happiness Way 271
76.   Plugged-In Happiness Hypnosis..275
77.   Hypnotherapy Of Pleasure 277
78.   The Hypnotherapy Of Luck 279
79.   The Conscious Smile Technique...281
80.   Hypnotherapy Of Laughter..283
81.   Stockwell's Hypnotherapy Of Persuasion...285
82.   Cosmically Maximize Suggestion 289

PART FOUR: HYPNOTHERAPY TECHNIQUES

83. Nothing-Need-Be-Done Hypnotherapy......................................293
84. Hypnotherapy Of Nothingness...295
85. Active Participation Hypnotherapy 297
86. Subconscious Hypnotherapist..299
87. Talking To Yourself Hypnotherapy 301
88. Stockwell's Subpersonality Approach 303
89. Hunter's Parts Hypnotherapy 307
90. The Slow-Down Clinic 313
91. Forget You Not Hypnotherapy 315
92. Computer Hypnotherapy 319
93. Infinite Smallness Hypnotherapy 325
94. Right Brain/Left Brain Hypnotherapy 327
95. Count Your Blessings Hypnosis 331
96. Your Little Theater Of The Mind 333
97. NLP Hypnotherapy 335
98. Stockwell-Nicholas NLP 337
99. NLP Movie Theater Techniques 347
100. Hypnotic Dream Work 351
101. Hypnotherapy Of Imagination 355
102. Aladdin's Arabian Hypnotherapy 357
103. The Hypnotic Seal 361
104. Abreaction Management 363
105. Stockwell's Ericksonian Hypnosis......................................367

PART FIVE: RELATIONSHIP HYPNOTHERAPY

106. Developing Personal Magnetism 375
107. Matrimony Hypnotherapy 381
108. Heart-Mending Hypnosis 383
109. Mind Trap Hypnotherapy 387
110. Stockwell-Nicholas Cognitive Hypnotherapy 391

PART SIX: MIND/BODY FITNESS

111. Mental Set Hypnosis 409
112. Mental Set Your Weight 411
113. Stockwell-Nicholas Joy Therapy 413
114. Coue's Autosuggestion For Wellness....................................417
115. Good Health Hypnotherapy 421
116. Anti-Aging Hunza Breath 423
117. Hypnotherapy Of Death 427
118. Common Sense Hypnotherapy...431
119. Stockwell's Hypno Wellness 433
120. Astral Hypno-Healing 441
121. Ellner's Neuro Linguistic Healing (NLH) 445
122. Reflexology Hypnotherapy 447
123. Stockwell-Nicholas Sleep Program.....................................451
124. Vitali's Hypnoaesthetics For Beautiful Skin 457
125. 3-D Hypnotherapy..461

PART SEVEN: ENERGY HYPNOTHERAPY

126. Hypnosis History And Energy Overview 467
127. Acupressure Hypnotherapy 473
128. Mesmerism/Hypnosis 477
129. Mesmer on Mesmerism 481
130. Mesmer's Fantasy & Facts 485
131. Bio Magnetic Hypnotherapy - Baron von Reichenbach 489
132. Magnetic Healing 491
133. Hypno-Reiki 499
134. Tapping Techniques 503
135. Vogel's Energized Hypnotherapy Couch 507
136. Light & Sound Hypnotherapy 509
137. Psycho Acoustic Hypnotherapy 511
138. Vitality Hypnosis 513
139. Stockwell's Biochemistry Of What You Feel 517

PART EIGHT: BE WELL NOW HYPNOSIS

140. Mental Anesthesia: Esdaile And Munro 531
141. Suggestive Therapeutics 533
142. Suggestive Therapeutics For Mastering Unwanted Habits 537
143. Waking Anesthesia 539
144. Mulder's Glove Anesthesia 543
145. Stockwell's Hypno-Anesthesia 545
146. Stockwell's Pain Management 551
147. Good Bye Headache 559

PART NINE: HYPNOTHERAPY SPECIALTIES

148. Pre-Birth Hypnotherapy 565
149. Stockwell's Happy HypnoBirthday 567
150. Hypnotherapy of Immortality 573
151. Thompson's Hypnosis For ADD & ADHD 579
152. Hypno-Creativity 583
153. International Hypnotherapy 587
154. Oates' Reverse Speech 589
155. Talent Hypnotherapy 593
156. The Long Hypnotic Sleep 595
157. Demonstrational And Stage Hypnosis 597
158. The Guardian Angel Hypnosis Show 607

PART TEN: REGRESSION SPECIALTIES

159. Regression & Hypnoanalysis 623
160. Fantasy Hypnoanalysis 625
161. Stop Stuttering 629
162. Evidence Of Previous Life Times 633
163. Previous Life Regression Hypnotherapy 641
164. The Question Of Karma 649

PART ELEVEN: HYPNOYOGA

165. England's Hypnoyoga 655
166. The Attention Technique 663
167. Yoga Nidra 665
168. Yoga Yama...671
169. Yogi Therapeutics..673
170. Holotropic Breathwork 677
171. Tantra Hypnotherapy 681

PART TWELVE: THE COSMIC CONNECTION

172. The Cosmic Connection 687
173. Enlightenment Hypnotherapy 689
174. Hypnotherapy Of Cosmic Love 691
175. Mastermind Hypnotherapy..693
176. Self-Realization Hypnotherapy 697
177. The Light Within Hypnotherapy 699
178. The Kundalini 701
179. Transpersonal Hypnotherapy 705
180. Guardian Angel Hypnotherapy Techniques 709
181. Spirit Depossession 713
182. Ten Giant Steps To Super Consciousness 719
183. Universal Mind Hypnotherapy 723

PART THIRTEEN: HYPNOMEDITATION

184. Thoughts On Meditation 731
185. Hypnosis Verses Meditation 733
186. Hypno-Meditation Formulas 735
187. You Are A Rainbow Self Hypnosis 739
188. Color/Chakra Balancing 741
189. The Ladder Of Colors: Stimulating Your Chakras..........................745
190. Hypnotherapy Of Infinity 749
191. Ancient Essene Hypno-Meditation...751
192. Essene Entering Darkness Meditation 757
193. Meditation Of The Violet Flame..761
194. Hypnotherapy Of Zen 765
195. Transcendental Hypnotherapy 769

PART FOURTEEN: EXTRA-ORDINARY PHENOMENON
196. Extraordinary Hypnotic Phenomenon 775
197. Out Of Body Hypnotherapy 779
198. Telepathy Experiments..783
199. Clairvoyance 785
200. Trance Channeling..787
201. Stockwell's Be More Psychic Hypnosis 789

PART FIFTEEN: 21st CENTURY TECHNIQUES
202. 21st Century Hypnotherapy 797
203. Bodhisattva Hypnotherapy: Wakefulness...801
204. Bodhisattva Hypnotherapy Continued 805
205. Metamorphosis Hypnosis 807
206. Epilogue: Your Mind Potential 811
207. About Ormond McGill 813

PART SIXTEEN: APPENDIX
Section I.   **Definitions/Index** 819
Section II.   **347 Scripts By Subject** 831
Section III. **153 Induction Scripts By Chapter**..................................835
Section IV.   **Resources/Hypno-Helpers**...837

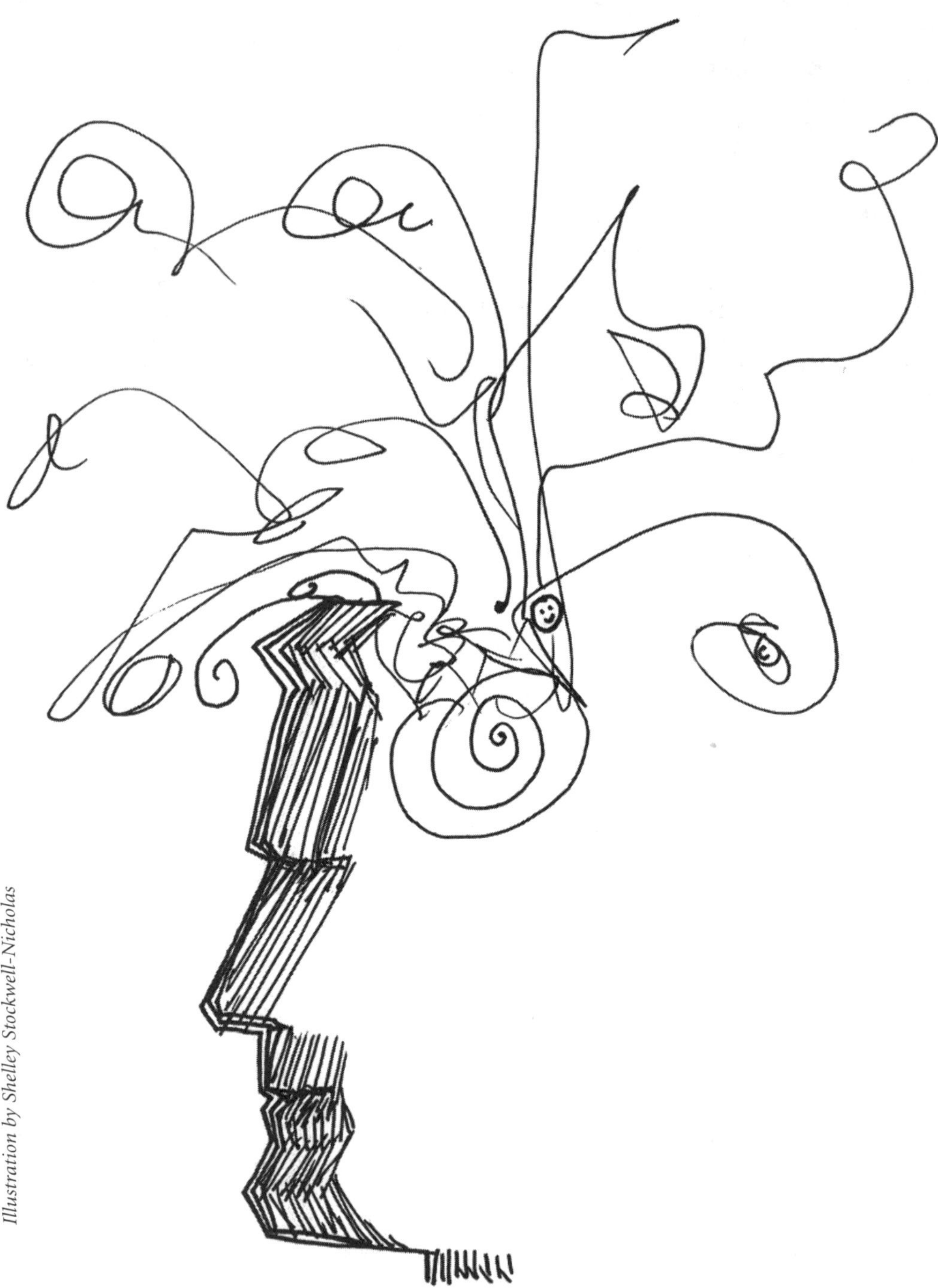

Illustration by Shelley Stockwell-Nicholas

Introduction

Most have lots of questions about hypnosis. Answering them clears confusion, educates and puts the conscious mind at ease. If these answers bring up more questions, ask yourself, "what is my implied statement behind my question?" Then you discover how much you already know.

WHAT IS MIND?

Mind is intangible. It is like walking. You know you have a mind just as you know you can walk. But after you walk, where is the walking?

It would probably be more understandable if mind were called "minding" for mind is a process for producing thoughts; an instrument for thinking. When properly under the control of consciousness it has tremendous power.

Mind operates on the interactive levels of what hypnotists call conscious and subconscious or unconscious. The conscious aspect is concerned with thinking by figuring things out and how to do things. It is self-evaluating and critical.

The subconscious aspect of mind deals with feelings and the automatic functions of the body, via the brain. Also with it are the prodigious memories of all that life has produced and (if you can expand that much) the memory of all the time you have existed as an immortal soul. The subconscious absorbs words, tones, actions, pictures and frequencies the way a sponge absorbs water. The subconscious mind, when activated with hypnosis and suggestion, bypasses critical conscious thought. That's why it is so effective a motivator.

No one knows where the subconscious mind lives or when it becomes operative. Some say it exists in utero, some say that it forms right after birth, and others say it is eternal.

WHAT IS THOUGHT?

Thoughts are things. Thoughts are forms that energy focused in a particular direction brings. In this book, as you direct your thoughts towards hypnotherapy, you are a vanguard of mind travel. Hypnosis provides a controllable mental state, which directly affects both your psychology and physiology. Mind and body are in constant interaction. Examples of this are easy to discover:

A mind filled with stress can reflect disease (dis-ease) in the body.

Conversely, a peaceful mind removes dis-ease.

Hypnotherapy provides a thought modality to stabilize both mind and body often in only one session! To paraphrase the great Psychologist, William James (who you will study in this book):

"Ideomotor action means that every thought you think produces an unconscious subconsciously controlled muscular action in the physical structure of the body."

Hold out your arm and make it strong while thinking happy thoughts. Have someone put pressure on it and it remains strong. You can easily resist any effort to move it. Now let your mind think unhappy thoughts and have some one push the arm. Somehow it has lost its strength and sags easily beneath the pressure.

Extend your arm and let a pendulum dangle from your fingers and hold your arm as still as you can while thinking of it swinging back and forth. Your thoughts alone, not consciously but subconsciously, cause the movement in your muscles which then moves the pendulum.

Ideomotor action is always there and your body as a muscular structure is always responding to it in varying degrees. Muscular structure is not only on the outside but also throughout your body. Even your vital organs are muscular structures. Subconscious mind controls it. Your subconscious mind can be its own analyst and present the correct therapy for the body it governs.

Renowned French Hypnotherapist, Emil Coue's generalized suggestion, **"Every day in every way, I'm getting better and better"** helped his clients in every way. The suggestion formula pretty well covers everything. Bernheim and Leibeault treated symptoms with simply telling the hypnotized person "Your symptoms will go away." And the symptoms often did.

Some probe the cause to remove it. Just tell the subconscious, **"Remove the symptom by curing the cause."** The subconscious is literal and does what it is told.

If you want the subconscious to do something, tell it what you want. If it is properly instructed, it will do beneficial things. Make your instructions clear and simple. Just remember that, while the subconscious follows instructions and does wonderful things, it doesn't produce instructions for itself. It functions like a computer with suggestion formulas as programs placed in it. This requires an outside operator to properly program it.

Hypnosis activates your bio-computer and then what has been programmed into it comes out automatically in your desired result. No computer is self-operating. An operator must program it. In the case of your biocomputer, the operator is your mind.

Your mind uses your brain to produce thoughts. And thoughts are forms of energy manifested through the body in 3-D space. In other words, thoughts produced by mind, manipulate and manifest via the physical organism in the dimensions in which you currently exist.

IF YOUR MIND PRODUCES THOUGHTS, WHAT IS BEHIND THE MIND?

Behind the mind is your SELF or your individual consciousness. Your SELF is absolutely unique and the only one exactly like itself in the universe.

In relation to your SELF, you stand at the very center of the universe and the whole "shebang" swirls about that center which is your SELF. Unique? Yes. Yet everyone has the same uniqueness. Wisdom comes from your awareness of your cosmic individuality. Awareness of your cosmic individuality is ENLIGHTENMENT. Being conscious of consciousness is a quantum leap to Cosmic Consciousness

Programming can come from your conscious mind or from outside. That is where the hypnotherapist comes in. A hypnotherapist carefully probes and digs up the source of problems and then promptly corrects them. Mind works like that. It can be corrected just as a computer application can be corrected. A short cut is to give the hypnotized person the suggestion **"On the termination of your hypnotic trance, the source of your problem will be clearly presented to your consciousness and when it is, any difficulty will melt away like dewdrops in the sun."**

WHAT HAS MIND GOT TO DO WITH IT?

Most problems people have stem from improper use of the mind. When mind under control of SELF is properly used it not only heals itself but it also heals the body and the life journey.

You will learn in this text various aspects of mind control to master your mind. A mind not under control of SELF has too much freedom and runs amuck with a mishmash of thoughts with little or detrimental value. A mind under control becomes silent until called upon to operate. Is your mind silent? Or is it constantly jabbing you?

Hypnotically instruct your clients and yourself to become master of mind rather than being mastered by mind. This makes you and your client a mastermind.

Suggestion formulas throughout this book present to the mind positive affirmations for what the client wants to occur. When used in conjunction with hypnosis, it becomes an effective and efficient way to modify behavior.

Once you get through to the subconscious, all you need to do is tell it what it needs to do. Then allow it the opportunity to discriminate on its own about what is the best treatment. Learn to appreciate that your client's subconscious mind knows more about what is right than your own conscious conjecture.

Believe it or not, computer technology is destined to become more and more associated with hypnotherapy in the 21st century. This simile is a handy way to look at things, but a human being has an element that no computer will ever have: via the subconscious it connects to Universal Mind, consciousness, and the VOID.

WHAT IS CONSCIOUSNESS?

Think of consciousness this way; attached to each particle of matter there is a particle of mind. Much the way fog can cause itself, by its moisture, to attach to particles of dust in the air. In this same way every little particle of mind stuff is attached to every atom in the universe and has its own particular "atom consciousness." When these atoms are bound together in the form of a starfish, you have starfish consciousness. If they are bound in the form of a bird they have bird consciousness. Or if bound together in the form of a man or woman, they have man or woman consciousness.

Everything in existence exists to the degree of being what it is in accordance to the consciousness for what it is. The more the consciousness becomes aware of self, the higher is the evolutionary form of the matter that composes it.

You can only understand consciousness in relation to yourself…it is your awareness of your being. That is to say, it is recognition of your self within yourself. It is not your outside self that you can see reflected in a mirror, it is your inside self which you cannot see at all, but which you know is there. And that SELF can directly create in the universe. It is God power.

HOW DO YOU CREATE?

Creative mind blends imagination and will.

An object is perceived, formed into the objective, and conceived by the creative mind. This is accomplished through visualizing (image or thought forming) what is desired to be created in the mind. In this process, the particles of "mind stuff" are agglomerated, forming the different units of consciousness. This concentration gathers more of these particles into one place. If it can be condensed into a point (just as a magnifying glass will focus the sun's rays) and you have absolute unity of concentration. It is through such concentration that the basis of matter (Akasha) can be molded by the creative mind to become reality in the universe.

Creation by mind takes energy. The basis of energy is the universal source of vibration and the vital energy of life is called Prana. Prana brings movement to the structure of all that is. It is manifested in gravity, electricity, magnetism, the rotation of planets, the solar system and the universe. Prana is the vitality that makes life possible…from the highest to the lowest forms. You may call it "the soul of energy." It is all pervading. The entire cosmos manufactures from its subtle material with the power of prana. Prana comes to you through breath and certain ways of breathing bring in greater quantities to you. This is exceptionally important when you're directing mental efforts to create in the universe that which you want for yourself. Your consciousness directs your mind with the purpose to produce thoughts and when energized by Prana becomes Creative Mind.

So there you have it! By an effort of will, projecting it upon the "Akasha" (physical or material form) and then vitalizing it with Prana (energy) creates, in a materializing form, the reproduction of that which your consciousness caused to be imagined in the mind.

Visualization + Affirmation + Projection (fueled by prana) = Creation

To effectively create in the universe you must use these three mental powers: visualization, affirmation and projection. This requires your ability to throw your mind blank, one-pointed concentration and a vivid imagination.

THE ILLUSIVE BUTTERFLY OF HYPNOSIS

I conclude this introduction with comments on the intangibility of hypnotherapy. If you grasp this ambiguous insight it will provide a quantum leap in this treasured science.

That which is intangible is something that seems not to be, yet actually is. As such, it is elusive and difficult to capture. Hypnosis produces an intangible state of mind and equally makes the intangible more tangible. All mental disturbances in humans are of an intangible nature.

A mental disturbance is that which disturbs the peace of mind of the individual and when mind then disturbs body. All mental disturbances originate with first pretending that something is wrong which develops into belief that something is wrong. It then advances to become reality in the behavior of the individual.

When this process is appreciated it can be reversed and disturbances corrected. Hypnotherapy provides the modus operandi to correct disturbances, which is why clients seek the hypnotherapist for help. The more intangibility advances to consciousness (awareness) the less intangible it becomes. However, it must be remembered that even consciousness has much about it that is intangible and is subject to constant change. Indeed the entire universe is intangible and is in a state of constant change.

Understanding these basic facts about the nature of the universe causes an understanding of yourself, as you are a miniature of the universe.

The secret of mastering intangibility is to appreciate that it IS and handle it in an organized manner rather than allowing it to become a mess inside oneself.

Helping your clients to organize their inner mess and allow their life to become an adventure in learning is the work of a master hypnotherapist. Beyond question, hypnotherapy is destined to be a leading process, for the more confused the outside world becomes, the more the inner world of the individual needs to find serenity.

All the diverse processes of hypnotherapy presented in this book are aimed to bring about this inner organization.

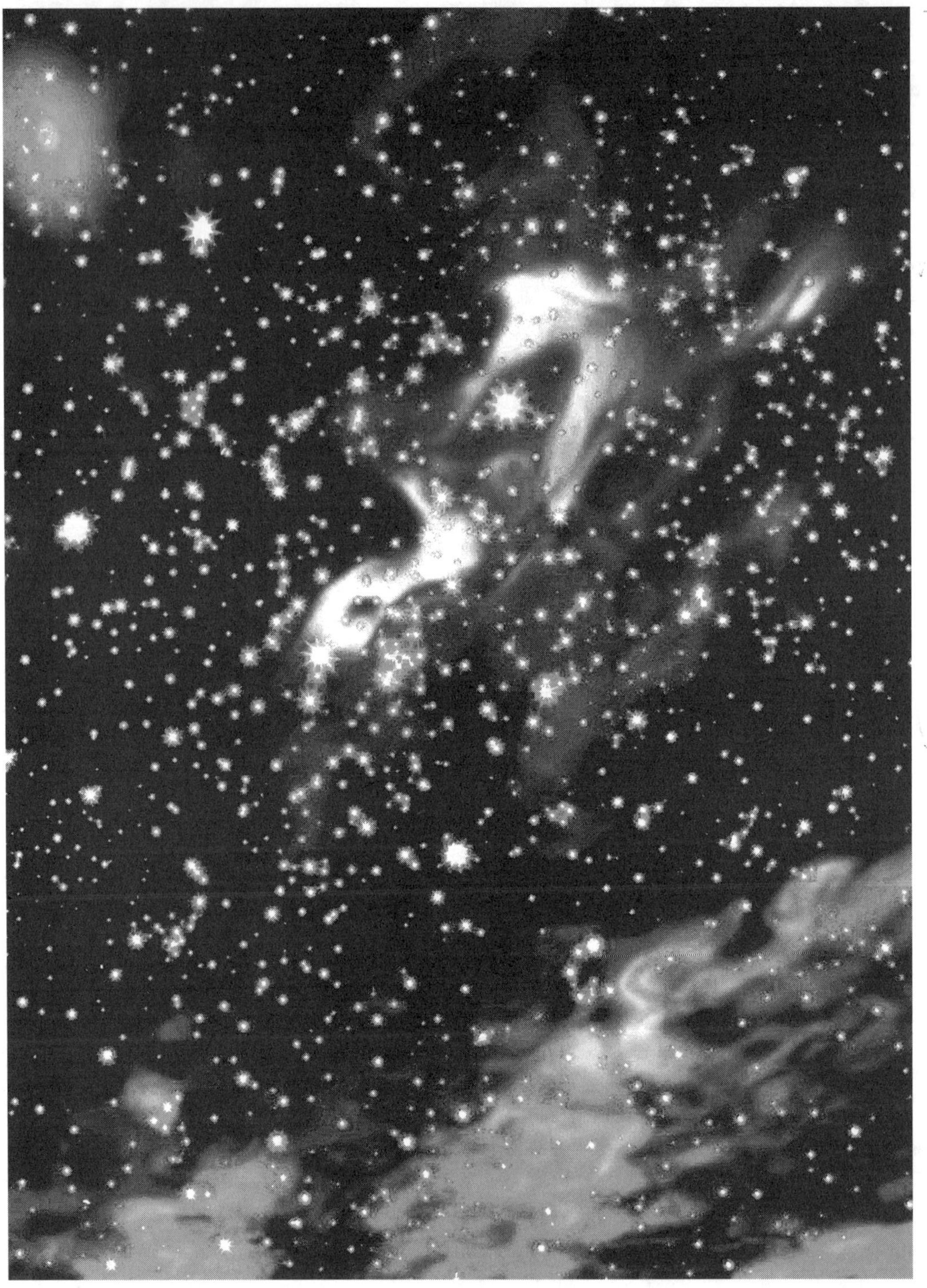
McGill's Hypnotherapy Encyclopedia

Preface

Encyclopedia: A course of general education; a work treating the various branches of learning or a particular branch of knowledge.
         —Webster

A book has to start somewhere. This book is called an encyclopedia because it is encyclopedic and deals with a specialty. The specialty is Hypnotherapy. Thus, I titled it "The Hypnotherapy Encyclopedia."

I have had an interest in hypnotherapy for a lifetime. My thoughts on the subject have been personal and cumulative. I have placed this conglomeration of my interest in this book. Extensive as it is, it can never be complete as hypnotherapy is a steadily advancing field. Indeed, advancing with every passing moment to fulfill a destiny of becoming a leading modality for the progressive future of humankind. This text will teach you many things about hypnosis, and the more you study and learn, the more you will come to realize that the potential of the human mind is so vast you will be awed by its wonderful study.

In this book you will master an array of hypnotic inductions, somnambulistic modus operandi, healing modalities, and innovative instructions. Don't just read this book, it has to be studied, conjectured upon and then applied.

To assimilate its maximum value, energize what you learn by the source of Cosmic Power, which is the energy behind all hypnotherapy work. George Lukas, in his Star War Trilogy called this Cosmic Energy THE FORCE. THE FORCE is not something your create yourself; it is Cosmic in origin. It is the creative energy of the universe that you channel into yourself from out of the VOID.

Plato called the VOID "logos." Jesus called it "my Father in heaven." Einstein called it "space." The VOID is emptiness, which is ever filled with the vibration of creation in which the unformed is formed into form. The VOID is space a vast energy filled with a myriad of planets, solar systems, stars and galaxies…so numerous as to be likened to the quantity of all the grains of sand found upon all the beaches of the world. Yet, even with this infinite quantity of created matter, the VOID is 95% emptiness. It is the crucible of creation.

The entire Universe has a sentience about itself. That is to say that everything created has enough consciousness to be what it IS. Consciousness means awareness and awareness means communication is possible. It is thus that you can ask the Force to come into yourself.

We know consciousness in our immediate here and now as:
1. Unconscious Consciousness as in Rocks
2. Simple Consciousness as in Plants
3. Dawning Self Consciousness as in Animals
4. Advance Consciousness as in Humans
5. Cosmic Consciousness as in Universal Consciousness

With Cosmic Consciousness we bring in the Force. Think of the FORCE as a warm personal friend. "Ask and it shall be delivered unto thee".

The Universe is a vast reservoir of energy and you, as a part of this Universe, may partake of it as much of that vital energy as you please. The supply is infinite. Energy follows thought, so use your mind to visualize (mentally picture) the energy of the Universe flowing into you. Then, use your body to experience the energy as it flows. It is especially useful when you need extra energy. If you use it each morning it will make your day. If you use it as you commence each hypnotherapeutic session, you will amplify the positive results. Here is how to bring in the FORCE:

MODUS OPERANDI: BRINGING IN THE FORCE
"Shake your hands vigorously and become the shaking.

Then allow your whole body to become the shaking. You will find that your whole body becomes alive with energy.

Now allow your hands to dangle down by your sides, but not touching your body. Close your eyes and direct your attention within. Let your thoughts come and go as they will. Just be there with yourself however you are. Your mind becomes silent and your body tuned to receive energy waves from the Force. Imagine within your inner space a column of brilliant white living light coming from out of the Void into your crown filling your head with light. Let this flow down your neck and shoulders and throughout your entire being. Take a deep breath and hold it. And say out loud,

'I bring the cosmic force into my mind and body for strength, guidance and protection.'
'I bring the cosmic force into my mind and body for strength, guidance and protection.'
'I bring the cosmic force into my mind and body for strength, guidance and protection.'"

As the cosmic energy comes into you, you will feel the Force. Charged with vital energy you are now ready to take in all the information that you will find in this book. This is foundational. NOW BEGIN THE STUDY.

—Ormond McGill
Palo Alto, 2003

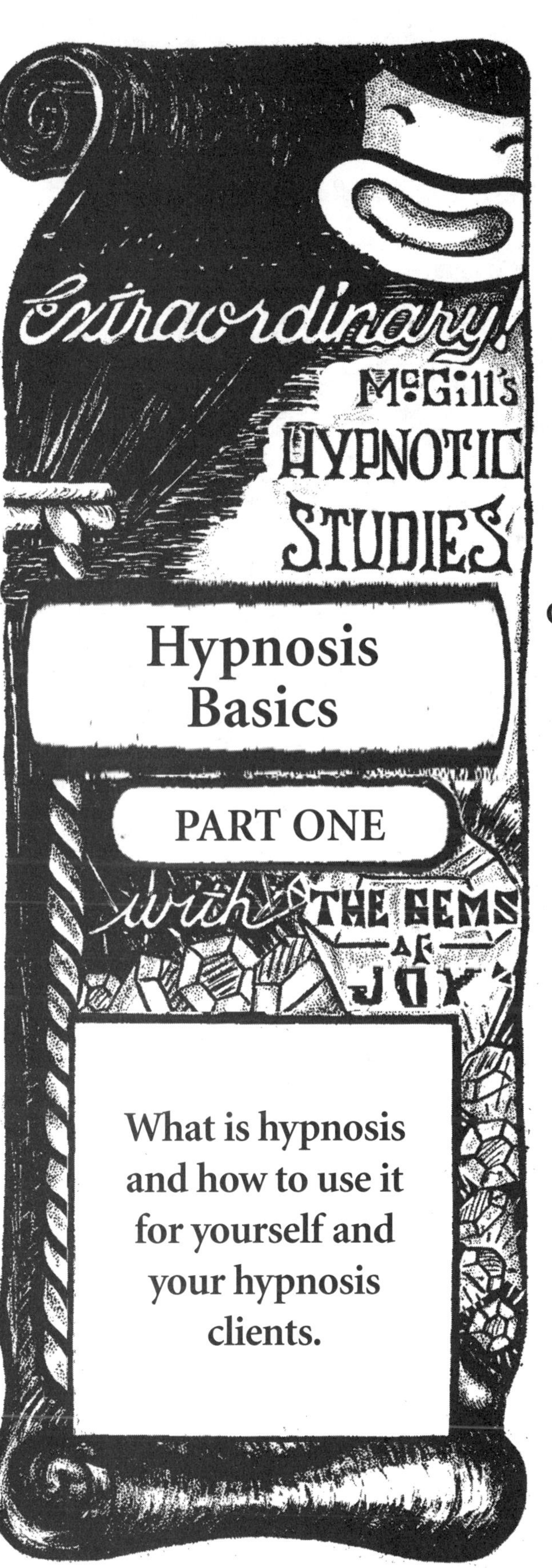

CHAPTERS IN PART ONE

1. What Is Hypnosis? ....page 1
2. Additional Thoughts On Hypnosis 5
3. The Power Of Belief 7
4. Healing Waters 9
5. Were You Hypnotized? 11
6. The Question Of Will Power 15
7. Five Hypnotic Mind Myths 17
8. Hypnotic Hodge-Podge 19
9. Basic Structure Of A Session 23
10. The Consultation 29
11. Pre-Hypnosis Hypnosis 33
12. Direct Mental Marriage Hypnosis 35
13. Thoughts To Play With 37
14. Answers For Clients 39
15. Professional Wisdom & Protocols 45
16. Stockwell's Legal Requirements 47

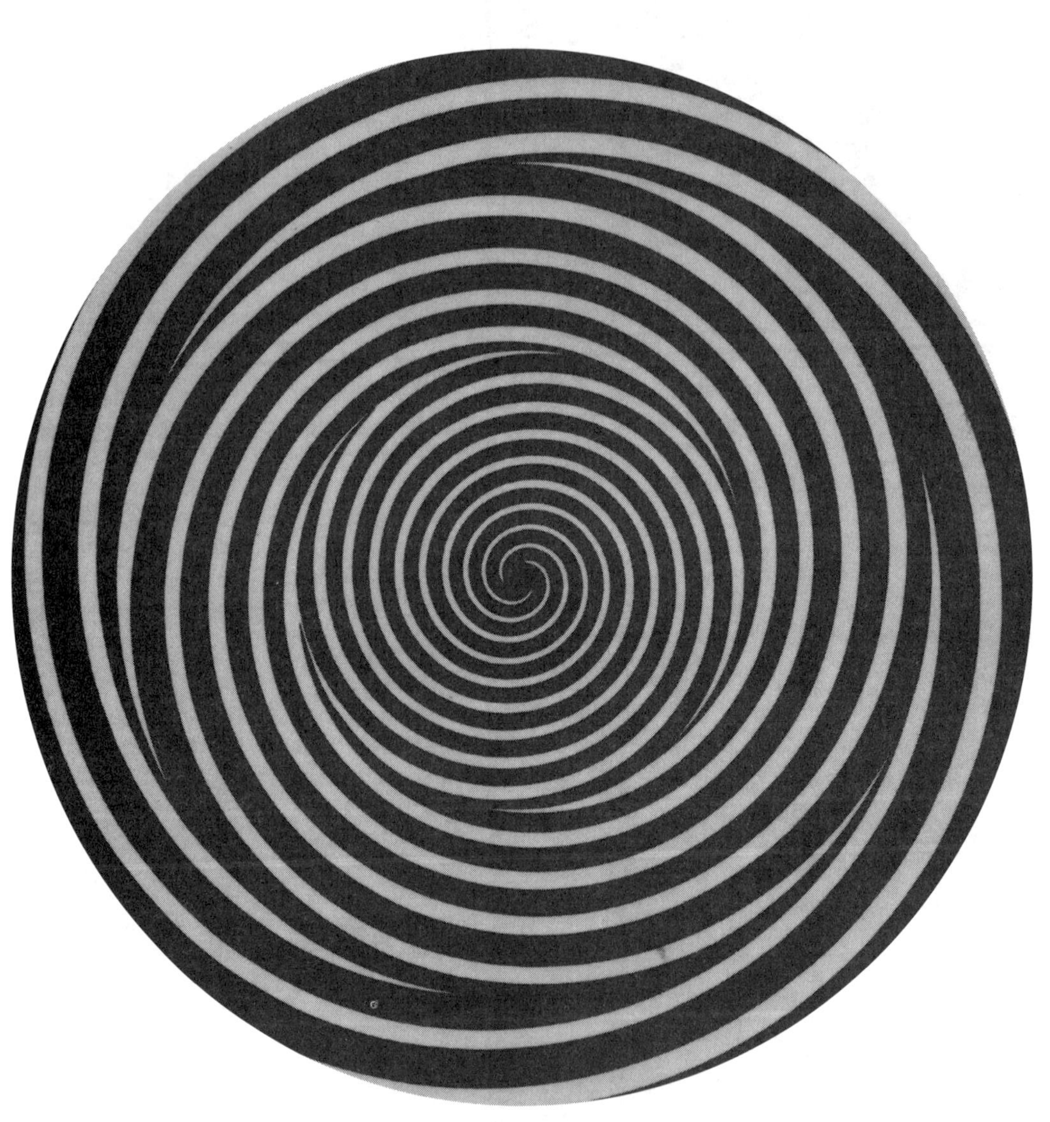

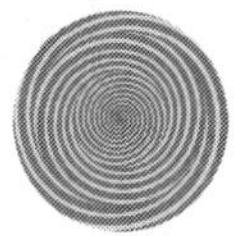

~ *Chapter 1* ~
WHAT IS HYPNOSIS?

Includes
Definitions of Hypnosis
The Characteristics of Hypnosis

Hypnosis and Hypnotherapy have been called everything from Yar-Phoonk to Voodoo. After Dr. Frederick Anton Mesmer's work, it was named "Mesmerism." Dr. James Braid called it "Hypnotism" and the name stuck.

DEFINITIONS OF HYPNOSIS

As a Hypnotherapist you will be asked, "What is hypnosis?" many times. There are nearly as many answers to that question as there are hypnotherapists. It is well to have an answer on the tip-of-your-tongue. Here are answers from various prominent people in the field:

"Hypnosis is an induced mental state that consists of bypasses of the critical mind and establishes selective thinking."
—Elman

"Hypnotism is the science and art of mentally controlling thoughts and actions."
—Cook

"Hypnosis is a reverie state of mind. It is much like day dreaming."
—Dunne

"Hypnosis, or hypnotic sleep, implies a mind condition in which mental action is under control of suggestion."
—Quackenbos

"Hypnosis is a state induced by suggestion and controlled by suggestion. It is a mental state in which suggestions are accepted and acted upon uncritically."
—Weber

"Hypnosis is a natural state of heightened awareness where you accept suggestion from without and within."
—Stockwell

"When the mind is under control, the mind becomes like pure crystal reflecting equally, without distortion, the perception, the perceiver, and the perceived. It is through such mind that consciousness is known."
—Patanjali

"Hypnosis is largely a question of willingness to be receptive to beneficial ideas and to allow these ideas to be acted upon without interference."
—Witzenhoffer & Hilgard

"Hypnosis is a state of intensified attention and receptiveness to an idea or set of ideas."
—Erickson

"Hypnosis is a process which produces relaxation, distraction of the conscious mind, heightened suggestibility and increased awareness, allowing access to the subconscious mind through imagination. It also produces the ability to experience thoughts and images."
—Krasner

"Hypnosis is a particular altered state of selective hyper-suggestibility brought about in an individual by the use of a combination of relaxation, fixation of attention and suggestion."
—Ansari

"Hypnosis is a state of relatively heightened susceptibility to prestige suggestions."
—Hull

"Hypnosis is an altered state of the organism originally and usually produced by repetition of stimuli in which suggestions have a peculiarly potent effect."
—Bowers

"Hypnosis is an aspect of conditioning."
—Salter

"The hypnotized subject evinces superior refinement and obedience to suggestion."
—Dr. J. Milne Bramwell, 1902

"In hypnosis, the subconscious, having no power of reason, accepts and acts upon any fact or suggestion given to it by the conscious mind."
—Caprio & Berger

"Oh magic sleep! O comfortable bird, that broodest o'er the troubled sea of the mind till it is hush'd and smooth."
—Keats (Endymion)

"The bypass of the critical factor of the conscious mind followed by the ability to accept suggestions."
—US Department of Labor

You may use one of these or intelligently form your own answer. If you wish you can simply say, *"No one knows exactly what electricity is yet we constantly use it just the same."*
—McGill

THE CHARACTERISTICS OF HYPNOSIS

"Though often denigrated as fakery or wishful thinking, hypnosis has been shown to be a real phenomenon with a variety of therapeutic uses-especially in controlling pain."
—Scientific American, May 2002

"Research over the last 40 years shows that such hypnotic techniques are safe and effective. Furthermore, a growing number of studies show that hypnotherapy can treat headaches, ease the pain of childbirth, aid in quitting smoking, improve concentration and study habits, relieve minor phobias and serve as anesthesia-all without drugs or side effects."
—Psychology Today, January 2001

"A trance state fosters heightened communication between mind and body…also used to diffuse anxiety and panic…for uncovering and healing psychological trauma, hypnosis is a technique that many therapists believe to be without equal."
—Lois B. Morris, New Woman, September 1993

"Major hospitals use trances for fractures, cancer, burns; speeding recoveries…"
—Michael Waldholz, Wall Street Journal, October 7, 2003

Hypnotic trance happens to everyone ever day naturally just before you drift off to sleep at night and upon awakening in the morning. We also drift into the hypnotic state of mind when bored, daydreaming, enthralled or excited. Here are the characteristics of a hypnotic trance:

Hyper-Acuity of the Senses

Hypnosis focuses the field of attention for perfect concentration. In this state, sensory perceptions are more accurate and active. Logical powers of mind are heightened. A narrowed field of attention and stimuli is determined by suggestions given. Smell and taste are easily enhanced with hypnosis. Eyesight is reportedly improved.

Hyper-Acuity of Memory

Hypnosis produces a prodigious memory. It is possible to revive and recollect circumstances and impressions from long ago that are lost to the conscious state of mind. Every sensation ever experienced, everything ever learned, can be recalled with hypnotic suggestion. Likewise you can suggest that something be forgotten.

Fixation of Attention

Hypnosis limits the field of attention until a concentrated and unvarying field results. How narrow the range of focus is strongly influenced by suggestions given.

Reflexes and Nerve Responses Are Easily Influenced

Pulse rate may be altered, areas anesthetized, blood flow and menses regulated, childbirth time determined and automatic body function controlled. You can stimulate a curative effect or produce a pathological one. A burn can go away or you can suggest a burn and redness of the skin will appear. You can change your temperature.

Less Autonomy As Perceptions Become Controlled by Outside Suggestions

Usually someone in hypnosis complies with suggestions. Hypnotized people do not awaken themself, choose their action, or prevent doing something, even if unpleasant, unless they counter something strongly opposed to their natural tendencies or moral nature; in which case they would refuse to act on the suggestion or terminate the trance.

Another Reality

A hypnotized person earnestly and sincerely believes the specific suggestions they receive. They actually believe that they are proud, humble, happy, sad, can sing, laugh, cry, dance or are relaxing in a forest glade. All sensations of the past, no matter how subtle, may be called forth to enhance hypnotic hallucinations. You've seen a stage show for example where someone really thinks that they are Elvis or the broom they are dancing with is a beautiful partner. A hypnotized person can eat an onion and believe it a peach. They can drink water and experience it as nectar of the gods.

Susceptibility to Post Hypnotic Responses

Suggestions given in trance are performed after the client awakens. Often the subject doesn't even remember the original suggestion.

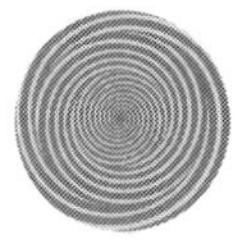

~ *Chapter 2* ~
ADDITIONAL THOUGHTS ON HYPNOSIS

From Waking To Trance:
WAKING = State of mind of daily awareness
TRANCE = State of mind while in hypnosis

Hypnosis provides a practical tool to change the mind. It creates an overwhelming desire to do what YOU want to do rather than being mastered by a desire to do what you don't want to do. In other words, hypnosis provides a directive that controls the mind. The subconscious mind, much like a computer, can be programmed to do remarkable things.

Hypnosis Just For Hypnosis
Hypnosis in and of itself is of real value to an individual. It provides an opportunity to penetrate the depths of yourself and take a little vacation from the world. How nice it is when hypnosis quiets mind's constant chattering and mind becomes silent for a while.

Additional definitions:
"Hypnosis is a deliberately induced state of hyper-suggestibility. The state of mind produced is extremely responsive to the subconscious realization of ideas. In hypnosis, mind moves beyond critical limitations of itself (objective) and the subconscious mind state (subjective) willingly accepts its potential to do what might normally be considered impossible. In this condition, behavior and bodily processes are modified to a remarkable degree and miracles occur."

And
"Hypnotic Trance is an intermediate condition between sleep and wakefulness characterized by disassociation, involuntary movements, and automatisms of behavior."

And
"Hypnosis is a deliberately created mental process for causing alterations in perception and behavior in the individual even to the extent of the bazaar."

In trance, the features of the face (physiognomy) are seen to change. Often a flush comes to the cheeks, the mouth becomes less firm, and the eyes become glassy, take on a faraway look, and occasionally roll upwards. A person's general demeanor becomes receptive rather than aggressive.

In hypnosis there is a willingness to accept beneficial instructions without question, even if such suggestions might seem impossible in a person's waking state. The critical conscious or objective mind limits what you think you can accomplish. The subconscious or subjective mind is unlimited and omnipotent.

Nothing is impossible to the inner mind.

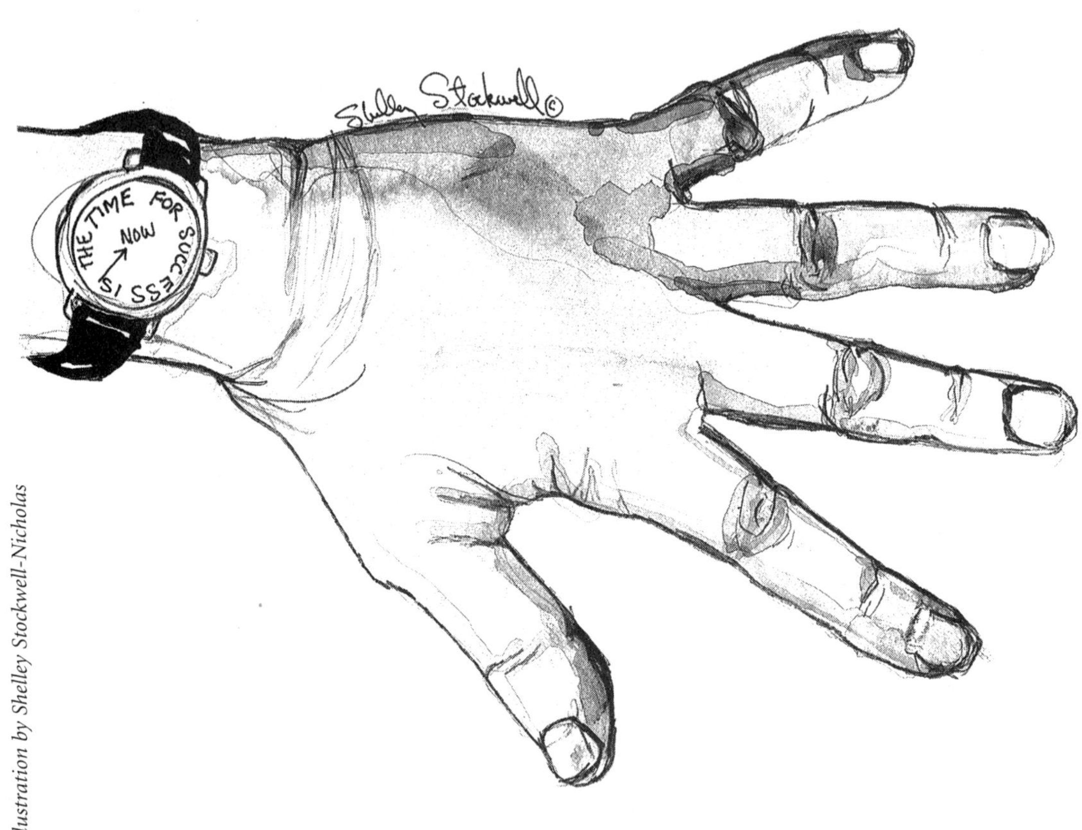

Illustration by Shelley Stockwell-Nicholas

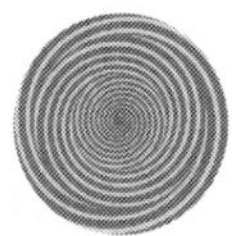

~ *Chapter 3* ~
THE POWER OF BELIEF

"Humankinds next great discoveries will be found within our own inner space."
—Charles Steinmetz

Belief makes humans objective and is a basis for successful hypnotherapy. The dictionary describes belief very simply as *"Acceptance as truth or actuality without certain proof that it is so."*

Belief can be positive or negative:
"I believe in God; I do not believe in God."
"I believe in angels; I do not believe in angels."
"I believe I will fail; I believe I will succeed."
"I believe that the waters of a holy shrine, such as Lourdes, has healing virtue."
"I believe that hypnotherapy can make me well."
"Now is the time for success.'

Belief is very powerful. The subconscious phase of mind readily accepts what you believe is helpful, without proof of any kind, and goes to work using that premise. When belief becomes strong enough, even the critical mind becomes non-critical. This is the magic power of belief.

MAYA: The Illusion of Belief
Much of what is created and accepted as reality is "Maya" or illusion.

Here are the three steps of belief:
1. Accepting an idea - Create conscious and subconscious acceptance of an idea.
2. Imagining and creating the idea as so – Pretend that it is so.
3. Belief becomes reality

BELIEF= Conscious/Subconscious acceptance of the idea= Pretending it is so= Enlisting the imagination and Creative Function of mind= the idea is accepted as REALITY

Hypnosis is Belief
Hypnosis is belief. It establishes, in the mind, deliberate, organized and desired BELIEFS. Believe this book will expand your consciousness and that hypnosis will change the world… and you will be correct.
Enlisting the conscious and subconscious mind to synchronize and work together in harmony is profoundly effective for establishing powerful belief and belief then becomes our reality.

"If the belief doesn't serve you, fire it. If the belief serves you well, promote it."
—Stephanie Rothman, CHt

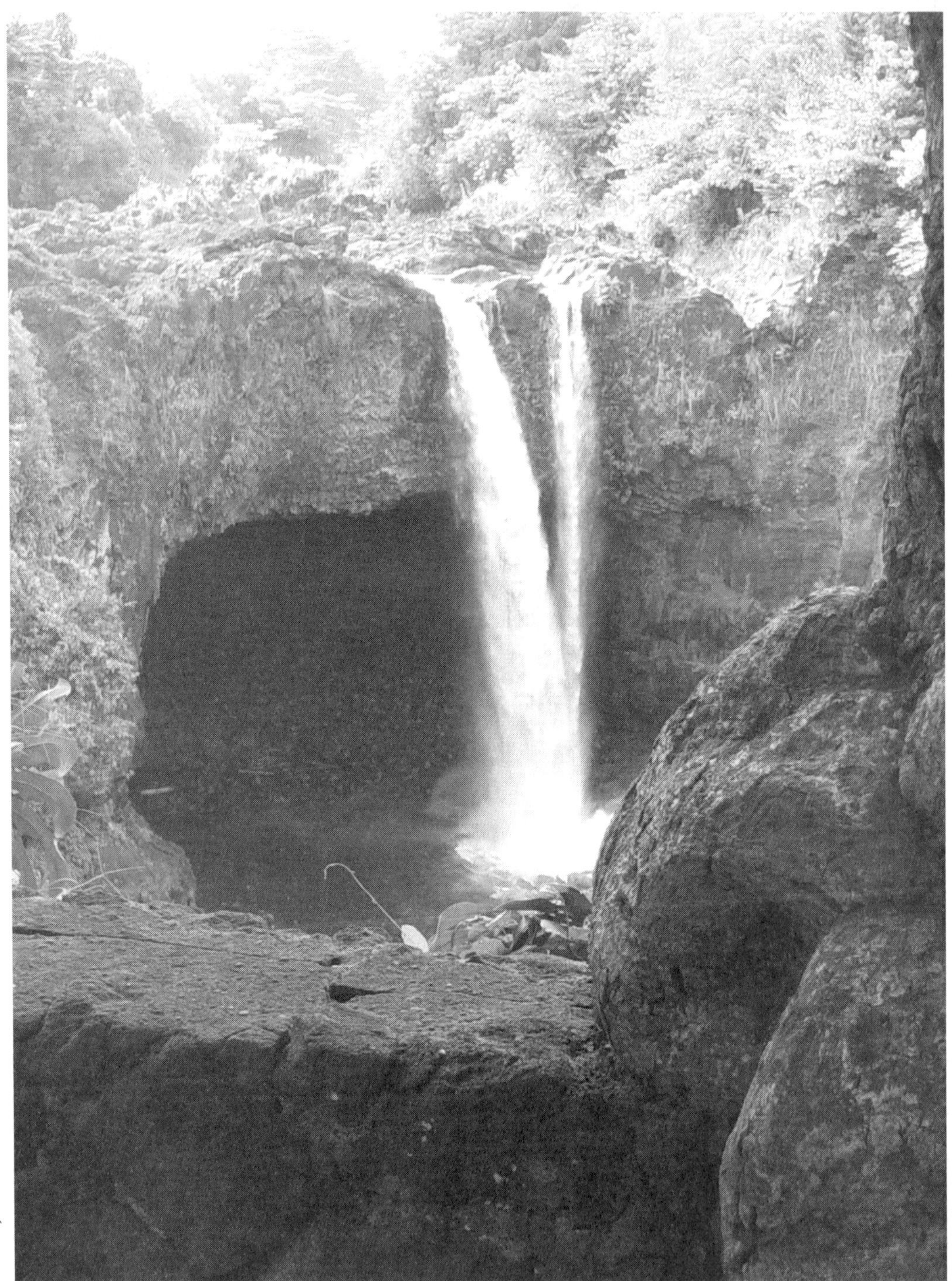

Photo by Jon Nicholas

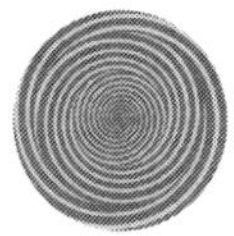

~ *Chapter 4* ~
HEALING WATERS

Includes
Healing Water Hypnosis
Holy Water Hypnosis

Healing Water is historically recognized in many forms:
*   Holy Water in religious ceremonies. Sprinkle water on your head and your sins are forgiven.
        BELIEF!
*   Sacred Water of Holy Shrines. Take a dip or sip and you are healed.
        BELIEF!
*   Love Elixir dropped on the tongue makes you loving and passionate.
        BELIEF!
*   You are told that an inert medicine will cure your illness. The placebo effect does the job.
        BELIEF!
*   A concocted "witches brew" curses you. If you believe it's true, the curse kills you.
        BELIEF!

Concentrated thought focused in a particular direction is belief. In the Holy Script: *"As a man thinketh in his heart, so is he."* Thinketh is to produce thoughts and thoughts are forms of energy that affect mind and body. Thoughts can heal or harm. This is "the power of suggestion" in operation. Or, as Henry Ford said, *"If you think you can or you can't, you are correct."*

History has long respected the virtue of "healing water." Why not include it into hypnotherapy? Good idea! Thoughts centered on something physical increases the power of suggestion. Healing water concentrates a suggestion by bringing something physically tangible that is taken in by the client.

HEALING WATER HYPNOSIS
    You Will Need:
    An Eyedropper Bottle of Pure Water (This is a gift you give your client who takes it with them when they leave your office.)

"This bottle contains HEALING WATER that you will use nightly to reinforce the beneficial effects of your session today."

Include these written instructions:

"Using the eyedropper, drop in six drops of the Healing Water into a glass of water. As each drop drops, repeat the suggestion you have been given. For example, if it was to stop smoking, each time a drop drops into the glass of water, the suggestion is repeated. 'I am so glad I smoke no more!'"

With each of the six drops, thoughts have been centered upon a tangible effect. THEN, **"With the completion of the six drops, and the affirmation, drink the glass of water. It will flood your inner self with great healing power."**

Make any sense?

History says it does.

The subconscious mind so believes. The hypnotherapist bypasses critical mind in producing hypnosis. Thank your lucky stars your critical mind chooses what suggestions you take in. Otherwise, what a mess! The power of inner-conviction, right or wrong, creates your reality.

HOLY WATER HYPNOSIS

The effectiveness of this hypnosis astounds.

While your client is in profound hypnosis, tell them:

"You are going to drink a glass of Holy Water…all water is holy. It brings you life. You would die without water. Drink the Holy Water slowly and as you do, it will cleanse, heal, and benefit you in every way. The water you drink will be a catharsis to both your mind and body."

Give them a glass of pure spring water to drink. And, as they drink it, instruct them:
"Sense the healing virtues of this Holy Water. As it floods your inner system, it permeates every cell."

The water is drunk. Pause some moments for the water to absorb within their body. Then arouse your client from hypnosis. Make no comment. Your client will go on their way, RENEWED.

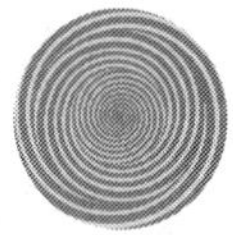

~ Chapter 5 ~

WERE YOU HYPNOTIZED?

Includes
The Old Susceptibility Scales
Weitzenhoffer and Hilgard Stanford Susceptibility Scales
The Davis-Husband Susceptibility Scales
The Older Depth of Trance Idea

The phenomenon of hypnosis is nothing new. At one time or another, in one form or another, your client has experienced it all. Yet even a profoundly hypnotized person (one in the deepest level) who performs even bazaar behavior on stage, when asked, "Do you think you were hypnotized?" Most often answers: "I don't know" or "I don't think so." That's because of the false concept that being hypnotized will be a dramatically new and novel experience, while actually it is a very ordinary and familiar.

The best way to get a positive answer from the client of "Yes, I know I was hypnotized" is to suggest to them in hypnosis, **"When asked if you were hypnotized you will say, 'yes, I know I was hypnotized.'"** This is frequently used to conclude a hypnotherapy session. It gives the client mental assurance that their session was successful. Tricky but it works. However, such a programmed answer is not really knowing; it is just a response to the post hypnotic suggestion to say that they were hypnotized.

The fact is, a person cannot actually know if they were hypnotized because hypnosis is not an isolated mental phenomenon. It is a very familiar experience. During the course of daily living, mind is constantly, automatically and spontaneously going in and out of hypnosis (even to the extend of occasionally causing amnesia). In other words, the so-called "waking state of mind" and "hypnotic state of mind" is continually combining to produce what is regarded as normal behavior. Thus, what mind has come to know as "normal" is often unrecognized hypnotic behavior. This formula sums it up:

The waking state of mind + hypnotic state of mind = all behavior.

Basically, hypnosis is a way (a process) to forcefully give directions to the mind to rapidly change and advance behavior patterns to those especially desired. The only way the client can actually know whether or not they were hypnotized is to objectively evaluate the success of failure of the hypnotherapeutic session.

The Old Susceptibility Scales

Early operators felt that hypnosis was of two types; light hypnosis, in which a train of consciousness was maintained throughout the trance state, and profound hypnosis, in which the subject was asleep and unconscious of what occurred during the hypnosis. Remarkably both are correct, for whether they are asleep or awake to the experience is irrelevant except to the degree that they take on suggestion.

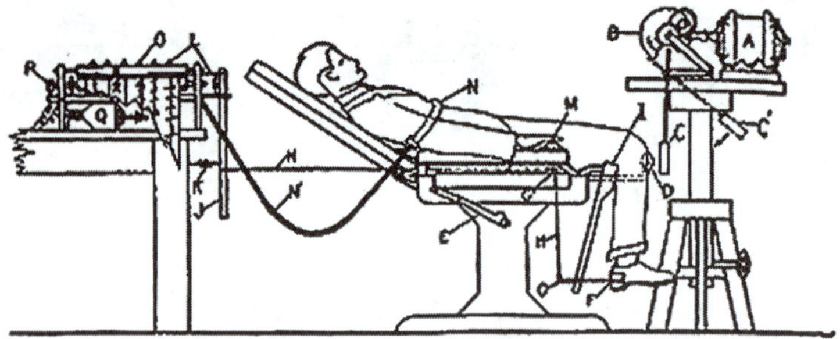

1930's gismo to distinguish between trance and sleep

Antiquated theories, used to "scientifically" measure how susceptible a person was to hypnosis, promoted the idea that a lengthy procedure and deep trance was necessary to induce hypnosis. In fact, successful suggestions are received and acted upon while a person is under light, medium and deep hypnosis.

The Weitzenhoffer and Hilgard, Stanford Hypnotic Susceptibility Scales

A series of 12 activities were given a hypnotized subject to determine the extent to which they "responded" to hypnosis. Tests included holding your arm outstretched and imagining that you were holding a heavy ball and sniffing a vial of ammonia after being told that they have no sense of smell. Those who responded to the most tests were said to be the most responsive and therefore a "good" subject. Most people scored five to seven out of the possible twelve and 95% of the people tested "passed' by responding to at least one test.

The Davis-Husband Scale of Hypnotic Susceptibility

This scale attempted to identify a correlation between hypnotic susceptibility with physical reactions. Here it is:

DEPTH	SCOPE	TEST SUGGESTION AND RESPONSES
	0	
Insusceptible	1	Relaxation
Hypnotic State	2	Fluttering Of The Eyelids
	3	Closing Of The Eyes
	4	Complete Physical Relaxation
	5	Catalepsy Of The Eyes
Light Trance	6	Limb Catalepsies
(Hypnoidal)	7	Rigid Catalepsies
	8, 9, 10	Glove Anesthesia
	11, 12	Partial Posthypnotic Amnesia
Medium Trance	13, 14	Posthypnotic Anesthesia
(Cataleptic)	15, 16	Personality Changes
	17, 18, 19	Kinesthetic Delusions
	20	Complete Amnesia By Suggestion
Deep Trance	21, 22	Ability To Open The Eyes Without
(Somnambulism)		Affecting The Trance
		Bizarre Posthypnotic Suggestions
	23, 24	Complete Somnambulism
	25	Positive Visual Hallucinations
	26	Posthypnotic
	27	Positive Auditory Hallucinations
	28	Systematized Posthypnotic Amnesia
	29	Negative Auditory/Visual Hallucinations
	30	Hyperesthesia

The Older Depth of Trance Idea

Jean Charcot from the mid 1800's said that there are five phases of "fascination" that gradually went to the greatest depth of trance:

1. Wakeful State
2. Somnambulism
   (Fascination enters here)
3. Catalepsy
4. Lethargy
5. Hypno-Lethargy or Coma

Each phase interlocks with each other into a gradual descending of hypnotic depth.

Dr. Luys describes the deeper states this way: "Imagine a subject suddenly plunged into a deep well; at the bottom his whole organism will be under the influence of the prevailing darkness. This is the lethargy stage or even sometimes a degree further, that of hypno-lethargy which is a phase so deep that even contact with the operator is lost and such is in a hypno-sleep with the subject entirely to themselves."

Hypno-lethargy is said to be produced by the clients themself and this "suspended animation." had great therapeutic value. On rare occasions a person may sleep for surprising lengths of time.

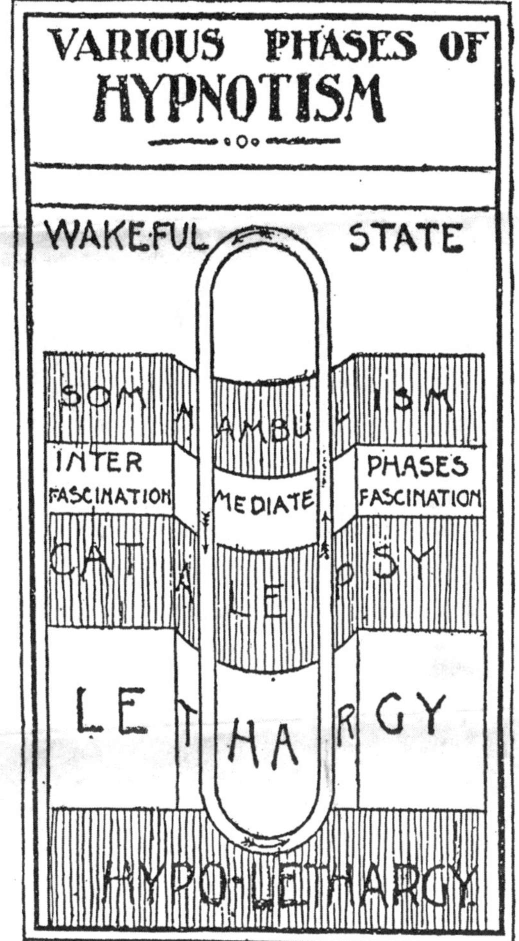

Illustration by Dr. Luys

THE VARIOUS STAGES OF HYPNOSIS.

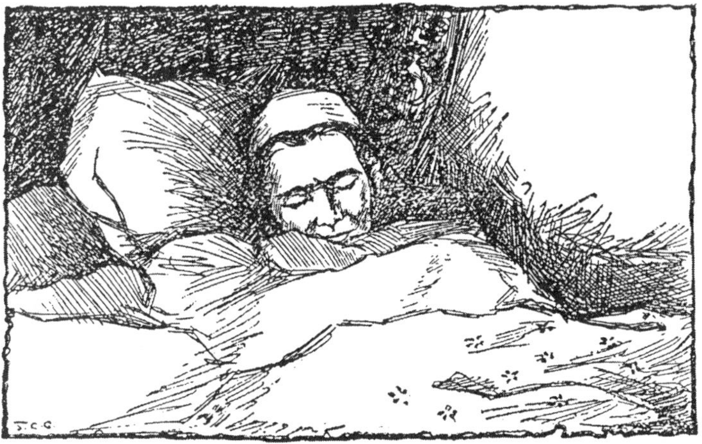

The Silence of Thenelles

In one long ago reported case, Margarite Boyenval, known as the "Sleeper of Thenelles" is said to have slept for 132,000 hours at one stretch.

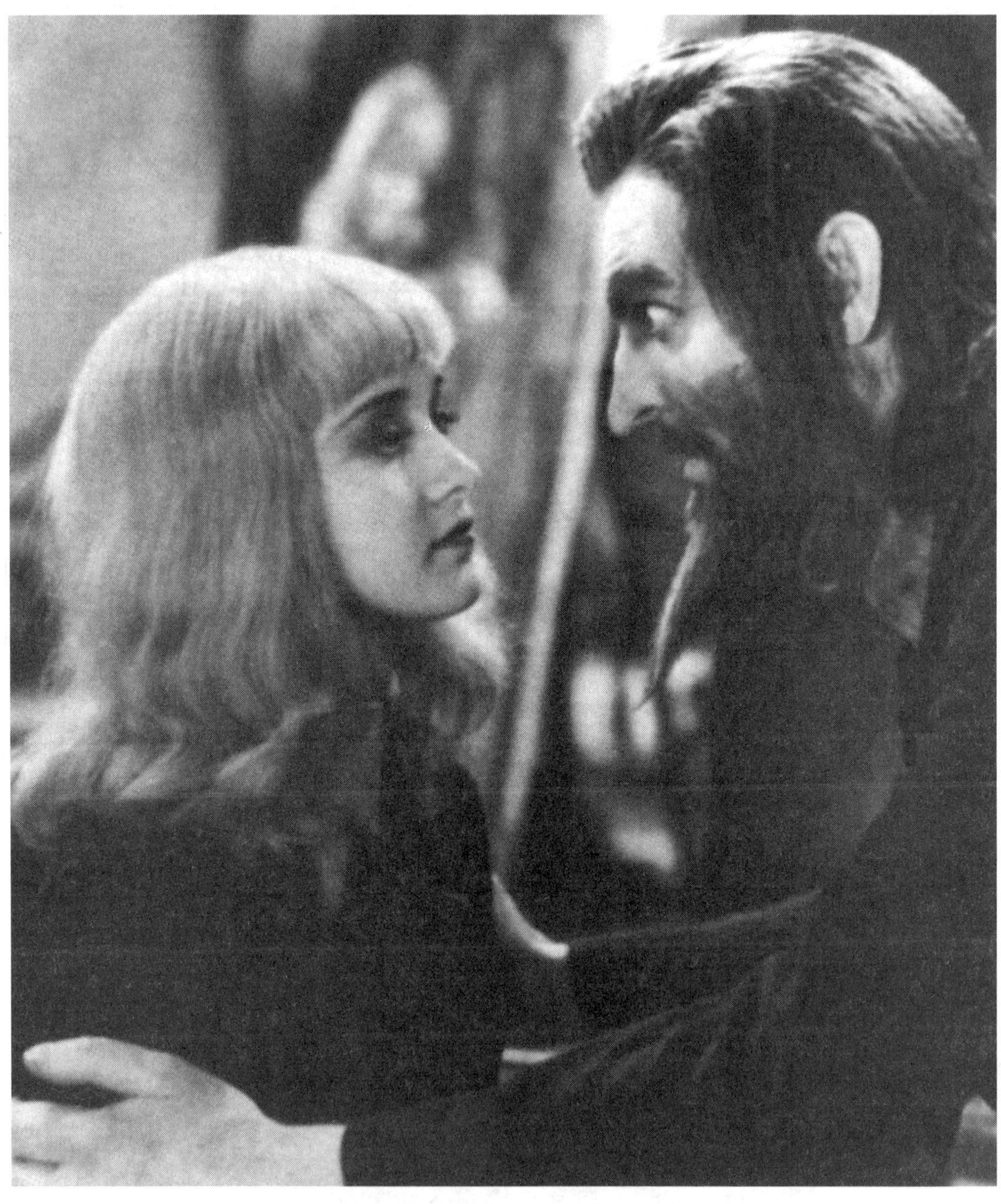

"Svengali", a movie from 1931, made many
believe that one would do ANYTHING with hypnosis.
Here John Barrymore entrances the hapless maiden.

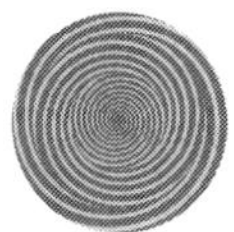

~ *Chapter 6* ~
THE QUESTION OF WILL POWER

Includes
Ideas Win Over Will
Imagination Over Will

A new client may ask the hypnotherapist, "What if I have too much will-power to be hypnotized?"

The answer to this question requires us to explore how mind operates.

Simply say, **"Will power has nothing to do with your not being hypnotized, as will power is used to assist you in entering hypnosis. You see, will power is conscious mind activity. Hypnosis, on the other hand, is a subconscious mind activity. When you get the subconscious to accept an idea, realization follows automatically."**

Thinking an idea is conscious mind activity. For a suggestion to carry power it must be accepted by emotions that live in the subconscious. Willing and/or will power can sabotage results; by making conscious mind more active and suppressing the subconscious.

A person, just using will to implant subconscious ideas, attempts the impossible. A sick person thinking over and over that they are not sick is still sick. By trying to will themself to health, they may feel worse because this idea and their critical mind constantly remind them that they are indeed sick. They contemplate the opposite of what they want and battle with their will to repress thoughts of illness. The more they struggle to hold illness thoughts in check, the more the thoughts possess them.

Hypnotherapy is not a question of will power or a weak mind verses a strong mind. It is the task of learning to operate your mind instead of your mind operating you. Hypnotize your client with the quiet assurance that they easily direct all parts of their mind to bring to them what they desire.

IDEAS WIN OVER WILL

Emile Coue', The master of autosuggestion, said *"Not only is the will incapable of vanquishing a thought but as fast as the will brings up its big guns, thought captures them and turns them against itself."* Or in other words, **whenever will struggles with an idea, the idea invariably wins!**

Prove this principle to yourself by putting a six-inch wide by twelve-foot long plank of wood on the floor and walking along it from end to end. Though narrow, you can do it easily.

The same plank, spanned between two tall buildings, is a different story. Timidity and the fear that you could lose your balance and fall may cause you to beat a hasty retreat.

Why?

The position of the board across a vast canyon of air arouses the suggestion of falling, colored with the emotion of that possibility! Your subconscious accepts the idea of a possible fall.

With will power you try to battle the impulse to fall. Says critical mind, "Of course you can walk along it. You proved to yourself you could do it, when you walked it before." Your subconscious assesses the risk and the more you think about "not" falling, the more the counter-idea is suggested. If you then stubbornly persist in taking the risk, you consider that you may lose your balance and topple into space.

Your precious will power is so helpless at times!

IMAGINATION OVER WILL

The pseudo-psychological Law Of Reverse Effect, created by French psychologist Baudouin said, *"When imagination and will are in conflict the imagination invariably gains the day."*

Or, *"The force of the imagination is in direct ratio to the square of the will. Thus the will turns out to be not the commanding monarch of life, as many would have it, but a blind Samson capable of either turning the mill or of pulling down the pillars."*

Hypnosis avoids the conflict between ideas and will. It replaces wrong thought by right; not by resisting or overpowering bad thoughts, but by bypassing critical mind and establishing selective thinking. Assure your client while in hypnosis **"You are excited to realize whatever you suggest to yourself. What you suggest to yourself now or with your conscious mind will be accomplished"** and they stimulate positive emotions to embrace will power as motivational tool that gets the conscious and subconscious mind to work together.

Hypnosis and properly presented suggestions then provide gardening tools to cultivate fertile subconscious fields of full crops for better living.

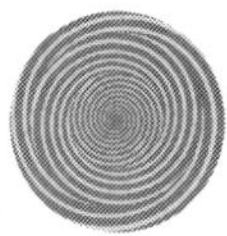

~ Chapter 7 ~

FIVE HYPNOTIC MIND MYTHS

Hypnotic suggestions have little value unless the client is willing to accept and realize them. The following points help dispel misunderstandings about hypnosis and underscore its potential:

Myth # One
The Hypnotist Exerts a Special Power Over a Subject

Unless the subject believes the hypnotist has that power, this is ridiculous. The subject chooses what suggestion they embrace or discard.

Myth # Two
Hypnosis Causes Unconsciousness

The subject is aware at all times, except when they willingly choose to accept amnesia, a deliberate interruption of the stream of consciousness. The hypnotized subject always freely decides what suggestions will be accepted or rejected. Suggestions in accord with regular pattern of behavior are the ones most readily accepted.

Upon arousal from hypnosis, most subjects are aware of what occurred. However, the shift in consciousness can cause spontaneous amnesia. Accepting suggested amnesia, of course, will make most consciously forget.

Myth # Three
The Hypnotist Controls the Trance State

In hypnosis, the client is in rapport with the operator and themselves. A client controls what suggestions they accept. They respond best to suggestions that are reasonable and pleasing. Negative things are accepted because they are *chosen* to be accepted.

Even in profound hypnosis, the client has control of all their facilities except one: "the critical facility." That's why if you give them a suggestion that pleases, they will accept it even if in their ordinary mind mode might discount it as "impossible." Examples of this are suggestions of mental anesthesia that erase pain and total recall of infancy and beyond. The critical faculty—who disbelieves fantastic things—if bypassed in hypnosis, allows suggestions to be installed.

The element of choice still exists in the hypnotic state. If a suggestion is disagreeable or contrary to the client's code of ethics, the person either rejects the suggestion or terminates the hypnosis. This is why hypnosis is such a safe therapeutic tool.

There is optimism in this opinion and it reflects the positive approach. However, appreciate that life has negative elements that inadvertently hypnotize us. The positive approach to life is to be commended; it is the happy way.

Myth # Four
Your Hypnosis Method is the Best One
It is amusing how therapists of all kinds regard their method as the best method. They are much like a preacher who "knows" that their way the only way to find God.

There is no "right" or "wrong" in hypnotherapy. There is only what IS, until it is changed. This Encyclopedia of Hypnotherapy gives you hundreds of effective techniques. Use the methods that make you most comfortable and you will become an expert in aiding your clients. The average hypnotherapist is not a scientist researcher so forget about theories. Be content with the effects and not the cause. Hypnotherapy is primarily concerned with effect.

Myth # Five
All Hypnosis is Self-Hypnosis
This blanket statement is very much like saying when we buy a car, "This car is mine because I bought and paid for it." In this, we overlook the salesperson who directly influenced the sale. Hypnosis is produced in two levels: hetero-hypnosis and self-hypnosis. In hetero-hypnosis, the salesperson is very much in evidence, and the practitioner is in intimate communion with the client.

Western thought accepts the idea that all hypnosis is self-hypnosis or self-contained concentration directing thought. Eastern hypnosis views it more as meditation with a cosmic connection expansion and not concentration.

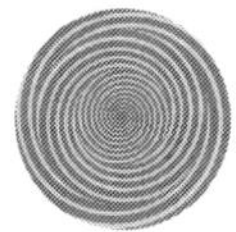

~ *Chapter 8* ~
HYPNOTIC HODGE-PODGE

Includes
An Adventure Of Structure
Agreement
Induction
The Dave Elman Pretend/Believe/Reality Induction
Suggestions
Arousal From Hypnosis

Most chapters of this book were written for you. This chapter is written for myself. It is a miscellany, hodge-podge, mixture, gallimaufry, jumble, farrage, mélange, mishmash, medley, conglomeration, olio, olla podrida, potpourri, and omnium gatherum. In other words, I write this chapter for myself just for the fun of it. You are welcome to share it, but for heaven's sake don't take it seriously. It is just stuff of my personal hypnotic thoughts.

Much of hypnotherapy deals with helping clients brighten up the dark side of their lives. To help them, I sometimes think I must develop the eyes of a cat.

Many clients who seek hypnotherapy are caught up in a spider web of neurosis, which is a mental illness characterized by irrational or depressive thought of behavior. It is like they live in a dark cave, into which my job is to shine a flashlight beam.

Being neurotic isn't so bad if one doesn't mind being unstable, disturbed, confused, irrational, disordered, maladjusted, distraught, oversensitive, overwrought, anxious, and nervous. As there is no organic reason for such mental disturbance, the neurotic person must somehow enjoy the distressful fun. If they come to me to clean up the mess, the first thing I must do is dump out the garbage, dust away the accumulated dust from the mind, and finally reach a mental state of emptiness inside. Only by becoming empty, is there room to become happily full.

Beyond neurosis is psychosis in which the person shows mental derangement, delusions, hallucinations, and loss of contact with external reality. In other words, they're crazy.

Ever think that maybe someone is not as crazy as they appear? In modern institutions for the insane, life isn't bad at all. There is constant pampering, attention, good food and lodging, and it's all for free. Why try to get well, when you've got it so good? And so, many remain in the institution. Although society today would never permit it, maybe the old way of flogging to get the "demon" out wasn't so dumb after all. With enough whipping, it becomes more disagreeable to stay in the institution than to get well and get out! Crazy thought!

Hypnosis can produce all the mental states of insanity- delusions, illusions, hallucinations, catalepsies, personality alterations, confusion and compulsion- but it is under control of the mind, and the craziness can be turned off like a faucet. The genuine psychotic has lost the control, and the craziness becomes the controller. Sometimes one wonders on how much of insanity is based in wanting to be insane: society takes care of you, the food may be better than you usually get, you remove yourself from personal stress, and the government pays the bills…it's not so bad a deal.

Beyond question, hypnosis could help many a psychotic person get well, *if they wanted to get well!* Effective hypnotherapy must be based on wanting to change. Then your work will be effective, as you motivate the desire to change.

Neurosis is often quite amenable to change.

Psychosis, on the other hand, can be very resistant, as it does not wish to change. The person retreats into a stupor or throws a fit, internally saying, "Leave me alone or I will kill you." A maniac has killed many a "Helpful Henry." Then the maniac is assured of his keep for life.

Enough stuff about the nuts.

In my personal chapter, I want to write about my experiment in the basic structure of hypnotherapy.

In this THE HYPNOTHERAPY ENCYCLOPEDIA a gamut (which is a whole scope of anything) of hypnotherapeutic techniques are given; yet as varied as these are, each follows a basic structure.

AN ADVENTURE OF STRUCTURE

I wanted to discover the basic structure of hypnotherapy. Here is my adventure…

I worked with my friend as my subject– someone who shares an equal interest in learning of the structures of hypnotherapy. We began with the consultation:

Quietly together, we went into my hypnotic session room. Lights were low; soft music played in the background. I asked my "client" to relax for a few moments while I organized our adventure.

In this case, I didn't need to find out my volunteer's presenting issue to ascertain what they want to accomplish in the session. We came together to investigate the structure of a trance. My client's relaxation afforded them time to think about what was about to happen.

AGREEMENT

Next on the agenda was the hypnotizing agreement. The client agrees to allow them self to be hypnotized by the hypnotherapist during the forthcoming session. In my adventure, the agreement is obvious as my friend volunteered to cooperate in the experiment. In a session the client allows hypnosis by the hypnotherapist and the hypnotherapist agrees to perform the best hypnotherapy for client.

INDUCTION

Next, I hypnotized my client. This begins with an induction. You may begin your induction during the interview or you may use a formal induction. The method use to hypnotize a client depends on what you, the hypnotherapist, prefers. In my adventure, I used a Dave Elman pretend, believe and reality induction. Here is what I did:

THE DAVE ELMAN PRETEND/BELIEVE/REALITY INDUCTION

For this…I told the cooperative subject;

"Close your eyes and place your right hand flat on top of your head and pretend that it is stuck there and that you cannot lift it off.

The subject did as was instructed.

I then suggested, **"Press your hand flat on top of your head and press it there firmer and firmer. Now, pretend you cannot lift it off, and let it happen."**

Done.

"Now, from pretending advance to <u>believing</u> you cannot lift your hand off of your head."

Done.

"BELIEVING is a step upwards from pretending." I let the suggestion of believing the hand was stuck on top of the head sink in.

Done.

"Now from believing it is stuck to the top of your head, let reality enter and you will find your hand so firmly stuck to the top of your head that you cannot remove it. Try as hard as you will."

Done.

The subject tries in vain to lift the seemingly stuck hand and I add the suggestion, **"The more you try to lift your hand from the top of your head, the more firmly it becomes stuck there."**

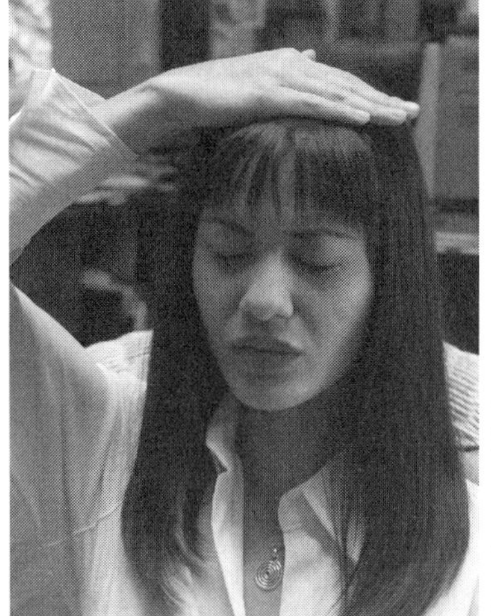

Pretend Your Hand is Stuck

The "Law of Reversed Effort" snaps in and the more the subject tries to remove their hand from atop of their head, the more firmly it sticks there. When this happens, you bypassed conscious mind control, which says, "of course you can lift your hand from your head" to subconscious mind control that says, "You cannot lift your hand from the top of your head."

Subconscious mind wins the day, just as habits win the day until they are reconditioned.

Done. All established.

If I allow the hand of the volunteer to remain stuck for several hours, even though it is uncomfortable, it becomes a habit of behavior. All habits take time to become firmly established in the mind. In this experiment, the lapse of time established a "mental set" in the subject.

Done.

Unwanted mental and/or physical behavior is "conditioned" into the mind in the same way. Hypnotherapy is a process of unconditioning.

In my example, I established a disagreeable situation in the subconscious of the subject, and enforced a time period to allow it to germinate and become established as a habit. I *induced experimental neurosis.* I set up an observable, disturbing, uncomfortable and unwanted situation in my subject that was so established in the subconscious that it moved beyond conscious mind control.

Usually in hypnotherapy you remove old unwanted behavior and replace it with the new (wanted) behavior on both intellectual and emotional level. To do this you have to determine the disturbance the client wants to change. In this experiment, the disturbance came from the hand on the head, a deviation from normal behavior. However, both are the same; an altered source of behavior has been established in the subconscious.

SUGGESTIONS

Now I presented beneficial suggestions and reinforced them.

Your suggestions result from what you ascertained as the disturbance (trauma) during the initial consultation. You can also learn about it by conducting the fact-finding interview while the client is in hypnosis. If you do, the information will be more subjective and less objective. You can also make this determination by analyzing a detailed intake form and/or any notes you have taken. Reverse speech analysis (see the chapter on it) can also be used.

Once you know what a client wants to benefit themselves, you place them into a receptive subjective state of mind (hypnosis), and give the proper suggestions (suggestion formula) to condition their mind for the desired performance.

All unwanted mental or physical behavior stem from having become conditioned into the mind. Hypnotherapy provides wanted behavior by unconditioning and reconditioning the mind of the client.

AROUSAL FROM HYPNOSIS

After the reconditioning suggestions have been given, allow the subconscious to take its time to grant acceptance, and arouse the client from hypnosis when the session is complete.

In the case of our very patient volunteer subject, who all this time has been sitting with their right hand stuck to their head, the suggestions are given. **"Close your eyes, relax, and drop down into a subjective state of mind in which your behavior leaves the realm of the subconscious and returns to conscious control. When you open your eyes, your hand will immediately be released from your head."**

It is done. This experimental session is complete.

As this is my chapter, and since I live in the Silicon Valley (surrounded by computers), I am favorably inclined to regard clients as having remarkable bio-computers within their head. These biocomputers can be programmed as is required and desired. The operator of the biocomputer is the SELF. The keyboard of the biocomputer is the MIND. The biocomputer is the BRAIN.

Do these personal conjectures make any sense OR are they just plain mad?

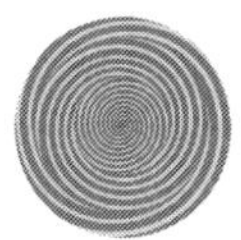

~ Chapter 9 ~
BASIC STRUCTURE OF A SESSION

Includes

The Ten Segments of a Beautiful Session:
> **First Meeting: Building Rapport**
> **The Consultation: Discover What the Client Wants To Accomplish**
> **Private Cognition**
> **The Hypnotizing Agreement**
> **Formal Hypnotic Induction**
> **Deepening Suggestions**
> **Presenting Beneficial Suggestions**
>> **Suggestion Formula For The Hypnotherapist**
> **Hypnotherapeutic Processes**
> **Arousal from Hypnosis**
> **The Encouraging Dismissal**

Whatever induction method you employ, a beautiful first hypnotherapy session can be divided into 10 segments, viz.:

1. FIRST MEETING: BUILDING RAPPORT

When client and hypnotherapist meet is the time to develop immediate rapport. The dictionary describes rapport as "a close relationship characterized by harmony." Before the session starts, look at your client while holding thoughts of warm friendship. You could invite them to "sit in silence for a few minutes" while gently looking upon them. Make your eyes soft by thinking kind thoughts. Some hypnotherapists think of sending them white light. The client, of course, is looking back. Five minutes of this intimate energy exchange is amazing.

An intimate level of communication between the hypnotherapist and client can be easily achieved with active listening; the art of mirroring and matching your clients words, phrases and body language.

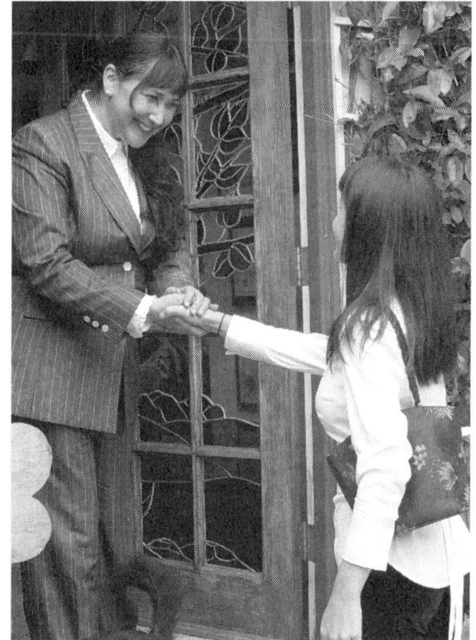

Greeting

2. THE CONSULTATION: DISCOVER WHAT THE CLIENT WANTS TO ACCOMPLISH

The dictionary defines consultation as "conferring." Actively listen while the client tells you their story and the reason for the visit. In this segment of the session, you ascertain what they desire to accomplish in their session. Consultation time varies with each individual. Allow full time. There is no hurry. Provide an opportunity for the client to express fully what they want to accomplish via hypnotherapy.

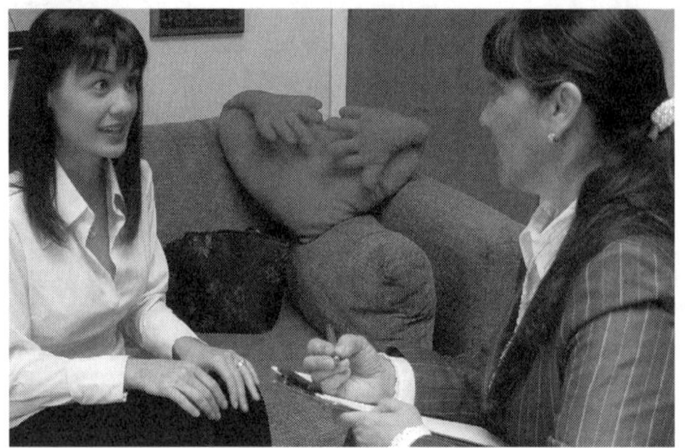

The Consultation

Photo by Jon Nicholas

3. THE HYPNOTIZING AGREEMENT

The dictionary explains agreement as "A harmony of understanding. A harmonious arrangement."

An agreement made between the hypnotherapist and client is threefold:

* You both agree the induction will proceed.

* The client agrees to follow instruction and allow hypnosis to occur.

* The Hypnotherapist agrees to use their full professional skill to benefit and aid the client to accomplish what they desire to accomplish.

This formalized agreement affirms that the client will cooperate fully allowing complete induction and the acceptance of beneficial suggestions. It removes obstacles to assure success. You can use the hypnotic contract as a deepening technique.

Your agreement can be simply verbalized between you. You could bring the lights up for this phase if desired. You might have the client write these words, **"I will do everything to positively assist my hypnotherapist to affect the changes I want for myself."** A written agreement, mutually constructed and signed by each party is powerful too.

THE HYPNOTIC CONTRACT

This contract constitutes a friendly agreement between myself and the hypnotherapist for self help for the specific purpose herein outlined.

_________________ (*Client*) henceforth known as Party of the First Part and
_________________ (*Hypnotherapist*) known as Party of the Second Part

The Party of the First Part agrees to be hypnotized by Party of the Second Part with complete willingness, cooperation and confidence for the purpose herein outlined (*Write the purpose of the session*)

____

____

Party of the Second Part agrees to use professional hypnotic skills to benefit the Party of the Second Part to obtain the mastering of this purpose with confidential protocol.
For the purposes and obligations herewith expressed, we affix our signatures and date this contract.

Client ____

Hypnotherapist ____

Date ____

---

4. PRIVATE COGITATION

The dictionary describes cogitation as "to quietly ponder."

Following the consultation, create a thoughtful period for the client. Invite them to, "Sit relaxed and comfortable in this special chair (a recliner is fine) and think about what you told me you want to accomplish." If your office lends itself to this, guide them into another quiet, darkened room or dim the lights. A violet light could be illuminated and soft meditation music played. Ten minutes is ample time for this period.

5. THE FORMAL HYPNOTIC INDUCTION

Dictionary defines induction as "to motivate the occurrence of the occurrence." An induction is the process used by hypnotherapists to bring about and stimulate hypnosis. It transforms your client's mind state from ordinary awareness to the trance. Inductions can take as long as 30 minutes. Rapid induction can be as short 30 seconds.

Have the client sit back into a comfortable chair, recliner, or lie down upon a couch. Lights are lowered. The *Serenity Resonance Sound* (alpha/theta sounds I created with Joseph Worrell) is helpful to play as background to the induction of hypnosis. Stand or sit close by your client while performing your preferred hypnotizing induction method.

6. DEEPENING SUGGESTIONS

Imbed a deepening suggestion into your induction like **"You are going deeper and deeper with each breath you take." "Every sound takes you deeper."**

7. PRESENTING BENEFICIAL SUGGESTIONS

The dictionary describes suggestions as an "act or intention to suggest a desired occurrence." Suggestion in hypnotic terms seems may be defined as "the subconscious realization of ideas."

Remove the <u>old</u> and replace it with the new. The suggestions you give are generally decided upon during the consultation. These beneficial suggestions may be presented to the client as waking hypnosis or while in hypnosis. Verbal suggestion uses the "art of semantics" directing verbalized thought toward specific helpful purpose.

Repeat suggestions directly into the client's ear. Such close up suggestions are implanted into client's subconscious. Use their name freely during this part of the session.

Post hypnotic suggestions are deferred suggestions that take effect after your client awakens from the trance state. These suggestions will unconsciously carry over into their future daily art of living. Hypnosis conditions and reconditions positive outcomes.

Hypnosis can be performed under almost any condition. It is best however to a have a private atmosphere free of distractions. A successful trance induction depends most on the attitude of the hypntherapist. If the hypnotherapist is calm, the client calms. If an unwarranted disturbance like a phone ringing is greeted with a suggestion **"The sound of the phone** (Or any outside noise) **takes you deeper and deeper into hypnosis."**

SUGGESTION FORMULA FOR THE HYPNOTHERAPIST:

"Fill your mind with the knowing that you are an excellent hypnotist. Come to know this deep within yourself. Know it completely. You are a professional and confident hypnotist. Every day in every way you learn more and more ways to be competent. Hypnosis is a skill that gets better with practice and you succeed and learn every time you hypnotize someone; getting better and better each time. You handle each client as unique. You honor each individual's responsiveness to trance. Learning these processes is like learning your 'A B C's…simple and easy. Because you are conscientious you succeed and are on your way to being a great hypnotherapist."

8. HYPNOTHERAPEUTIC PROCESSES

A myriad of popular techniques, often included in a hypnosis curriculum, include: Affirmation, Aversion, Behavior Modification, Biofeedback, Brainwave Entertainment, Breathwork, Brief Therapy, Catalepsy, Cell Demand, Chakra Balancing, Cognitive Shift, Coaching, De-Hypnotizing, Demonstration, De-Programming, Depossession, Desensitizing, Elman Method, Eye-Movement Desensitization & Reprocessing (EMDR), Emotional Release, Enneagram, Energy Balancing, Ericksonian, Fantasy, Forgiveness, Gestalt, Guided Imagery, Hypnoanalysis, Hypnoanesthesia, (Non-pharmacological Analgesia), Hypnocatharsis, Education, Hypno-Yoga, Ideomotor Response, Induction, Inner Child, Joy Therapy, Life Strategies, Magnetism, Memory Chain, Mental Rehearsal, Mesmerism, Metaphor, Mind Mapping, Mind Mastery, Motivation, Neurolinguistic Psychology/Programming (NLP), Neurypnology, Nocebo Effect, Parts or Sub-Personality, Pinpoint Method, Placebo Effect, Posthypnotic Suggestion, Progression, Projection, Re-Alerting, Reality Therapy, Rebirthing, Reframing, Regression, Reinforcement, Release, Reparenting, Reprogram, Reversal, Reverse Speech, Ritual, Scripting, Self-Hypnosis, Sensory Distortion, Sleep-Learning, Soma-Psychic Integration, Somnambulism, Suggestion, Squish Method, Tantra, Tapping (EFT), Time-Line Therapy, Trance, Trance Channeling, Quantum Focus, Visualization and Wellness vs. Illness. A rose by any name still smells sweet. All these labels should accomplish the same thing: bringing your client mind/body/spirit well-being and inner harmony and joy. You will explore many of these in this encyclopedia.

9. AROUSAL FROM HYPNOSIS

Also called re-alerting or re-awakening, arousal brings someone from the hypnotic state to the waking state. The dictionary describes arousal as, "a thought to awaken from sleep."

In awakening the client from hypnosis you accomplish four things:

1. You reinforce suggestions and implant a final suggestion for more rapid and deeper hypnosis in the future.
2. You can further deepen the hypnosis in progress during the awakening.
3. You help the client to be more refreshed and revitalized.
4. You have an opportunity to immediately re-hypnotize the client with increased depth of trance.

The arousal should always be a gentle process, just as you would want it if someone were to awaken you from a deep sleep. In inducing trance you presented your suggestions slowly and with care so apply this same gentle and calm approach to the removal of hypnotic sleep. Remember as a hypnotist it is your obligation to arouse the client feeling fine and well in every way. Arousal from hypnosis removes the often-drowsy state of hypnosis, as the client becomes **"fully awake, alert and feeling well and fine in every way."**

Allow time for the subconscious to make its own decisions when successful hypnotherapy has been accomplished.

Since hypnosis is often induced by suggesting the idea of going to sleep, it stands to reason that the reverse suggestions for awakening from sleep or trance removes the hypnotic condition. A good wake-up suggestion is, **"You are deep in hypnosis now and it has been a wonderful experience. When you come back to room awareness in a minute you will awaken feeling wonderful and well. I will count from one to five and with every number you will slowly awaken. At the count of five feeling wide, wide-awake as if you have awakened from a wonderful healthful nights sleep. In the future, whenever I snap my fingers, you will immediately go into this deep wonderful hypnotic state.**

I am starting to count so get ready to awaken now. One. Two. You are beginning to wake up. Three. Your eyes are opening; you want to move about and stretch. Four. You're waking up. Five. Wake up. You are wide awake and feeling fine!"

Under the influence of these suggestions, your subject will gradually open their eyes, move about, stretch and awaken feeling fine. Hypnotherapy has been accomplished.

Re-Hypnotizing

Interestingly, arousal from hypnosis can also be used as a deepening technique of the hypnosis. Immediately after arousing them from trance, suggest that they repeat the hypnosis and this time they will drop even deeper. **"You come back to room awareness refreshed and feeling fine and then, when you close your eyes, you go even deeper."**

Using this important psychological moment of heightened suggestibility is called "re-hypnotizing." It allows time for subconscious more time to reinforce previous suggestions. When you are done restating the suggestions, you can then let the sub-conscious make its own decisions as to when hypnosis is successfully complete by saying, **"You have done very well. Come back now when you desire feeling wonderful and well."**

Or you can bring them back by suggesting "This has been a very good session for you and has done much good. You feel deep inside yourself how improved you are in every way and you will continue to improve from this time on. When you awaken now from hypnosis you will feel wonderful and well."

Or if you would like to instill somnambulism you could suggest **"When you awaken, you will have no memory of anything in this session and the good and powerful suggestions will have made a deep permanent impression on your thoughts and actions. It will be as if you dozed off for a minute."**

10. THE ENCOURAGING DISMISSAL

Let the session end right here and do not discuss it further. To do so brings the critical faculty to mind. The client will take some moments for reorientation. Be sociable. Remember to that they are still highly suggestible to what you say, so be positive.

When the client is fully awake and back into their stream of normal consciousness, make the next appointment and recount any specific instructions you may have.

The dictionary describes dismissal as "to be on your way." An effective dismissal from a hypnotic session is the Buddhist affirmation, "The one who came into my office is not the one who leaves my office." A change in the individual has taken place. What was requested has been achieved.

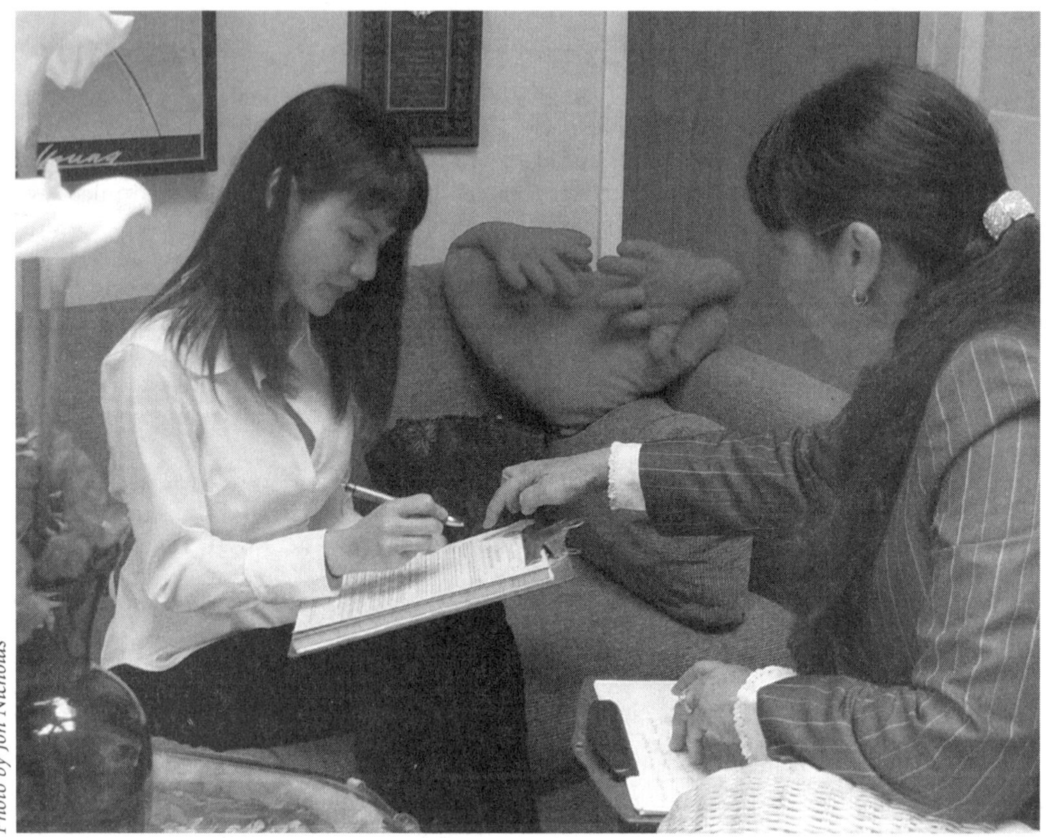

The Consultation

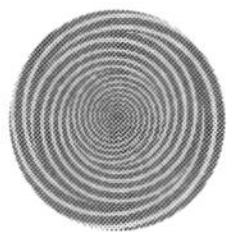

~ Chapter 10 ~
THE CONSULTATION

Includes
Consultation Forms
The Interview
Listening
Expectation
How To Establish Empathetic Rapport
Boundaries

Your consultation is as important as the hypnosis session itself. Some seek help solely for a sympathetic ear. Telling someone your problems can be quite cathartic. Between your sympathetic listening ears must be wisdom as well. During your consultation you need to:

1. Understand why the client seeks your help.
2. Bring out information of value to use during the hypnotherapy session.

CONSULTATION FORMS

Write down your client's name, address, telephone number, age, marital status, children, business or profession, the date, any referring doctor's name, address and telephone number. Keep these records for each client. (Some states require a written disclosure form at the first visit to a hypnotist and this would have the client's information on it. More about this in the chapter 16.)

You may use the acronym "SOAP"

S = Subjective information, facts given
O = Objective information, what induction or procedure is used
A = Assessment, affirmations and post-hypnotic suggestions used
P = Plan, future processes you are considering using

To save time you could present your client with a written consultation form that fill out before actually meeting with you. This gives them a chance to carefully assess their personal concerns. Written words are so precise and permanent. Spoken words can be lengthy and fleeting. A written consultation saves time and makes your plan of action clear.

THE INTERVIEW

Your interview begins when you ask the client **"Tell me about yourself. Why have you come to me today?"** and you listen without comment to what they say.

You want the client to talk about him or herself. Your client's greatest interest is their problem and how to feel better. Let the client air their problem. Get the details. It is good for them. The success of the session depends on the rapport you establish during this listening.

LISTENING

Listen from the point of view of the speaker. This lets you "stand in their moccasins." What words impact them or engage their imagination? What are their values? What is their mission and belief? What do they need to be happy? How do they experience the world? When you discover what it's like to be in the other's skin you learn how to speak to them in their language.

Be a sympathetic listener, but do not take what is said over-seriously. This is good psychology. The chances are, the client has come to see you because they take them self very seriously, and this seriousness has gotten them into trouble. Treat problems with respect and assure them that: **"With hypnosis you will be surprised at how un-serious your concerns become. Most problems are solved when someone changes their attitude about themself and their problem. Hypnosis is a wonderful changer of attitudes."**

Facilitate your client to be comfortable and at ease. Subjective information comes forth best when the body is relaxed. A relaxed body is conducive to a relaxed mind.

Zippy Consultation Tip: The Entrancing Interview

To speed up your consultation, hypnotize the client prior to your interview and suggest that when they "return" or while still in trance, they will tell you the real purpose of their visit and how you can best help them. Or you can actually interview them in the trance state.

EXPECTATION

Your consultation helps build expectation that the hypnosis process is easy.

With such expectation, you can successfully hypnotize in pantomime without a single word being spoken. This makes hypnotizing someone who speaks a foreign language possible. Generally of course, it is best that both the hypnotist and subject speak (and think) in the same language or to have a translator standing by.

Expectation is created in everything you put out to your client. Your business card, your phone message, your office, the way you are dressed, how you greet them and the words you use to communicate. Your consultation must convey the idea that they you can help them achieve what they came for.

HOW TO ESTABLISH EMPATHETIC RAPPORT

Rapport is benchmark of good relationships between people and determines the success of your session. Characterized by harmony and trusted communication between you. Rapport helps clients deal effectively with change and develop their own resources to overcome emotional blocks. Another word for rapport could be sameness.

There three basic qualities of rapport:

1. Duo Rapport
"They don't care that you know until they know that you care."
   —Zig Zigler

Duo rapport is most commonly used in hypnotherapy. The Hypnotherapist listens with a sympathetic ear to the story of the client. It is a confidential communication. The Hypnotherapist understands and offers their assistance, but the rapport is not complete, as duality is there; there is not a direct connection. The communication is like looking at a work-of-art, in a gallery. The painting is appreciated in being observed, but there is no personal connection between the painting and the observer. In relation to hypnotherapy, the client is the painting and the hypnotherapist is the observer. It has value, but not the value of Oneness Rapport.

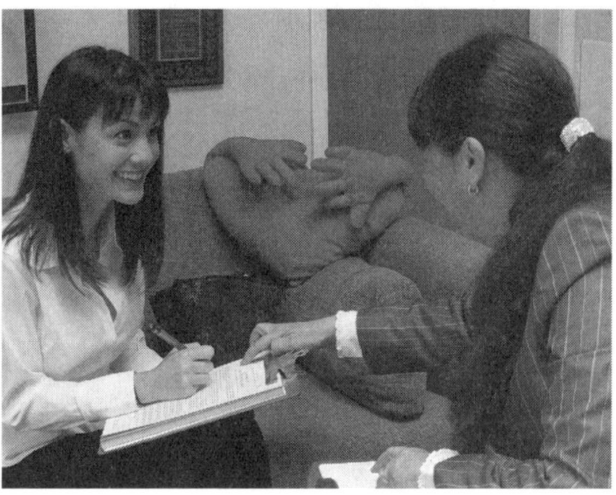
Rapport

Photo by Jon Nicholas

2. Oneness Empathetic Rapport
"Love your neighbor as yourself."
   —Jesus

Oneness rapport is also called presence, compassion or empathy. This is the ideal type of rapport between client and the hypnotherapist. In such closeness, you become the artist who helps repaint the client. It is a dynamic relationship between the client and you. A natural bond of friendship develops when your client feels your interest in helping them help themselves.

With such empathy you almost experience what the client experiences inside them.

The connection becomes so close that even bodily sensations are felt together. For instance, if the client feels thirsty the therapist equally becomes thirsty and vice versa. One drinks the water and both feel equally satisfied. It is a biofeedback connection. It helps the client accomplish their goal sometimes. The client may not realize it, but rapport is a subtle secret kind of hypnosis. Of course, the client came for hypnosis so you'll want to formally hypnotize them too. When it happens the best formal hypnotherapy is performed.

Your experience will teach about such empathy. It can happen instantly or build over time. With instant empathetic rapport, you instinctively know what is going on inside the client, even before a formal interview begins. Instant rapport is instant TRUST. Some people are naturally empathetic while others have to cultivate it. To cultivate empathy, accept that the other person is as important to the universe as you are. Feel this sincerely and deeply inside yourself.

The more expert you become as a hypnotherapist, the more you create Oneness Rapport with your clients. Hold a strong intention for this human art form and watch/feel it develop on its own. As your consciousness advances in yourself, so does your mastery of Oneness Rapport advance.

Editor Stockwell's Comments

Research shows that ninety-three percent of the way we communicate is based on something other than words. For six months, telemarketers at a major credit card company matched speaking patterns and energy with the person on the other end of the phone and increased their sales by 254%, while complaints dropped 90%! Behavioral hypnotists teach business managers to motivate others with rapport.

3. Selfless Consciousness

"Feel the consciousness of each person as your own consciousness. So leaving aside concern for self, become each being."

     —Shiva to his consort Devi,
     5,000-year-old sutra

In love, rapport happens spontaneously. Two become one and flow together as one consciousness. Lovers feel a oneness of life-flowing together. Once you love, rapport is easy. Friends adapt similar patterns smoothly, unconsciously and naturally. Practice blending your consciousness with a beloved or friend. Lose yourself in them. When you lose yourself in them, they lose themselves in you. To love, you leave aside concern for self. This high state will develop your talent of empathy. This is rapport of the highest level.

BOUNDARIES

What I am about to say may seem paradoxical yet it is equally as important as establishing selfless rapport: When you hypnotize a client always stay within your own space. Never intrude upon their space. Hold these five virtues:

1. Detachment
2. Continence
3. Forgiveness
4. Contentment
5. Humility

Because of the deep rapport between the client and hypnotherapist the client may feel a co-dependent connection to the hypnotherapist:

1. They may depend on you rather than themselves and believe that their "control" is out of their hands and in yours. To override this illusion, include suggestions that increase the clients control over themselves and the recognition of their own responsibility in making themselves what they want to be.

2. Some clients develop "transference" where they project their own feeling on to you. They can even think that they are in love with you. To counteract such an illusion you can hypnotize in a more impersonal manner and minimize contact with the client. Some hypnotherapists record all sessions for a complete record and some have a witness to the sessions.

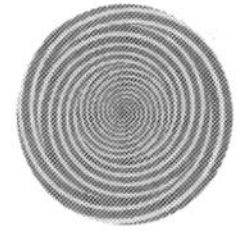

~ *Chapter 11* ~
PRE-HYPNOSIS HYPNOSIS

Includes
Explaining Hypnosis To The Client
Suggestion Formula For Pre-Hypnosis
Hypnotic Amnesia: Will You Remember?

Now that you have establishing rapport with your client, they have confidence in you as a professional hypnotherapist and helper. You've chitchatted about how you can help them with hypnosis. The interview includes a good understanding of what hypnosis is and how hypnosis works. Now ask them, "Have you been hypnotized before?" Listen well to their response. If they say "yes" ask them what it was like for them. If it was favorable do it the same way. If they did not like the other experience ask why and honor their preferences.

EXPLAINING HYPNOSIS TO THE CLIENT

If they have not been hypnotized before ask, **"What do you expect to happen?"** They may have no idea of expect or they may expect a deep trance where they will be almost unconscious. Some will say, "I think it is like going to sleep" and others may say. "I think it feels greatly relaxing." Each reply is correct for the experience will be much like the client expects it to be.

After you've heard what they expect hypnosis to be, tell them, **"Hypnosis is a state of mind in its own right where the conscious mind steps aside and the subconscious accepts good and beneficial suggestions. Some feel that that they are wide-awake and merely relaxed while they take on suggestion. Others are unconscious of what occurs in hypnosis. Your hypnosis experience will be what you create for yourself.**

Whichever experience you prefer, you'll naturally advance your awareness in that direction. In fact, the form hypnosis takes today will have nothing to do its effectiveness in correcting the problem you came to solve. Your results will be terrific."

Make sure that they understand this concept so that they come out of hypnosis feeling that they were indeed hypnotized. The mental set you establish in advance of the hypnosis regulates, to some extent, the form the experience takes on.

Use everything the client tells you to enhance their session. Your client expects to succeed as a result of hypnosis. Guide them to experience hypnosis the way they expect to experience it.

SUGGESTION FORMULA FOR PRE-HYPNOSIS

Another way to explain hypnosis especially to someone who has no idea what to expect is this this: **"Some say that hypnosis is related to sleep. Others say it is related to wakefulness. The truth is that hypnosis is related to both and is neither. Hypnosis is a state of mind in its own right. It is an altered state of consciousness in which the critical faculties of the conscious mind are placed aside and the subconscious mind is brought to the fore. In hypnosis, subconscious behavior becomes more active, while the conscious steps aside.**

The more you understand how the subconscious operates, the better you will understand hypnosis. In hypnosis, the subconscious easily accepts ideas and acts upon those that agree with your beliefs.

In hypnosis, you will be fully aware at times, relaxed and highly responsive to suggestions. Whether you feel awake or asleep, either way, you easily respond to suggestion. Suggestion is the "key" to how and why hypnosis works.

The form your hypnosis session takes has nothing to do with its effectiveness in correcting your problem. You may feel deep asleep or lightly relaxed, it's up to you. The key thing is that you just relax to set your mind for hypnosis."

Make certain that your client understands these points. Otherwise, some who are keenly aware in and out of trance come out of the experience feeling they were not hypnotized because they thought they were supposed to lose consciousness. Some, deeply asleep, don't remember and therefore think that nothing happened. And then,

"The important point for you to understand is that you enter into the hypnosis you create for yourself."

HYPNOTIC AMNESIA: WILL YOU REMEMBER?

Whether or not you remember your experience after coming out of hypnosis depends on the depth of trance, whether or not the subject expects amnesia to occur, and if amnesia is suggested. Explain to your clients that, **"Being hypnotized will be much like a dream. Sometimes dreams are vivid and the memory of them persists before fading away. Other dreams are less vivid and not recalled at all, and some dreams are so striking that they are never forgotten. Hypnosis is like that."** This *dream concept* provides a good explanation of the phenomenon of hypnotic amnesia.

Explaining these aspects of the hypnotic occurrence to your client places the experience in their lap. Their mind will create their journey as it wishes to be. Be completely unconcerned as to where they go during the process. All you want is for your client's conscious mind to step aside so you can direct your suggestions directly to the subconscious. There, they are accepted uncritically.

The really important thing is not the personal experience of being hypnotized, but the desired hypnotherapeutic results.

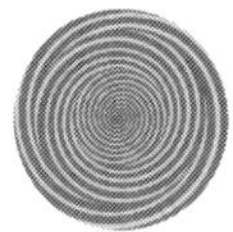

~ *Chapter 12* ~
DIRECT MENTAL MARRIAGE HYPNOSIS

Includes
Direct Hypnosis In A Nutshell
A Holistic Mental Marriage Contract

Customarily, we think of hypnosis as "bypassing the critical conscious mind" to establish selective thinking in the subconscious. We say that the critical mind requires hypnosis because it is limited and directly connected with the world.

True...

But critical mind, when positively engaged in the hypnosis process, becomes a powerful ally uniting all mind states. Direct hypnosis, instead of bypassing the conscious critical mind, implants beneficial suggestions there so that it, in turn, implants them into the subconscious.

In truth, the subconscious phase of mind is in a perpetual state of hypnosis, so it readily accepts and reacts upon suggestion without going through any bypassing rigmarole. The subconscious mind is unlimited and directly linked with the infinite or Universal Mind.

Direct hypnosis motivates the critical, conscious mind to be the opposite of critical. It directs it as a companion mind to the other mind modes. Direct Hypnosis simply implants beneficial suggestions directly into the Conscious Critical Mind, which, in turn, implants them into the subconscious, thereby activating the universal mind. This is easy to do and very powerful.

Mind is a process for producing thoughts. Mind functions on three levels:
1. Conscious Critical Mind (objective, your perception of the world)
2. Subconscious Mind (subjective, inner perception of yourself, the pathway to universal mind)
3. Universal or Superconscious Mind (connection with the cosmos and pathway to the universal mind)

The subconscious is filled with many suggestions and eagerly accepts and reacts upon new suggestions. If suggestions are good, they are helpful. If suggestions are bad, they are hurtful. Hypnosis produces a state of mind that is open to react to and accept suggestions. All it needs is good instructions. Direct hypnosis lets your conscious mind give good instructions.

DIRECT HYPNOSIS IN A NUTSHELL
The conscious critical mind implants suggestions directly into the subconscious and activates superconscious awareness as the pathway to UNIVERSAL MIND. It is a holistic approach.

Let this remind you of what it is all about:

MIND IN WHOLENESS = SUPER PERCEPTION

MODUS OPERANDI: A HOLISTIC MENTAL MARRIAGE CONTRACT

Talk directly to your client,

"Open your mind as a whole with no part bypassed. No more criticism. Let your conscious and subconscious mind recognize your whole MIND'S infinite capacity. Both conscious and subconscious mind come to recognize MIND'S infinite possibilities. You now open the pathway to your universal mind."

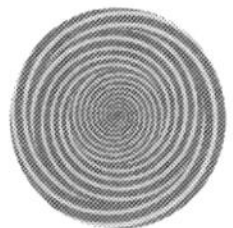

~ *Chapter 13* ~
THOUGHTS TO PLAY WITH

Scientific studies confirm that our thinking and our interpretations affect the world around us by actually creating our physical reality!

Your neural networks are the beating wings of the mysterious butterfly of your soul.

The more we understand about the brain, the more it appears to function like a physical transmitter and receiver, decoding and encoding information between our body and the outer world. It's an intricate system of bioelectrical activity producing energy frequencies and brain wave patterns.

Your body is obvious. It is a visible amazing form that via its brain performs in a 3-D here and now.

Your brain is less obvious. It functions like a bio-computer and learning to use it to full capacity, *a la* the thoughts it can produce, is a great purpose. Mind is intangible. It is a process for producing thoughts. It can elevate to genius or descend to insanity based entirely on how it is used. The universe does not care. Up or down, both provide practice in the using. Most are in the middle.

The biocomputer brain is not immortal. It is a mechanism and will die. The mind cannot die, for it is not a mechanism. It is simply a process of self.

Your SELF is CONSCIOUSNESS. It is that which you recognize existing behind your eyes when you look closely at your reflection in a mirror. Your SELF is your individual consciousness, of which there is no duplicate in the entire Universe. It is immortal. It is timeless. It is perpetual as mind belongs to its functioning, mind too is immortal.

The entire universe is a vast consciousness. The more you connect with that vast consciousness, the more you become a master. How do you make that connection? Hypnosis, of course, is the special process that produces desired thoughts.

Goodness, gracious, golly…so much to do and so much to understand.

Not really. Just let it take care of itself.

"Make life a playground not a battle field," said Shiva.

"Go with the flow," said Lau Tsu.

"Nothing need be done," said Buddha and

My dear wife Delight said, "Just be like a log drifting down the stream, and among the things you bump into will be found the real treasures of your life."

A paradox of course…the entire Universe is a paradox. A paradox is much like a puzzle. Do you have fun trying to solve puzzles? If you do, have fun!

Just always remember, as Shiva told Devi as she sat on his lap, "Don't take what I say about it seriously Gal, or you'll miss the truth."

Have fun and appreciate the miracle that you are.

P.S. take your time about it all. You have eternity and there is no time in eternity.

Illustration by Shelley Stockwell-Nicholas

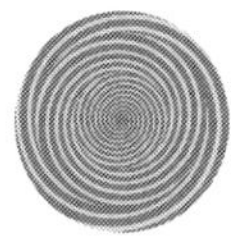

~ *Chapter 14* ~
ANSWERS FOR CLIENTS

By Shelley Stockwell-Nicholas, PhD

From the book "Hypnosis: How To Put A Smile On Your Face & $$$ In Your Pocket"
Creativity Unlimited Press

Includes

Can Everyone Be Hypnotized?
Who Can Do Hypnosis?
How Does Hypnosis Feel?
Were You Hypnotized Convincers
Why Do Some People Have Doubts About Hypnosis or is it Dangerous?
Do You Need Hypnosis or Hypnotherapy?
Can You Really Resolve Physical Problems With Your Mind?
What Happens To The Hypnotherapist's Information About Me?
If You Can't Solve Your Problems Without Help Do You Have A Weak Will?
How Does Hypnotherapy Work?
What Happens To The Hypnotherapist's Information About You?
What Happens If You Don't Come Out Of Trance?

These questions and answers placed in the waiting area of your office can be very helpful to your clients:

CAN EVERYONE BE HYPNOTIZED?

Yes, of course! Everyone goes in and out of trance, the basic hypnotic state, throughout the day. You, dear reader, have been in trance several times *today*. You just may not have called it hypnosis.

Daydreaming, runners high, before sleep, upon awakening, reading, watching TV, video game playing, movies, a boring meeting, shopping or a freeway drive, can and do naturally entrance you. Anytime you move from an outward perception to an inner awareness you enter trance. Words you use induce trance too; "wonder," "imagine," "amaze," "puzzle," "understand," "curious," "dream," "mesmerize," "turn inward and notice," "mindful" and "hypnotize," cause you to go inside to make them make sense.

Hypnosis techniques put you in charge of your natural ability to enter trance. Hypnosis is a skill, like reading or writing that anyone can easily learn.

WHO CAN DO HYPNOSIS?

Anyone who has the mind to, and even those who don't, can and do, do hypnosis. Anyone who can concentrate for a few moments can easily learn the steps it takes to induce a self-hypnotic trance. You practice hypnotism every day with the things you say to yourself and others. You hypnotize yourself with repetitive actions and thoughts. This is called autosuggestion.

Mothers and fathers are master hypnotists and their verbal and nonverbal conditioning often stick for life. Advertisers use hypnosis in all their work and so do religions.

Professional hypnotists receive special training in the technique and use of hypnosis before they achieve certification. Professional groups offer training and opportunities to keep skills updated. Visit hypnosisfederation.com to see a list of well trained hypnotists, many have also been trained in a wide range of other mind, body, and spirit disciplines.

A psychologist may have only attended a lecture or a one-day class in hypnosis and then present themself as a hypnotist. If you want psychology, go to a psychologist. If you want hypnosis, go to a professional hypnotist specifically and thoroughly trained in hypnosis. Hypnosis is their main focus and training.

HOW DOES HYPNOSIS FEEL?

Familiar! The by-product of all hypnosis is relaxation where muscles, nerves and mind relax. Some describe it as feeling "passive, placid and mellow," others as "filled with light or surprised by new perception." One client said, "I saw strange pictures for the first time, felt new feelings, thought new thoughts and understood things I never could before. It's difficult to find the words to describe the hypnotic experience."

When in hypnosis there is often a distinct experience of automatic, spontaneous or involuntary thought or action as compared to the feeling you get with conscious thought. Returning to regular "room awareness" makes everything more peaceful. One friend says that after a hypnosis session, "My heart went around grinning all day."

Hypnosis is definitely a common and varied experience. Each hypnotic trance may be different from what you expect, or from the last one you experienced. This makes sense considering you are not the same person you were the last time! Your *experience* of trance will differ from another's. In all cases a person feels relaxed, calm and passive, as if in a wonderful dream. Senses are heightened and you are aware of everything going on around you.

Sometimes part of us can be hypnotized while another part is not. For instance, if you are driving a car and having an animated conversation with your passenger, the part of you driving may be unaware and hypnotized and the part of you talking, fully conscious.

Hypnosis, like sex, looks different than it feels. From the observer's point of view, the subject might appear caved in or passed out and, therefore, we might presume that the subject is unconscious. Actually, subjects are super-conscious and keenly aware of everything going on around them. This keen focus may leave the subject feeling like they aren't doing anything particularly unusual.

MODUS OPERANDI: HYPNOTIC CONVINCERS
HOW DO YOU KNOW IF YOU ARE HYPNOTIZED?

Convincers or suggestibility tests are a fun way to convince someone that something extraordinary has occurred. Here are some fun convincers:

1. **Balloon & Lead Weight**
    "Put both arms out in front of you and close your eyes…very good. Now imagine that I have tied a gorgeous balloon gently on your left wrist. The balloon is filled with high-octane helium and it easily lets your hand and arm lift and rise and float. Up it comes, lifting, rising and floating…lighter than air. Want it to happen, let it happen, watch it happen. It feels so good. Excellent. Now imagine that on your other hand we have placed a very heavy lead brick…it is so heavy. Wow, it just pulls that other arm down it is so heavy. OK just open your eyes and notice where your hands are. That is the power of hypnotic suggestion. You did very well."

2. Fingers Coming Together
    "With your eyes open, outstretch your arms and clasp your hands in front of you…very good. Interlock your fingers. Now stick out your two pointer fingers separated about an inch. Imagine an invisible thread pulling those two fingers together. And as you look between the fingers say to yourself 'fingers coming together, fingers coming together'. When they finally touch just close your eyes and drop gently into hypnotic relaxation. Excellent."

3. Hands Coming Together
    "Put your hands out in front of you, palms facing each other. Look between them. It is like a giant magnet is pulling your palms together; hands coming together…hands coming together…When they touch, you drop into deep hypnosis."

4. Eye Roll
    "Close your eyes and roll them back into your head. Very good. It is as if you could see right out of the back of your skull. Now try to open your eyes only to discover that they just don't want to open. The harder you try the less they want to open so now that you convinced yourself stop trying and drop deeply into hypnosis. Very good."

THE INWARD SIGNS OF HYPNOSIS

Relaxation/Peace and Calm A Feeling of Total Well Being

Tingling Sensation in the Fingers, Toes or Limbs

Goose Bumps (pilomotor response)

Chills Down the Spine

Light Pattern With closed eyes many see flashing lights, patterns or vivid colors.

Lightness or Heaviness of Limbs Sensational awareness of floating or rising up. Others feel heavy and unable to budge.

Detachment Some say they feel like they leave their body.

Passivity Feeling like you just don't want to move or exert any effort.

Relief Feeling happier, brighter, with fewer problems.

Real Time Distortions Time seems to slow down or speed up. An hour session usually feels like ten minutes. Yet the moment of now can seem to last forever.

Increased Body Awareness In trance, your senses become finely perceptive and you become more aware of these senses. Some swallow more or are more attuned to body processes. There are often changes in body temperature

Deep Breathing

Rapid Eye Movement

THE OUTWARD SIGNS OF HYPNOSIS

Yawn, Sigh, Laugh, Cry
"What did the grape say when he was squished?"
"Nothing he just let out a little wine"

—Jon Nicholas

Entering or deepening trance may evoke a deep sigh, yawn, laugh or even cry. This energy release heralds the opening to the door of deep relaxation.

Deep Breathing In trance, breathing tends to be deep and shallow, much like regular sleep. You'll notice subtle changes in breathing.

Relaxation The by-product of all hypnosis shows in the relaxed muscle tone of the limbs and face. You can lift up a subject's hand, and it dangles loose and limp and lazy like a loose rag doll. Feet splay apart if the subject is resting on their back.

Rapid Eye Movement The eyes have it when it comes to trance. With closed lids, the eyes often go back and forth or flicker as they do in dream or REM (rapid eye movement) sleep. Some folks experience extra tearing and most have a temporary redness in the whites of the eyes or a glazed look for a few minutes after opening the eyes following trance.

Changes In Body Temperature If you touch the palm of the hand, you'll discover that the temperature, while in trance, is either hot or cold and sometimes very moist.

WHY DO SOME PEOPLE HAVE DOUBTS ABOUT HYPNOSIS?

Since hypnosis looks different than it feels it is often misunderstood. Once you feel it, the apprehension goes away. The media cliché "Look into my eyes you are in my power" and the stage performance "Cluck like a chicken" have sometimes misrepresented the value of hypnosis.

Unknown Quantity

Some doubt the value of hypnosis because they themselves have not experienced its benefits. And there is a tendency for the conscious mind to harshly judge new, unfamiliar ideas. Once someone experiences hypnosis for themself, they know how safe and rewarding it is.

Fears and Superstition

Some folk's fear that hypnosis will force them to "go out of control" and then they'll reveal some buried truth that they're "not supposed to" or that they'll lose control. Or, even worse, look foolish.

While in trance your inner wisdom is your guide and that wise part of yourself will tell you the truth. Such truth offers insight and a tremendous relief. And, you needn't worry; your subconscious mind will only reveals what you choose to reveal.

In a trance, any suggestion that violates morals or self preservation is greeted with a natural "Cancel, cancel, cancel."

Shelley: A True Hypno-Tale

The first time I was hypnotized, I was 21 years old. I went to see Pat Collins (the "Hip hypnotist") at the Celebrity Club in Hollywood. After watching one show I was doubtful: "Where those subjects set-ups?" I thought. So to prove something to myself, I stayed for the second show and bounded on the stage when Ms. Collins called for volunteers.

During the show I followed her instructions so as to "not to embarrass the nice lady." After all, she was an entertainer. I noticed that every time she exclaimed, "Sleep" I felt an irresistible urge to cave in on top of my neighbor and even to the floor! But I definitely "was not hypnotized."

When the audience chose me to be suspended between two chairs (my neck on the back of one chair and my heels on the back of another); I found myself supine and staring at the ceiling stage lights for many minutes.

"Maybe I'm hypnotized," I said to myself. "Just maybe, because I don't think that I'd normally do this."

CAN HYPNOSIS BE DANGEROUS?

Hypnosis is no more dangerous than natural slumber. Practiced by yourself or with a qualified hypnotist, it is safe, satisfying and self-empowering.

Not learning hypnosis can be dangerous. If you allow all suggestions to accidentally enter your mind during your natural trance states, you may buy things you don't want and act in ways that harm you. Advertisers use hypnosis to sell products. If you are hypnotized to smoke, for example, you could kill yourself smoking. If you are "hypnotized" by parents, teachers, mates or your own self-talk to believe you are "less then," incompetent, or a failure, that harms you too.

Self-hypnosis lets you decide which suggestions to embrace or discard. It puts you in the driver's seat of your behaviors and emotions. When you learn to choose which suggestions you receive or act upon, you take back control of your life. If you don't control your subconscious mind, it will definitely control you.

It's ironic that some folks worry that hypnosis will make them lose control, because hypnosis gives them back control.

There was a young man of the Clyde,
who went to a funeral and cried.
When asked who was dead,
he stammered and said,
"I don't know, I just came for the ride."

DO YOU NEED HYPNOSIS OR HYPNOTHERAPY?

If you want to use your natural resources to your best advantage, get the most out of life, be your full potential, and have great relationships, then hypnosis is perfect for you. There's nothing to lose but tension, depression, fear, fatigue and pain. You gain relaxation, joy, peace of mind, energy and feel great.

If you have hurtful patterns, habits and behaviors or limiting beliefs, hypnosis can change them into helpful habits, peaceful patterns and beneficial beliefs. If you want to improve your golf game or up your libido, hypnosis is the ticket. Hypnosis offers creative options, updates your mental files and makes you an unlimited human.

CAN YOU REALLY RESOLVE PHYSICAL PROBLEMS WITH YOUR MIND?

Many physical symptoms have an emotional basis. Come to think of it, it's not really so strange that emotional strain or worry would produce physical symptoms. After all, every organ in your body is connected with your brain by nerve channels. Crisis or conflict upsets your nervous system and therefore your body. When you learn to relax the mind/body, your central nervous system returns to homeostasis and wellness.

IF YOU CAN'T SOLVE YOUR PROBLEMS WITHOUT HELP DO YOU HAVE A WEAK WILL?

Of course not. It is sometimes a struggle to work out emotional problems yourself because you're too close to see clearly. More and more, even those with a great deal of psychological knowledge, hire someone to "hold the mirror" for them. Hypnotists help people overcome emotional symptoms, increase abundance and creativity, and better personal relationships. Hypnosis strengthens the part of you that chooses growth.

HOW DOES HYPNOTHERAPY WORK?

Unresolved inner conflicts cause nervousness and unhappiness. Hypnotherapy helps you relax, understand and constructively resolve these conflicts.

WHAT HAPPENS TO THE HYPNOTHERAPIST'S INFORMATION ABOUT YOU?

Professional hypnotists agree to keep records that clarify problems and generate solutions confidential. They do not show your records to others unless subpoenaed by a court of law.

WHAT HAPPENS IF YOU DON'T COME OUT OF TRANCE?

Some worry that if they go into trance, they won't come out. Ormond McGill says, "Where would you go?"

You have been going in and out of trance since you were born. It is the most natural thing in the world to dream, relax, sleep and return to critical thinking. Your body naturally cycles in and out of trance. You easily terminate any trance when you choose.

In trance you naturally awaken as you would after any nap. If there were an important reason to return to room awareness during the trance (like someone calling your name or a baby crying), you would easily detach from trance state and attend to any business that needs attention.

It's easy to forget linear time when you relax deeply. If you have time restraints. If you practice self hypnosis or listen to a hypnosis tape at home, it's a good idea to set an alarm clock before you enter trance and to give yourself a timely suggestion like, "I choose to relax for half an hour," or "At 2:30 I will come back to my regular awareness."

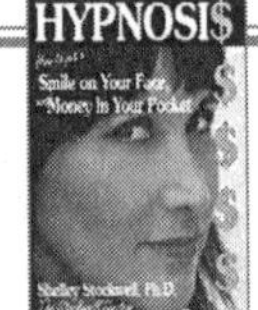

Hypno-Helper
"Hypnosis: How To Put A Smile On Your Face and Money In Your Pocket" by Shelley Stockwell is available on the order form at the back of this book and answers many more questions.

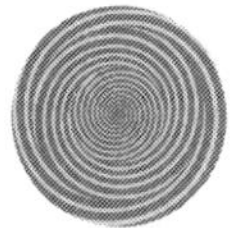

~ *Chapter 15* ~
PROFESSIONAL WISDOM AND PROTOCOLS

Includes
The Twelve Wisdoms For Professionalism
Hypnotherapy Ethics

Wisdom One: "Clients" not "Patients"
There are strict laws against "diagnosing, prescribing or treating" someone without a medical license. Avoid the term "patients" unless you are a medical doctor or nurse. People you work with are not "physically ill," they have "behavior challenges" they want to master with hypnosis.

Wisdom Two: Maintain Neutrality
Witness a session without personal opinions.

Wisdom Three: Reeducate Behavior Patterns
Hypnosis provides the way to change the mind. Reeducation of behavior patterns frequently means changing attitudes. Changing attitudes is surprisingly basic. Life's most disturbing problems stem from attitudes. Changing attitudes from a negative to a positive often causes trouble to evaporate. Help all clients take responsibility for their own thoughts and actions.

Wisdom Four: Maintain Confidentiality
Your exchange of information is a professional exchange. Keep their information to yourself.

Wisdom Five: The Golden Rule
"Do unto others as you would have them do unto you."

Wisdom Six: Do Everything for the Greatest Good of Your Client
Make the physical and mental well-being of each client your prime consideration. Keep them safe and be respectful of them. Provide help of equal value to all clients.

Wisdom Seven: Be Professional
Handle every session with the dignity and professionalism worthy of your profession. Never violate your client in any way. Be appropriate! Have the highest moral standards. Furnish services in accordance with the highest standards applicable to other therapy professionals and within the limits of your competence.

Wisdom Eight: Continue To Improve Your Hypnosis Skills
Study. Attend classes. Share ideas with other professionals. Join a hypnosis association.

Wisdom Nine: Learn From Others, But Do Not Copy Others
Hypnosis is an art form. Create your own masterpiece. An original Van Gogh sells for millions, a copy for $50.

Wisdom Ten: Publicly Promote Hypnosis
Proudly advertise yourself as a Certified or Clinical Hypnotherapist. Encourage and promote public interest and confidence in your practice of hypnotherapy. Hypnosis is a legitimate, valid area of human endeavor, research and application. Honor it.

Wisdom Eleven: Refrain From Misleading or Exaggerated Claims
Tell the truth. Hypnosis is so profound and results so valuable there is no need to exaggerate. Never misrepresent yourself as being what you are not. Do not imply or state that your hypnotherapy services are superior to another's.

Wisdom Twelve: Look Upon Each Person as a Trinity of Body, Mind and Spirit
The body/brain combine together in activating the physical body in 3-D space; it is not immortal. The body is the outer form you wear for a limited space and time. It is mortal and in time will die, as you advance on to live within another body. Think of the body as a suit of clothes. Mind and spirit combine together, and dwell within your body as your soul, which is the individual you. Mind/spirit together form your immortal self or consciousness. There is no other consciousness precisely the same as yours in all the universe.

These two quotes say it well:
"The soul is the unit drop in the ocean of eternal spirit which dwells in the body as the knower, seer and doer. It experiences all sensations and actions. It alone is the power in the body that reacts to any mode of application of therapy. Your soul is the immortal part of you for all eternity."
—Dr. Randolph Stone

"As the embodied self continually passes in this body from childhood to youth to old age, the self similarly passes into another body at death. A person who has realized their spiritual identity is not bewildered by such change."
—Bhagava Gita –2:13

HYPNOTHERAPY ETHICS
Render services in an ethical and professional manner
Treat others with respect and courtesy
Honestly clarify all costs and conditions pertaining to the services offered
Benefit your client, community and profession
Always improve your knowledge, skills and awareness of state-of-the-art findings
Enlighten and instruct the public about your profession
Induce confidence and respect for your profession
Never mislead or misrepresent yourself
Maintain information shared by a client as private and confidential
Comply with national, state and local laws and the regulations of your hypnosis organization

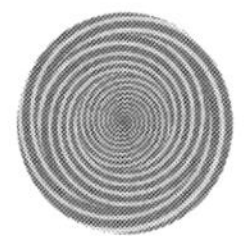

~ *Chapter 16* ~
STOCKWELL'S LEGAL REQUIREMENTS

By Shelley Stockwell-Nicholas, PhD
Founder/President of the International Hypnosis Federation

Includes
What's In A Name
Professional Training Requirements
Professional Hypnosis Organizations
Code of Ethics
Referrals
Florida Abuse
Protected By The Love Of God
Legal Disclosure Forms
Advertising
Liability Insurance
Turf Wars: Follow The Money
      Spiritual Prowess
      Academics vs. Non-Academics
      Professional Jealousies: Hypnotist vs. Hypnotist
Legislation
The Business of Hypnosis
Fees
Health Care Reimbursement
Promoting Yourself

Hypnotato

Hypnosis is freely used by advertisers, religious leaders, motivational speakers, parents, teachers, politicians, and, of course, by and for yourself. It is fun and easy to learn and belongs to all of us. It came with the package of your consciousness. You regularly hypnotize yourself with self-talk. You can easily learn to hypnotize (or de-hypnotize) yourself or another in less than ten minutes and of course can learn from exceptional books such as this.

WHAT'S IN A NAME?

The post nominals most commonly used by hypnotherapists is "CHt" meaning "Certified Hypnotherapist" or "CHI" for "Certified Hypnosis Instructor." In most states, anyone can call himself or herself a "psychotherapist" "counselor" or "therapist" as these are unlicensed titles. In Colorado a psychotherapist is either "registered' or "licensed." The state's current 2200-plus "Registered Psychotherapists" are mostly Hypnotherapists.

Generally you cannot, call yourself "Psychiatrist," "Psychologist," or "Clinical Social Worker" unless you have specific licensure. Psychiatrists are medical doctors and therefore can write prescriptions. A "psychoanalyst" has been trained in analytic techniques and may or may not be licensed. If you work in Canada in the Northwest Territories, The Yukon and Nunivat Territories you may call yourself a psychologist with no licensure.

Your title is important in some states of the USA. After you find out what your country, state and city requires, choose a designated title based on the laws, your training and desires: Hypnotist, Master Hypnotist, Hypnotherapist, Advanced Hypnotist/Hypnotherapist, Alchemical Hypnotherapist, Assertive Behavioralist, Assertive Behavior Hypnotherapist, Behavioral Hypnotist, Childbirth/Midwifery Hypnotist, Clergical Hypnotherapist, Clinical Hypnotherapist, Cognitive Hypnotherapist, Deprogrammer, Developmental Hypnotherapist, Educational Hypnotist, Ericksonian Hypnotherapist, Forensic Hypnotist, Guided Imagery Coach, Health Care Hypnotherapist, Higher-Self Hypnotist, Holistic Hypnotist, Humanistic Hypnotherapist, Hypno-Advisor, Hypnoanalyst, Hypnoanesthesiologist, Hypnobirther, Hypnocoach, Hypnocounselor, Hypnodontist, Hypnodoula, Hypno-Healer, Hypno-Integrationist, Hypno-Kinesiologist, Hypno-Life Coach, Hypnologist, Hypno-Metabolic Specialist, Hypnomotivator, Hypnopsychologist, Hypnopsychotherapist, Hypnoresearcher, Hypno-Technician, Hypnosis Instructor, Jurisprudence Hypnotist, Marketing & Motivational Specialist, Medical/Dental Hypnotherapist, Motivational Hypnotist, Motivational Speaker, Naturalistic Hypnotist, Neurolinguistic Programmer, Neurolinguistic Psychologist, Pastoral Hypnotherapist, Performance Hypnotist, Past Life Therapist, Past Life Regressionist, Psycholinguistic Specialist, Psychotherapeutic Hypnotherapist, Relaxation Therapist, Re-Patterner, Repatterning Counselor, Re-Patterning Hypnotherapist, Re-Programmer, Shamanic Hypnotherapist, Sports Hypnotist, Spiritual Hypno-Counselor, Stage Hypnotist, Substance Abuse Hypnotherapist, Suggestion Specialist, Surgical Hypnotherapist, Time Line Therapist, Transformational Hypnotherapist, Transpersonal Hypnotherapist and Wellness Wizard are some possibilities.

PROFESSIONAL TRAINING REQUIREMENTS

Hypnosis is a legal self-regulated profession, meaning that, in fact, you can practice with no formal training at all. However, concentrated instruction is very important in my opinion.

Requirements for professional hypnosis practitioners vary from country, city and state. Always find out what the legalities are in your place of business and do what is necessary to satisfy those regulations. For example, New York statutes requires "some form of formal education" to practice hypnotherapy.

Hypnosis and self-hypnosis training is offered by hypnosis societies, post-secondary schools and individuals at colleges, seminars, in meeting rooms, homes and through long distance learning. Some offer certification and others do not.

There are no agreed upon standards for the number of hours required for certification or a certificate of completion. They vary from one weekend to three years. Schools receiving federal monies for "occupational rehabilitation training," must adhere to federal rehabilitation funding act, require as much a 1000 hours of in-class and long distance learning. Certification fees range from a few hundred dollars to $25,000.

COPHO (the organization of professional hypnosis organizations) has had many hot debates on this subject and currently recommends at least 100 hours for certification with a distance-learning ratio of 40 hours of distance learning combined with 60 hours of in-class instruction. All hypnosis organizations encourage or require yearly continuing education.

The International Hypnosis Federation® (www.hypnosisfederation.com) requires 150 hours of training to be a certified Hypnotherapist. In the first 50 hours, and upon passing an exam, you become a certified "Hypnotist," after 100 hours a certified "Master Hypnotist" and after 150 hours a "Certified Hypnotherapist." The International Hypnosis Federation charges $600 for members for each 50-hour certification course and includes textbooks.

PROFESSIONAL HYPNOSIS ORGANIZATIONS

You are not required to join any affiliate hypnosis organization or union. However, most hypnotherapists join organizations, agree to a code of ethics, spend hundreds of hours learning and practicing hypnotic techniques, are certified and regularly attend conferences on the subject. I personally enjoy networking with like-minded people, the ability to purchase malpractice insurance and keeping informed as to the latest information in the field. But, to satisfy local and state laws, belonging to a hypnosis organization is not necessary. You have many options when you choose an organization and the benefits vary. Remember that each organization is a business. Choose one that supports your business.

ORGANIZATIONS FOR LICENSED & COMPLEMENTARY HYPNOTHERAPISTS

ACADEMY OF PROFESSIONAL HYPNOSIS ALUMNI (APHA)
Academy of Scientific Hypnotherapy (ASH)
American Association of Professional Hypnotherapists (AAPH)
American Association of Professional Hypnologists
AMERICAN BOARD OF HYPNOTHERAPY (ABH)
AMERICAN BOARD OF NLP (ABNLP)
American Counsel of Hypnosis Examiners (ACHE)
American Hypnosis Association (AHA)
American Society of Clinical Hypnosis (ASCH)
ASSOCIATION OF PROFESSIONAL & THERAPEUTIC HYPNOSIS (APATH)
CALIFORNIA PROFESSIONAL HYPNOTISTS ASSOCIATION
Canadian Hypnotherapy Board (CHB)
Clinical Care Network Professional Group (CCNPG)
GULF SOUTH HYPNOTHERAPY ASSOCIATION (GSHA)
Hypnosis Education Association
Hypnosis For Health
HYPNOSIS SOCIETY OF PENNSYLVANIA (HSP)
Hypnotists Local Union 472
INTERNATIONAL ASSOCIATION OF COUNSELORS & THERAPISTS (IACT)
INTERNATIONAL HYPNOSIS FEDERATION (IHF)
INTERNATIONAL HYPNOSIS HALL OF FAME (IHHF)
INTERNATIONAL MEDICAL & DENTAL HYPNOTHERAPY ASSOCIATION (IMDHA)
International Association for Regression Research & Therapies (IARRT)
Milton Erickson Association
NATIONAL ASSOCIATION OF CERTIFIED HYPNOCOUNSELORS (NACHT)
NATIONAL ASSOCIATION OF TRANSPERSONAL HYPNOTHERAPISTS (NATH)
National Federation of Hypnotists Union Local 104
National Federation of Neurolinguistic Psychology (NFNP)
National Forensic Hypnotherapy Association (NFHA)
National Guild of Hypnotists (NGH)
New Orleans Hypnotherapy Group (NOHG)
NATIONAL SOCIETY OF HYPNOTHERAPISTS (NSH)
National Society of Clinical Hypnosis (NSCH)
NEW YORK STATE HYPNOTHERAPY ASSOCIATION (NYSHA)
North Coast Hypnosis Society (NCHS)
Society for Clinical & Experimental Hypnosis
TIME LINE THERAPY ASSOCIATION (TLTA)
World Conference of Professional Hypnotists

(Council of Professional Hypnosis Organizations- COPHO -members are in bold capital letters)

CODE OF ETHICS

A member of an organization agrees to abide by certain ethics. International Hypnosis Federation members from a broad range of disciplines agree to conform and be accountable to the following ethical principles or risk suspended or cancelled membership.

Commitment To Human Welfare: Each member promises to honor the holistic well being of the individual and respect every human's innate ability for personal expression, introspection, wellness, enlightenment and joy. Any abusiveness is strictly prohibited.

Positive Programming: Each member agrees to provide verbal and nonverbal positive programming and related techniques in hypnosis and in any of their other respective specialized professions.

Modality Interaction: Each member agrees to work together with others to broaden and improve all uplifting mind, body, spirit and joy modalities.

Legal Conformity: Members shall observe the professional ethics of their conscience, specific affiliations, training standards and the laws of their city, state and country. Legal alternative health care providers will disclose that they are not licensed health care providers.

Truth In Advertising: Hypnotists and other legal self-regulated and regulated professionals agree to proudly proclaim the good results of their fine work. Members shall be truthful in their advertising and not overstate credentials or make unsubstantiated claims.

Confidentiality: Members agree to maintain the confidentiality and privacy of information shared during client sessions as is acceptable under the law.

REFERRALS

According to statistics released by the New England School of Medicine, over half of people seeking health care, go to practitioners like hypnotists. Professional hypnotists are now part of the permanent staff at major hospitals.

Qualifying California based hypnotherapists, (along with massage therapists, yoga instructors, and dieticians) are recommended by Blue Cross of California in their "Healthy Extensions Network" list mailed to their 40,000 members twice a year. To qualify, according to the programs administrator, you must have "well over" 150 hours of documented training, liability insurance and a business license.

More and more licensed medical doctors, nurses, psychologists, psychiatrists, physical therapists and dentists value alternative health care and refer clients for complementary services. They know that a patient who learns specific non-medical techniques can relieve pain, fear, panic, anger, stress, change negative patterns and habits into positive attitudes, sleep better, lose weight, become more motivated, optimistic and joyous and stimulate the body's innate ability to heal. Just what the doctor ordered!

Some hypnotherapists ask for a doctor's referral before assisting someone. Asking a specialist for a written referral makes them your "wellness partner" and often generates lots of referrals. A simple referral note for a doctor to sign might say: **"I have no objection that _________ use self-hypnosis and hypnosis to help __________ alleviate or eliminate mental and physical discomfort."**

Florida law currently requires such a referral and says that you may practice hypnosis...for non-therapeutic purposes, but... not hold yourself out to the public as possessing a license "or use a title protected by this chapter."

Sample Referral Letter
Put this on your letterhead with your address and phone number and include a return envelope:

Dear Dr. Johnson,
I am a hypnotherapist certified by the International Hypnosis Federation *(name your certification training; it gives credibility)* and a member of the International Medical and Dental Hypnotherapy Association *(name an organization you belong to, to give credibility)*.

Your patient ___________________ *(client's name) (or their parent/guardian)* has requested my assistance in _________________ *(managing stress, overcoming addiction, losing weight etc)*. Hypnosis is a legal self-regulated alternative health care modality that uses the mind's natural ability to create a positive attitude to support medical care, reduce stress and relax the nervous system. Your signature below authorizes me to use hypnosis techniques like visualization, progressive relaxation, suggestion, reinforcement, mental rehearsal and more to enhance their natural resources for a more positive outcome.

Thank You,
(Your Name, CHt)

Doctor ___________________
Patient ___________________
Parent/Guardian ___________
Date ___________________

FLORIDA ABUSE

Florida rulings say it is illegal to practice hypnosis "for therapeutic purposes" unless you are a "practitioner of the healing arts, as herein defined, or acts under the supervision, direction, prescription and responsibility of such a person"…"Healing arts shall mean the practice of medicine, surgery, psychiatry, dentistry, osteopathic medicine, chiropractic medicine, naturopathy, podiatric medicine, chiropody, psychology, clinical social work, marriage and family therapy, mental health counseling and optometry."

In other words, Florida legislators think that a foot or eye doctor's referral makes your practice "legal." Can you imagine if the tables were turned and a podiatrist could only see patients if referred by a hypnotist! Chiropractors, social workers, drug and alcohol counselors, I've been told, enjoy this mandated partnership and form financially rewarding alliances with hypnotists to satisfy this law. Think about this the next time you're asked to support licensing or registration legislation.

In June 2002, a woman called Florida based Hypntherapist, Jose Cartagena saying she wanted to "lose 20 pounds with hypnosis." She arrived at her scheduled appointment accompanied by a man. Cartagena filled out his standard intake form and asked the woman "What are your hypnosis goals?" The couple asked odd questions like, "Do you offer medication?" "Of course not" he replied, "I'm a Hypnotist."

Shortly afterward, the man stepped out to "use the phone." When he returned, the woman left saying she "wanted to use the restroom." She returned with seven men in street clothes wielding drawn guns, followed by television cameras and reporters. "I thought I was being robbed," said Cartagena, "until they handcuffed me and said, 'We are police officers and you are under arrest for practicing medicine without a license!'"

Cartagena, is a reputable, high profile hypnotherapist who appears on television talk shows (weeks earlier he appeared on a TV debate with a hostile psychologist). He worked as a "Psychotherapist and Hypnotherapist" at Columbia University in New York City where he counseled state prosecuted sex offenders and he taught hypnosis courses for third-year students at Cornell University.

He said to the officers "I have been practicing Hypnosis in Florida for the seven years and I have a legal and current Miami/Dade occupational license issued with 'Hypnotherapy' on it."

A policeman responded, "It doesn't matter. We are going to close down all the hypnotists in Miami." Cartagena was taken away in a police car, charged with a felony for "practicing psychology without a license" and detained for 3 hours. "It was the most traumatic experience of my life, I was forced to hire an attorney at great expense to represent me for these serious accusations. The felony charges were subsequently dropped when I showed documentation that I was an ordained minister with the Universal Metaphysical Ministry…Ministerio de Metaphysica Universal…who has 'used hypnosis in my ministry for over 12 years.'"

PROTECTED BY THE LOVE OF GOD

Which brings me to the next point: in any restrictive environment, it seems wise to have your client sign a legal disclosure form (see next section) and define yourself as both a hypnotherapist and a "minister who uses hypnosis for spiritual counseling."

You can become a minister on line with the "Universal Light Church" or call the "Crown of Life Fellowship" in San Jose, California (408-353-5666). Both organizations of worship offer ordination as a "Spiritual Minister" at no charge. The Crown of Life Fellowship "allows Pastoral Counseling to address psychic and emotive issues with the use of practices including hypnosis, past life regression, past life therapy, soul retrieval and all that is meditative." Applicants must submit evidence of their service area (like a copy of a hypnotherapy certificate) and a specific statement of the counseling purpose that includes 'for the spiritual well being of all sentient creatures.'

LEGAL DISCLOSURE FORMS

California law, as of January 1, 2003, requires that client's of all "non-licensed practitioners" sign a written disclosure form at their first visit. One copy is to be given to the client & the other is to remain in your records for three years. This form is said to protect you from "being cited, penalized or fined for violating the Medical Practice Act of California." Other states are considering similar legislation. It is a good idea to use such a form in all states as legal protection.

Stage hypnosis volunteers can sign the disclosure before the show begins. If you are video taping the show for resale, demonstration or teaching purposes, that the person signs both the disclosure and a written permission (waiver) for you to use their image.

The International Hypnosis Federation offers a printed "Alternative & Complementary Health Care Provider's Form." They are an attractive, positive, professional and promotional two-page-duplicate that defines and delineates all mind, body, spirit and fun modalities not requiring state licensing. Hypnosis and other self-regulated (and often self taught) holistic specialty treatments identified are; Coaches, Counselors, Hypnotists, NLPers, Spiritual Counselors, Pastoral Counselors, Therapists, Nutritionists, Naturopaths, Bodyworkers, Energy Workers, Skincare Specialists & Movement Therapists and more. Each could potentially be held in violation without this form. The form can be ordered by calling (310) 541-4844 or from the back of this book.

ADVERTISING

Advertising claims are important too. The California code is good everywhere: "A person who advertises such lawful (alternative) services must say that he or she is 'not licensed by the state as a healing arts practitioner'" and I would add: "but has fulfilled the state requirements in their field of expertise"

Or better yet, let your advertising read, "_______ **(Your Name) is a Legal Alternative Healthcare Provider and not a (California) licensed healing arts practitioner.**"

LIABILITY INSURANCE

Malpractice and Professional Liability insurance is something you might consider. It is available in the United States to Hypnotherapist members of various hypnosis organizations (www.hypnosisfederation.com is one place you will find it). It is required if you are referred by Blue Cross as I am. Some rental offices require that you have insurance. For a few hundred dollars you are covered for millions of dollars in the unlikely event that someone sues you. Insurance is available to stage hypnotists through other specialized agencies. Weigh premium rates against potential risk and decide if this is something you want to do.

Jillian LaVelle of the International Association of Counselors and Therapists recommends that you purchase pre-paid legal insurance.

TURF WARS: FOLLOW THE MONEY

Some put hypnosis down because they are uneducated about what hypnosis really is or they think hypnotists take away their business, or because they want to be elite, powerful or own the light.

Spiritual Prowess

Some Evangelists whose income comes from veiled hypnosis techniques sometimes preach fear-based suggestions against hypnosis. It's fun to watch a skilled "faith" healer use rapid hypnosis inductions so the faithful (literally) fall into a deep trance and powerful healing suggestions work wonders.

Academics vs. Non Academics

A "lay hypnotist" is a derogatory term coined by academics to discredit non-licensed hypnotists as not being "educated" or qualified in hypnosis. Ironically a licensed doctor, dentist or mental health professional (like a psychiatrist, psychologist, social worker, nurse, and marriage and family therapist) usually has little or no hypnosis instruction. Yet, for the sake of more business, many of these folks initiated legislation attempting to eliminate competition and suggest that only "licensed" practitioners, or those with at least a master's degree, practice hypnosis. "Lay" practitioners are not qualified to make a "medical assessment" they say. Conversely, licensed practitioners are not educationally qualified to make "hypnosis assessment" or practice hypnosis either.

A hypnotist is not usually a psychologist or doctor and a psychologist and doctor is not a hypnotist. Hypnosis is a distinct and separate wellness modality and profession. For professional hypnotists, hypnosis is a well-studied main therapeutic method.

An occasional doctor, dentist or psychologist makes it their business to go to hypnosis school to be certified as a professional hypnotherapist. Yet, most of these well-versed professional, do not have time to practice hypnosis. That is why so many hypnotically educated licensed professionals regularly refer patients to certified professional hypnotists.

Professional Jealousies: Hypnotist vs. Hypnotist

Bizarrely, some hypnotists put down other hypnotists and some hypnosis schools put down other hypnosis schools. Occasionally a clinical hypnotherapist will sneer at stage or spiritual hypnotist.

Some hypnosis organizations quest for power, revenue and/or exclusivity. In 2003 a group of ten highly trained, licensed and non-licensed members of the New Orleans Hypnotherapy Group were invited and joined the New Orleans Chapter of American Society of Clinical Hypnosis (ASCH) and when they attended the society's hypnosis conference they were invited to leave because the speaker refused to "address anyone with less than a master's degree." (This same hostile posture is reportedly held by a few other societies.

Beware of any organization that claims to be the only "legitimate" one. A few national groups have forbidden members to attend other conferences and refused to recognize continuing education from other groups. Some have outright deceived by claiming that you cannot legally practice unless you belong to their group. Avoid any affiliation that implies or blatantly claims that their standards are the only thing to keep you exempt from the law. It is not so. Many reputable groups support each other and offer ways to protect the integrity of hypnosis.

There is room and abundance for all who offer nourishing and positive service to humanity. We must work together for the good of everyone in our profession and avoid putting self-serving interests of any person or organization ahead of that goal.

LEGISLATION

A few states have faced the scourge of psychology, psychiatry and/or hypnosis organizations attempting to control the fine business of hypnosis with legislation. Such bills have thus far been killed in Iowa, Louisiana (3/26/01 Richmond HLS 1332 House Bill #78), Massachusetts (Bill S580, 1999) and California. There are no restrictions in Alabama, Alaska, Arkansas, Arizona, Connecticut, Delaware, D.C., Georgia, Hawaii, Idaho, Iowa, Kentucky, Maine, Maryland, Massachusettes, Mississippi, Missouri, Michigan, Nebraska, North and South Carolina, North and South Dakota, Ohio, Oregon, Pennsylvania, Tennessee, Vermont, Virginia, West Virginia, Wisconsin, and Wyoming. I've listed those states that have something going on.

California

As of January 1st, 2003, clients must sign a form disclosing a definition of your special modalities, your hours of training and experience and the announcement that you are "not a licensed health care practitioner" but an "alternative health care provider." (See section above for more information on acquiring these forms.)

Colorado

In the late 80's Steve and Connie Andreas started the "NLP Comprehensive" and the "Colorado Association of Psychotherapists" with the purpose of getting "unlicensed professionals the same rights as licensed ones." 1998 a disclosure law came into effect that requires all unlicensed psychotherapists to take the "Jurisprudence Workshop" a one-day class in legal and ethical issues for therapists and hypnotherapists must now "register" in the state data base as "unlicensed psychotherapists or they are fined. To date there are some 2200 unlicensed registered psychotherapist, most of whom are Hypnotherapists and NLP practitioners. There are now meeting underway with paid lobbyists to create a "governing body" and rewrite the state's Mental Health Code to serve various interest groups. To have a hypnosis school, you must get approval and post a $10,000 to $20,000 "surety bond."

Florida

Regulates "therapeutic" use to licensed providers. It is legal to use hypnosis for "non therapeutic" purposes.

Illinois

There are no restrictions. A once limiting "American Psychology Act" was sunsetted and not renewed in 2002.

Indiana

Restrictive legislation was passed in Indiana requiring 350 hours of training for one of only a few approved schools, a state exam, and a licensing fee and now two apposing lawsuits are pending and another bill has been filed to severely restrict the terms of this legislation. There is no restriction on hypnosis stage shows.

Kansas

Restriction on stage hypnosis.

Louisiana

Currently there is no restriction. A licensed post secondary school that teaches hypnosis must post a $10,000 bond. A bill now proposed by a hypnotist would require at least a Bachelor's Degree to practice and advertise oneself as a "licensed hypnotherapist." Such proposals have been tabled several times.

Nevada

Forensic hypnosis restriction.

New Hampshire

Legislation pending.

New Jersey

New Jersey Hypnosis exemption legislation (in 1994) requires that hypnotists call themselves "Hypno-Counselors" or "Hypnotists" but not "Hypnotherapists." A business card in New Jersey can read: *"Hypnocounselor-New Jersey, Hypnotherapist."* They can freely offer smoking cessation, weight management, study skills, sports and creative activities. Anything related to "mental or health disorders" or diseases require a doctor's referral and "Hypnocounselors" must avoid using the words "depression" or "insomnia."

New York

An active registration in 2005 is scheduled for presentation to the governor and state legislature.

Ohio

Hypnotherapists must avoid using "medical terms" like "anxiety" and "depression." Hypnosis schools must be a licensed vocational school or risk paying a $10,000 a day fine.

Oregon

Oregon's licensing bill (house bill 2625 Kruse Y2001) was defeated and scheduled to come up again in 2005.

Pennsylvania And Unions

In 1963, the Hypnosis Society of Pennsylvania introduced a Pennsylvania bill licensing hypnotism as a legal profession. It eventually passed the House and Senate. Then in 1971, then Governor Schapp, held a news conference and announced that he would "not only veto the hypnotism bill" but he "would do all in his power to see that hypnotism would be banned forever in Pennsylvania." Several attempts to do just that were introduced as amendments or attached to other bills. This pending threat of extinction made the bill's proponents wonder if they were "better off leaving sleeping dogs alone."

Unionizing was their solution. Twenty-five local hypnotists pitched in $100 each to make the required $2500 bank account and agreed to pay the $4 monthly dues and in November, 1971, they were charter as the first hypnotism union, Hypnotist Union, Local #467 OPEIU AFL-DIO-CLU. Local charters in Philadelphia, New Jersey and California followed. OPEIO Union lobbiests asked legislators, "Do you want to go on record as the congressman or lobbyist that put a union worker out of work?" The bill banning hypnosis was defeated and several legislators sent letters of apology.

Texas

Texas hypnotists call themselves "hypnotist," keep accurate records, and avoid using "psychological terms"; use "sadness" not "depression"; "not sleeping well" instead of "insomnia"; "stress" not "anxiety"; "bad habits" not "compulsions"; and "fear" not "phobia." seeking exemption from the "Psychology Licensing Act" which says that hypnosis is a "tool for psychology."

Canada

Canada has the same self-regulated status for hypnotherapy as most states of the United States. As of November 2001, medical doctors are now allowed to refer patients to hypnotherapist for hypnosis. The Northwest Territories and the Yukon and Nunivat Territories of Canada allow you to call yourself a psychologist with no licensure. There is an attempt by current proposed legislation to restrict the use of the word "emotional" by unlicensed practitioners. You can, however, become a "licensed holistic practitioner." This registration process has been sanctioned by the governor and is codified until 2013.

THE BUSINESS OF HYPNOSIS

Hypnosis is a rewarding career that helps a lot of people and brings you satisfaction and abundance. It is a terrific career for men and women of all ages and backgrounds, is easy to learn and belongs to everyone.

FEES

Money is a playful thing abundant as fresh air.
Every time I breathe some out, I find that more is there.
Coins in towering mountains dwarf my tiny size
And pathways thick with green backed notes stretch before my eyes.
Abundance fills my every pore: I give so much away
Knowing that the more I give the more will come my way.
It's really just a playful game: money's heaps of fun.
I have more than I'll ever need and so can everyone!
> —Winifred Morice

Hypnotists charge private clients anywhere from $75 to $350 an hour for a private session. If you are a medical doctor practicing hypnosis, of course your fees will be commensurate to what your fees usually are. If you charge what a doctor or chiropractor charges, you will be fine. Some hypnotherapists offer a sliding scale based upon the client's income.

If you're not accustomed to asking for money, you'll need to get over it. People are thrilled to pay for your hypnosis services and they value more what they pay for. By not charging, you do them a serious disservice!

When a person asks for an appointment tell them on the phone how much it will cost. If you charge $100 an hour for example, say: "My fee is $100 an hour and your first session might be about an hour to an hour and a half, so your first session will be $100 to $150."

I usually add, "You'll leave my office with an audio tape that you play at home. This gives you a chance to re-enforce your session." (My tapes are prerecorded and available to hypnotists or you can make your own.)

Some hypnotherapists charge in blocks of time. "Usually five sessions, at $100 an hour, are $500 so if you pay for five sessions up front the fee is $450 and you save $50."

Forensic hypnotists testify in court. An accident case pays approximately $700 for as little as a 10-minute appearance. In the 1950's, law enforcement like the Los Angeles Police Department trained officers to help prod the memory of witnesses. One hypnotist I know is hired by his special state public defender for "hypnosis contact visits" at $1500 and hour to help the accused remember facts so they don't get flustered under cross-examination.

Hypnotists who work on the movie sets with actors for stress reduction or consult for movies often join the Screen Actor's Guild and are paid handsomely.

Individual Programs

Before you offer long-term discounts, make sure that your client realistically requires many visits. Weight control and addictions often do. Remember your goal is to get clients in and out as soon as possible so they can successfully use the tools and insights that you offered to live their life. A great deal of work can be done in one hour and results will astound even you.

If you do think a long term individual program is a good idea, $995 to $1700 per person for a three-month program is standard. Such programs include one to seven personal sessions. One woman I know offers a three-hour initial session, plus two sessions a month (in person or on the phone) for a total of nine contact hours. She charges $1350. This breaks down to $150 an hour.

I sign up someone, who needs to release a large amount of weight, for a six months program at $995 plus $99 materials fee. For that, the client receives one or two private sessions with me, a once a week group program, their own set of four audio-tapes, ("Lose Weight", "No More Sugar Junkie", "I Love Exercise" And "Peace & Calm") my video and book, "Stockwell's Great Shape Hypnosis: 10 Easy Steps To A New You."

Long-term commitments help a client permanently improve their quality of life. Positive Changes Hypnosis®, the high priced ($27,000 to $50,000 for a "franchise territory" plus a monthly fee for each client and paid advertisement) weight loss business, charges clients $1200 to $1700 for a three-month program. Prices are often negotiable and may be as little as a $1000 a month. Their advertised "free hypnosis evaluation" is actually a meeting with a commissioned sales person who pitches the program which includes six to seven "private sessions" (where the client wears eyeshades with blinking lights and is read a script). These sessions are twice a week for two weeks and then once every three or four weeks. As often desired, the client can also come in to view a thirty-minute nutritional video followed by an "accelerated" double induction audio tapes (again with the dark blinking eye goggles). A receptionist turns on the tape machines every half hour for anywhere from six to ten clients at a time and may also be called upon to read hypnosis scripts. These reinforcement sessions are recommended twice a week. Some programs include a monthly yearlong follow up group meeting where a video and group hypnosis takes place.

HEALTH CARE REIMBURSEMENT

I don't take insurance but am happy to fill out forms for a client after they pay me for the session. Some company health benefits deduct money from employee paychecks and put it in a tax-free fund that can be used for hypnosis. "UniAccount" for example offers group health insurance coverage to employees under a "Flexible Spending Account" (FSA) that "may" reimburse "hypnosis for treatment of illness."

Hypnotherapists on staff at medical care facilities are paid employees with a written financial agreement or may have an arranged "fee for service" agreement with a hospital. If you charge via a hospital inpatient or outpatient insurance system, billing is by "unit," usually meaning a 30-minute session. Fees are billed under "hypnotherapy" or "relaxation."

Paul Durban, PhD, the on-staff salaried Director of Hypnotherapy at Pendleton Memorial Methodist Hospital in New Orleans, Louisiana, is paid part of the regular patient's bill.

Some hospitals give "independent hypnosis contractors" an office and their patients. The patient pays the hospital $65 or $70 an hour and the hypnotist invoices the hospital for compensation. Reimbursement can take a week or two. Some hospitals bill insurance at a rate of approximately $70 an hour and then pay the hypnotist sixty percent ($42). Reimbursement can take as long as 45 days.

TREATMENT CODES

Diagnostic and Statistical Manual of the American Psychiatric Assoc.
–4th Edition (DSM-IV-R) Codes are:

General Stress	300.02
Anxiety	300.02d
Adult Depression	300.40
Somatization	300.81

The International Classification of Disease – 9th Edition (ICD-9) Codes are:

Fatigue (acute or chronic)	780.7
Relaxation Therapy	780.7
Insomnia	780.52
TMJ	524.6
Obesity	278.0
Smoking	305.10

Expert Advice V-Codes. Codes are:

Relationship Problems	V 62.81
Bereavement	V 62.82
Academic Problems	V 62.30
Occupational Problems	V 62.20
Spiritual or Life Passage Problems	V 62.89
Acculturation (New Place Adjustment)	V 62.40
Request for Expert Advice	V 68.20

Place of service is "O" for office.
The current procedural code for "hypnosis service" is CPT90880 or write "Hypnotism."

If you teach a class at a hospital you can negotiate a percentage of the individual fees paid. If fees are $45 for a 4-hour class you may be able to negotiate as much as 90% of the gate. This percentage is negotiable.

Hypnotherapist Zoilita Grant, says that national health insurance companies like "Humana" and "United Health Care" reimburse for "the use of hypnosis for positive change psychotherapy" "with a referral and under the supervision of a licensed psychologist, psychiatrist, marriage and family therapist or social worker." You simply have them sign the appropriate form (available at www.selfhealing.com) using the referring healing art's practitioner's state license number and billing it under the psychological code for anxiety- 300.02, adult depression- 300.40 or somatization- 300.81. Otherwise use "expert advice V-Codes" that defines "human" not "medical" challenges. Do not make a "diagnosis."

PROMOTING YOURSELF

As Ormond says, "Doing business without promoting is like winking in the dark. You know what you are doing, but nobody else does." The goal of marketing your services is to give the public the perception of your perfection. Help the public perceive you as valuable for them or they will go elsewhere. Your image dominates your content. Everything is energy. Create a positive open posture as a successful crowd pleaser. Pay attention to how you look, the way you dress, your voice, word choices, your presence. Walk your talk. Great marketing includes:

POSITIONING: Position Yourself as Outstanding in Some Special Way
- ❑ Get there first
- ❑ List of the top three who are "there" and make it your goal to join them
- ❑ Let people know how you are unique and different from the others
- ❑ A prestigious address makes you sound important

PUBLICITY:
- ❑ Know who you are selling to and speak their language
- ❑ Motivate these people to come to you
- ❑ Tell them over and over again why they should come to you: sell benefits
- ❑ Hook 'em right away with your first words, your headline, your presence.
- ❑ Use short sentences and simple language
- ❑ Create juicy mental images
- ❑ Make words active, not passive "I'll Help You Slim Down Now" not "Weight Class"
- ❑ Make your literature professional. Hire a writer or graphic artist if necessary
- ❑ Time your publicity. January and August are the best times for weight loss clients

ADVERTISING/PROMOTION
Advertising CHECK LIST:
- ❑ TV, Radio and Webcast Talk Shows
- ❑ Trade Shows
- ❑ Newsletters
- ❑ Newspaper Columns
- ❑ Public Speaking
- ❑ Teaching
- ❑ Demonstrations and Free Seminars
- ❑ Web Promotions
- ❑ Offer excerpts of your book to magazines and newsletters
- ❑ Offer a seminar on your book subject

Many hypnotherapists believe that the better they become at hypnosis the more clients will show up. Yet if a client doesn't know about you, how can they come? Advertising and promotion gets the word out about the good work you do! To succeed, marketing expert Joe Hammer's "Stealth Marketing Program" includes these Marketing "Bill of Rights":

1. Right Audience–Who?

Who wants your services? Appeal to what they WANT. Address only the people you seek . What options are available to reach them? Do a little homework. It pays off. A caption like: "Isn't It Time You Visited An Alternative Health Care Provider?" may bring in droves.

2. Right Message–What?

The one they hire,
Fills desire
Match what you do
to what they think is true
> —Shelley Stockwell

Create your advertising to match your target customers knowledge and experience. Talk their language. The right massage tells your customer "I can assist you to ___________." You become their ticket to dreams and desires. Buyers do not make the best decisions; they make emotional choices based on what they want. Platitudes don't touch attitudes. Client centered advertising is "all about the client," and evokes an immediate and direct response; the phone will ring and you'll get results. The ad or promotion proves itself. Don't leave your advertising message to advertising or media reps. Sales people are trained to play to your pride and ego so they can hypnotize you to buy. They are not oriented to make you successful. A sales reps motivation is a sale's commission. Advertising agents have an award and quota mentality. Agency driven ads require repetition so that the agency makes money and the investment seems worthwhile to the corporate client. Institutional company centered ads emphasize a corporate image. Ads may be cute, creative and win awards but do they bring results?

Joe Hammer says that when you sell hypnosis you are really selling uncertainty, confusion and misconceptions. One hypnotherapist took a survey asking, "What do you think of hypnosis?" and a large percentage responded, "It doesn't work." So they ran an ad captioned: "Hypnosis Doesn't Work!" agreeing with the preconception and moving emotionally to the advertiser's way of thinking. Truth in advertising is nothing more than the thought in the customers mind. Join the unspoken conversation going on in another's mind.

3. Right Media & Placement–Where?

Put your advertising where your customer will see or hear it. If your clients are women, advertise in the media that women enjoy. Advertising pimple cream at a retirement community or hypnosis at a fundamentalist church may not work too well.

4. Right Timing–When?

Timing is everything. The World Trade Center skyline after September 11th won't make it. A fireman might.

5. Right Resources & Information–How?

Make the cost of advertising a fixed element of your business. The more effective your message the more you leverage these expenses.

Publicity Events

Send out news releases and get as much publicity as possible. Newspapers are always eager to print things of interest so think about a slant that would be newsworthy:

"Hypnotist Helps Relieve Holiday (High Alert Day…Test Anxiety, Etc) Stress"

"Children Excel (Get Better Grades) With Hypnosis"

"Hypnosis: First Aid for Flood Victims"

Don't Chicken Out: Seize Opportunity

Since ancient times, promotional events brought business. Franz Mesmer, Milton Erickson, De Waldoza, Rexford North, and most old timers practicing today performed "hypnotic seances." Gerald Kein staged friends to picket against himself and invited the press. Ormond hypnotized women in department store windows to remain still in "window sleep."

I inadvertently became internationally famous for doing a hypnosis demonstration that included hypnotizing chickens. My face was on the front page of newspapers, and page three of USA Today. I was on television stations around the world, David Letterman showed my picture and even USA Vice President Al Gore, I'm told, was so entranced he announced that he too knew how to hypnotize chickens.

It all started as a delightful New Hampshire radio interview when I told the announcer "I hypnotized a chicken when I was teaching a hypnosis certification course in Bali, Indonesia." "How did you learn that?" asked Ken Gidge, the announcer. "I learned it from an Ormond McGill book I bought at a convention in your town." I told him. "As a matter of fact, I'll be there again next summer to speak with Ormond." "Terrific!" said the host, "Why not hypnotize twelve chickens for the Guinness Book of World Record?"

The Mayor of Nashua, Bernie Streeter, called the show and told me on the air, "When you come, I'll do the invocation." A fellow called and offered to bring the chickens, a lady named Dot called and said she'd bake cookies and several people called up and volunteered as "chicken handlers." It turned out to be a terrifically fun event. Ken Gidge supplied everyone with memorial rubber chickens and his warm personality. Ormond and I had a great time and even the chickens seemed to enjoy it…but the most fun was hypnotizing the television reporters and children and explaining that "…while we are having a lot of fun here today, hypnosis is a powerful tool that helps people lose weight, quit smoking, get better grades and love themselves more."

I got wonderful letters asking how someone could learn more about hypnosis, dozens of clients and I was able to give out hundreds of referrals to other Hypnotherapists.

When Ormond wrote in the March 1995, Journal Of Hypnotism, "A consideration of Animal Hypnotism will give you a far better understanding of hypnotism than any text book ever could." He well might have added "and will have clients flock to your door."

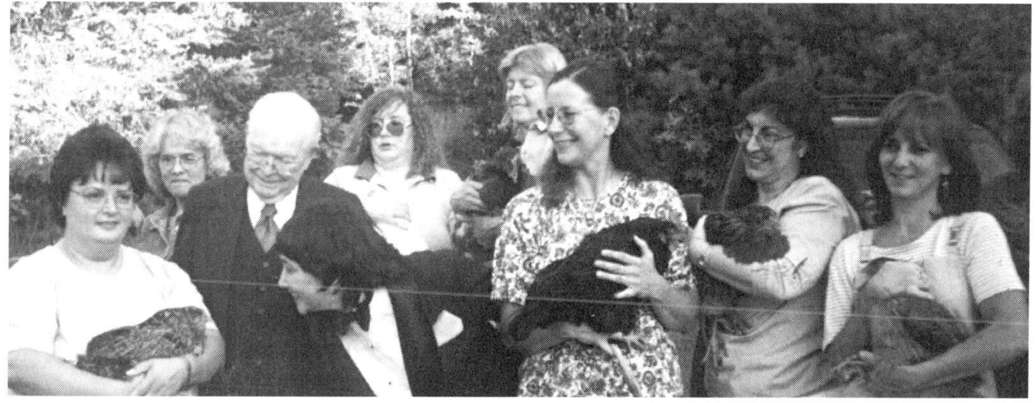

Photo by Jon Nicholas

Hypnotizing Chickens for a bid at the Guinness Book of World Records

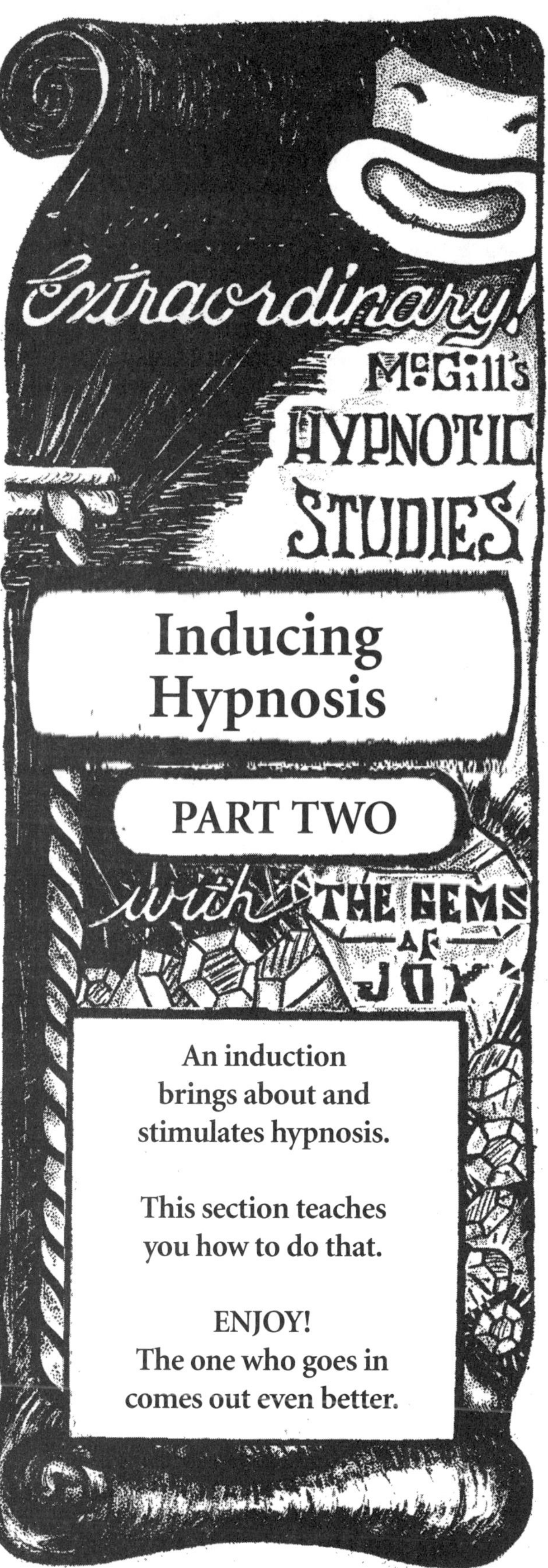

CHAPTERS IN PART TWO

17. Inductions.....................................page 65
18. Hypnotic Sleep 75
19. Producing Somnambulism 79
20. Elman's Hypnotic Coma 83
21. The Art of Waking Hypnosis.................87
22. From Waking To Trance.....................91
23. Establishing the Hypnotic Mood 93
24. Waking Hypnotic Inductions
    & Convincers 95
25. Rapid Induction to Profound Trance..103
26. More Rapid Inductions 105
27. The Relaxation Method 109
28. William James: Let's Pretend.................113
29. I Can, I Can't Rapid Inductions 117
30. Let's Pretend Some More 121
31. Acting Out Hypnosis For The
    "I Can't Be Hypnotized" 125
32. The Ideomotor Induction 129
33. The Sandy Beach Induction 131
34. Serenity (Symbiotical)
    Resonance Sound 133
35. Magnetic Mind Toning 137
36. The Holistic Method 141
37. Quotation Induction 143
38. Elman's Rapid Induction 147
39. You Are The Star Hypnotherapy 153
40. Bale's Outside/Inside Method.............157
41. England's Rag Doll Induction..............159
42. Hypnotizing Children 163
43. Candy Induction.....................................171
44. Blum's Singing Bowl Induction 173
45. Transpersonal Induction 175
46. Hypnodance 177
47. Otto's Vertigo Induction 179
48. Whirling Dervish Induction................181
49. Instant Gamma Hypnosis 185
50. Oriental Hypnotherapy Inductions....189
51. Oriental Cobra Method.......................193

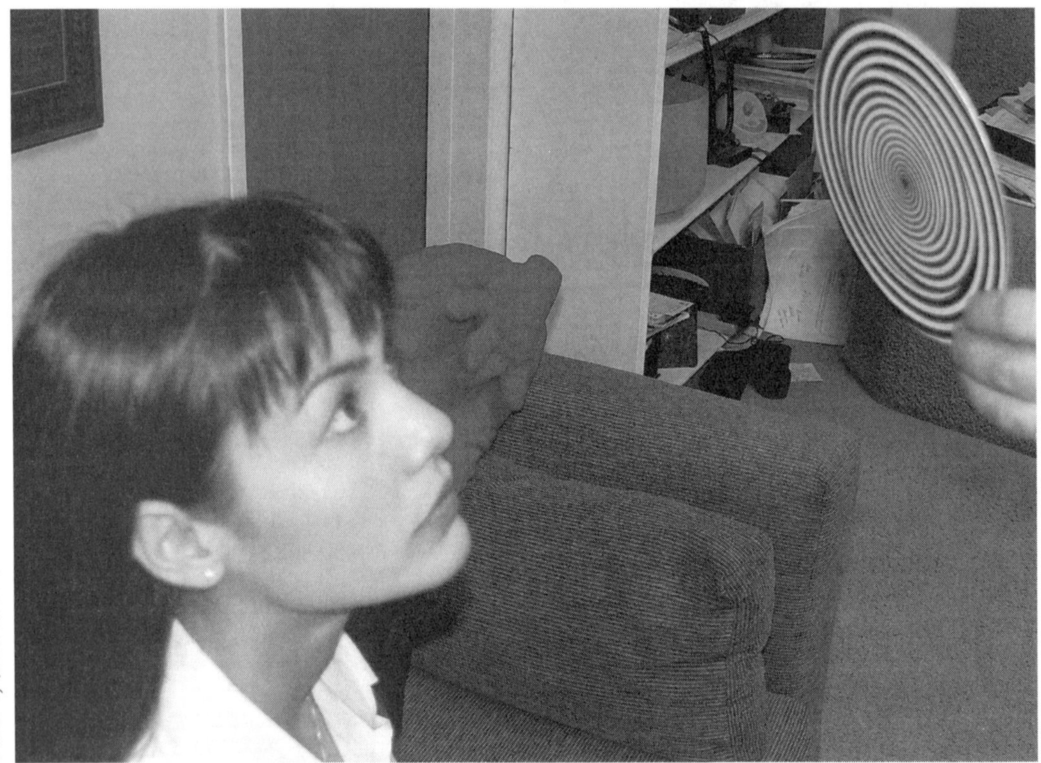

Hypnodisc

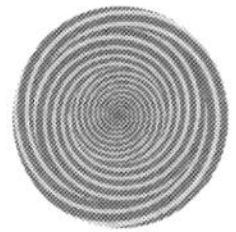

~ *Chapter 17* ~
INDUCTIONS

Includes
The Four Requisites To Enter Trance
Fast or Slow Inductions: Which Is Best?
Different Ways to Induce Trance
The Four-Fold Induction Approach
Fascination of Attention: Twenty-Two Inductions
>**To Fascinate Sight**
>>**The Stick Induction**
>>**The Penlight Induction**
>>**The Penlight Self Induction**
>>**Watch The Watch Induction**
>>**The Clock Dial Induction**
>>**Look at your Spine Induction**
>>**Using A Hypnodisc**
>>**Using A Pendulum**
>>**Hands Over The Eyes Induction**
>>**The Hypnotic Gaze**
>**Fascination of Hearing**
>>**The Ticking Watch Induction**
>>**Hands Over The Ears Induction**
>>**The Hypnotic Voice**
>>**The Buzz Induction**
>**Fascination of Smell**
>>**Perfume Induction**
>**Fascination of Taste**
>>**That's Delicious Induction**
>>**Sip The Water Induction**
>**Fascination of Touch**
>>**Focused Feeling Inductions**
>>**Bite the Cork Induction**
>>**Hold Your Tongue Induction**
>>**Hot Money**
>**To Fascinate Imagination**

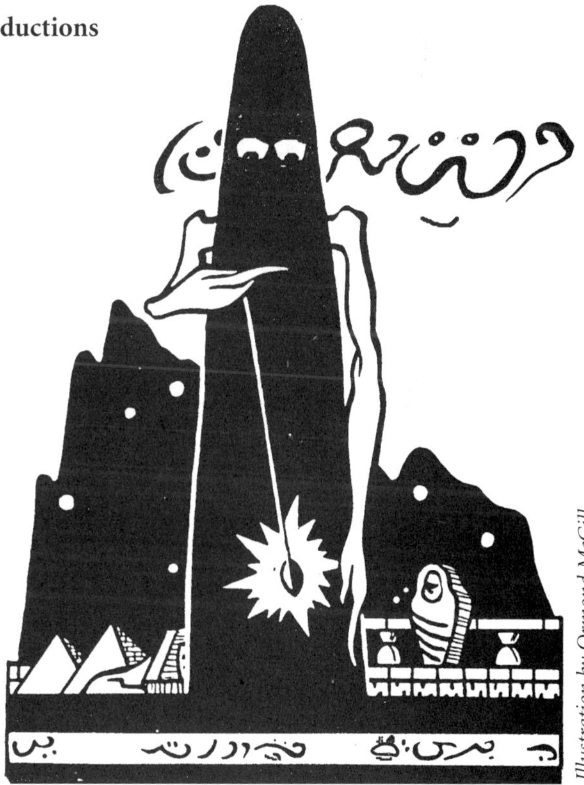

Using a Pendulum

Illustration by Ormond McGill

Hypnotic inductions stimulate hypnosis. They guide someone from the ordinary state of mind into the hypnotic state of mind. Hypnotic induction and the power of suggestion, both induce the hypnotic state of mind and control the mental state it induces.

HYPNOSIS + THE POWER OF SUGGESTION =
A SUBCONSCIOUS REALIZATION & CONTROL OF IDEAS

Profound deep hypnosis is accomplished only by making the effort without effort. To enter you must bypass critical mind (wakeful awareness) and drop into the realm of reverie (like dreams and sleep). Too much effort to be hypnotized keeps consciousness awake in performing the process. It is like going to sleep at night. If you try hard to go to sleep, you lie awake hoping to go to sleep. The only way to go to sleep is to make the effort (purpose) of going to sleep without effort. Do that and you go to sleep. It is the same with entering hypnosis, one just has to let go and GO.

THE FOUR REQUISITES TO ENTER TRANCE
There seems to be four requisites that invite the mind to enter hypnosis:
1. **Trust in the Operator: "You and I understand each other."**
    In other words you have built a feeling of rapport
2. **Expectation for Hypnosis: "I am going to hypnotize you."**
3. **Communication Between Operator and Subject: "If you follow my simple instructions you will be easily hypnotized. This is what is   going to happen to create your hypnosis experience…"**
4. **Consent or Agreement for Hypnosis: "All right. Are you ready to begin?"**
    The consent of the subject (willingness) to be hypnotized is basic to the successful induction of hypnosis. This can be either a conscious acceptance or an unconscious acceptance. The operation can be summed up in the word, expectancy.

There is no way you *can't* hypnotize a person if you use these steps.

FAST OR SLOW INDUCTIONS: WHICH IS BEST?
Rapid hypnotic inductions can be done in the snap of a finger and they can give more time during the session for beneficial "suggestions formulas." Slower hypnotic inductions give more time for an intimate relationship to develop between hypnotherapist and client. Which is best depends on the particular client and time restraints. The skilled hypnotherapist knows both approaches. During the consultation, decide which approach to use.

One induction technique or a combination works well. Using more than one induction is known as "layering inductions."

THE FOUR-FOLD INDUCTION APPROACH
This four-fold pattern works to induce trance:
1. **FASCINATION OF ATTENTION:**
    Example: **"Focus your attention on the spiral…"** (or something that engages Sight, Sound, Smell, Taste, Feeling and imagination.)

2. **RESPONSE TO SUGGESTION:**
    Example:**"These effects are an optical illusion and you will find that they make your eyes tired, very tired and heavy. Soon when I tell you to close your eyes you will become aware of the after image created by this design which will gradually become confused and blurred and finally fade away…"**

3. **GENERALIZING:**
    Example:**"…your eyes are stuck together and don't want to open…"**

Example:"**...close your eyes now and as the after image fades disappears, you will slip down deeply into hypnosis.**
Example:"**...let eyelids relax even more than before and let that relaxation flow down over your entire body.**"

4. SLEEP SUGGESTION:
    Example:"**...so you stop trying and go into deep hypnotic slumber.**"
    Example:"**...deeper and deeper you go into profound hypnotic sleep and remarkably you hear every word I say and yet you are sound asleep...**
    Example:"**This makes you very sleepy and drowsy, so just drift away into sleep. Sleep. Sleep. Go to sleep.**"

> **"A few seconds after reading this you will be sound asleep. You are going fast asleep. Go to Sleep NOW."**

DIFFERENT WAYS TO INDUCE TRANCE
1. **Verbal Suggestions** Monotonous words or sounds, direct instruction, confusion
2. **Mental Suggestions** Imagining things that relax you, autosuggestion
3. **Energetic Suggestions** Sweeping contact or non-contact passes over the client
4. **Eye Fixation/Fatigue** Gazing a spot or bright, flashing or spiraling object
5. **Startling Sounds** Unexpected loud noises
6. **Soothing Sounds** Soft Music, Alpha Theta Frequencies

FASCINATION OF ATTENTION: TWENTY-TWO INDUCTIONS
Here are a series of inductions that fascinate attention on sight, sound, smell, taste, feeling and imagination:

TO FASCINATE SIGHT
Instruct your client to look at the base of their own brain, the tip of their nose, their favorite color, a candle, a crystal ball, an imaginary spot on the ceiling, a light, a marble, a pencil, a pendulum, a ring, a spiral, hypno-disc, your eyes, someone else's eyes, the drawing of an eye, their own eyes in a mirror, a finger, a dot on your finger, a pocket watch, the word "sleep" written on a piece of paper, the imaginary word "sleep" written in the page of a book, or a photo of a "famous hypnotist," Saint or loved person from history.

The Stick Induction
You Will Need:
A Small Stick

Hold an object like a small stick eight inches at eye level in front of their eyes and tell them **"Stare at the tip of this stick and follow it with your eyes no matter how much I move it."** Then grip the back of their neck firmly so that they can't move their head and must move their eyes, as you move the stick up. When they cannot follow it further they will automatically blink shut. Do this six times and on the sixth time say **"When your eyes blink shut this time keep them closed"** and place the stick on the top of their skull pressing downward as you say, **"Your eyes are locked they cannot open no matter how hard you try. Stop trying and go deeply into hypnosis."**

The Penlight Induction
You Will Need:
A Low Powered Penlight

Have your subject sit in their chair and place the palm of your left hand over their right eye. Shine the penlight directly into their left eye about an inch from the eye. The dim light will not bother their eyes **"Keep staring into the light and relax your body completely. You will close your eyes when I tell you to."**

After about thirty seconds forcefully say **"Close your eyes tightly together. You will see inside your closed eyelids a very bright spot of light. This spot will change color as you watch it. It will fade away and reappear. Watch the spot of light closely inside your eye. Concentrate your full attention upon the spot. As you do, you will begin to feel yourself become very sleepy and drowsy."**

The Penlight Self-Induction
You Will Need:
A Low Powered Penlight

Hand your client a penlight. It is a small flashlight with a place to press that causes the light to shine. Tell them to **"Grip the button firmly so that the light is on and stare at the light as you hold it before your eyes."**

As they gaze at the light suggest, **"Your eyes will quickly become tired and as they do your hand will relax and finally when the light goes out you will close your eyes and go into sound sleep. The hand is becoming heavy and is dropping in your lap while you sleep in hypnosis.**

You may see the light come and go as bright spots behind your closed eyes and if you do your eyelids will become stuck together."

As soon as they drop the pen say **"You go deeper into hypnosis with each breath."**

Watch The Watch Induction
You Will Need:
A Watch With A Second Hand

"Look at the second hand of this watch for thirty seconds and then close your eyes for thirty seconds. Then open your eyes and do it again until your eyes refuse to open. When this happens you will let them remain shut and go deeper." As they do this repeat the idea that **"It is becoming increasingly difficult to open your eyes."**

The Clock Dial Induction
You Will Need:
A Drawn Clock-Face With No Hands

On a round cardboard, draw a circle and write the numbers one through twelve around the inside periphery like a clock face. Make the numbers easy to read. You, the hypnotherapist, are standing behind them and as they perform these breaths. Have the client hold this before themselves and instruct, **"Concentrate on the number one and, as you do, inhale deeply. Then say 'sleep' out loud. While, still looking at the number one, exhale and say 'deep sleep.'**

Now look at the next number, the number two, and inhale twice and say the word 'sleep' two times. Then exhale twice and say out loud 'deep sleep' two times. And on to the number three take in three inhales saying the word 'sleep' three times and then three exhales and say 'deep sleep' three times…and so on with each number."

You now barrage them with a stream of words whispered in their ear as they attempt to carry out your assignment. This confusion technique evokes trance. **"Your eyes concentrate upon the numbers as your eyes move along ahead from number to number around the clock dial, as you inhale and exhale deeply and repeat the words 'sleep' and 'deep sleep' it sends you down to sleep in deep hypnosis. It is more and more difficult for you to see the numbers, they begin to blur before your eyes. The numbers are blurring and your eyes are becoming tired and are so tired they are closing. You are getting very tired of doing this whole thing and you just want to get it over with. So just close your eyes now and let the card drop from your hand as you drop into sleep, hypnotic sleep. Go to sleep…"**

Clock With No Hands

They proceed from number to number. By the time they would reach twelve they would be required to breath in twelve times, say sleep twelve times and exhale twelve times and say 'deep sleep' twelve times. Each number becomes increasingly more difficult. Very few make it past number five or six before closing their eyes and drifting to sleep.

Look Into Your Spine Induction

"Close your eyes and drop your head forward upon your chest and imagine that you are looking through your body to the base of your spine. (Let this happen for about two minutes) **"How sleepy this makes you so your just relax all over and go to sleep."**

Using A Hypnodisc

You Will Need:

A Spiral Disc (A metallic spiral is available by calling (800) 366-7908) Mechanical versions that rotate electrically may be found on line.)

Hold a disk like the one shown here about four or five inches from the subjects eyes and have them concentrate their attention on the center of the spiral as you move it in a circular manner.

Continue the movement as you say, **"Look into the spinning disc. These effects are an optical illusion and you will find that they make your eyes tired, very tired and heavy. Soon when I tell you to close your eyes you will become aware of the after image created by this design which will gradually become confused and blurred and finally fade away…your eyes begin to feel tired and they are becoming heavy, heavy, heavy. They are so tired that they begin to blink. They are closing now. Go ahead and let them close right down and relax all over."**

Another version: **"The revolving spiral is designed to closely hold your attention. Keep your attention fixed on it. Look at it in an easy, relaxed fashion. As you watch it, you will soon find your eyes going slightly out of focus. Let them go. Let the spiral soften and flow…just watch it…the center will seem to draw you into itself or push you out. Make believe that I am talking to someone else and hear me as a murmur in the background with your full attention on the spiral. The effects become more and more pronounced and ingrained in your mind."**

Hypnodisc

Using A Pendulum

You Will Need:

A Pendulum (Numerous styles of pendulums are available. You can use a watch, weight or crystal on a chain, or a necklace as a pendulum). Fixation on a pendulum is hypnotic.

"As you sit comfortably in the chair, dangle this pendulum before your eyes" Have them hold the pendulum up high enough to strain to look at it. **"Fasten your attention upon the highlights on the pendulum and as you watch it, it will soon begin to swing back and forth before you. As soon as it does you will begin to feel very sleepy and will close your eyes. When your eyes close your upraised hand that is holding the pendulum becomes very heavy and drops into your lap. When this happens, you will promptly go to sleep in hypnosis."**

In another version of this, the Hypnotherapist dangles the pendulum that is held aloft before the client's eyes. **"As the pendulum begins to sway back and forth, back and forth, follow the movement with your eyes and notice that your eyes are growing tired, will close and you will go to sleep…"**

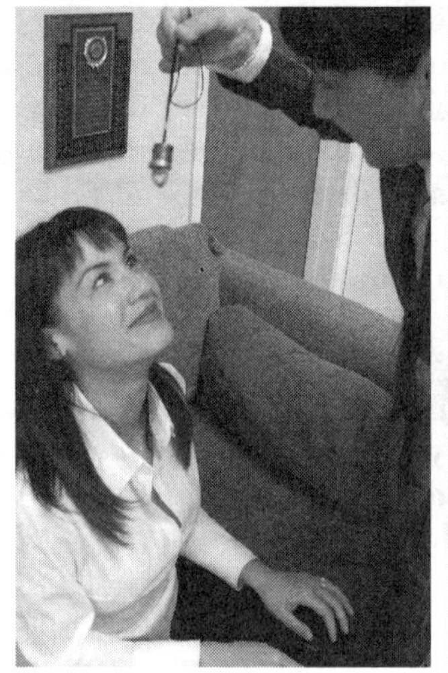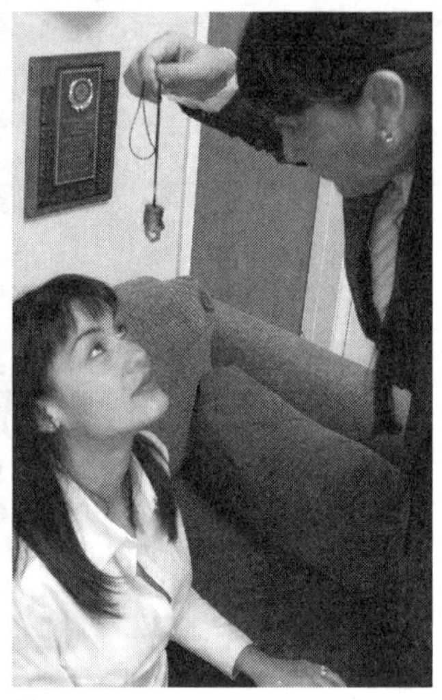

Pendulum

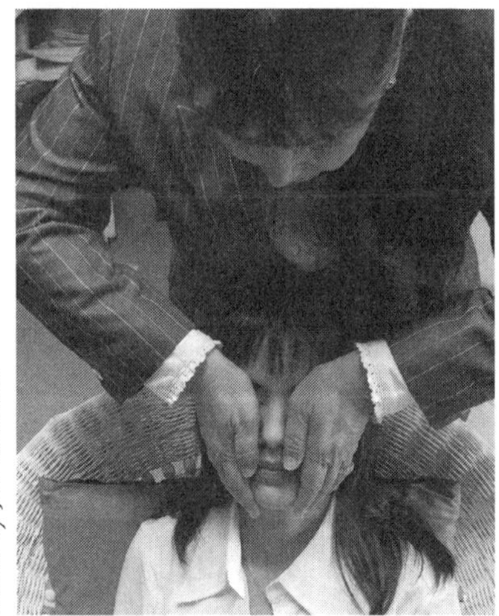

Cupped Hands Over Eyes

Hands Over The Eyes Induction

Have your client sit comfortably and **"Close your eyes and place your cupped hands over them. In a few minutes you will become so relaxed that your hands will just fall into your lap and when they do you will immediately go to sleep. When you remove your hands your eyelids will be so relaxed that they just don't want to open."** Leave them to do this for three to five minutes and they will go deeply into trance. You can also use your own cupped hands if you prefer. When you remove your hands, do it quickly and suggest, **"Sleep. All the way down."**

Another version of this also fascinates hearing. Have your client place the thumbs of each hand closing off the ears and their fingers closing their eyes. You place a gentle hand on their head while they do this. After a few moments take down their hands and rest them in the person's lap as you say **"Sleep now."**

The Hypnotic Gaze

The use of the eyes with the hypnotic stare is traditional in hypnotizing. Very few people can hold their eyes steady and unwinking the necessary length of time without practice. To perfect a steady eye, stand in front of a mirror and look at your eyes. Look at them steadily,

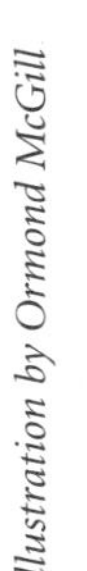

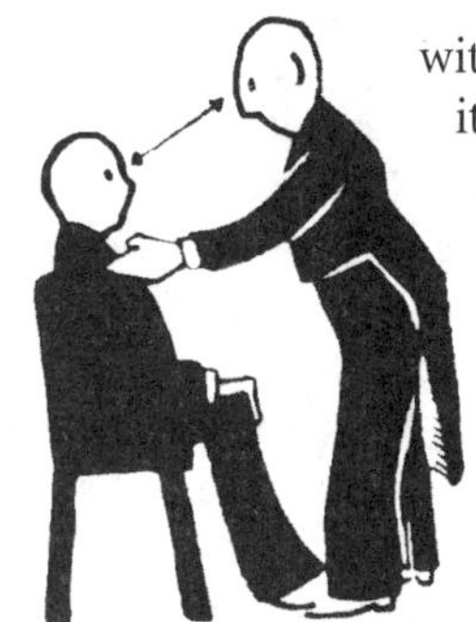

without letting your eyelids blink. Hold your gaze as long as you can stand it. About a minute is about right for the first trial. The second time you practice, you will find that you can look at them longer without blinking. Practice for a few days until you can stare at yourself for at least five minutes steadily. Having mastered staring at your eyes in the mirror, focus on an imaginary point six inches in back of the glass.

In hypnotizing, you'll apply this practice by centering your attention on the root of the client's nose (between the eyes). Then focus your gaze at a point on the back of their head. This gives the appearance that your eyes are starring directly into their eyes, looking within their very brain and is wonderfully effective in holding attention.

FASCINATION OF HEARING

Instruct them to hear the sound of music, a bell, a singing bowl, sounds in the room, sounds outside the room, a metronome, the sound of your breath moving in and out, the sound of my voice…

The Ticking Watch Induction
You Will Need:
A Ticking Watch or Metronome

Have your client sit comfortably with their eyes closed. Tell them **"I am going to hypnotize you today by having you give your attention to sound."**

Hold the ticking watch (or metronome) close their ear and say, **"Give your complete attention to the ticking. Concentrate fully upon it so the ticking completely fills your mind. I will remain silent. After some moments it will begin to feel as if the ticking is becoming fainter and fainter and farther and farther away in the distance. As the sound recedes you will be dropping deeper and deeper to hypnotic sleep."**

Now let them listen for some moments, as you remain silent. Then move the watch gradually away from their ear and when you have moved it entirely say **"The ticking is all gone now and you are going fast asleep."**

Hands Over The Ears Induction

Have your client sit comfortably and **"Close your eyes and place your cupped hands over your ears. When you remove your hands in a few minutes you will drop deeply into trance."** Leave them to do this for three to five minutes and they will go deeply into trance. You can also use your own cupped hands if you prefer. When you remove them do it quickly and suggest, **"Sleep. All the way down."**

The Hypnotic Voice

A good hypnotic voice is essential to bring about trance. A squeaky, uncertain voice carries no conviction, while a resonant, strong voice compels. A voice that starts in your head is tinny and weak. Bring your voice up from your diaphragm.

Practice this exercise: Stand in front of a mirror and, speaking directly to yourself, give that reflected "self" these positive suggestions: **"I easily succeed as a hypnotist. I speak with a deep, clear, resonant voice. My voice is becoming better and better. My voice is getting deeper and deeper. My voice is getting stronger and stronger. My voice is clear, deep and resonant."**

Practice this seriously, repeating the suggestions over and over. Speak in an even tone. Do not vary the pitch. Talk to yourself just as if you are conversing with a friend. No need to feel funny talking to yourself; after all no one sees or hears you and it's a splendid exercise. In a few days you will notice the results.

Continue this practice conscientiously. A voice with a nice, even tone can accomplish wonders. Above all else, learn to speak positively. You have, perhaps, heard an officer say to a company of soldiers: **"ATTENTION!"** Notice how the Sergeant says it. It's positive! It is a command! The soldiers straighten up immediately, almost automatically. The thrill of that command goes through you if you were there listening. A suggestion of "sleep," properly given, is equivalent to such a command. Practice getting positive authority into your suggestion-commands. Of course, not all suggestions must be so commanding. Some are done subtly and gently. Learn many ways to use your voice as an instrument for motivation and you assist your clients to easily enter into a trance.

Go into the privacy of your room and look at a chair or any piece of furniture. Imagine that the article is alive and address it as though it were a living person. Talk to that "person" with kind forceful commands, as; **"You WILL do as I tell you! It's no use; you MUST do as I say! You CANNOT resist me!"** Repeat such forceful commands over and over.

Practice this exercise and it will amaze you how soon you unconsciously develop a positive quality in your voice. Of course, when you actually hypnotize someone you will not use or give such bombastic orders but the practice imparts a ring of authority that calls for obedience even in gentler phrases. This authority coupled with heartfelt compassion works miracles. Practice it well.

The Buzz Induction
"Place the tips of your thumbs into each ear. With your middle and forefingers, lightly close your eyes to keep out light. Press your nostrils with your ring fingers. Hum with your mouth closed and feel the vibration. Now, open your lips while pushing your tongue against your closed front teeth and make a buzzing sound. Relax and go to sleep."

TO FASCINATE SMELL
Perfume Induction
> You Will Need:
> **Something Aromatic to Smell** (perfume, fresh baked bread, or ammonia)

"Close your eyes. The smell that you notice does not produce sleep itself yet it causes you to become drowsy and your eyes will not be able to open."

TO FASCINATE TASTE
That's Delicious Induction
> You Will Need:
> **Something Presumptuously Scrumptious** (fresh baked cinnamon rolls, a hard candy…)
> Instruct them to enjoy the scrumptious taste and go to sleep.

Sip The Water Induction
> You Will Need:
> **A Glass of Water**

"Take a sip of this water and you will discover how it induces a deep hypnotic trance. With each sip you swallow say to yourself 'this is putting me to sleep'. You taste end feel it spreading relaxation through out your mind and body. Pause between each sip and when the entire glassful has been taken in you will find that you go into a very deep trance."

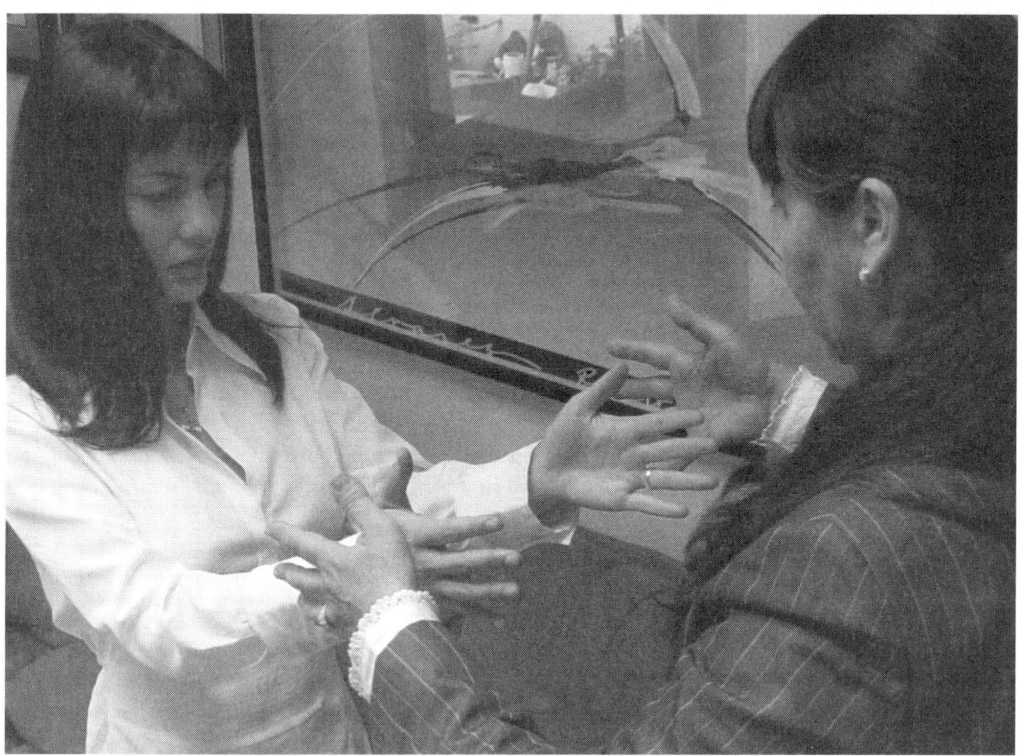

Touch

TO FASCINATE TOUCH

Instruct them to **"feel this soft cushion," "roll a ball in your hand," "feel a string with knots," "…the texture of their breath,"** their pulse, heartbeat, the magnetic pull between the hands (fingers)…"the big toe on your left foot."

Your touch is also hypnotic. You can tap their third eye, tickle their face with a feather, put your hand in ice water and stripe their face and nose with coldness, You can stand behind them and place your interlocked fingers against their forehead as you exert pressure against the sides of the head inward and rest their head on you or the chair back as you suggest **"Close your eyes now and the pressure you feel now makes you very, very sleepy."**

Focused Feeling Inductions

Example 1	**"Turn your attention to your eyelid and let them relax…"**
Example 2	**"Focus your attention on the bottoms of your feet and feel the bottoms of your feet completely relax. Let your feet become loose and limp and lazy. Now feel this relaxation of your feet gently creep up into your legs…"**
Example 3	**"Yawn, Yawn, yawn…the yawning sensation engulfs your entire body as you drop into sleep."**
Example 4	**"Find the pulse beats in your wrist and when you do count the beats to yourself. At this same time will your heart to grow slower and slower. Your heart rate slows in response to these thoughts and you sink deeper and deeper to sleep."**

Bite the Cork Induction
You Will Need:
A Cork

This one fatigues the muscles and causes profound relaxation. The jaw of the head transfers fatigue to all parts of the body. Suggest, **"Place this cork between your teeth and close your eyes and bite firmly into the cork with your might. When you notice how tired you are, that is the feeling of hypnosis coming on. How very much you want to drop off into slumber so you relax your jaw and go to sleep."**

Hold Your Tongue Induction
Another version of the bite the cork induction instructs your client to, **"Sit comfortably with your eyes closed and hold your tongue back in your mouth as far back as you can. You can hold this position more easily by pressing your tongue against your palate. How tired you are becoming and go directly to sleep and just relax all over."**

Hot Money Induction
You Will Need:
Two Coins

Suggest, **"Hold one coin in each fist and rest your fists on your hips. Now close your eyes. The coins are becoming warmer and warmer in your hands. Warmer and warmer…they are getting hot! The coins are hot, hot, hot you want to drop them but you cannot because your fingers are stuck tightly around them. Take a deep breath forget all about the coins and now your eyes are stuck together and you cannot open them so take a deep breath relax and go deeply into hypnosis."**

TO FASCINATE IMAGINATION
Have the client close their eyes and take an imaginary trip…around the country…or to the ocean…or a park…or their favorite place in nature. After four minutes of vivid verbal suggestions or having them report their own graphic inner world. Go to an eye fixations suggestion and suggest sleep.

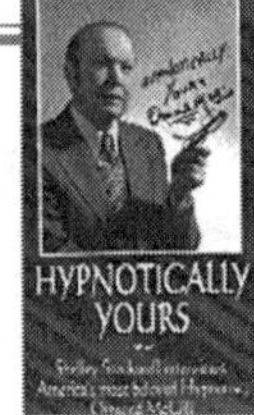

Hypno-Helper
"Hypnotically Yours" video by Ormond McGill shows several inductions and discusses how they work.
"How To Hypnotize in 30 Seconds" video by Shelley Stockwell-Nicholas demonstrates rapid inductions.
Both are available from the order form at the back of this book.

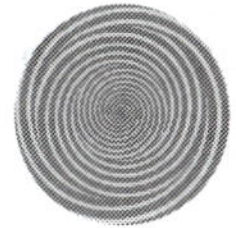

~ *Chapter 18* ~
HYPNOTIC SLEEP

Includes
What Is Hypnotic Sleep?
How to Induce Hypnotic Sleep
Hypnotic Sleep Test
Hypnotic Sleep Suggestions

WHAT IS HYPNOTIC SLEEP?

"Sleep" is a classic word used by hypnotherapists. Both sleep and hypnosis are brought about by relaxation. The suggestions of "sleep" and "go to sleep" are common in hypnotic inductions and slumber. Yet, though the outward signs of sleep and hypnosis appear to be the same, inwardly they are different. During natural sleep attention is diffused and the body relaxed. In hypnotic sleep, attention is concentrated, intensified and productive, and the body is often alerted and active. During hypnosis your attention is similar to wakefulness.

The hypnotic command "go to sleep" is very effective in inducing trance but not a necessity. Mentioning sleep simply establishes a familiar focus, which motivates the hypnosis. Without the mention of sleep another causation focus like "you are spell-bound," "in a deep meditation" or having "an out of body experience" motivates the subject into the hypnotic state.

Hypnosleep is natural somnambulism intrinsic to human nature and often attached to regular sleep. Research finds that an average person breathes 8 to 16 times a minute during their waking hours and 7 to 10 times per minute during sleep. This slowed rate represents hypnosleep. More study of these breathing and brain wave patterns might show us the exact correlation of these patterns and hypnosis.

When you suggest to a hypnosis subject "Your hands are locked together and you cannot take them apart" they obey the suggestion. Their hands are locked until the suggestion is removed. If such an "off beat" suggestion is obeyed, why not expect the suggestion "Go to sleep!" to be obeyed? One goes to sleep every night of their life. There is nothing unusual about going to sleep in response to a suggestion of "Sleep!" is there?

Every sound-minded human being is hypnotized every day.

The hypnotist evokes a state of trance where a person talks and walks. Somnambulism is the state of profound hypnosis from which the awakened subject seems to be aroused as if from sleep. Approximately one in five people are natural somnambulists and have the ability to enter profound hypnosis on a first trial.

Sleep and hypnosis are much the same as natural sleep. Both sleep and wakefulness alter us. Wakefulness can become reverie, reverie sleep, and sleep somnambulism. Sleep produced in hypnosis is not a natural sleep but an altered sleep. Normal sleep is produced by diffusion of attention; hypnotic sleep is produced from focused attention. This hypnotic accentuation of attention makes it easy to take in beneficial suggestion.

In regular awareness your conscious mind hears what you are saying. In somnambulism your conscious mind often "sleeps" and no longer hears what is being said.

Hypnotic sleep is the trance state of hypnosis. It is the state that many people regard as "really" being hypnotized. Hypnotic sleep takes you to a deeper level of hypnosis and is characterized by hyper suggestibility. The effectiveness of suggestions given when awake is like a pop-gun compared to the shotgun of hypnotic suggestion. In the depth of trance, suggestions go right to the target!

MODUS OPERANDI: HOW TO INDUCE HYPNOTIC SLEEP
You Will Need:
A Pencil or Other Object

Putting someone in a trance calls for smooth handling. This methodical hypnotic technique is a good one to practice. Seat your client comfortably in a chair with any lights coming from behind the client and directed at you. Have them place their feet flat on the floor and rest their hands on their thighs.

Suggest, **"Make yourself comfortable and relax your muscles."**

Then take a pencil or other object, it makes no difference. It makes this lesson clearer using a pencil with a shiny tip. Stand in front of the seated person, on their right side and hold the pencil about five inches from their eyes and up high enough so that they will have to open their eyes wide and look upward. Hold the pencil between their eyes so that their pupils will converge as much as possible as they stare at the tip of the pencil. They may look cross-eyed. You will get the point, if you look at the tip of your nose. It fatigues the eyes rapidly. Tell them, **"Look with both eyes at the shiny tip of the pencil and at nothing else, until your eyes get so tired you cannot keep them open any longer.'**

Hold the pencil quite still and at the same time, direct your own gaze at the root of their nose and concentrate your mind on the idea that they will go to sleep. Tell them, **"Think of going to sleep but do not close your eyes until you simply cannot keep them open any longer."**

Shortly their eyes will start to blink and water as they stare. Soon they close them. You can facilitate this by saying the following when you see them blink, **"Your eyelids are getting heavy. They commence to blink. You cannot keep them open any longer. Your eyes are watering. They are tired. They feel heavy and are closing now and you are becoming sleepy…very, very sleepy. When I count from to ten your eyes will close and you will be asleep…fast asleep."**

Count slowly from one to ten in a low even tone. In many cases, your client's eyes will be closed by the count of ten. If not, gently close them by passing your hand over them. As soon as the eyes close, place your left hand on top of their head and with your right hand make passes across their forehead from the left to the right temple as you say,

"You are so sleepy…sleepy, drowsy… sleepy…drowsy. Your head feels heavy sooo sleepy …sooo drowsy… sooo tired. You cannot keep awake any longer. You are so sleepy. You hear nothing but the sound of my voice. You are going sound asleep, fast asleep, sound asleep. Sleep. Sleep. You are fast asleep…sound asleep. Everything is dark before you." (As you say this lay the palm of your hands over their eyes).

Change your position and stand directly in front of your client. Without touching their body now spread your fingers and make downward sweeping passes at least an inch over their body from the top of the head towards the feet with both hands while keeping your gaze on their forehead between the closed eyes.

Make the passes very slowly and when you get to the knees, turn palms outward (away from the body) and bring them in an upward motion to the top of the head again with half circles "fluffing them" from knees to head and then start the downward passes again.

"You cannot move your arms because they are so heavy. You cannot move your legs they are like lead too. Your whole body feels numb. You hear nothing but my voice. When I count ten you will be fast asleep. One. Two. Three. Four. Five. Six. Seven. Eight. Nine. TEN. You are fast asleep. FAST ASLEEP." (Say this last "fast asleep" in a commanding tone.)

Continue with these passes for about five minutes in silence and then softly give the sleep formula again. As soon as their head drops you will find that hypnotic sleep has been produced. Now insist **"You cannot awaken until I tell you to and you listen keenly to the sound of my voice. You hear only the sound of my voice."**

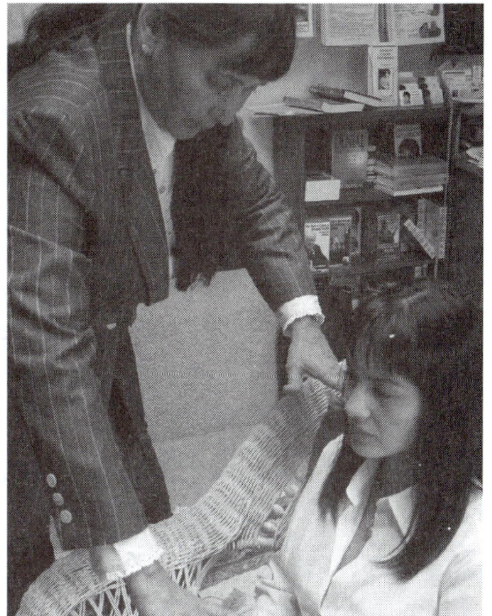

Sweeps

HYPNOTIC SLEEP TEST

When you think that your client is in hypnotic trance and sleeping soundly, lift up their right or left hand to a horizontal position and say to them, **"Your arm is suspended up and you cannot drop it. Try as hard as you will. Try. Try. Try hard. Try as hard as you will you cannot move it at all."**

If it remains up, it is a good indication of hypnotic sleep.

You can also use this to deepen trance by saying, **"You cannot move your arm because it is so stiff but you will find it begins to feel so tired it commences to slowly drop down to your lap and, as it drops down, you will go deeper and deeper into hypnosis and when it finally reaches your lap you will be deeply asleep in profound hypnosis. You will be profoundly hypnotized."**

HYPNOTIC SLEEP SUGGESTIONS

Hypnotic sleep in itself provides tremendous therapeutic value. The easiest way to do this is:

1. Determine during the consultation what your client wants to help with hypnosis and then suggest that **"Rest in hypnosis with the thought that this hypnosis will completely heal your problem."** And the second approach is

2. While in hypnotic sleep make this suggestion **"As you sleep in hypnosis, think about going into profound hypnosis as your mind and body are refreshed and revitalized. In every way you are becoming absolutely perfect. Remain hypnotized until you know fully of your own perfection."**

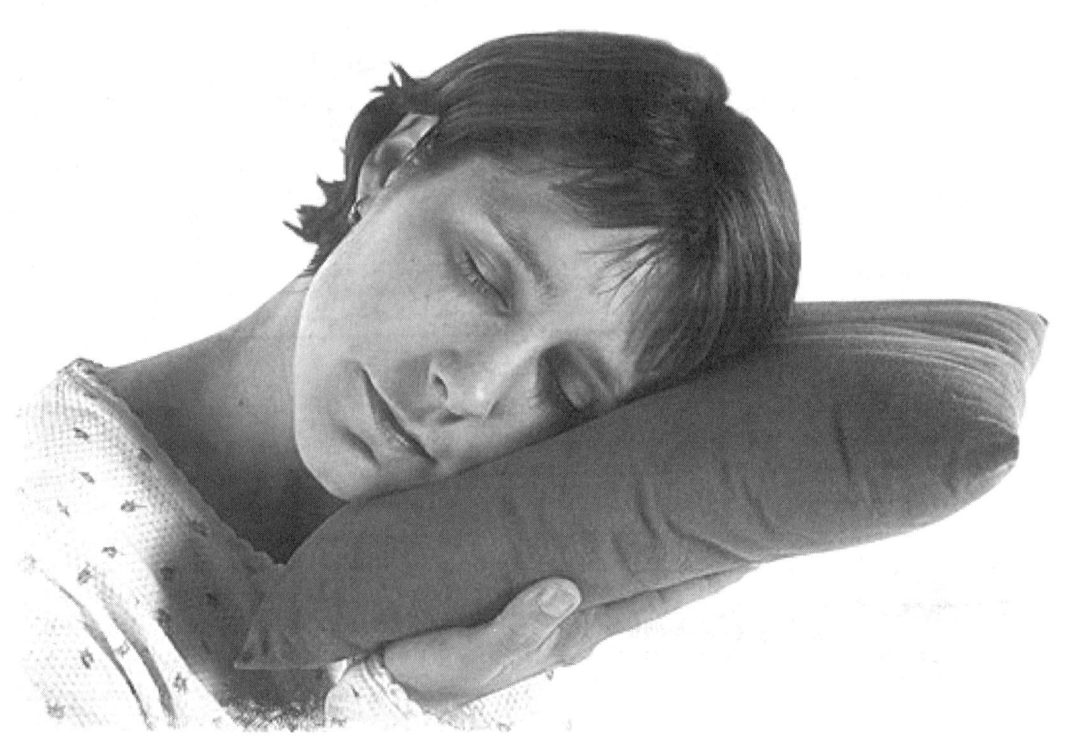

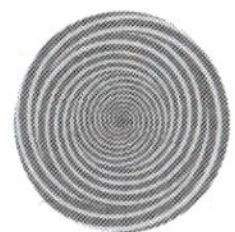

<h1 style="text-align:center">~ Chapter 19 ~
PRODUCING SOMNAMBULISM</h1>

Includes
PRODUCING SOMNAMBULISM

Somnambulism according to Charcot in the mid 1800's was the lightest state of trance. In more recent times it is best known as a quirky state in which a person will walk or talk in their sleep and when they awaken, have no memory of what they did. Consider it the "attic of relaxation of the mind" that makes you subjectively responsive to suggestions.

Somnambulism is an interruption in the stream of consciousness where you do things without being aware of the doing. Not unconsciousness, just an interruption. About one-fifth of the population enters the somnambulistic state when hypnotized. Some immediately, others after repeated trials and some never reach it at all.

In somnambulism many of the most striking hypnosis phenomena occur, e.g. posthypnotic suggestions followed to the letter, hallucinations, loss of memory (amnesia) or pain sensitivity removed may be induced.

"Somnambulism" old texts say, "is a very deep state of hypnosis where remarkable achievements are easily accomplished. This state is often sought and rarely obtained. The operator has to be satisfied working in the lighter states of hypnosis." Despite these printed words, somnambulism is EASY to achieve when properly evoked. It is actually a rather common mind state we enjoy everyday or it may even be annoying. After all, somnambulism is often characterized by loss of memory, or absent-mindedness.

Frequently somnambulism comes unbidden. Have you ever been doing something at your desk, possibly tending to some important paper when something interrupts you? *"The papers seem to vanish into thin air. And where is that darn pen? I just had it."* You look and look, getting more and more frustrated. Suddenly the paper and pen reappear right before you – almost like magic. What a relief. Now you can get back to work.

Have you been driving along the freeway, and in the monotony of driving your mind wanders? Suddenly you jerk back with a start, and for a moment you are disoriented. *"Where am I?" "Darn it!"* you say to yourself, *"I've gone past the turnoff I wanted to take."* Suddenly you realize you must have driven miles on the busy highway without being aware you were driving. *"Brother,"* you say to yourself, *"I'd better pay more attention while I'm driving, and not daydream."*

Dangerous?
Yes and No.

You weren't consciously paying attention to your driving but subconsciously you were. Thankfully, your subconscious is conditioned to protect YOU. Survival is the number one directive of life. The danger comes not so much from yourself, as it does from other drivers to whom you are not giving attention. Safe driving is always defensive driving and should you have an accident, it is unlikely the Highway Patrol would have much interest in your explanation that you were temporarily in a state of somnambulism. The officer would probably say, "Tell it to the judge!" Generally speaking, it is best not to become somnambulistic when driving. It is a time to be objective not subjective.

Have you ever misplaced your keys? *"I should know where I put them, but somehow I've forgotten."* It almost drives you crazy, as keys have a way of becoming very important to smooth living. *"Those keys… where are those keys? I know I had them."*

You look and look, and the more you look the more the loss becomes. Want to find your keys? Stop looking and allow the state-of-loss to submerge. Stop worrying and suddenly they appear. You say to yourself, *"Funny, here they are. Wonder how that slipped my mind?"*

And then you rationalize, *"Oh well, the important thing is that I found the keys."*

Amnesia does not belong exclusively to hypnosis and does not always occur when a person is hypnotized. However, it can be produced and when it is, it facilitates the deeper hypnotic state of somnambulism. If you want someone to remember what happened during their hypnosis session tell them to remember. If they insist "I don't think I was hypnotized," re-hypnotize them and give them the post hypnotic suggestion that they will "get all the positive results but not consciously remember the session at all." That amnesia suggestion convinces some people.

Stage hypnotists remove effects induced during the show by suggesting, "All effects now fade and vanish like a dream and are entirely forgotten when you awaken."

Dave Elman had a way of obtaining somnambulism in counting numbers backwards from 100 until the numbers drop away. Here is a variation using numbers in an even more personal way.

MODUS OPERANDI: PRODUCING SOMNAMBULISM

When you hypnotize a person, the first thing you do is invoke relaxation of the body. Relaxing the body is an early stage in reaching hypnotic depth. Begin by suggesting, **"Your eyes muscles relax until they become so relaxed they will not work to open your eyes, even when you try. Then the relaxation from your eyes moves down over your entire body to produce total relaxation."** (Certainly that is not the only way to relax the body, but it is one way that works quite well).

To go deeper and obtain somnambulism you must also relax the mind. Remember, somnambulism is characterized by the production of amnesia. By having the subject relax sufficiently, for a fragmentary pause in time, you can cause the mind to become blank concerning specific things. It does not matter what the "thing" is. You have produced amnesia. Tell the subject, **"Now your body has become relaxed, next you will relax your mind and produce somnambulism. As your mind relaxes, amnesia will occur, and you will forget familiar numbers that you normally know."**

Then suggest that they have forgotten their Social Security Number (this is a good number to start with as many people can't remember their Social Security Number anyway). **"You cannot recall what your Social Security Number is! The numbers have completely dropped out of your mind. Understand? If you agree lift your left forefinger."**

Wait for agreement signal. Then…

"Tell me the first digits of your Social Security Number." There is no answer. The mind goes blank. This first test successful, then…

"Now you will find that your telephone number has likewise dropped out of your mind. You can't for the life of you remember your telephone number. What is your telephone number?"

There is no answer. The mind goes blank. Then…

"All numbers drop away from your mind. You can't even recall your home address, where you live. You can't recall it. It has vanished from your mind. What is your home address?" There is no answer. The mind goes blank. Step-by-step you have lead the mind into amnesia, and that is the same as leading the mind into somnambulism…success thus far. Then try: **"You can't even recall your own name. You can't even remember who you are."**

Blank! Blank! Blank! You have produced somnambulism. If you were to pinch the subject, there is no response. Their mind is now ready to manifest all manner of somnambulistic phenomena, in response to your suggestions. In this state, you can suggest to the subject, **"Open your eyes, and as you do so you will go even deeper into hypnosis. With eyes open, you can observe the indicators of hypnosis everywhere."**

All manner of medical and dental procedures will find this state advantageous. It works brilliantly well for surgery and when the session is over and the operation is completed without pain, do not be surprised if some patients say, "How could I have been hypnotized? I was wide awake and watching you during the entire treatment."

The somnambulistic state awakens a person to the wonderful powers within the depths of mind. What does the hypnotherapist do if the client refuses to go into somnambulism? Nothing. Quit trying. After all, it is not your responsibility if the person chooses to turn critical mind against using the remarkable potential of their subconscious.

Appreciate that somnambulism is a euphoric state, in which the client gains an appreciation of him or herself. And, while it can cause amnesia, it never produces unconsciousness. Somnambulism does not bring on a zombie-like state. The client does not lose consciousness. Instead, they gain awareness. Some researchers claim that a person's awareness surprisingly quadruples while in somnambulism.

You can conclude the session here, or you can proceed on taking the subject clear down into "the basement of relaxation," the Hypnotic Coma.

Before you bring them back to room awareness reinstate their "memory." **"You have an excellent memory and easily recall your name, your social security number, telephone number, address anything you would like to remember."**

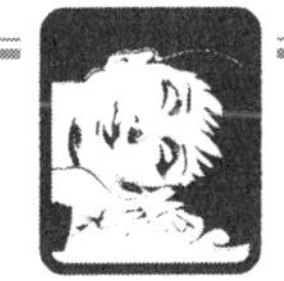

Hypno-Helper
"Sleep, Beautiful Sleep" by Shelley Stockwell-Nicholas
"The Sleeping Pill" tape by Ormond McGill

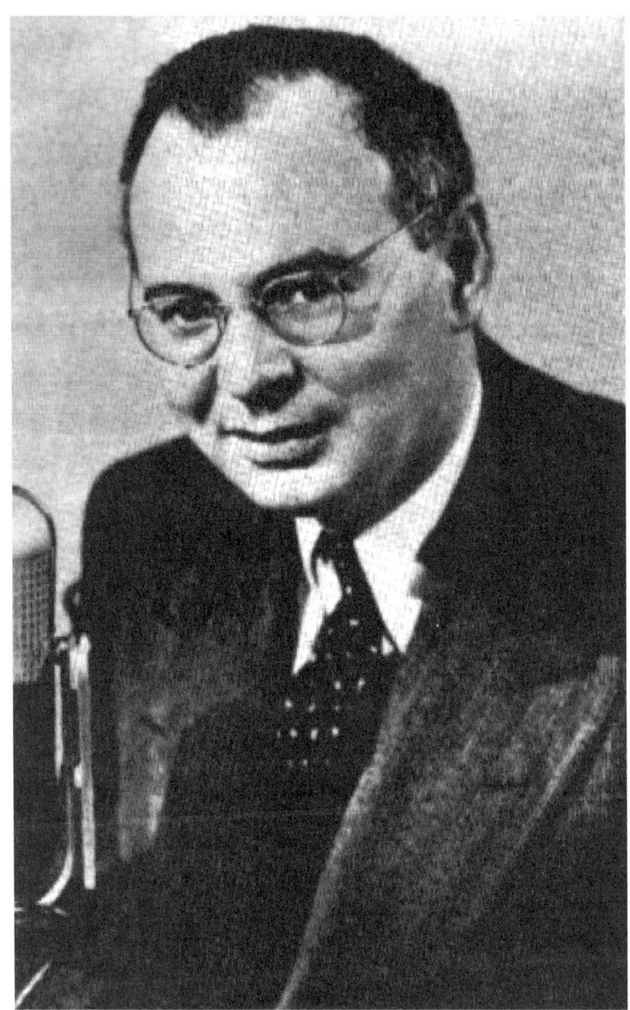

Dave Elman

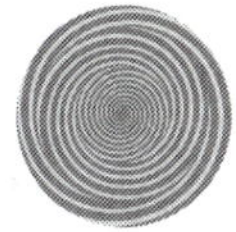

~ *Chapter 20* ~
ELMAN'S HYPNOTIC COMA

Includes
What is Hypnotic Coma
How To Evoke The Coma
Awakening Someone From The Coma

Dave Elman was a rebel soul.

Rebel souls are quite rare. Every so often they come along to advance our knowledge. They each seem to have their specialties. Dave's specialty was hypnosis.

Everyone has a soul…it is the seat of individual immortality. But most souls are quite content to accept things just as they are, and mind their own business. They avoid challenges. Rebel souls not only do not avoid challenges, they create them. Rebel souls have a restless nature and look for things to challenge to make new discoveries. One such challenge for Dave Elman was THE HYPNOTIC COMA.

The Hypnotic Coma is rarely mentioned in hypnotic literature and, when it is, it is discounted as "too rare to be concerned with." Somnambulism was touted as the deepest useful depth of hypnosis. Only a rebel soul like Elman or a kindred rebel soul like Esdaile would bother to give this state its due attention.

WHAT IS HYPNOTIC COMA?

The Hypnotic Coma is a state so deep that the subject loses contact with the hypnotist, and drops into an abyss of themself. It is such a pleasant and peaceful state that the person literally would be content just to remain in it, and let the world go by. In the coma, one just doesn't want to be bothered by outside contact. Like Garbo saying "I vant to be alone"…alone, but not lonely, for you can never be lonely when you are truly with your SELF. In the coma, the dust that seems to have gathered about the mind is wiped away and mind becomes like crystal. Stress of mind and body vanish as both mind and body just coast and rejuvenate.

The coma state is harmless, pleasant and a boon to your being.

For the unwell, it is an excellent state to recover in. Very possibly that is its purpose. Being in such a profound depth of hypnosis just for the state itself sans any specific suggestions is excellent hypnotherapy: like coasting in catatonic neutral gear.

Doctors find it to be particularly good for surgery, as their patients seem to automatically anesthetize themselves without special suggestions being given. And though clients in the coma seem incapable of taking physical suggestions that require bodily movements, they follow mental suggestions for organic functioning. Suggestions such as removing a migraine headache are immediately responded to.

In the state of coma, the hypnotist seems to have lost guidance control of his subject and the subjects seems to take off on their own. They seem particularly self-centered and truly independent. The rapport between hypnotist and subject appears to be lost. The "I just don't care" feeling of the hypnotic coma, in time becomes "I wish that everyone would shut up…especially the hypnotist." To an operator who does not understand the coma, this can be a concern. What if the person never returned to the here and now? This puzzle causes many to avoid it.

Dave says:
"Worry. Worry. Worry. How the hypnotist worries when his subject goes so deep into hypnosis he will not follow suggested commands. For heaven's sake, stop worrying and be thankful you have made things so pleasant for the subject that the coma state is achieved…
The coma is the most profound state of relaxation mind/body can reach. In the coma state, such a deep phase of relaxation has been obtained that the subject does not want to be disturbed. And so he turns off the hypnotist, so he can fully enjoy by himself the euphoria he is in. He drops within himself, and to heck with the hypnotist outside. That is HYPNOTIC COMA…
The Coma is not so difficult to understand when you examine the reactions of yourself at times. For example, you are relaxing in a hammock, a little breeze sways it gently, it is a lazy balmy day, you enter a state of peace with yourself. It is so nice you just want to be left alone. If anyone intrudes upon your reverie you are annoyed, and your inner mind says to itself, 'Please go away and leave me alone so I can just enjoy my being, as I am right now.' And so you withdraw and remain very quiet, and hope they will go away."

For a hundred years, it was believed that the coma occurred accidentally in only one of a thousand cases. Antiquated textbooks said that should it happen, it is best to leave the subject alone, and that in time they will pass from coma into natural sleep, and will awaken of their own election. Nonsense.

In the first place, few people, if any, find it possible to fall asleep in the hypnotic state. From the coma the subject does not pass into and arouse from natural sleep; the person simply arouses themself when they know it is best for them to come back from the coma. If asked "Were you asleep?" they will simply say "No I just didn't want to come back from where I was…it was so nice to be there." A person can be quickly aroused from the coma when the proper suggestion is applied.

This most maligned hypnotic state is really not a coma at all, as the person has complete awareness, and can recall everything that occurred when returned from it. Amnesia rarely occurs in the coma state. Even amnesia is not unconsciousness. It's sub consciousness– that is in the moving from one stream of consciousness to another, a lapse can occur in the continuity of memory. Elman contends that even in profound hypnosis the client has the element of choice. Freedom of choice is always there in both the objective and subjective states of mind. Only habit can tie you up.

MODUS OPERANDI: HOW TO EVOKE THE HYPNOTIC COMA

Intentionally induce the Hypnotic Coma by promising, **"How pleasant it will be. Those who experience it say it is the best hypnotic experience they have ever enjoyed. It's wonderful."**

Then, hypnotize the client into wonderfully relaxed somnambulism using your favorite induction. Then affirm, **"You are deeply in hypnosis now and wonderfully relaxed. You enjoy the relaxation so much that you crave to go yet deeper and become even more relaxed. You know within yourself that you can go into a depth of relaxation far deeper than the relaxation you are in right now. You want to go into the very basement of relaxation inside yourself. If you are ready now to go into the basement of relaxation nod your head."**
(Client nods their head.)

"Good. Get ready now to descend into the basement of yourself. Imagine that you are in a spacious house of your very own. It has an attic, which is the space you are in right now. And below the attic is FLOOR A… below Floor A is FLOOR B… below Floor B is FLOOR C, which is the basement to your house. There is an elevator in your house that will take you down to these floors lower and lower inside yourself. We are going to take this elevator and go down in it to these lower floors, and in each floor you reach you will become twice as relaxed as you are right now here in the attic of your somnambulistic self until you reach the very basement of relaxation. How eager you are to reach that basement of relaxation. Understand? Nod your head."

(Client nods their head.)

"Good. Fine. Get into the elevator now and we are going to start down. All ready. Good. Ready. Set. Go! Down we go to FLOOR A in which you become twice as relaxed as you are right now. Down…down we go and we have reached FLOOR A now. Enjoy the relaxation for a few moments -of this floor which is twice as deep as the relaxation you enjoyed while you were in the attic of your house."

(Allow the client some quiet moments to enjoy the relaxation of floor "A".)

"When, you are ready to go down the elevator now to FLOOR B even deeper, nod your head."

(Client nods their head.)

"Good. Back in the elevator now, and down we go to FLOOR B. Down. Down you go and reach FLOOR B where you enjoy twice the wonderful relaxation you enjoyed on FLOOR A. Enjoy some moments of this great relaxation you have now that you are on FLOOR B. Are you ready to go down to FLOOR C now, which is the basement of relaxation inside yourself. If you are ready, nod your head."

(Client nods their head.)

"Okay, back in the elevator we go… down and down we go… into the basement of languorous relaxation inside yourself. You are in the basement of relaxation now. Get out of the elevator and enjoy the delicious space you are in… down in the basement of relaxation."

(Observing the hypnotized client, you will notice what seems like absolute contentment settles about them. This is HYPNOTIC COMA.)

Somehow the person has become self-contained and it appears you have lost contact. You try to communicate and there is no response. Even a suggested command; there is no obedience. In the Hypnotic Coma the person becomes in rapport with themself. They are not unconscious and they hear you and know that you are there. But they have become so pleasantly withdrawn within themself that they can't be bothered to do anything but just ENJOY. They are so far withdrawn that even outer noise or pain sensations are not reacted to.

Then the interesting phenomena of catatonia sets in. You lift up an arm of a person in Hypnotic Coma, and it just remains where it has been placed. The person has become like wax. Lift up a leg and it stays lifted. If left for some time, it will gradually descend to the floor… but for the most part arms and legs just stay where they are moved. Bend them at the waist and they stay bent at the waist. It appears most strange. A psychiatrist would call it an abnormal state of "waxy flexibility."

An abnormal state? In a sense it is, as it certainly differs from what we expect of what we call "normal behavior." But it is not abnormal as far as Hypnotic Coma is concerned.

The inner mental mechanism, really is not too difficult to understand: In the basement of complete relaxation, there is at last complete freedom from all stress and tension. The body feels good; so good that the person doesn't even feel like wanting to move their own body. If an outside person, such as the operator, wants to bother to move them OKAY... but being in the coma is so enjoyable all attempts at voluntary muscular movement seem just too much bother. A complete withdrawal sets in. Yet, all the while, the comatose person knows what is happening, They just prefer things to be as they are. Their "mental set" is "Don't bother me. I don't want to come back yet. I like it here."

AWAKENING SOMEONE FROM THE COMA

What if you tell the client to come back out of coma and there is no response whatsoever? First attempt to bring them back by counting up from the basement to floor C then B then A, into somnambulism and back to room awareness. Be calm and collected so as not to give the impression that they are difficult to arouse. Your confidence is necessary to remove the trance you have produced. You could say, **"I want you to wake up now. I know that you are sleepy and tired but you MUST wake up now. You have slept long enough. Tell you what I'll do, I'll count you back up very slowly from the basement up to FLOOR C then to FLOOR B and finally up into the attic of your mind when you will wake up feeling great. Fair enough. Will you awaken when you get to the attic?** (Persevere until you get a response) **All right here we go C, B, attic WIDE AWAKE FEELING GREAT. EYES WIDE OPEN. WAKE UP. WAKE UP. WAKE UP."** You may make upward passes with your hands or clap your hands loudly. Don't worry about a startling noise re-inducing trance because this subject is lethargic in nature.

If all else fails, a very direct and simple way to bring the person back from coma, and very quickly too is the way Dave Elman showed to his doctor students. Just tell the person in Hypnotic Coma, **"If you don't come right out of it now, you will never have another opportunity to enjoy this euphoria again in the basement of absolute relaxation."**

The arousal from Hypnotic Coma is almost like a threat (a threat gets attention), and the coma subject will arouse on the instant.

Why does this work?

Because being in coma provides freedom from all stress and bodily aches and pains. It feels so good. It is euphoric. The client very much looks forward to being given the opportunity to enjoy it again.

If the client still remains in self-centered rapport and not with you, just relax and say, **"Go ahead and do whatever you wish. I will pay no more attention to you."** And go about the business ignoring them. You will be surprised how quickly they will come back on their own.

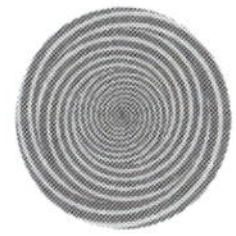

~ *Chapter 21*
THE ART OF WAKING HYPNOSIS

Includes
Non-Verbal Waking Suggestions
Verbal Waking Suggestions
Medical Waking Suggestion
Accidental Waking Suggestions
Three Waking Group Hypnosis Experiments:
      Spritzed-Not-to-Be-Mist Experiment
      A Rotten Yoke
      Dress Distress

A hypnotherapist needs to use waking hypnosis in their work as much as formal hypnosis. With experience, waking hypnosis becomes inherent to your nature and seems to literally become the way you express yourself when using hypnotic skills.

Half the value of hypnotherapy occurs before any formal hypnosis is applied. It starts with deciding to visit the hypnotherapist, to get outside unbiased help to deal with whatsoever is requested. And then a sympathetic ear listens to the telling of the trouble. That alone can be a great help, especially with the intelligent use of hypnosis in the waking state.

Suggestion is the subconscious realization of ideas. Waking hypnosis goes beyond critical mind and establishes the subconscious realization of ideas without any formal hypnotic induction. A great time to use it is when a client is resistant to the trance state, or when you want to save time.

What is especially unique about the hypnotic "power of suggestion" is that suggestions are effective both in the waking and hypnotic state, as long as they are accepted and established in the subconscious. Both waking hypnosis and trance hypnosis offer fine short-range results. The same mental mechanism is present in both, but trance hypnosis with suggestion seems to turn up the power. When time is plentiful, always include the benefits of trance state suggestions.

Your mind is always ready to function on two levels. One level, the conscious mind is like parents who can be awfully critical of what can be or cannot be done. The other level, the subconscious is a child-like Samson with great, unlimited power just waiting to be told what to do by its parents. If the parents (your conscious mind) are wise and do not bring in limitations, all is well and fine, but if they are very critical, they distort the power of the child (your subconscious).

Hypnosis provides a way to bypass critical parents and get right to the power of the helpful child within. That little you is eagerly freed when properly directed. Waking hypnosis is the informal way to release the little giant. Have you ever thought about it this way?

NON-VERBAL WAKING SUGGESTIONS

Waking hypnosis can be non-verbal. For example, Mommy kisses a young child's hurt place or "booboo" and stops the pain. Try these non-verbal suggestions:

1. Take a lemon and poke a hole in it. Suck the lemon and remark on how sour it tastes. All watching will commence to experience saliva flowing into their mouth. A mental idea (suggestion) of something being sucked that is sour causes a physical reaction.
   Or...
2. Tell someone to think of itches upon their body, as they watch you scratch. Soon you will have them scratching.
   Or...
3. Yawn or say, "yawn...yawn...yawn." They will commence to yawn– a physical reaction to the suggestion of yawning.

VERBAL WAKING SUGGESTIONS

Examples of waking hypnosis in the medical field are many. An accident victim is rushed to the hospital. He seems to be in bad shape. He's a mixture of shock and panic. In the emergency room, he hears the reassuring words: "Not too serious. He'll be first rate again in no time." Those magic words: "not too serious" calms and heals him. Such fine words have saved many lives. Conversely, what happens if they say, "I doubt if he'll make it." Or, how about the document you have to sign before surgery that describes, in detail, all of potential negative outcomes? How many lives has that effected?

Has something like this happened to you or someone you know? A person in pain goes to the doctor or dentist to get an opinion. Somehow while in the office, when asked to explain the pain, they can hardly describe it any longer. Why? The person fears what the doctor or dentist will say about the pain more than they fear the pain. Waking hypnosis.

MEDICAL WAKING SUGGESTIONS

Medical doctors do well to learn the fine art of waking suggestion and semantics (or suggestions if you prefer) to produce mental/physical ease and healing:

A radiologist considers the barium enema his most unpleasant procedure, but is hesitant to use hypnosis to prepare patients for one. He thinks that if he hypnotically tells his patient that the procedure is "comfortable," he would deceive them. The result: it is a real pain! So to ease the pain a little, he tells a patient, "I have to put you through a process that isn't very comfortable but I'll make it as painless for you as I can." There is little point in going half way like this.

I suggested to the radiologist. "Why not make the process comfortable by using the proper semantics? Why not tell the patient, **'You are fortunate to be here today. The doctor who referred you tells me that she needs some X-rays. In order to get them painlessly, I am going to coat the lining of your stomach with a wonderful soothing and gentle medication. You will be comfortable.'"**

The radiologist refused to say anything so "absurd" until one day he had to work on a man who was already in terrible discomfort. Out of desperation, he tried this recommended approach. The patient was relieved, and actually enjoyed the barium enema treatment!

The radiologist now uses this approach consistently. The only problem he has encountered is that some patients so thoroughly enjoy the "soothing medication," that they retain the barium and refuse to let it go. He solved this by telling them **"It feels as pleasant leaving as it did entering."**

Another doctor learned a variation of this "waking hypnosis" and the art of semantics. He tells a patient, **"A new preparation just arrived from Europe– a form of local anesthetic especially designed for such examinations."** Then he swabs the patient with a bit of scented Vaseline. After waiting a few minutes for the placebo effect to result, the examination proceeds without difficulty. The placebo suggestion in waking hypnosis, just like a trance suggestion, takes a few minutes to go into action. It works perfectly!

A dentist applied "waking hypnosis" simply by stating to patients: **"As I press a certain nerve spot on your gum it will deaden all sensation and make it numb. As I press in, you will feel the numbness come."** Sure enough, the numbness comes, and the dental operation proceeds. Most dentists today have been trained to use the word "numb" when a needle is poked in the gum.

Truly the "power of waking suggestion" is remarkable. A physician reports: "It works great with patients, but my office staff gets nervous when they see me do a biopsy and I cut in with semantics as the only anesthetic used."

ACCIDENTAL WAKING GROUP SUGGESTIONS

Accidental waking hypnosis happens to us throughout life, especially in the early years. Prenatal thoughts from mother go the infant during pregnancy, birth and things that mother and others say are often instantly taken in and accepted. What, where, when and how you interpret it can convey powerful and lasting hypnosis. What you say to yourself can also be waking hypnosis.

In all cases waking hypnosis bypasses critical judgment and is automatically conveyed to the subconscious mind.

MODUS OPERANDI: THREE WAKING HYPNOSIS EXPERIMENTS

Here are a few experiments in group waking hypnosis you can try when the opportunity affords. They bring you an appreciation of the technique:

1. SPRITZED-NOT-TO-BE-MIST GROUP EXPERIMENT
You Will Need:
An Atomizer Bottle Containing Water

Bring out the atomizer labeled "perfume" and say, **"I am going to perform a test to determine who has the keenest sense of smell. This atomizer contains a delicate fragrance perfume from France; and I am going to spray some in the air, and as you smell it, hold up a hand. The order in which hands go up, will determine who has the keenest sense of smell."** Then, squirt the "perfume" into the air in various directions, so the room is well covered. **"When you smell the perfume, raise your hand,"** you emphasize. Hands go up about the room. Some even tell you what odor the perfume most resembles.

What is amazing is that you have only squirted plain water into the air. Of course, animals can smell water miles away but most humans can't.

2. A ROTTEN YOKE
You Will Need:
An Egg and A Dish

Here's one you can try with a group. Crack open a perfectly fresh egg before them and make a wry face exclaiming: **"Wow, smell that egg. It's rotten. I wouldn't eat the egg for a million dollars. Oh boy, what a stink! Here, smell it."** Now, pass the egg around for people to smell. Person after person will say: "That egg smells bad, all right." Some may even say: "Why it even looks bad."

These people have been hypnotized with waking hypnosis have bypassed their critical mental factor and established in its place subjective thinking.

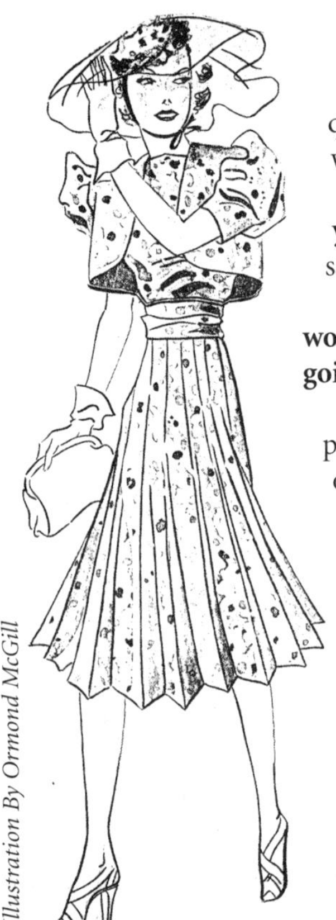

Illustration By Ormond McGill

3. DRESS DISTRESS
Imagine yourself nicely dressed and someone you respect quizzically looks you over as though they have noticed something wrong with your outfit and then they say:

"Do you mind turning around once? There's something about your clothes that puzzles me." They gaze at you critically for a moment saying:

"Hum, turn around the other way, won't you please? I was wondering what was wrong. Thank you so much. Sorry, but I must be going now. Good-bye."

When they walk away without further comment they have precipitated waking hypnosis. Despite assurances that you are quite okay, you will somehow think that your clothes are not right: too long, too short, too small, too big, or that it bulged or didn't bulge in the wrong or right places. It makes you uncomfortable and questioning your own judgment. You have substituted what you believe for their implied judgment. This is a form of waking hypnosis.

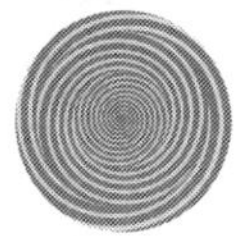

~ *Chapter 22* ~
FROM WAKING TO TRANCE

Waking Hypnosis is often all your client requires. Of course, a formal hypnosis session is included as it is expected so the client feels they are getting their money's worth. Still, it is well to experiment with Waking Hypnosis to gain an appreciation and understanding of its effectiveness…its skillful use is powerful.

MODUS OPERANDI: FROM WAKING TO TRANCE INDUCTION

This disguised hypnotic technique hypnotizes without ever once mentioning hypnotism. It is a subtle method, and catches your client unawares that they are being entranced. Tell your client, **"I will show you how to relax using the power of suggestion. Would you like that?"**

You bet they would. Everyone appreciates the value of relaxing. And the more a person is led into relaxation, the more their critical mind is moved to one side, and the threshold of the subconscious is exposed. Hypnotic influence is caused by compounding suggestion upon suggestion, and this case, piling unmentioned hypnosis upon hypnosis.

"This method offers relaxation throughout your body. It is wonderful, as in just a few moments of concentrated relaxation you can obtain the equivalent of a full hour of rest. Sit comfortably in your seat. Think of nothing special. Just let your mind drift. To obtain this complete relaxation, just listen to my voice and do just as I tell you.

Ready, set, go. Now, close your eyes as you relax comfortably in your seat. All comfortable! Your eyes closed! Fine. Now keep your eyelids tightly closed and roll your eyeballs up just as if you are looking right into the top of your head; right inside your brain. Eyes closed, looking right up inside your head. Relax, comfortably relaxed and thinking of nothing but what I tell you.

I am going to count from one to six, and while I am counting you will find it is impossible to open your eyes. You are relaxed all over, with your eyes closed, looking right up inside your head…eyes tightly closed.

One. You cannot open your eyes because the more you try the tighter they keep shut.

Two. Your eyes are so tightly shut, looking up into your head that, try as you will, you cannot open them. Try. Try hard, but it is impossible for you to open them because they are so tightly shut.

Three. You cannot open your eyes. They are glued shut. You are relaxed and comfortable all over. You hear nothing but my voice. You think of nothing but what I tell you. Your eyes are tightly closed.

Four. You still cannot open your eyes, and you don't want to now, for it is so comfortable sitting there, comfortable and relaxed, with your eyes shut, hearing nothing, thinking of nothing but my voice. Eyes shut, shut tightly relaxed and comfortable.

Five. You cannot open your eyes because you are sinking into such a comfortable, pleasant deep relaxation that it makes you feel sleepy. You feel like dropping into a deep, deep sleep. You are so nice and relaxed all over, dropping into a deep sleep, into the realm of sleep. Thinking nothing, hearing but my voice; all comfortable and relaxed. Dropping into the realm of sleep. Sleeping. Going deeper and deeper into sleep.

Six. You are now so relaxed and comfortable, as your drift and drift down into the realm of sleep. Sleep. Sleep. Go deep to sleep, and as you go deeper and deeper into the realm of sleep, and as you drop down ever deeper and deeper into sleep, let this become your reality."

Now give them the suggestions for success that they came to you to receive. If you choose to take them even deeper, you may layer more induction techniques saying:

"When you come back and are again wide-awake we are going to try together some experiments in relaxation. You will respond to each and every one with marvelous effect.

All ready now, I will bring you back from this deep relaxation so you can enjoy other wonderful success in performing relaxation experiments. I will count from one to five…and by the count of five you will be wide-awake and eager to perform these experiments together experiencing the power of suggestion.

One. Two. Begin to stir and come back now. Three. You are coming back from the realm of sleep and entering the realm of wakefulness now. Four. You stir and move about, and your eyes open. Five! You are wide-awake now. You feel wonderful and well in every way, as we perform these experiments together."

This method has a powerful, very subtle effect. It has produced a hypnotic condition of mind without mentioning hypnosis in any way. It conditions the mind for spontaneous responsiveness to the next "experiment" and to more fully take on your beneficial suggestions.

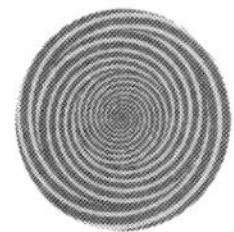

~ *Chapter 23* ~
ESTABLISHING THE HYPNOTIC MOOD

Includes
Hypnotic Prelude Before a Consultation
Hypnotic Prelude After a Consultation

Let your client come to a happy place in space and time. The hypnotic mood is so apparently simple that many overlook its value. It's so simple, yet so fruitful for producing profound hypnosis.

Make every effort for the client to feel relaxed and comfortable. Make your office bright and pleasant. Have fresh flowers. No mystique or medical clinic approach. The hypnotherapy office is a place of strength, guidance, and protection. Greet your client with warm friendliness.

In this approach, the clients create for themself an atmosphere of receptivity for profound hypnosis. This is done through autosuggestion. Autosuggestion is self-hypnosis or suggestions that the client gives themself.

Request that your client go alone to an adjoining room. If there is not a separate room available, step out of the room and leave them there. The room is pleasantly warm and dimly lit (With a violet light when possible). Play music softly in the background. The Serenity Resonance Sound is recommended. A comfortable recliner chair is excellent.

The following Hypnotic Preludes remarkably enthrall. Both are done before a formal hypnotic induction is presented.

MODUS OPERANDI: HYPNOTIC PRELUDE <u>BEFORE</u> A CONSULTATION
You Will Need:
Soft Music (Preferably the *Serenity Resonance Sound* available at the back of this book)
Reclining Chair (If available)

In this first approach, you use the prelude session first and then conduct the consultation or interview.

"Sit in the chair, close your eyes, place your hands over your ears, and repeat out loud these suggestions…over and over…for five minutes, 'I want to be profoundly hypnotized for my personal benefit. I allow it to happen.'"

When the minutes have passed, invite the client to return to the session room (Or you reenter the room) saying, **"We can now begin our consultation and formal hypnotic induction."**

MODUS OPERANDI: HYPNOTIC PRELUDE AFTER A CONSULTATION
You will need:
Soft Music (Preferably the Serenity Resonance Sound)
Reclining Chair (If available)

In this approach, you conduct your consultation first and then hypnotize the client.

"Now that we know what concerns you, we are going to use hypnosis to remove that concern. Before we start, go in my adjoining room. You will find it silent.

Take a seat. Relax comfortably. Close your eyes, if you wish. Sit quietly for ten minutes while you think to yourself how you feel the experience of being hypnotized will be. Give your full attention to this. Do not allow your mind to wander from that purpose. I will come in in ten minutes and begin. Do you understand?"

Or, if you haven't two rooms, explain to your client;

"I am going to dim the lights and leave you alone in your chair to relax for 10 minutes while you think to yourself how you feel the experience of being hypnotized will be. Give your full attention to this, and do not allow your mind to wander from that purpose. Do you understand?"

(Client agrees)

Give them no hint as to what the hypnosis experience will be. Such conjecture is entirely what the client thinks the experience will be. The instruction to "give full attention to thinking what the experience of being hypnotized will be" and the command that "your mind must not be allowed to wander from that purpose" are literally impossible suggestions to follow. For how can the client experience an experience that is pure conjecture?

How can attention be kept upon such an entanglement? The command to not "allow mind to wander" causes the mind to wander more.

Ever present in the client's mind are the hypnotherapist's instructions with which they wish to comply. Thus, attention swings from going away to not going away. Back and forth the pendulum of attention to inattention swings. A paradox has been created. A paradox cannot be logically solved. It bores the mind. A paradox causes the mind to go blank.

So what?

The client's alone period in the quiet darkened room, prior to returning to your office (Or your return to the room) to be hypnotized will seem like an hour.

Finally, when the period of aloneness in the dark room thinking of how it feels to be hypnotized is over, the client's attitude towards hypnosis has developed. Will it work or will it not work? Mind has become indifferent. Like in going to sleep, indifference is the best way to go to sleep. Hypnosis follows the same pattern. Mind is now eager to get busy and do something, and that "doing something" is going to be profound hypnosis.

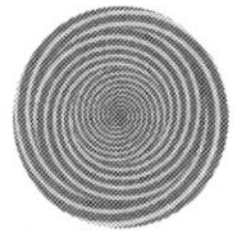

~ *Chapter 24* ~
WAKING HYPNOTIC INDUCTIONS
& CONVINCERS

Includes
Sensory Effects
Eyelids Experiment
Hands Locked
Fingertips Glued
Hand On Your Head Test
The Fist Lock
Hands Stuck To A Stick Experiment
The Arm Rising Experiment
The Falling Backward Experiment
The Falling Forward Experiment
The Memory Experiment
Making Yourself Light And Heavy
The Anti-Gravity Body Lift Group Demonstration

Waking hypnosis feels like body magic to the client and stimulates surprise. Surprise stimulates imagination and imagination stimulates the subconscious. The more genuine hypnosis appears to be; the more someone accepts the beneficial suggestions you give them. Confidence begets confidence. As long as confidence is there, it is good hypnotherapy.

Some hypnotists use such susceptibility to trance tests before beginning the more formal hypnotherapy work. Waking hypnosis starts with conscious doing and then moves into subconscious acceptance. Your body's activity stimulates your mental activity via the power of suggestion.

Painless surgery is a profound convincer.

You administer these techniques while the client is seemingly fully awake. They can be used as inductions, convincers and even deepening techniques. Some erroneously believe that they actually demonstrate "trance capacity." The last two convincers in this chapter, "Making Yourself Light and Heavy" and the "Antigravity Lift" can be used as group convincers during a public hypnosis demonstration.

Waking hypnosis convincers include:
"Your arm is so stiff and rigid you can't move it."
"Your eyes are stuck together so tightly, you can't open them"
"Open your mouth wide open and you can't close it."
"You can't stand up."
"When I pinch your arm you won't feel a thing."

SENSORY EFFECTS

Sensory effects you can produce using Waking Hypnosis:

1. Gustatory Effects
   "Taste your fingertip and it will be very, very salty."
   "A sip of this water and tastes as sweet as sugar."
   "This piece of candy is become completely tasteless."

2. Olfactory Effects
   "Smell the aroma of roses."
   "The room smells exactly like lavender."
   "You smell a pungent odor."
   "This perfume on a handkerchief takes you deeply into hypnosis"

3. Visual Effects
   "See a (suggested) color."
   "The room illuminated by the color blue."
   "Visualize a scene."

4. Tactile Effects
   "This object you hold is iced cold."
   "You feel very warm all over."
   "Suddenly you experience a tickle."

When producing sensory alteration via waking hypnosis, there is no need to restrict yourself to only one effect. Include two or more in your suggestions and each suggested effect compounds the next. Here are a number of waking hypnosis experiments you can perform that greatly increase the response to your suggestions.

EYELIDS EXPERIMENT

Speak softly in a confident tone, **"Relax completely as you close your eyes. In this experiment, you will discover that your eyelids are so tightly fastened together, you will be unable to open them as hard as you try. All right, your eyelids are becoming stuck together so tightly that you cannot open them try as hard as you will. They are fastened firmly together, and will not open until I tell you they will. Try. Try hard to open your eyes, but you cannot do so."**

The client tries to open their eyes, but finds them fastened tightly shut. Their eyes will not unfasten until you give say, **"Your eyes become unfastened now. Open wide your eyes."** Or if you would like to use this as an entry to more formal hypnosis you can continue, **"OK close your eyes and go deeper. That feeling you had when your eyelids did not want to open, that is the feeling of hypnosis. But hypnosis is a state of mind not a state of eyelids so let us proceed into formal hypnosis…"**

HANDS LOCKED

This induction is a classic. Your client, can be seated or standing. Instruct them, **"Look into my eye as you them clasp your hands together, interlocking the fingers in a firm grip. You are going to lock your hands so firmly together that you cannot separate them (until I release them for you). You will not be able to take them apart no matter how hard you try."**

Take their interlocked hands in yours and press firmly, as you suggest, **"Listen to me and concentrate upon what I say. Your hands are becoming locked tightly together…tight… very tight. They are locked tightly. Concentrate on how tightly they have become locked together. Concentrate on being unable to pull them apart until I release them from you.**

They are locked. Locked. You cannot get them apart try as hard as you will until I release them for you. Try. Try. Try with all your might. You cannot separate your hands. They are locked together!"

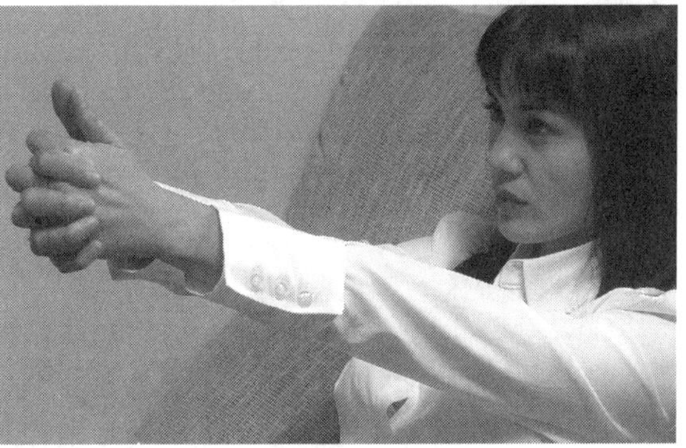
Hands Locked

Photo by Jon Nicholas

Your client will try in vain to unlock their hands. After proof of the response has been established, state, **"Alright, now, your hands are relaxing, the fingers are separating. You can easily take them apart now."**

FINGERTIPS GLUED

Stand in front of your client while looking at them squarely. Tell them **"Touch your fingertips together in front of your chest. Press them firmly and pretend that they have become stuck together. Pretend that they are stuck so tightly that you cannot pull them apart, no matter how hard they try. You are not to jerk them but exert a steady pull. Pretend, pretend, pretend. Your fingertips are stuck together so firmly that you cannot separate them. Try as hard as you will."**

The suggested effect is powerful and the client will find it impossible for him or her to pull their hands apart. It is best to have all fingers stuck together but even one finger will do the trick.

Here comes the topper…

After the person, still pushing their fingertips together and holding them against the chest, has found it impossible to pull them apart say **"How tightly your fingers have become stuck– via the power of suggestion– now the fingertips will be impossible to pull apart."**

Then you grip their wrists and try to pull, pull, pull their fingertips apart. If you are doing a demonstration, have a strong man from the audience come up and try to pull the fingers apart by clasping the wrists. This leverage is such that even a child can resist a man. Your subject's fingers will not separate and will resist all pulling. In your office this experiment goes a long way in convincing the client how much influence their mind has over their body. On stage, both parties will be astounded.

Then instruct the hypnotized person **"When I blow on your fingers they come apart easily."** And they do!

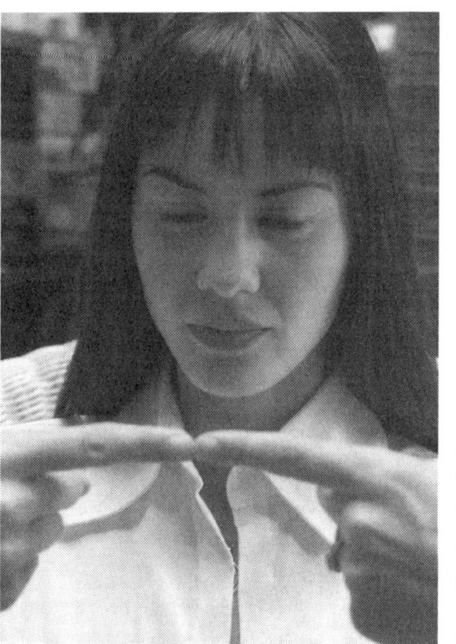
Fingertips Glued

Photo by Jon Nicholas

HAND ON YOUR HEAD TEST

You can use this same principle by having someone **"Press the palm of your left hand on top of your head. Press firmly and pretend you cannot move your hand from your head try as hard as you will. Pretense becomes reality. Pretending makes it so. Your hand remains stuck. Even a strong man cannot lift it off your head. Yet, a command from me that the adhesion is gone and all is free."**

THE FIST LOCK

Have the client stand before you, double up his fists, and place one over the other and pushes them firmly together as tightly as you can.

Suggest: **"This demonstration, shows how an affirmation of power, just like hypnosis, can benefit yourself. Make two fists and place one over the other and push them firmly together. You are going to bring strength into your fists by concentrating your mind upon them and they become super strong, and no one will be able to knock your fists apart no matter how hard they try. You clamp them together with all your might."**

Then proceed to try to pull them apart clasping the wrists and they won't budge!

"Now using the power of my mind I will knock your fists apart."

Then, using only the forefinger of each of your hands, you knock their fists apart. Their confidence in you mounts as they see how strong your mind has made your fingers. Paradoxical, the harder they attempt to hold their fists together the more easily you can knock them apart.

There is nothing to it– you just do it! You will even surprise yourself at how easily you can knock their fists apart by a sweep of your two forefingers in opposite direction.

Should your client challenge you saying that they can do it to you, you make it impossible for them because you have a little secret. As you clamp your clenched fists together, one on top of the other, you secretly grip your left thumb firmly in your right fist. This action, of course, must be done unnoticed by the client. You can do this easily, by keeping your fists in motion a little, as you clamp them together.

With your left thumb so gripped inside your left fist, no amount of finger pushing will separate your hands.

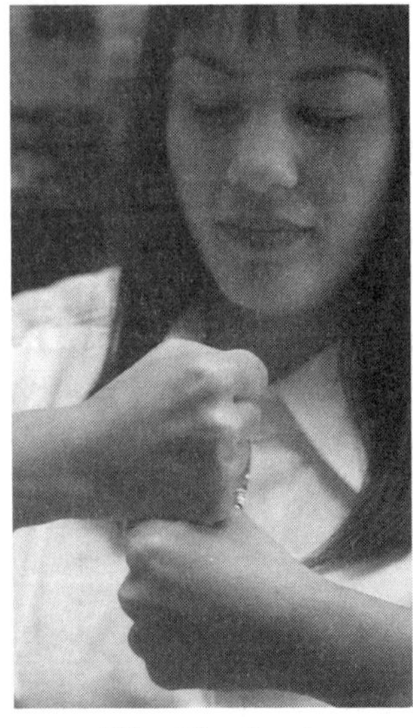

The Fist Lock

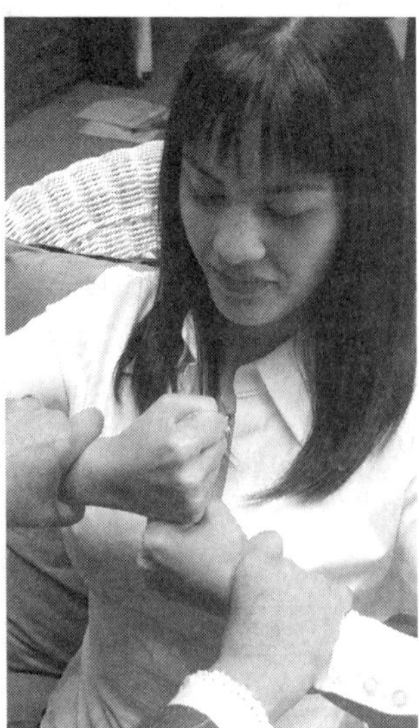

The Fist Lock Pull Apart

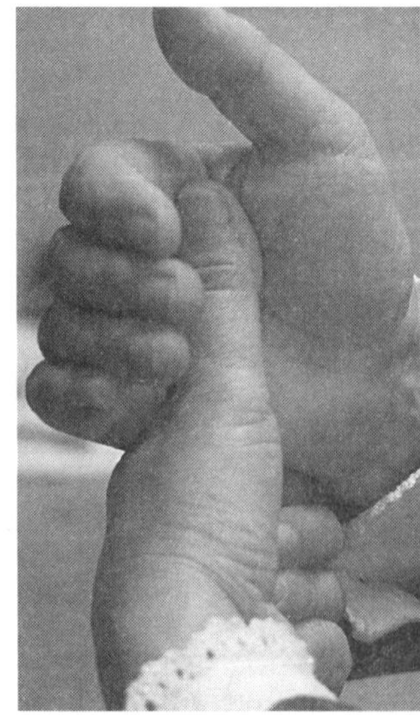

Thumb & Hand

HANDS STUCK TO A STICK EXPERIMENT

You Will Need:
A Stick

Have your client stand before you, make eye contact as you tell them **"In a moment I will have you grip this stick in your outstretched hand and when I count to ten, it will be impossible for you to release your grip on the stick."**

Commence to count slowly: **"One, you are gripping the stick tightly…Two, the stick is becoming stuck to your hands, and you cannot release it…Three, you are concentrating very hard…Four, concentrating on your hands being stuck tightly to the stick…Five, your grip on the stick is becoming tighter and tighter. It is impossible for you to release it…Six, tighter and tighter becomes your grip on the stick…Seven, tighter and tighter ever becomes your grip on the stick. So tight it is impossible for you to release it…Eight, it is impossible for you to release the stick from your hands…Nine, the stick is stuck so tightly to your hands, it is impossible for you to release it try as hard as you will…Ten, try, try hard to throw the stick away from you. It is impossible because the stick is stuck so tightly to your hands!"**

After they have tried in vain to free the stick suggest, **"When I snap my fingers, immediately the stick will be released, and will drop to the floor."**

Snap your fingers. The stick is released and drops to floor. The induction/experiment is complete.

THE ARM RISING EXPERIMENT

Have your client sit in a chair, arms relaxed with hands resting on their knees. Ask, **"May I borrow your arm for a minute?"** If they agree, take one of their arms to a horizontal position and draw your hand slowly and respectfully down the arm from the shoulder to the tops of their fingers. Do this several times. Then place the tip of your third finger on the subject's other hand. Press firmly for a few seconds, and then suggest: **"As I release my pressure you will feel a compelling desire to follow my finger."**

Gradually release the pressure, bring your third finger slowly upwards and away from their hand. As this is done, suggest: **"That's right. Follow my finger. You can feel your hand rising following my finger. That's right, right up. Up, up, up higher still… following my finger all the way up."**

The subject will raise their arm to follow your fingers up as high as you wish it to go. To end the test: **"You have done fine. Relax now, and let you hand drop back to your lap."**

THE FALLING BACKWARD EXPERIMENT

Have your client stand with their feet together, arms at their sides, head erect and bent slightly back. Stand behind them or behind them and the hypnosis chair saying, **"Close your eyes."** Then pass your hand in a backward drawing action gently across the side of the face backwards towards yourself while you suggest:

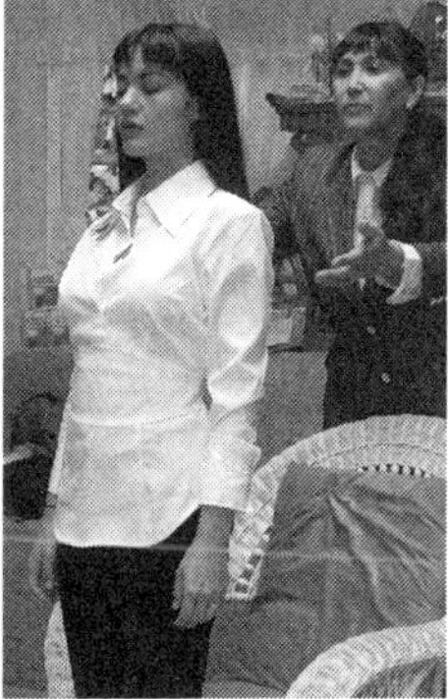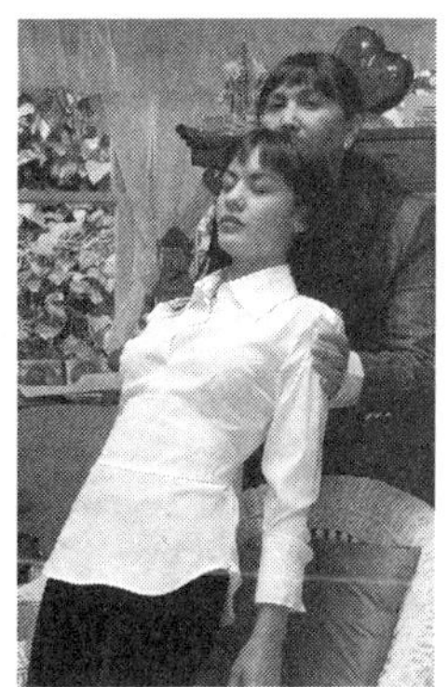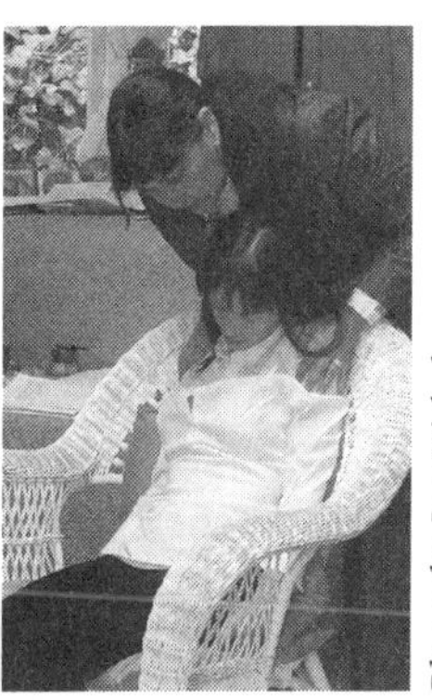

"As I draw my hands across the sides of your face, you will feel a strong sensation pulling you backwards. You will come backwards. Just let yourself go, and I will catch you as you fall. That's it. Let yourself fall and I will catch you. I am directly behind you. That's it…coming back…right back into my arms (or the chair). I am here to help you."

Continue the suggestion of falling backwards until the subject falls back into your arms. Make sure that you are really there to catch them and return them to a standing position.

THE FALLING FORWARD EXPERIMENT

This is similar to the previous subtle induction, but this time you stand in front of subject whose eyes are kept open. Ask them to **"Look intently into my eyes."** Concentrate your gaze at the bridge of your client's nose. Give similar suggestions as you did in the falling backward experiment, **"You will feel a strong sensation pulling you forward…just let yourself go and I will catch you. That's it, coming forward, right here."**

Catch the subject and return them to a standing position.

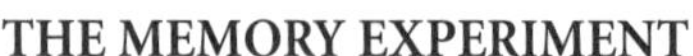

Illustration By Ormond McGill

THE MEMORY EXPERIMENT

Have your seated client gaze into your eyes for a few moments. Then tell them, **"Close your eyes very tightly…we are going to do an exercise that activates your memory. We will begin by temporarily de-activating it. Listen now, as I count slowly from one to ten."**

Count slowly from one to ten.

"Now, you count from one to ten, just as I did. And as you count, the numbers will drop out more and more from you mind, and by the time you reach number ten it will be impossible for you to say that number, as number ten is gone from your memory. It has become completely forgotten. In fact, when you get to number nine, it will come out after a struggle; when you get to ten it will be impossible for you to say ten as you cannot remember it at all. You understand? If you understand nod your head."

Watch for nod of head, it signals a subconscious agreement. Your client indeed will find it a struggle to say number "nine" and number "ten" will not be spoken at all.

If you are using this exercise to enhance memory proceed with this suggestion,

"Now you have learned how easily you can drop something from your mind. It is because you have told yourself it is so. It is just as easy to enhance your memory. So take a deep breath and take back the number ten. In fact you are terrific with numbers. Numbers and other things that you find important to remember are easily memorized and come to you easily whenever you want or need them."

This is a nice transition from waking hypnosis into formal hypnosis. You can continue compounding inductions and induce the client now into a formal hypnotic trance. Practice experiments in Waking Hypnosis so you can perform them well. The more you become master of Waking Hypnosis the better hypnotherapist you will be.

MAKING YOURSELF LIGHT AND HEAVY
You Will Need:
A Third Strong Person Present

This feat immensely builds confidence in one's own powers. It is terrific to use as a demonstration in front of many as you need a third person for more impact.

Hypnotize your client, and directly suggest "I am going to teach you how to make your body light or heavy, under the control of your own mind. Stand up nice and tall with your feet flat on the floor. Think of yourself as becoming light in weight. And as you do we will have someone lift you from the floor."

Then have a strong person grip them around the waist, and lift them from the floor. The lifter will be able to do this easily. Then have client returned to floor and suggest:

"You will go deeper and deeper into hypnosis, as you now stand on the floor."

This first lift at a "light weight" is performed easily and naturally. The strong lifter stays nearby as you continue:

"Now stand up nice and tall again and think of yourself becoming so powerful and solid that you won't budge. This gives you great confidence in yourself, you can now make your body so heavy with your will power that the strong man cannot now lift you from the floor at all."

To effect perfect results, you place your right hand on the wrist of the lifter and the index finger of your left hand upon the side of lifter's neck, and press in.

By pressing simultaneously upon these body points, the strongest man can be defied to make the lift. It works perfectly. Try as the man will, the client has made themself so heavy they can't be lifted from the floor.

"So you see, you have learned how to make yourself light or heavy, at your own mental command."

THE ANTI-GRAVITY BODY LIFT GROUP DEMONSTRATION
You Will Need:
Four Helpers

This is also for a demonstration in front of a group since it requires four helpers. One of the greatest mysteries of "body magic," it has puzzled even scientists. When performed, the hypnotized person sits in a central chair, and instruction given will be performed precisely. The client is told **"This test lets you gain remarkable control over your entire being."**

Tell the four persons to **"Stand around the person seated in this chair. Place your closed fists together with the backs of your hands upward, and extend your two forefingers."**

Instructed one of the four to, **"Place your two extended forefingers under the seated person's left armpit"** and a second person to **"Place your two forefingers under the right armpit."** The third person is told to **"Place your fingers under the left knee"** and the fourth to place his fingers **"under the right knee."**

Tell them **"It is impossible for you to lift the seated person with your fingers only held in this position. Try and see for yourself."** They do not succeed.

You now tell the group, **"Now that you have proven to yourselves how heavy the person actually is and how lifting them on your extended fingers is so very difficult, I will show you how to do it easily. It is a magical way to lose weight, the anti-gravity**

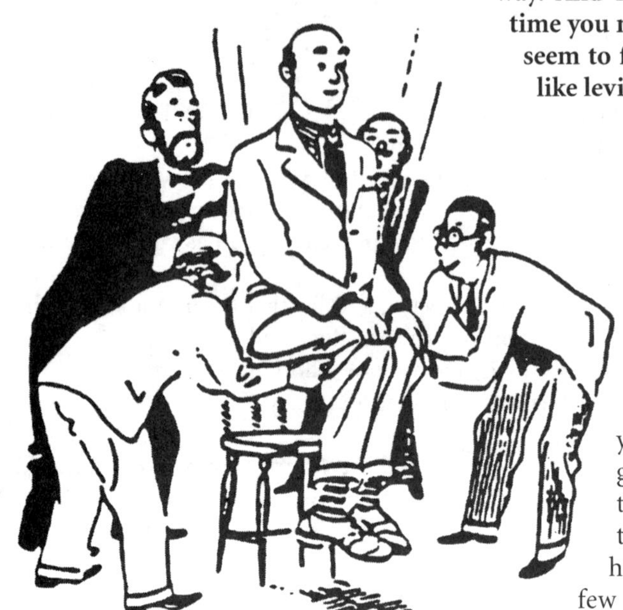

Illustration by Ormond McGill

way. **And following my instructions, the next time you make the lift, the person will literally seem to float up into the air, it almost seems like levitation."**

Taking their respective positions around the seated person, they are told (including the seated person) to **"all take three deep breaths inhaling and exhaling in unison, and on the third breath you are to hold that breath in your lungs, and when you I say, "Go! you make the lift."** All will do as you have instructed, and when you give the command, **"Go!"** they all lift together and up goes the person into the air, light as a feather. They hold him thus surprisingly supported for a few moments, and then return them downward to their seat. The effect is astonishing.

Study now From Waking To Trance in the following chapter.

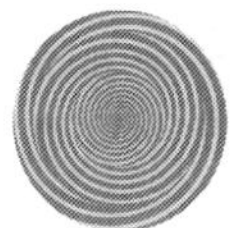

~ *Chapter 25* ~
RAPID INDUCTION TO PROFOUND TRANCE

Includes
Rapid Induction From Wakefulness To Profound Trance
Entering Waking Hypnosis
Moving From Waking Hypnosis Into Profound Hypnosis

The mind works swiftly to bring about hypnosis. Once you have hypnotized your client offer the post hypnotic suggestion, **"When I do _____** (their name) **you will immediately go into hypnosis even deeper than you are now."**

MODUS OPERANDI:
RAPID INDUCTION FROM WAKEFULNESS TO PROFOUND TRANCE

Here is a rapid hypnotic induction to move your client from waking hypnosis to trace.

Start in the waking state. Stand before your seated client and demonstrate the process as you explain how to do it. Tell them, **"Extend your hands and arms in front of you, with your palms facing each other. Next, bend your hands so the palms face you and the tips of your fingers are opposite each other.**

Now, spread your fingers apart and bring your hands together so that the fingers interlock and touch as the base.

Rotate your interlocked hands so that you see the back of your hands, as you raise them above your head.

Finally, stretch your hands upwards as far above as possible. Arms are outstretched with fingers interlocked and palms of your hands turned upwards."

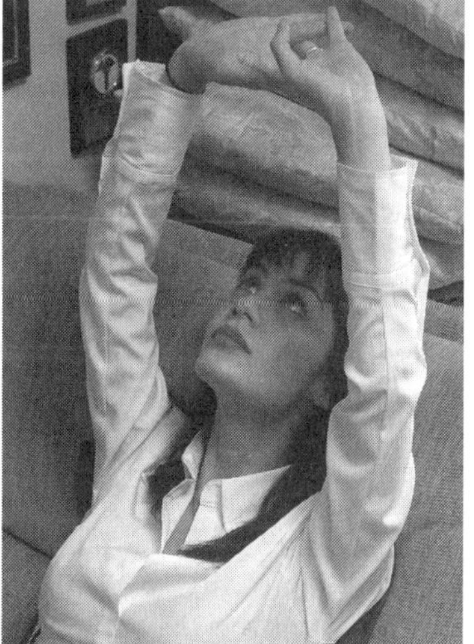

Photo by Jon Nicholas

Push Your Hands Upward

ENTERING WAKING HYPNOSIS:

"Concentrate your attention on your eyes and listen carefully. Keep pushing your hands upwards above your head with fingers interlocked. Your arms are stiffening and your hands are becoming tightly locked together. The muscles of your hands and arms are becoming more and more stiff and your hands are locked together so tightly you cannot unclasp them. They will continue to get more and more tightly locked together.

I am going to count from one to three and, at the count of three, you will find your hands are so tightly locked together that you cannot unlock them no matter how hard you try. One…your hands and arms are getting tight…very tight…so you will not be able to take them apart. Two…your hands and arms are getting stiff…very stiff…so stiff you cannot move them. Three! Your hands are stuck fast. You fingers are locked together. You cannot take your hands apart no matter how hard you try. Try…try hard…but you cannot get your hands apart!"

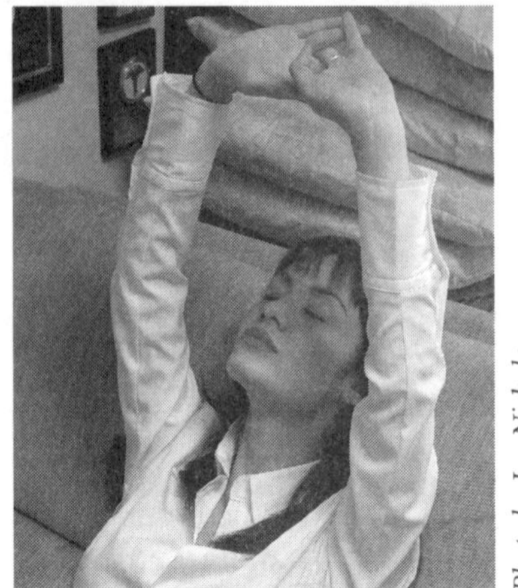

Trance is Induced

The client will try in vain to separate their hands held high above their head. It seems to have become impossible. In this you have bypassed critical mind and have established response to the suggestion in the subconscious. You have induced Waking Hypnosis.

MOVING FROM WAKING HYPNOSIS INTO PROFOUND HYPNOSIS:

Tell your client to **"Close your eyes and think of just letting your mind drift and just go into the realm of sleep."**

Now give these suggestions: **"As I push your locked hands down from above your head to your lap, you will drop down, down right along with your hands into the realm of sleep…into hypnotic sleep. By the time they rest in your lap, you will immediately relax all over and be in trance."**

Slowly push the client's stiff arms downward into their lap, while repeating:

"Down, down you go to sleep in profound hypnosis." Finally, hands rest again in client's lap.

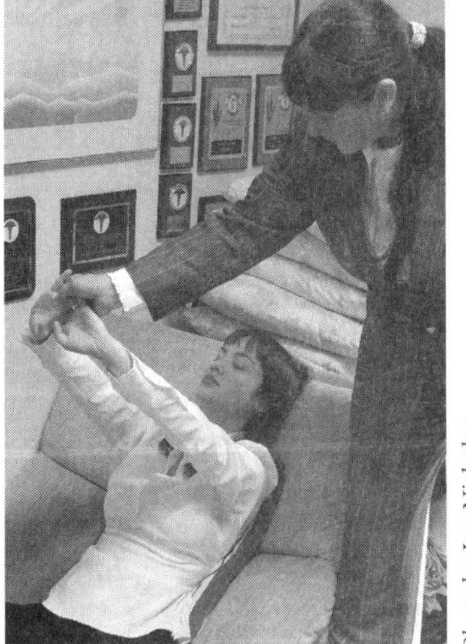

Pushing Hands Down

Suggest: **"Instantly relax now and go to sleep. That's it! Go way down! Go way down deep to sleep! Your head falls forward upon your chest, and you are in Profound Hypnosis."**

The client's head falling forward to their chest indicates trance has been induced and you are ready to proceed with the hypnotherapeutic session. Suggest, **"Subconscious mind open wide your vistas and let these beneficial suggestion I will now give you become reality in your life. You will accomplish to perfection what you have come to me to accomplish."**

Proceed with the session.

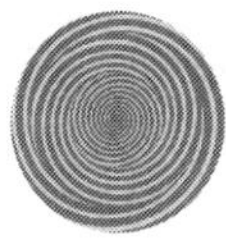

~ *Chapter 26* ~
MORE RAPID INDUCTIONS

Includes
McGill's Concentration/Relaxation Technique Version #1
McGill's Concentration/Relaxation Technique Version #2
Stockwell's 30 Second Zap
Bale's Finger Induction
McGill's Forehead Flick
Kerr's Cockroach On The Bar

Rapid Inductions are ridiculously easy to learn and there are more of them than you or I could possibly imagine. They prove to the subject that they are hypnotized (testing).

MCGILL'S CONCENTRATION/RELAXATION TECHNIQUE VERSION #1

This associates hypnosis with relaxation, concentration and following your instructions. Have your client take a seat. Begin with the statement:

"Many people think that they know how to relax while actually they do not. This self-hypnosis process trains you to easily relax. Let's begin. Raise your left arm to a right angle in front of their chest, then extend your right forefinger and place it under the center of your left palm.

Concentrate on relaxing your left hand and arm entirely so that the only thing supporting them is your extended forefinger. Your left hand and arm are completely relaxed. (Make sure it is). **At the count of three withdraw your forefinger and see what happens."** (If they followed your instructions, the moment the finger is withdrawn, their left hand will fall into their lap.)

If the hand does not drop repeat the instruction again until you get the desired relaxation.

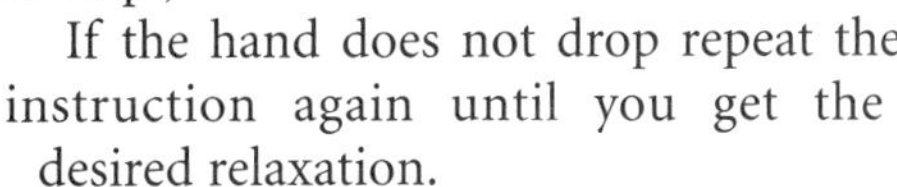

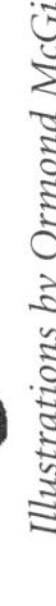

MCGILL'S CONCENTRATION/RELAXATION TECHNIQUE VERSION #2

"There are two necessary things for the trance state: concentration and relaxation. When you learn this you'll be able to do hypnosis for yourself. Concentration. Relaxation. Raise your left hand, elbow bent at a right angle, in front of your chest. Now, extend your forefinger and place it in the center left palm."

Your forefingers get stiffer and stiffer. This is concentration and supports your left hand.

Now, the relaxation…your hand is relaxed and limp as loose rubber bands. The limp hand on top of the rigid forefinger just hangs there, completely supported. Concentration. Relaxation.

Notice how heavy and relaxed your limp hand feels as you concentrate on the opposite being stiff and rigid.

In a moment, at the count of three, very quickly pull your stiff and rigid hand and finger away and your limp hand should easily fall to your lap, your eyes will close and you will go easily into hypnotic sleep…one, two, three, remove your concentration hand and sleep."

If they did not drop their hand say:

"You have mastered one part, concentration, but not relaxation. If you had, your hand would have dropped. Let's try it again…"

STOCKWELL'S 30-SECOND ZAP

Dr. Stockwell's simple, straightforward, and can be done anywhere. Within 30 seconds it brings on a sense of peace and calm. She teaches this as "self-hypnosis" the first day of her Hypnosis Certifications Course or the first time she sees a new client.

"Before we begin look around the room and see how the world looks with your regular perception…very good. Now let's begin.

I'm going to say the word blue three times and with each blue I will give you a different assignment.

The first blue, 'blue,' let your eyes close down. That's right just close your eyes and think of a big blue sky, or a deep blue lake. That's right just let the color blue wash through your body and mind.

Your eyelids are so relaxed they don't feel like opening. Your eyelids are loose and lazy. Your lashes gently kiss your cheeks.

When you've done a good job of relaxing your eyelids, test them and discover that they just don't want to open. The harder you try the less they want to open. They just don't want to open. They are loose, limp and lazy. Stop testing them. And relax.

Two, say the word 'blue' again and this time let the blue wash over your body and take you deeper. Blue as an ocean or a beautiful blue sky. Feel the calm and peacefulness within your mind, accepting this feeling. Give yourself a positive suggestion; something you really desire for yourself. In hypnosis you are the most important teacher. You decide what you want to learn.

If you would like to deepen this trance you can count down from 5 to 1 and go deeper with each breath and each heartbeat. 5-4-3-2-1. All the way down. Here in this deep state of hypnosis you can easily listen to the profound wisdom that lives within you. Stay here as long as you like and when your are ready to return you will count back 1-2-3-4-5; ready to open your eyes and return to room awareness, Say your third blue 'blue' and you'll open your eyes, feeling refreshed and invigorated and come back to room awareness feeling terrific.

Each time you do this process, you go deeper and deeper into hypnosis…very good. And now your third blue, 'blue,' open your eyes."

Have them note the difference in their environment from before they did the Zap and after. Have them notice how everything is a bit brighter and that colors are more vibrant.

BALE'S FINGER INDUCTION

Hypnotherapist Dwight Bale created this ultra fast induction that involves eye fixation, deep breathing, direct suggestion and surprise.

Extend your pointer finger, on which you have painted a red dot, about 18 inches in front of the client's face. The other fingers on your hand are clenched. The client can be sitting standing or lying down.

"Watch the red dot and keep looking at the dot at all times. Inhale whenever I raise my finger and exhale whenever I lower my finger. Keep your eyes on the dot."

Now raise your finger about 9 inches above eye level but still within their range of vision and at the same time say, **"Inhale."** Then quickly say **"Exhale"** and lower your hand to about 9 inches below eye level, but still within their visual range.

Raise your finger slightly faster than a normal inhalation.

"Look at the dot."

Watch to be sure that they are following your finger with their eyes and breath. Breaths will be very deep after three or four passes with a maximum of 6 breath cycles. Get them breathing deeply. When they do, bring on three more inhalations and exhalations and then stop in the upward position, suddenly open your hand, cover their eyes and say, "Sleep!"

Place your index finger in the center of their forehead, cup your hand and place your fingers on the right temple and your thumb on their left temple. The back of their head is either supported by where they rest or by your hand.

Slowly turn their head from side to side in a rolling motion with intermittent and not predictable movements. They learn they must let you do it and they let go.

Next say, **"When I remove my hand, you will go 10 times deeper"** and then quickly and decisively remove your hand and say **"10 times deeper."**

To deepen you could say, **"When I turn off the overhead light and you will go 10 time deeper."** Then turn off the light and say, **"10 times deeper."**

MCGILL'S FOREHEAD FLICK

Put your two thumbs or your fingers side-by-side on your client's third eye (between their eyebrows) and rapidly flick your thumbs or fingers apart saying, **"sleep."**

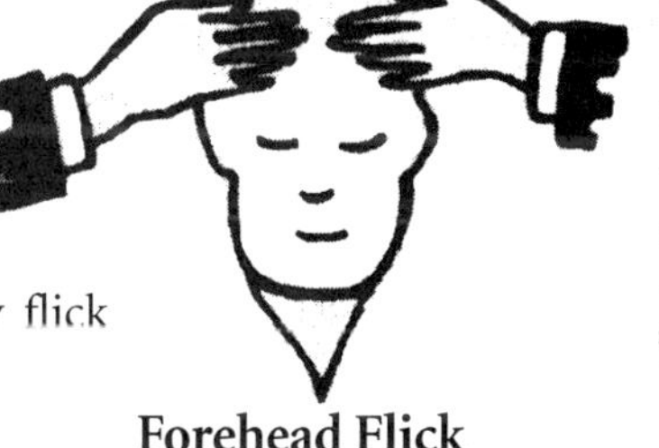

Forehead Flick

KERR'S COCKROACH ON THE BAR

Thanks to Dewey Kerr for this one: **"Place your chin and nose on this surface** (counter or bar) **and follow my hand with your eyes."** Now walk your fingers in front of their eyes saying **"watch the cockroach, he's getting sleepy"** then suddenly collapse your hand on the bar and say **"sleep."**

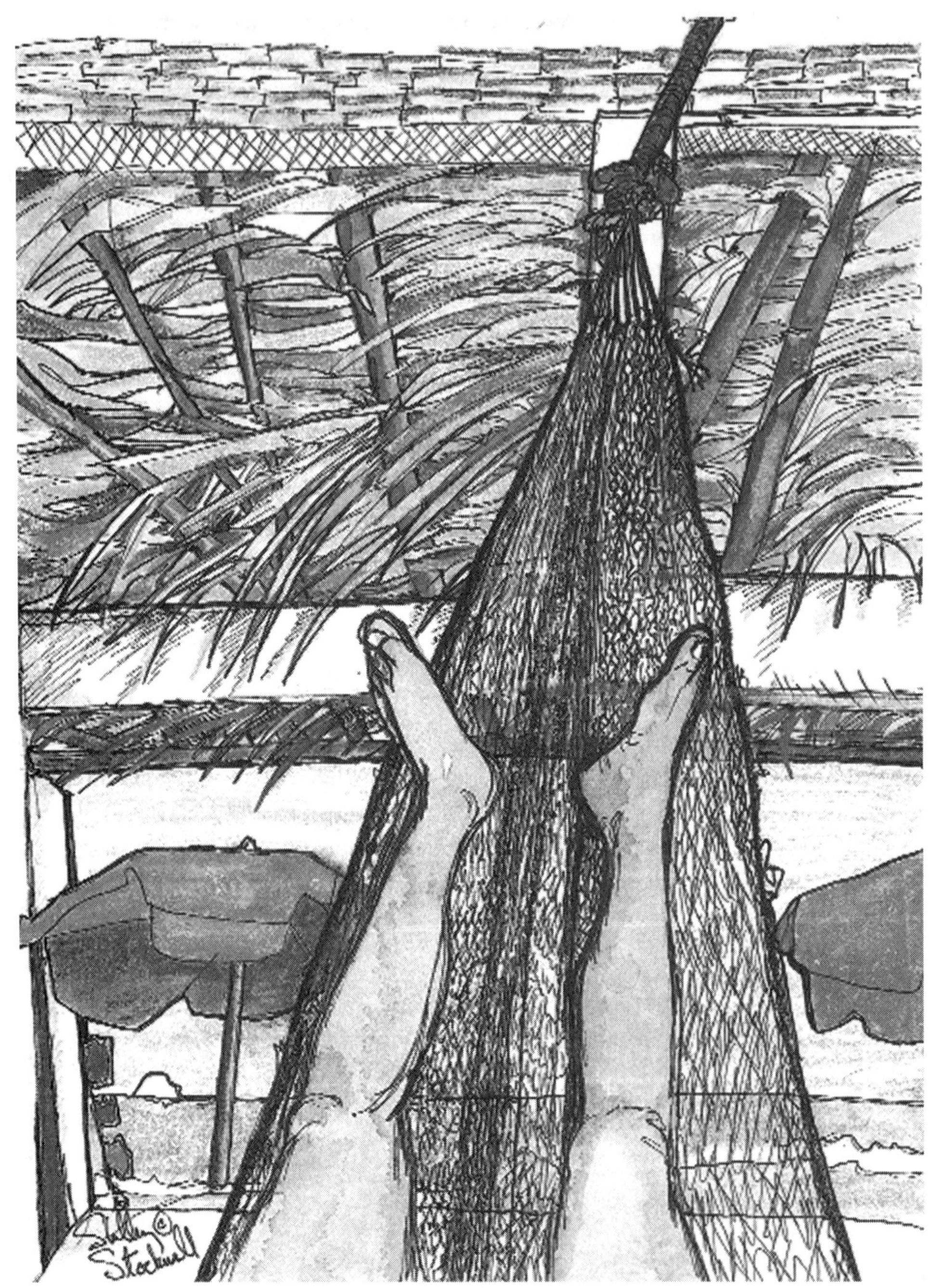

Mazatlan, Mexico

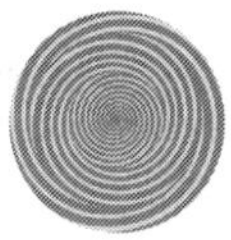

~ *Chapter 27* ~
THE RELAXATION METHOD

This is a very subtle method of hypnotizing. It is so subtle that the client is often unaware that they are hypnotized. It is performed entirely without suggestion of sleep and with only a casual mention of hypnosis. Attention is directed towards physical and mental relaxation, while a somnambulistic level of hypnosis is induced.

Your client's attention is directed toward achieving physical and mental relaxation. It is excellent with those who object to *going to sleep,* which they think means a loss of consciousness.

MODUS OPERANDI: THE RELAXATION METHOD OF HYPNOTIZING

Sit comfortably opposite your client and chat about hypnotism. Remember to communicate, build rapport and receive a go ahead before you proceed. Comment this way:

"I will show you a most pleasant way of relaxing that will make you feel so good! Doctors use this method to relieve tension. Very likely a doctor would define it as 'concentrated relaxation' of mind and body. It will make you relax and feel fine. Would you like to try it?"

Obtain the subject's consent and continue:

"Okay then. Make yourself comfortable and relax. Just relax your hand as I hold it for a moment. (Take their hand in yours and note their response) **Relax your hand so that it is completely loose and limp.** (Subject does as requested) **That's fine. You are doing excellently."**

Take their hand in yours and you can immediately determine their relaxation and how well they are following your suggestions. When you sense that their hand is entirely relaxed, proceed…still holding the hand:

"Now, take a deep, slow breath. Good. Hold it for a moment and now let it out slowly. Very good! Now, once again take a deep breath. Hold it, and let it out. It relaxes you.

Now, let your eyes close and think of relaxing any and all tension from your body.

You are doing just fine and feel better already, don't you? Relax the muscles around your eyes so completely that they feel loose and limp and lazy. When your eye muscles are so relaxed that they just don't want to open, try to make them work and you find that they will not work at all. You cannot open your eyes because your eyes have become so relaxed. Now stop trying and go deeper. You are now obtaining real deep relaxation. You can open and close your eyes at will. But because you are relaxed they just don't want to open."

At this point the subject has bypassed their sense of judgment that consciously would tell them that they can open or close their eyes at will. If your client was to open their eyes, tell them, **"Very good. You have just proven to yourself that you have not completely relaxed your** eye muscles yet. Of course, you can open or not open your eyes as you choose. Hypnosis is a state of mind, not a state of eyelids. So let's concentrate further on the relaxation of those muscles so that they become completely relaxed and will no longer function. All you need to do is pretend that your eyelids just don't want to open and as you concentrate further, your eye muscles become completely relaxed and no longer function." (Have them test their eyes, and if they remain closed proceed):

"Now that your eyes are closed and the muscles of your eyes are completely relaxed, you will find that you can now relax your whole body, much deeper than ever. The relaxation that started in your eyes lets you relax your whole body. You go deeper than you have ever gone before and you feel wonderful. That same feeling of bathes your whole body from your eyes to the very tips of your toes. What a nice feeling to relax like this. You enjoy it.

Now, here is something quite interesting. When I ask you to gently open and close your eyes you will find that you do it easily and it you relax more than ever. In fact, you will be ten times more relaxed than you are right now. All the muscles of your body completely relaxing only your eyes will open and close gently when I tell you to.

All right? One, two, three…open your eyes gently…now close them… and relax ten times as much as you were before. Notice what a wonderful surge of relaxation this brings over you. Now, when you do that again, just double your relaxation this time, and you will feel like you have a blanket of relaxation covering you from head to toes.

Ready again…one…two…three…now open your eyes and now close them, and become so much more relaxed than you were a moment ago Feel that blanket of relaxation covering you from head to toe."

You are still holding the subject's hand in yours and you continue:

"When I release your hand, it will drop like a limp rag doll into your lap, as you completely relax."

Release the hand and let it fall into their lap. You are now ready to deepen hypnosis by suggesting:

"You have learned to physically relax, and now you will learn to relax mentally as well. As you do, you will feel a hundred times better than you do right now. Here's how to do it: in a moment you will start counting backward, beginning with the number one hundred. With each number you will double your mental relaxation. By the time you get to number ninety-seven, the numbers will have been relaxed right off your mind. They'll simply fade out and disappear, and you won't be able to find any more numbers. Now, relax deeply, say that first number, double your relaxation, and notice what happens. All right begin by saying out loud, 'one hundred'" (Do not tell them that they can *not remember* numbers. Say that they cannot *find any more numbers.*)

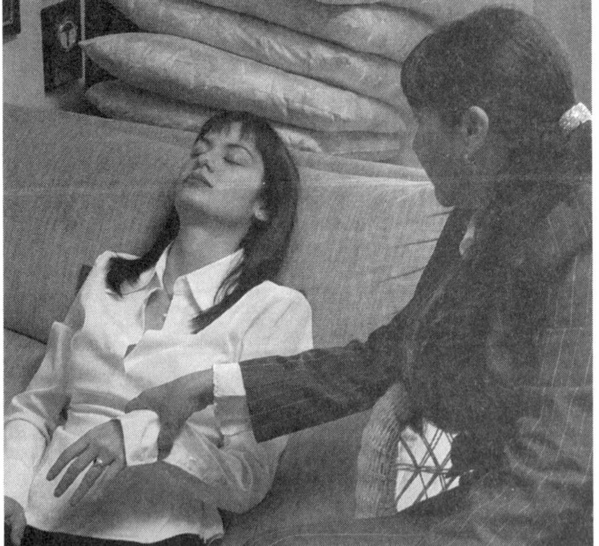

Relaxation Method

Client says, "one hundred."

"That's fine! Now double your relaxation as the numbers begin to fade away. Say the second number now."

Client says, "ninety-nine."

"They'll soon be gone. You won't see any more numbers in your mind. They just fade away and are all gone. That's fine. Now relax more with each breath and notice how relaxed and wonderful you feel. Your mind as well as your body is now relaxed."

If they continue to count backwards, stop them with the suggestion: **"That's fine. Relax between the numbers and let them stop all together. Relaxation makes them disappear. As I pick up your hand and drop it, the numbers drop away at the same time."** (Pick up their hand and drop it in their lap.).

"The numbers are gone. They've dropped right out of your mind. You can't find any more numbers. The numbers are gone and your mind and your body completely relax."

The subject will be in deep hypnosis and commenced amnesia with the "lost numbers." Then continue, **"You are now so completely physically and mentally relaxed, that you easily take on the beneficial suggestions I give you and you remember all numbers completely and fully. Your memory is excellent.**

The suggestions I give are seeds, which I will plant in the garden of your mind and they will grow into flowers of well-being. Your subconscious mind is now wide open and receives and acts upon suggestions of health, well-being and perfection. Relax and receive."

Proceed by giving your beneficial suggestions.

Illustration by Ormond McGill

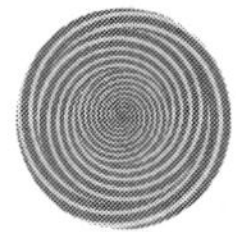

~ *Chapter 28* ~
WILLIAM JAMES:
LET'S PRETEND

"Imagination is the beginning of creation. You imagine what you desire. You desire what you imagine, and, at last, you create what you will."
　　　—George Bernard Shaw

"Thought is everything. You'll see it when you believe it."
　　　—Dr. Wayne Dyer

Psychology was not taught in American Universities before William James began to teach the subject in 1875. James, himself, had never taken a course in psychology because there was none to take. He once jested, "The first lecture in psychology I ever heard was the first I ever gave." James is the founding father of psychology and an educator most everyone admired.

Like Einstein, he was always open to the mysterious. How did Einstein put it? "Out of the mysterious we discover the undiscovered." Mysterious. Suppose you were to tell Einstein that something isn't so. What would he do? He would probably smile and say, "Is that so?"

James was more interested in a study of human inner space. Albert was more interested in outer space and would go out on a still and silent night and gaze up at the stars, and shout, "God it is all so wonderful!"

William James gets the credit for creating the ideas behind "Let's Pretend Hypnotherapy." He looked upon it as a form of conscious play-acting psychotherapy. The term "Hypnotherapy" did not come along until much later, when we learned to motivate the playacting instead of playing it as a conscious role.

Kindergarten children deserve credit too. For who can pretend better than kindergarten children? Their world is filled with fantasy: Peter Pan and Wendy, fairies, goblins, super heroes and sheroes and things that go bump in the night. We all pretend so well before our imagination is impaired by being told over and over that it isn't so.

Via "Let's Pretend Psychology" you can change behavior. Formerly negative ways can be transformed into the positive behavior you desire. In other words, you act out the positive and this role-playing brings mental imagining into a physical performance and becomes your truth.

Childish?

Goodness, gracious. Imagining brings you to what are you in your heart. Imagining and performing a desired behavior via deliberate actuated physical performance makes it a reality no matter your age.

William James "acting out psychotherapy" approach proved very helpful for many people. Here's how James applied his process.

MODUS OPERANDI: JAMES- LET'S PRETEND APPROACH

Let's say a client came into the office with a desire to overcome stage fright and lack of confidence so that they could give a speech. James would first ask,

"Think for a moment and truthfully ask yourself if you would really like to stand before a group of people, or, do you think you would really feel more comfortable keeping quiet and remaining in the background?"

If, after thinking it over carefully, the person might say that he was actually happier in being quiet in the background. Then James would say, **"For heaven's sake, don't learn to do something that makes you uncomfortable when you are comfortable just as you are. We usually behave best in ways that makes us feel contented with ourselves."** This was expert psychological counseling for many who then went on their way. But, suppose the client asserted: "Yes, I definitely want to get over my feelings of stage fright and feel confident in myself when I address an audience."

Then James would say,

"Very good. Then let's pretend you are doing exactly that. Stand before that mirror and let's pretend you are standing on stage addressing an audience. Who do you see in the mirror? You see only yourself and certainly you are not afraid to address yourself. Most people talk to themselves a good part of the time, as you know. Imagine that self you see in the mirror is your audience. You have nothing to be afraid of, you are just pretending as there is no stage, no audience, just you and me in this room together, and I don't even count, for I am not even visible to you. All you can see is yourself in the mirror. If you have a special speech you plan to give to the group, repeat it here and now while pretending just as you are."

Then James had the client give their speech before his or her image in the mirror. It was a rehearsal of the speech to oneself while pretending that oneself is the audience.

The method worked. The client went from his office preconditioned to feel free of stage fright, and filled with confidence to face an actual audience. James used the method often.

Whatever the negative condition, James would have the client pretend to be master of the problem by actually performing (acting out) the positive of the negative. The very act brought into physical reality that which is imagined in the mind. Imagination has moved from the negative form of behavior to the exact opposite– reversing the behavior patterns.

Imaging the desired behavior through an actual performance of the pretended preferred behavior produces a "mental set" of the desired behavior.

Professor James said, "Whistling to keep up courage" is not a mere figure of speech.

On the other hand, if you "sit all day in a moping posture, sigh, and respond to everything in a dismal tone of voice, your melancholy lingers. To conquer undesirable tendencies, we must assiduously and, in the first instance, cold-bloodily go through the outward movements of those contrary dispositions, which we wish to cultivate. Smooth the brow, brighten the eye, contract the back rather than the front of the body, and speak in a positive tone, pass genial compliments and your heart must indeed be frigid if it does not gradually thaw."

And further, "Can you fancy the state of rage without a picture of a sudden violent outpouring of emotion in the chest, the flushing in the face, the dilation of the nostrils, the clenching of the teeth, the impulse to vigorous action. Imagine a state of rage with limp muscles, calm breathing, and a peaceful face in their stead."

There is sound psychology behind "acting a part" in connection with visualizing. See oneself as acting-out the part, as going through the motions, as expressing in outward form the desired personal quality. Visualize first one desired characteristic, and then another… until all have been acted out in your mental vision. Further, whenever you think of yourself in connection with anything associated with or related to the characteristic in question, think of and visualize yourself possessing and manifesting that characteristic.

Get into a mode of thinking and seeing oneself manifesting in physical reality that inner state. In this way, you will establish a psychic path over which one can freely travel when it goes outward into action.

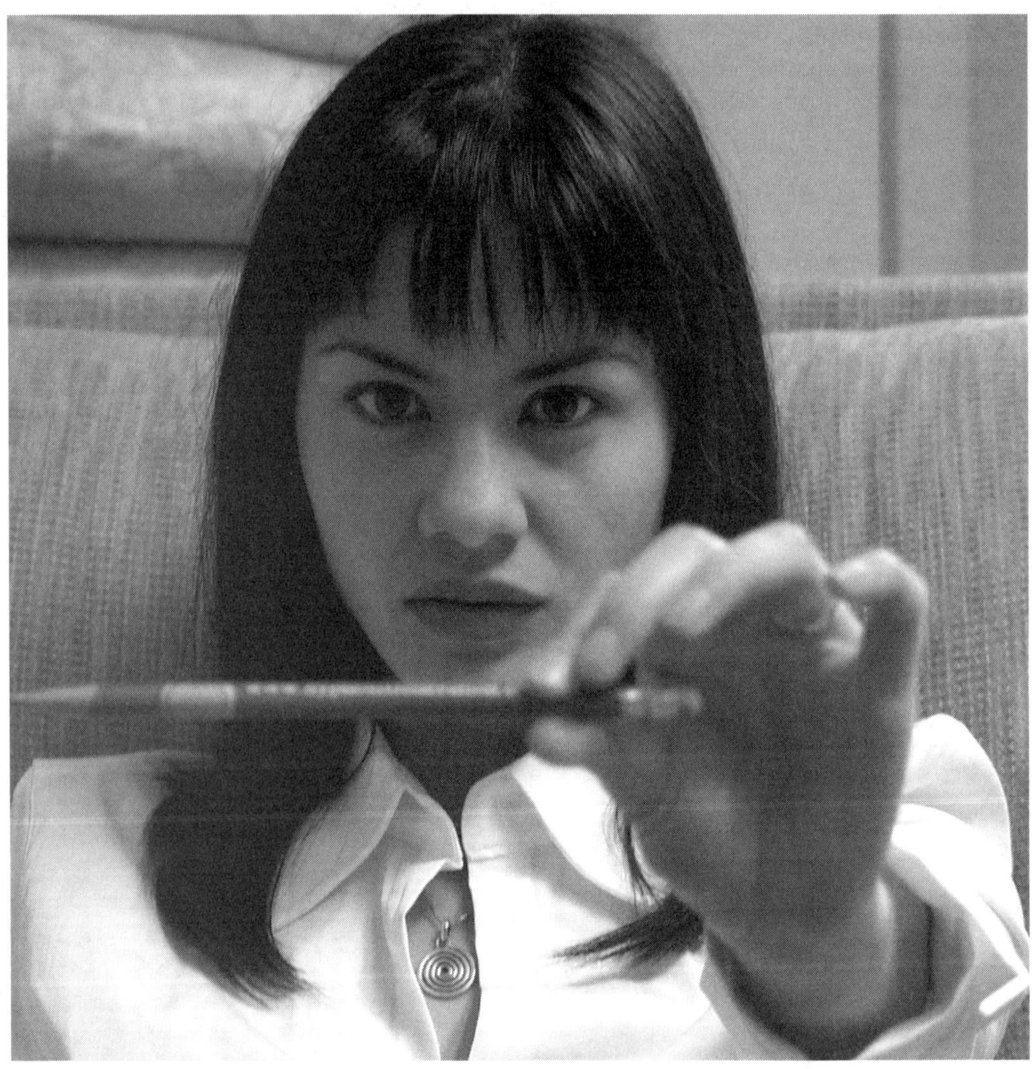

Pretend Pencil Drop

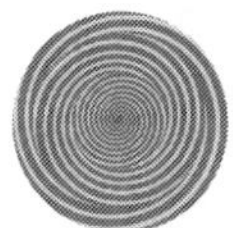

~ *Chapter 29* ~
I CAN, I CAN'T RAPID INDUCTIONS

Includes
I Can't, I Can Pencil Drop 1
I Can't, I Can Pencil Drop 2

How would you like a rapid induction method using the Let's Pretend approach? With it, you can hypnotize your subject while they stand or sit.

MODUS OPERANDI: I CAN'T, I CAN PENCIL DROP 1

Hand your client a pencil to hold. Tell them, **"grip it tightly and pretend that you cannot release it from your hand no matter how hard you try. While you are pretending that you cannot drop the pencil, try to drop it."** They can fling and flip their hand anyway they please to try and drop the pencil, but it is impossible for to do so while they are pretending that they cannot. Tell the person repeatedly to **"Try, try, try to drop the pencil, while pretending you cannot!"**

This provides a very objective means of determining the client's state of mind. It the pencil drops, it indicates that their critical mind is still in operation. In such an instance, a slower method might be used with that person. If on the other hand the suggestion "holds." it indicates that the client is responding subjectively to suggestions and that this method worked perfectly. This simple procedure causes mental confusion amenable to suggestion and the client is ready to move on to the next induction.

"Now allow will power to come in that says you can, while still pretending you cannot." An inner conflict can develop that causes some discomfort, as will and imagination have a struggle, but imagination wins out over will every time.

Proceed:
You state, **"Cease the conflict now. Close your eyes and pretend that you are drifting down into the realm of sleep where all is peaceful and serene. No longer do you need to pretend…for you are relaxed snug and cozy in every way…and at peace with all that is. And, as this deep relaxation enters you, the pencil drops from your fingers and your hands fall into your lap, and with the dropping you drop deep into profound hypnosis where everything you pretend to be becomes actualized as reality.**
This very moment now in space and time test this inner power of concentrated mind over your body for yourself. Extend your right arm straight out in front of yourself now. Make it stiff and rigid. Pretend that it has become so stiff and rigid that you cannot bend it at all, try as hard as you will. Try. Try. Try hard…but you cannot bend it at all. What you

pretend has become actualize as your reality. And so it will remain until I say it will relax and drop into your lap…and as it drops you will drop with it deep in hypnosis.

You are freed from pretending that your arm is stiff and rigid and that you cannot bend it…your arm becomes relaxed, and now drops down into your lap and you drop with it into profound hypnosis."

Profound hypnosis, very possible your client's conscious mind has not the slightest idea where that is or even what it is. But the subconscious knows. Your client/patient has entered a hyper suggestible state of mind where critical mind is bypassed and selective thinking is readily established in the subconscious. Advance now into somnambulism.

The entire process is accomplished inside of five minutes, and profound hypnosis has been established.

You could now take the pencil from them and stroke their eyes downward closing them and say, **"Now that your eyes a closed, shut them tightly and pretend you cannot open them. Your eye muscles have become so relaxed they cannot open your eyelids. Test them and see and you will find you cannot open your eyes now, try as hard as you will."**

A transference from pretending to actuality has occurred in these few minutes.

Continue suggestion; **"Now let that relaxation from your eyes flow down over your entire body and it makes your entire body relax all over."**

MODUS OPERANDI: I CAN'T, I CAN PENCIL DROP 2

It can take less than three-minutes to use from start to completion when you use this induction:

Give the subject a pencil to hold between thumb and forefinger, of either hand. Tell them: **"Grip this pencil firmly between your thumb and forefinger and pretend that you cannot drop it from your fingers, no matter how hard you try. While you pretend that you cannot drop the pencil, try to drop it."**

This causes a conflict in the mind between critical consciousness that says "Of course I can drop it while I pretend I cannot drop it." Trying to drop it is objective; pretending "cannot drop" is subjective. In other words, it is will power versus imagination. This causes a mental confusion amenable to suggestion.

If they have not dropped the pencil, take it from them and stroke your hand downward motioning them to close their eyes. Tell them, **"Now that your eyes are closed, shut them tight, and pretend you cannot open them. Your eyes will not open because your eye muscles have become so relaxed they cannot open the eyelids. Test and see, and you will find you cannot open your eyes now, try as hard as you will. Now, let that relaxation from your eyes flow down over your entire body, and it makes your entire body relax all over."**

Proceed on to deepening relaxation in the body: **"Having relaxed the body…now we are going to equally relax the mind."**

You are in the realm of waking hypnosis and ready to plunge the subject into hypnotic somnambulism. Proceed on relaxing the mind. Forgetting numbers is an effective way. **"You will count from 1-10 and the number four will fall off your mind. You just can't find it. Try as hard as you like and the number four is just gone."**

When they respond to this suggestion, you have produced amnesia, which is characteristic of somnambulism. A few deepening suggestions and your subject will be in somnambulistic state; profoundly hypnotized. This rapid form of induction can easily stay with a three minute time frame from start to completion.

Use this state and all beneficial suggestions will be readily accepted and implanted (non-beneficial suggestions tend to be rejected) into the client's subconscious.

Consciousness can be considered as parallel streams flowing along, side by side. You can jump your awareness from stream to stream, as each is complete in itself. Let mind jump from stream to stream to stream in an upward progression, and reach for the knowing of super consciousness (Cosmic Consciousness)– which is somehow an instinctive knowing of what it is all about.

Play that game. It's fun, and often can turn up some darn clever ideas.

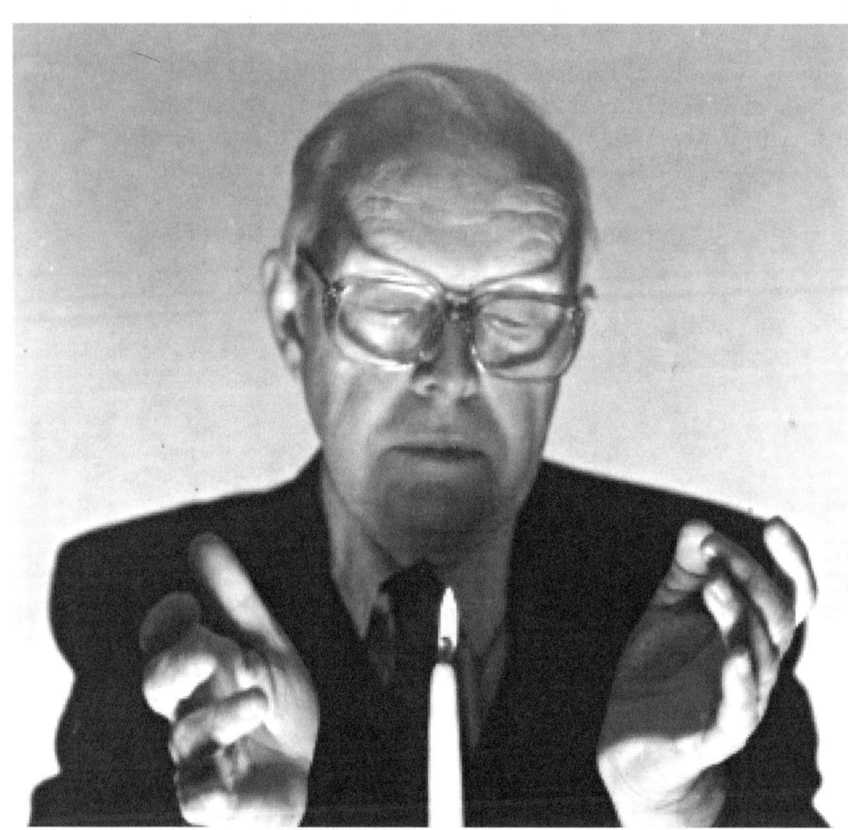

Ormond with Candle

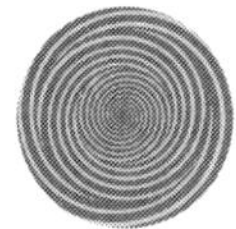

~ *Chapter 30* ~
LET'S PRETEND SOME MORE

Includes
The Four Stages Of Let's Pretend
Let's Pretend Candle Induction
Let's Pretend You're Not Pretending Induction
Let's Pretend You Sleep Soundly
Let's Pretend You Hate Smoking

"If you think you can or you can't, you're correct."
　　　　　—Henry Ford

Everything you create in the world starts in imagination and pretending is the start of imagination. Imagination is the creative function of the mind. Mental creativity transforms into physical creativity. If you pretend and firmly believe and imagine that you are destined for success, it will be so, in direct ratio to the power of your belief…believe it or not.

Conversely, if you are convinced that you will fail, failure will stalk you no matter where you go. The universe is like a great echo chamber. Sooner or later, what you send out, comes back. Let's Pretend Hypnosis is important to successful hypnotherapy. It can lead to miracles of mental healing.

1.　**Critical Mind = Conscious Mind Decides What You Want To Pretend**
2.　**Imagining Kicks In**
3.　**Selective Thinking = Directs Pretend Suggestions To Enter Into The Subconscious**

Think of pretending as the starter of the car and imagination as the motor. You press the starter and it starts the engine and then the car is ready to run…anywhere you wish to drive it. Prahna and, if available, the technology of the Serenity Resonance Sound provide the gasoline.

Any suggestion, which enters the subconscious phase of mind, must come through the conscious phase of mind. All "Let's Pretend" suggestions originate in conscious thought.

Consciously pretending bypasses critical mind in a very subtle (almost sneaky) manner. Because to pretend, you have to first consciously decide what it is you wish to pretend. Having made that decision, you quickly advance to "Let's Pretend"– which is subconscious in operation. Let's Pretend is imagination in action, which moves on to become created into the reality of behavior. Pretending is a subjective phenomenon.

"Let's Pretend Hypnosis" combines Dave Elman with William James' approaches. It is very effective in working with children. They quickly, almost spontaneously, move into deep hypnosis and somnambulism…No deepening techniques need be applied to young minds.

Let's Pretend Inductions

Pretending is a terrific induction for everyone, especially those who are (consciously or subconsciously) resistant to being hypnotized. With the "Let's Pretend" technique there is no resistance. After all, the person feels that they are just pretending.

An image is defined as a "mental representation of an actual object." The stronger the image, the more it approximates the actual object, the more it will materialize into "reality." The remarkable thing about the image is that it is capable of producing the same response as the actual object. For example:

"Imagine your hand submerged in a bucket of ice water" causes you to feel the chill creep up your arm. Imagining holding your hand over fire can produce a rise in temperature in the hand. A classic experiment in hypnosis suggests to the subject that a hot iron is being placed on the bare body, and a blister will form, on that spot. The implications are vast. If you believe something strongly enough it becomes real to you. And if you believe it you will conceive it.

The Four Stages Of Let's Pretend

Handle "Let's Pretend Hypnotherapy," in four stages:

1. Consult with your client and find out what their conscious mind has to say. You'll hear what the conscious mind has brought into the subconscious via pretending. And you'll learn what they have decided desirable and no longer desirable to pretend.

2. Hypnotize your client using the "Let's Pretend Hypnotizing Method" It is easy to use and effective for both client and by hypnotherapist.

3. Reverse the "Let's Pretend" of what is now unwanted into a "Let's Pretend" of what is wanted.

4. Arouse client pleasantly from hypnosis back to the here and now.
    Let's Pretend Hypnotherapy is complete.

MODUS OPERANDI: LET'S PRETEND CANDLE INDUCTION

You Will Need:
A Comfortable Chair
A Table
A Lighted Candle

This induction is terrific for those who want to achieve profound hypnosis.

Have your client take a seat in a comfortable chair, relax, and stare into the flame of a candle on a table placed in front of them. Suggest:

"Keep staring, staring, staring deep into the candle flame, and pretend you are becoming as one with the flame. Allow it to grip your entire attention.

Now I will count from one to three and at the count of three take a deep breath and hold it in your lungs. One…two… three…inhale…hold the breath. Now exhale slowly. And as you exhale, pretend that it is making you relaxed all over and very sleepy. And all this while you are staring, staring, staring and are pretending to become one with the candle flame.

Now, again, at the count of three, take another deep breath and hold it in your lungs. One…two…three…inhale…hold the breath.

Now exhale slowly, and as you exhale this time, pretend that your eyes are becoming heavy, and you want to close them and go to sleep. But don't close them yet, just keep staring, staring, staring and continue pretending that you are becoming one with the candle flame.

Now, just one time more, at the count of three you can close your tired, heavy eyes and relax all over, and pretend you are dropping way down into a deep, deep sleep. Ready, One…two…three…inhale…hold the breath. Now exhale slowly, and as you exhale close your eyes and relax all over, and pretend you are dropping down, down, down asleep.

Sleep…deeply sleep. Pretend that you are relaxed all over, and that the muscles of your eyes are so relaxed you cannot make them work to open your eyes try as hard as you will. (Client tests their eyes and finds it so.)

Now pretend the relaxation from your eyes is flowing down over your entire body, and you are becoming relaxed all over, and in this wonderful relaxation, pretend that you are going fast asleep. You are asleep in deep dreamless healthful sleep. Pretending takes you there. (Hypnosis has become client's state of mind.)

You are beyond the realm of pretending now, and everything that you pretend becomes an actuality in your mind and body. Anything that you pretend becomes actuality. Pretending is your reality. Your critical mind is fast asleep while your subconscious mind is wide awake ready to create whatever is suggested to it to become transformed into reality."

The "Let's Pretend Hypnotizing" process is complete and whatever is suggested for the subject/client/patient to pretend becomes automatically transformed into reality in their mind and body.

How Does It Work?

Tell someone merely to "pretend being hypnotized." While they pretend that you are hypnotizing them profound hypnosis is often achieved. Pretending removes the effort from hypnosis. Too much conscious effort to achieve hypnosis makes it difficult for mind to achieve hypnosis. It is like going to sleep, if you make great effort to go to sleep (knowing that you must go to sleep) you will not go to sleep; as the effort to go to sleep keeps you wide awake. Sleep is achieved best by drifting into it effortlessly. The only way to go to sleep is not to try to go to sleep, but just go to sleep. It is the same with going into hypnosis. If you try hard to be hypnotized you will not achieve hypnosis. Only by allowing oneself to drift into hypnosis effortlessly can it easily be accomplished. Let's Pretend provides the easy path.

LET'S PRETEND YOU'RE NOT PRETENDING INDUCTION

Dr. Alan Eastman, the Founder of the Canadian Board of Hypnotherapy says it this way:

"Pretend that you are hypnotized. Good. Then pretend that you aren't pretending…"

LET'S PRETEND YOU SLEEP SOUNDLY

Suppose the habit the client has developed is insomnia. Somehow their critical mind has brought in a "let's pretend you can't sleep" to the person, the result of which is insomnia. How do you correct this? Just reverse the pretend. Open mind to selective thinking and suggest:

"Let's Pretend that the moment you go to bed from this time on, you will immediately drop off into perfect sleep…and enjoy wonderful sleep all night long…and you will awaken in the morning refreshed and eager to face the new day with a bounce in your step and a sparkle in your eyes."

Let's pretend that you can use this same direct approach to correct everything that has been established in the mind. Seems almost too simple to be possible? Try it and see. It is a shortcut way to perform hypnotherapy. After all, how long does it take your computer on your busy desk to operate on a command? Your personal computer, inside your head, is a far greater computer than is the one upon your desk.

It is the classic principle of making effort without effort that produces mastery. Can you conceive of a great musician presenting a virtuoso performance by making great effort to play his instrument? If there is effort in doing, the performing is not true artistry. Artistry is only obtained when the effort to do what is done is effortless in being done. Using hypnosis is artistry.

The venerable Hindu Sage, Patanjali (128 B.C.), offers these words of wisdom:
"If you would achieve artistic success in any endeavor, make the effort to achieve the endeavor without effort to achieve the endeavor."

Great art in any field is created effortlessly. Pretending hypnotherapy is the way to achieve profound hypnosis without effort for either client or hypnotherapist.

Hypnosis is an induced state of mind in which critical mind is bypassed and selected thinking is established in non-critical (subconscious) mind. Here ideas are accepted and acted upon uncritically. This was a principle the famous Hypnotherapist Dave Elman taught to his doctor students.

Critical mind is limiting to the individual while non-critical mind is ever expansive. That is to say, your critical phase of mind allows you to do what you think you can do…your non-critical phase of mind allows you to do what you feel you can do…and your real capacities are far beyond what you think they are into your vast reservoir of subconscious wonderland.

Critical mind can be doubtful of what you can achieve. It can even imprison you. Use Pretend Hypnotherapy as a non-critical shortcut that directs the subconscious beyond doubt to marvelous freedom.

The subconscious has little selective power as to what is best for the individual, and behavior patterns, both wanted and unwanted, can become established in the subconscious seemingly on their own and manifest both psychologically and psychosomatically. Negative conditioning such as phobias and bad habits may be accepted when you are not even aware, until conditioning manifests as a seemingly spontaneous occurrence. The job of the hypnotherapist then becomes the task of seeking out basic causes of unwanted behavior and establishing, that which is wanted.

MODUS OPERANDI: LET'S PRETEND YOU HATE SMOKING

Living is survival. At its roots, the subconscious is directed for your survival, and to bring you the most pleasure. However, since it is nonselective, if your critical mind presents harmful ideas, they can be imprinted and hurt you. To understand, consider smoking versus not smoking: Let's say, conscious mind has found that smoking brings pleasure, and so a habit of smoking is established. The subconscious accepts the "Let's Pretend" of pleasure for smoking, and that's the habit.

When a person shows the good sense to want to break the habit, a hypnotherapist can be a direct help. How is the best way to correct an unwanted habit? You guessed it: Let's Pretend Hypnosis!

Pretending originated the habit and reversing it with Let's Pretend then removes it.

Put your client in a trance and suggest,
"Let's pretend that you hate smoking now. It is vile to you. Pretend that you will never smoke again."

Nothing more is needed. Let's Pretend Hypnotherapy is a shortcut hypnotherapy. Too simple you say? Complex really, but on the surface it seems simple. You break the smoking habit almost instantly when you reverse the Let's Pretend.

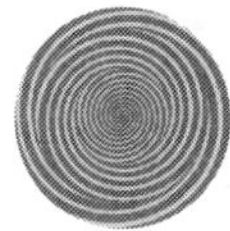

~ Chapter 31 ~

ACTING-OUT HYPNOSIS FOR THE "I CAN'T BE HYPNOTIZED"

Acting Out Hypnosis is similar to the "Let's Pretend Hypnosis." It gifts a "show me" client who comes for help and then RESISTS by saying, "I CAN'T BE HYPNOTIZED." Resistance to hypnosis is often an ego-matter. Some like to feel that they are in conscious control of everything they do. Of course, they are not, but they like to feel that way. Critical mind says, "I can't be hypnotized."

Agree with them and then simply have them "act out" the role of being hypnotized without being hypnotized. This bypasses the critical mind and selective thinking is established in the subconscious so results are accomplished. This is a subtle method, and the mind is tricked in doing exactly opposite from what it is told consciously to do. It is the same thing that happens when you tell a client "do not go to sleep" and they doze off.

MODUS OPERANDI: ACTING OUT HYPNOSIS
You Will Need:
A Reclining Chair (if available)
Cushioned Earphones Connected To A Microphone

In your client consultation, clearly establish their goal: what they want. Then agree with them if they say they can't be hypnotized.

Use a recliner if you have one. Big-cushion earphones connected with a microphone are to be worn by the client so that the hypnotherapist speaks in a microphone directly into ears of the client.

Begin with a verbal Hypnotherapist/Client agreement:

"Since you can't be hypnotized, there is little point in using hypnosis to solve your problem. To use hypnosis, the person has to allow themself to enter a passive state of mind, which is highly subjective. Since you cannot be hypnotized, it's obvious that you want to remain alert and conscious at all times. So, today, we'll use a technique where you act out the hypnotic state. When acting out something, a person is fully alert and conscious of the role they play. You understand this.

While you cannot be hypnotized, you can play act a role and pretend to be hypnotized. Doing this causes you to be more alert and more conscious than ever. It is the opposite to being hypnotized. Is it agreeable for you to deliberately act out the role of being hypnotized without being hypnotized, so that I can help you with what you want to accomplish? Is it agreeable?"

Get the client's agreement.

"Okay, let's begin. Sit comfortably in this recliner. There is no need to relax or anything; just be alert and fully conscious of everything. Above all do not go to sleep. Put on these earphones, which will give you a feeling of privacy, and I will coach you on your acting role. You will be alert and conscious all the time, which is just the opposite of being hypnotized."

Client dons the earphones and reclines in the recliner. Present these instructions in a WHISPERING voice to the client, via the microphone-to-earphones.

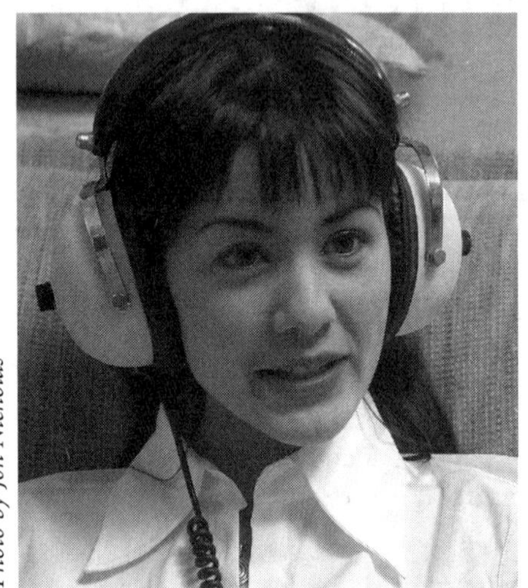

Photo by Jon Nicholas

Headphones Awake

"Okay, just rest comfortably without trying especially to relax. Remain fully alert and conscious at all times. Remember, you are not to go to sleep. Let's now start acting out the role of being hypnotized. Be alert and conscious at all times, of the role of being hypnotized that you are playing.

Recline back and close your eyes and become conscious of your breathing. Take a deep breath…hold the breath…then exhale the breath. That's right. As you do this, become fully conscious of the breath going into your nostrils, into your lungs, and on down deep inside yourself. Continue this deep breathing, and as you do so, become fully conscious of your breathing."

Allow the client some moments to himself or herself to act out this role of being conscious of deep breathing.

"You may find that being conscious of your deep breathing makes you kind of sleepy. In this role that you are playing, do not go to sleep.

Now, continue playing the role of being hypnotized. You are doing a great job of acting out the role. THINK of how every breath is causing you to become more and more relaxed and is sending you down into hypnosis. Continue right on acting out the role of being hypnotized. It is lots of fun playing this acting role. Enjoy every moment.

Now comes the real test of your acting the role of being hypnotized. The part you are playing calls for you to take sixty-nine rapid breaths – in and out – as the consecutive numbers are called. I will call the numbers, so all you have to do with each number is breathe rapidly in and out. I will allow you a moment between each number called, during which time think to yourself the word, sleep. THINK sleep in anyway you please. Just enjoy the experience. All ready to start this acting role? Ready, set, GO!

One…take a rapid breath in and out. Relax a moment. Think, "sleep" to yourself.

Two…do the same again.

Three…Do the same again. Do the same with each number I count, thus from one to sixty-nine.

Four…I will keep right on counting on to sixty-nine. Somewhere along the line of counting, it may be that you lose track of the counting, and will act out the role of being hypnotized."

Continue counting in the same rhythm – number by number on to sixty-nine, allowing a pause between each number while the client thinks of sleep. Having reached the sixty-ninth breath, very likely you will find your client has dozed away into hypnosis, but make no comment about it. Just continue right on:

"You have done a great job of acting while breathing in the role of being hypnotized. Now, let's continue playing the role of being hypnotized in relation to solving the problem (whatever has been requested in the advance consultation) **you came here to solve. Act out your part in solving the problem, as I give your subconscious these beneficial suggestions…"**

Present whatever suggestions are needed to solve and correct the problem. When you've done so, let the suggestions sink in. Then directly ask the subconscious to arouse the client when what is desired has been accomplished. As the client arouses, comment…

"You did a great job in acting the role of being hypnotized. Without the need of being hypnotized, you mastered what you came here for. You go on your way now, well and fine."

The session is thus concluded.

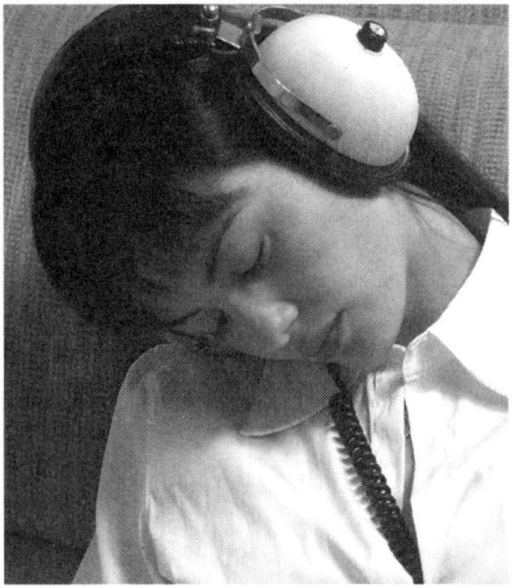

Headphones Asleep

Photo by Jon Nicholas

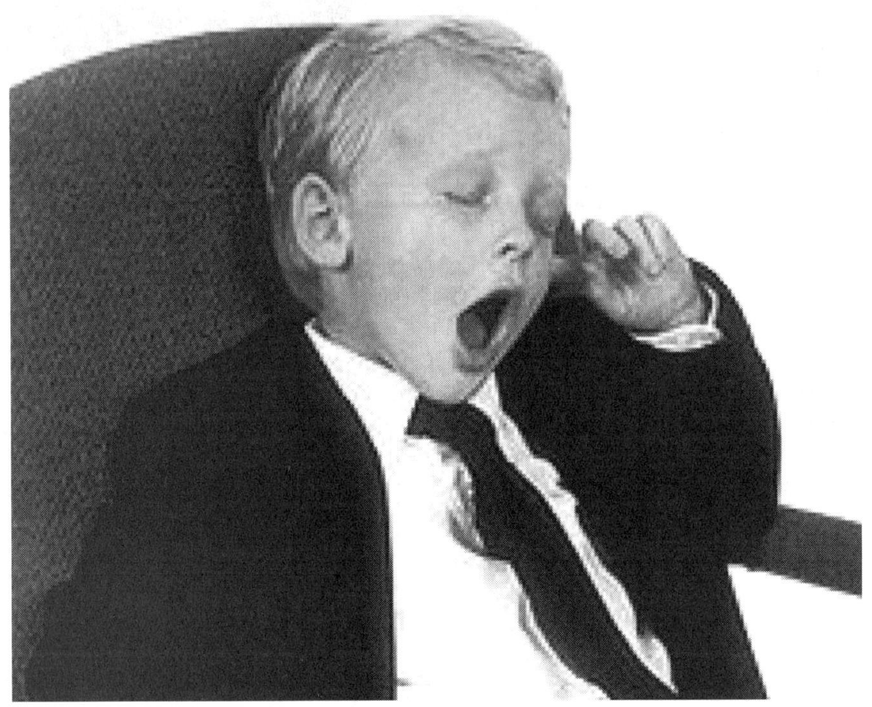

Think about yawning.

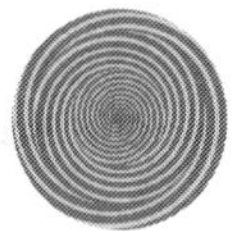

~ *Chapter 32* ~
THE IDEOMOTOR INDUCTION

William James is credited with discovering ideomotor (idea/motor) action. This principle says that the thought of physical action automatically produces a subjective physical response. The ideomotor response is terrific for fact-finding and a virtually automatic method of inducing hypnosis.

The "key" to success is to give your client an action to think about. This conscious thought affects the body's unconscious muscular action and brings about hypnosis. The state of hypnosis it brings about is related to sleep, and sleep is psychosomatic (mental and physical).

Perform this method in eleven deliberate steps. Each step gives the client something to think about. All thoughts are of comfort, relaxation and the pleasantness of preparing to sleep. This leads them from voluntary action to involuntary action and hypnosis. The act of preparing to "go to sleep" spontaneously releases muscular tensions in the body so sleep occurs. It is a circling method, commencing with mind affecting body and body, in turn, affecting mind.

Ideomotor hypnosis is easy to use. All you do is tell the client what to think about and the hypnosis occurs on its own.

MODUS OPERANDI: THE IDEOMOTOR INDUCTION
You Will Need:
A Comfortable Chair
A Pendulum (weight attached to the end of a string…given to the client to hold, during the course of the induction.)

Have your client sit in chair and stand before them. Time your instructions to afford client full opportunity to think of the physical processes to which their body is responding. Allow each step to occur prior to the next step being presented.

Have them follow these eleven sequential steps. Begin with this instruction:
"Relax and follow the instructions I will present. It is simple, just think about what I tell to think about."

Step 1 "Comfort"
Ideomotor action starts in this first direction.
"Think of how comfortable your body is as it relaxes in the chair." (Give them time to think about it).

Step 2 "Yawn"
"Think about yawning and now yawn." (Deliberately yawn right along with the client. Yawning sets the body in the direction of becoming relaxed and sleepy.)
"Good. Now rest a minute and yawn again."
"Think of another yawn. Yawn. Complete the yawn. (Pause)
"Good. Now think of another yawn. Yawn. Complete the yawn."

Step 3 "Pendulum"
Hand the pendulum to client. **"Hold this pendulum, dangling from your fingers with your arm outstretched before you. Center your eyes upon it and think of it swinging."** (Ideomotor action starts the swinging.)

Step 4 "Tired Eyes"
As the client watches the swinging pendulum, instruct: **"Think of how tired this makes your eyes. Close your eyes when they become tired. Think of how tired the swinging pendulum is making your eyes. This ideomotor reaction causes your eye muscles to become tired, and soon your eyes close."**

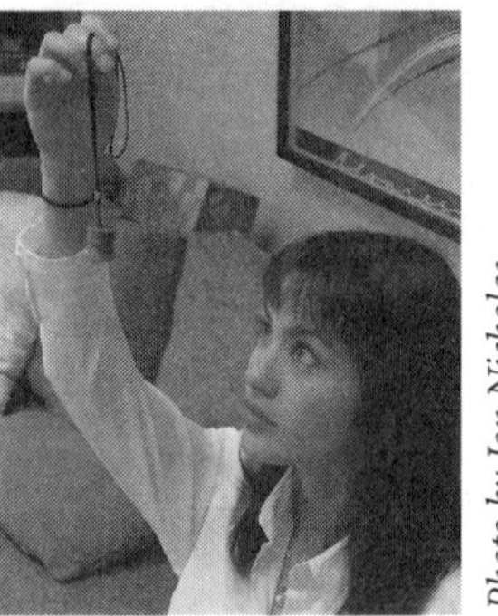

Pendulum

Step 5 "Tired Arm"
"Think of how increasingly heavy your arm is becoming. It is getting so tired you can no longer hold it up, and that it is dropping into your lap. When it drops into your lap, you'll think of going to sleep." Thinking of "going to sleep" starts the mind/body ideomotor action in that direction.

Step 6 "Dropping Arm"
"When your arm hits your lap, think of your hand relaxing and the pendulum dropping from your fingers to the floor." Ideomotor action causes the pendulum to be released from his fingers.

Step 7 "Relaxing to Sleep"
As the pendulum drops to the floor, **"Think of your whole body being as relaxed as your hand. Think that you are slumping down in the comfortable chair and going to sleep."** Ideomotor action produces the effects.

Step 8 "Breathing Fully"
"As you think of going to sleep, your breathing becomes full and regular." Ideomotor action causes the response. Watch the client's breathing deepen.

Step 9 "Breathing Relaxed"
"Think of your breathing slowing down to the breathing rhythm you have while sleeping." Body knows this rhythm and the action occurs as an ideomotor response. **"You think of how your 'sleep rhythm' of breathing is causing you to go to sleep in hypnosis, Every breath you take causes you to go deeper and deeper into the realm of sleep…deeper and deeper into hypnosis."**

Step 10 "Slip Into Hypnosis"
"Think of yourself slipping down into deep hypnosis." Ideomotor action produces sleep– in this instance hypnotic sleep, as that is the basic "mental set" to which the client is responding.

Step 11 "Be in Hypnosis"
"Think, 'I am in hypnosis.'" The subconscious mind in now receptive to put the beneficial suggestions that will be given into bodily action.

This productive induction renders the client receptive to whatever therapeutic suggestions you want them to manifest as behavior.

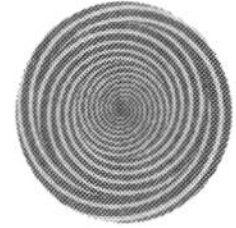

~ *Chapter 33* ~
THE SANDY BEACH INDUCTION
From the audio tape by Ormond McGill

This hypnotic journey into relaxation is so refreshing that clients request it time and time again.

MODUS OPERANDI: SANDY BEACH INDUCTION
You Will Need:
A Quiet Space (where you can dim the lights)
A Couch or Recliner
A CD player
CD with Ocean Wave Sounds

GETTING READY FOR THE JOURNEY
Use your private office or any quiet room in which you can dim the lights. Have a couch or recliner in the room for client to relax upon. The client enters into the room, sits down and leans back. You take a seat beside them, so you can whisper the Hypnotic Induction into their ear.

Have a cassette or CD with sounds of Ocean Waves and Rolling Surf to play in the background behind your voice as you take the client on a journey along the sandy beach.

Have dim lights in your hypnosis room as the journey begins.

Give your initial instructions to the reclining client in a soft singsong voice. Let your voice rise and fall in a drifty dreamy lulling manner. Sit by client's side, whispering into an ear. Often, by the time you are ready to start, the client will have already been lulled into a state of reverie. Now, commence the journey into hypnosis.

"Close your eyes, relax outstretched, and breathe deeply and freely. Allow your mind to drift and merge pleasantly into the background sounds of the ocean surf."

While they pleasantly relax, explain, **"This hypnotic experience will use your imagination while you are sinking down into a wonderfully deep level of relaxation. The experience will be so pleasant and refreshing you will want to return to this place and time over and over. We are going to take an enchanting journey walking along a sandy beach together close by the in-and-out flowing surf. Let your imagination take flight and picture in your mind a warm sandy beach down in the tropics.**

Now, let your imagination go a step further, and imagine that YOU are that sandy beach, stretched out at full length along the seashore with the warm sun shining down on you.

And there are seabirds soaring lazily overhead...and the ocean waves are rolling in and out... in and out... in and out covering you and uncovering you..."

Sound of ocean waves for some seconds. Then continue…

"Now, imagine that these ocean waves are great waves of relaxation, and, as these waves of relaxation billow onto the warm sandy beach you feel that relaxation flowing over your body from the top of your head all the way down to the tips of your toes, because you are that sandy beach."

Ocean sound.

"Now, take a deep breath Ahhh as the tide goes out. And as you exhale Ahhh a great wave breaks and rolls over the sandy beach, carrying relaxation to it farthest limits."

Ocean sound.

"Now, inhale Ahhh as the tide recedes, mobilizing its water for the next inward rush; and, as you exhale Ahhh feel the healing relaxation wash over your entire body, bringing in rest… bringing in peace."

Ocean sound.

"Now, take another deep breath Ahhh as the waters drain outward, and again as you exhale Ahhh bringing refreshing energy into you body and serenity to you mind. All is beautiful, peaceful, and serene, and you feel happy and good all over."

Ocean sound.

"Now, take another deep breath Ahhh as the waters drain outward, and again as you exhale Ahhh feel the waves of relaxation roll over the sandy beach which is YOU. Absorb this freshness into your BEING completely."

Ocean sound.

"It is high tide, so for a short space of time the sandy beach will remain under the ocean waters…this warm blanket of waters, which protects, soothes, and refreshes the little sandy beach.

How peaceful and calm you feel all over, all covered over with the warm waters of relaxation. A sense of languor steals over you. Your mind is still. Your mind is at rest.

Now, think of the sandy beach as the conscious aspect of your mind, which has become completely submerged under the warm healing waters, and the sandy knoll in the center of the beach is your subconscious, which has emerged and is now ready with its fertile uncritical soil to receive all beneficial suggestions which will lovingly be given you to become part of your life.

While drifting and dreaming let these wonderful suggestions enter deeply into you subconscious and become your very own."

Insert your desired clinical hypnotic session here.

Finally, arousal your client from hypnosis slowly against background of ocean waves and "You awaken from hypnosis now to the sound of the rolling surf, happy awakening, feeling wonderful and fine."

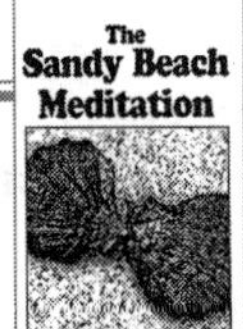

Hypno-Helper

"The Sandy Beach Meditation" by Ormond McGill on audio cassette is available on line at www.hypnosisfederation.com or from the order form at the back of this book.

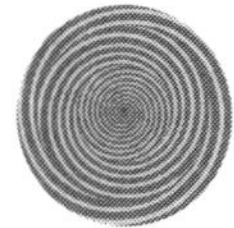

~ *Chapter 34* ~
SERENITY (Symbiotical) RESONANCE SOUND

By Shelley Stockwell-Nicholas and Ormond McGill

Includes
How To Make Digital Hypnotic Audio tapes And CD's

Everything can be equated with vibration or frequency, colors, sounds, matter and humans. Each cell radiates its own significant sound and reacts to environmental sounds. Rhythm, timber, pitch, breath make for each of us a pattern, which resonates as brain wave patterns.

Sound to influence mind has been used forever. For example, Handle's "Hallelujah Chorus" arouses passion for many. You certainly have observed how music can change your moods and emotions. Actually, it is not the music that moves you; it is, at its roots, the vibrational matrix that resonates and harmonizes with your inner matrix that results in e-motion (energy in motion). Nada Brahma is what the Hindus call a constant state of sound vibration or the "fundamental reality of sound."

Gabriel Blow Your Horn

Ancient Egypt, China and Japan used sacred instruments to receive spirit.

Babylonians blew the royal trumpet, the Tibetans, the shofar or rams horn. In the South Pacific it was the conch shell. Bells, drums and the beating and tapping of percussion instruments all advance subconscious acceptance. That is why they are used in religious and spiritual practices. The subconscious mind automatically comes forward when aroused by loud vibration. In rapid hypnosis inductions the sharp command of "sleep" produces instant trance. Ever wonder why TV commercials are on high volume?

Chanting, singing, mantras, prayers, ritualistic songs, Gregorian chants, OM, and the Tibetan "O OH AH EH EH E" all expand consciousness. Hawaiian's rhythmic tones saying "Let myself come down upon me like a mist." Legend says that the locals on Molokai stood on the shore singing it at the top of their lungs and successfully warded off invading Tahitians.

THE SERENITY RESONANCE SOUND
Theta/Delta Frequencies= The Hypnotic State

Hypnotism has advanced from the occult, to psychology and now to technology. The SERENITY RESONANCE SOUND is the hypnotherapy breakthrough of today's Technological Age. Thoughts come best when the mind is relaxed. Hypnosis and the sound easily relax the mind.

Brain wave patterns of theta and delta produce the subjective state of mind we call "hypnosis."

Ormond McGill, computer expert Joseph Worrell and sound technician Rolf Wyler created the serenity sound by artfully blending and repeating the computer-calibrated alpha to theta/delta range vibrations. They named it the "Serenity Resonance Sound." It is terrific for all mental activity where concentration and relaxation are of value. Use it for yourself and you'll understand.

HUMAN BRAIN FREQUENCY LEVELS (How frequent the vibration is called "frequency")

BRAIN CYCLES/SECOND		STATE	CHARACTERISTICS
GAMMA	40-60 HZ	Stimulated beta-endorphins & anxiety	High level processing,
BETA	39-14 HZ	Wide Awake	Alerted outer evaluation
ALPHA	13– 8 HZ	Relaxing	Tranquil More Serotonin
THETA	7– 4 HZ	Resonance Reverie Tones	Inspiration, Intuition
DELTA	3– .5 HZ	Resonance Sleeping Tones opiates, pituitary releases growth hormones	Renewal, endogenous

---

Some nickname the Serenity Resonance Sound the "miracle sound" because it aids relaxation in every situation. We have found this CD is an effective background at work, home or play to enhance studying, romance, meditation, sound sleep and reduce stress and pain and of course hypnotherapy.

When used in hypnotherapy it has proven effective for:

1. Relaxation
2. Induction
2. Opening And Stimulating The Subconscious For Heightened Suggestibility
3. Condensing The Time Needed For Suggestions Formulas
4. Relaxing And Inspired The Hypnotherapist
5. Rapport Building

HOW TO USE THE SERENITY RESONANCE SOUND

The Serenity Resonance Sound is an excellent background for all the hypnotherapy methods in this book. Its raw energy has no purpose in itself. Its value comes when directed with purposeful thoughts. Played softly, its oscillating beat becomes a drone-like sound mist pleasantly lulling the mind into a state of relaxed reverie; enhancing each process.

When your client concentrates attention on the "meeting point" of the sound, the sound drops away and they will scarcely be aware of any sound at all. Then you do your subconscious training.

Meditative music and Serenity Resonance Sound can be used together. We recorded two such versions; *Hypno-Music* which is overlays a soothing, melodic music and *Entrancing Music* which adds lilting piano and the human heartbeat.

DIGITAL SUGGESTIONS

Words have, through long usage, been used in communication (conscious mind) and become conditioned in us to convey feelings (subconscious mind). Examples are everywhere. Say "love" and you feel a warmth of closeness. "Joy,""happiness," "good," and "gladness" make you feel good. Say "hate" and you feel anger and danger. Words like "fear," "awful," "ghastly," "terrible" make you feel bad. All words convey emotional feelings some more than others and some are more or less neutral.

There are thousands of words. A hypnotherapist has to be choosy of the words they use or they can cause trouble. Words become conditioned in the mind and subconsciously effect behavior. Pavlov's experiments in conditioned behavior of dogs showed the principle. One bell was rung and the dog was given dinner. Another was rung and the dog was given a shock. The experiment brought on neurosis in the dogs. They did not know whether the immediate bell stood for steak or a hot-foot.

And there is more:

The dogs did not understand that the bells were only sounds; empty symbols with the event. A bell is neither dinner nor an electric shock. A bell is only noise. But you can't tell that to the dog. They were not sophisticated dogs and consequently could not make an intellectual evaluation of mere sounds. That shouldn't happen to an intelligent person.

It does though...

Dr. David Pink says, "Words are triggers to action." Words are to people what Pavlov's bells were to his experimental dogs. Habit patterns spring into action at the stimulus of a word. Habits may be compared with electric appliances like a light bulb, washing machine, radio, television, or VCR. The word is the switch that starts any of these appliances into use. You have energy within you to do all kinds of things. The right word releases this energy and directs it into appropriate channels. Many clients come to the hypnotherapist using the wrong words, which muddle them up, confuse and cause interbrain misbehavior and the jitters. The use of the right words (suggestions) can get the client back on track. The proper use of words (semantics) is vital to successful hypnotherapy.

Words carry power. Words trigger action. Similar to a pistol, pull the trigger and the gun goes off. Something is shot forth that could cause joy or even cause death. The right words spoken in the right can change a world.

Hypnosis is a state of mind, which is hyper suggestibility so the responsibility of good hypnotic word usage is obvious. Suggestion formulas are combinations of words designed with great care to benefit the client.

The power of words moves in two directions, the physiological and psychological. On the surface words convey feelings, which are psychological. But at their roots words are vibration or physiological. Every spoken word and sentence is a series of special frequencies of vibration.

Thus far our coverage has focused upon the psychological. So now lets consider the physiological element of words. Digital suggestions combine these formulas with vibrational frequencies to amplify the power of words.

What does that mean...

It means that through technology you can more powerfully influence suggestion. But enough theorizing...let's get down to the nitty-gritty to teach you how to produce Digital Hypnotic Suggestions that combine mental, physical and the Serenity Resonance Sound.

MODUS OPERANDI: HOW TO MAKE DIGITAL HYPNOTIC AUDIO TAPES AND CD'S
You Will Need:
Recording Equipment
Oscilloscope
Computer
The Serenity Resonance Sound
Whatever Helpful Script You Choose

There are thousands of hypnotic tapes on the market. Their manufacture and sale has become an important part of hypnosis. Work with any hypnotic tape you please; it makes no difference, as long as the message it conveys is helpful. Words greatly influence the thoughts we think and any recording is of real value if well psychologically designed.

But, such recordings only scratch the surface of the power of words, as they do not take advantage of physiological power. Combining the psychological with the physiological takes us into the hypnotherapy of the Twenty-First Century. The Serenity Resonance Sound amplifies hypnotic induction and combined with "digital suggestions" greatly increases the power of suggestion. Digital hypnotic suggestions concentrate on the specifically targeted frequencies of words and language.

Here is how to make a masterful digital tape:

1. As you record your words speak simultaneously into an oscilloscope. This will make one track as spoken word and another track capturing the underlying vibrations. You will see the words appear on the screen of the oscilloscope and both recordings will be perfectly synchronized. They have to be for they are a part of each other.

2. The computer transforms these visual vibrational images to sound vibrations. Technology!

3. Now bring in the Serenity Resonance Sound as a soft background behind both your words and vibrational sound and record them together in stereo so that the verbalized words go into the left ear and the vibrational sound plays to the right ear of headphones. They mix within the brain.

There you have it. The hypnotic power of such suggestions offer!

In time, yet another device will combine SRS and DGS forever increasing power for hypnotic suggestions. A device of such nature is being developed here in Silicon Valley in the same laboratory where we created the Serenity Resonance Sound. It will provide quantum advancements in suggestion formula recordings.

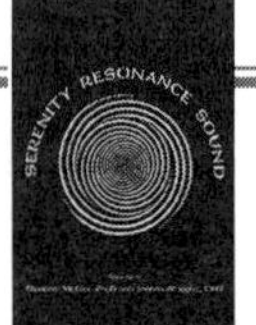

Hypno-Helper
"The Serenity Resonance Sound" by Ormond McGill and Joseph Worrell entrains the mind into receptivity of trance and suggestion and can be used as ambient sound for all you do.

"Hypno-Music" overlays soothing, melodic music with "The Serenity Resonance Sound" "Entrancing Music" adds lilting piano and the human heartbeat to the "Serenity Resonance Sound."

Both are available on cassette and CD at www.hypnosisfederation.com or from the order form at the back of this book.

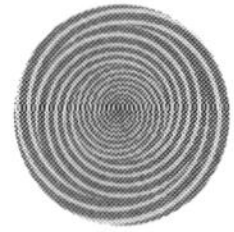

~ *Chapter 35* ~
MAGNETIC MIND TONING

Includes
Magnetic Mind Toning
Five Main Functions Of Mind

MODUS OPERANDI: MAGNETIC MIND TONING
You Will Need:
Serenity Resonance Sound
Echo Effect (if available)
Soft Music

This process lets your client create right action and master thoughts. It uses the Serenity Resonance Sound most effectively. I used this script for the Magnetic Mind Toning audio cassette:

Music In: (Voice over music with strong echo effect if available.)
"Relax and listen… listen… listen…
This is the process for toning your mind. Toning your mind will make you Master of Your Mind. Becoming Master of Your Mind makes you a MASTERMIND."

(Echo effect fades out… music remains behind the voice.)
"You can tone your mind wherever you are or however you are. You can lie down or sit comfortably in a chair. It makes no difference. Just position yourself so you are at ease… listen and follow these instructions.
Now, close your eyes and let your mind drift. Become silent inside yourself and absorb yourself in the SERENITY RESONANCE SOUND, which will now be given you. Just relax, listen, and become as one with the sound. That's all you have to do. Relax and listen… listen… listen…"

(The Serenity Resonance Sound comes in softly at first, then gradually rises. The music can continue along with the sound.)
"Listen and become as one with the sound. It drifts your mind pleasantly into the Theta and Delta state of subconscious reverie. Just relax, listen and go deep into the sound."

(The Serenity Resonance Sound rises up to loud volume for five minutes. Then softly again behind voice.)
"Now, lift your hands high up into the air, pointing towards the ceiling. Now, take a deep breath and repeat this affirmation out loud: *'I bring the cosmic force from out of the void into myself.'*

Wait a moment and you will experience it. Experience THE FORCE entering your hands as electric-like tingles.

Repeat it again. Take a deep breath and affirm out loud, 'I bring the cosmic force from out of the void into myself.' Feel THE FORCE come in even stronger now.

Now, one more time, take a deep breath and affirm, 'I bring the cosmic force from out of the void into myself.' You will sense it coming in stronger than ever now. Feel it. Experience it. Lower your hands to rest in your lap or by your sides. Relax... relax... relax and experience THE FORCE continuing to buzz in your resting hands."

(The Serenity Resonance Sound goes softer and music goes up more.)

"Now, place your hands over your ears and press in gently and affirm out loud to yourself: *'I am obtaining a peaceful mind. I am friendly towards the successful. I am compassionate but not miserable towards the miserable. I appreciate the virtuous.'*

In reverie, let these affirmations for a peaceful mind sink deep into your subconscious. Let these wonderful affirmations sink deeply into your subconscious.

Now, again, repeat these affirmations for obtaining a peaceful mind: *'I am friendly towards the successful. I am compassionate towards the miserable. I am compassionate towards the virtuous.'*

Now, rest quietly and let your hands drop down from your ears and rest while the Theta and Delta sound sets them into your subconscious mind.

Again, place hands over ears and affirm out loud, "I am obtaining control over my mind, as I affirm these truths for myself. They become reality. *'I make my mind think what I want it to think. I make my mind stop thinking when I do not want it to think. I am a witness to my thoughts and I view my thoughts passing before me as though I were viewing a movie upon a screen. I am gaining perfect control of my mind. I am master of my mind. I am becoming mastermind.'*"

(Go silent for a few moments while The Serenity Resonance Sound rises up and then fades behind voice. Repeat above affirmations two more times.)

"Relax... relax... relax and let this CONTROL OF YOUR MIND become your reality.

Lower your hands over your ears and rest knowing you have gained control over your mind. You are now going to gain KNOWING of the five main functions of your mind."

THE FIVE MAIN FUNCTION OF MIND

(The Serenity Resonance Sound becomes softer and the music comes up a bit.)

"I know my mind has five main functions of operation. These are my mind centers.

One is the Center of Right Knowledge in which I instinctively know what is truth.

Two is the Center of Wrong Knowledge in which all mistakes are made. It is the center of pessimism.

Three is the Center of Imagination, which I know as the Creative Function of my Mind. I will always use my Center of Imagination constructively to produce beautiful and wonderful things.

Four is my Center of Sleep. I will use my Center of Sleep to refresh and revitalize me in mind, body and spirit.

Five is my Center of Memory. I use my memory to gain from it useful knowledge that I have learned but I fully realize that memories are of events that have happened in the past, which will never happen again. I equally realize that the future may never happen at all. There is only the here and now..."

(Repeat these affirmations three times…The Serenity Resonance Sound rises up between each time… then lowers behind the voice each time. Rest and intone these thoughts into the background of The Serenity Resonance Sound.)

"I relax quietly now and allow this wisdom to become my very own. 'I allow my mind to drift and drift, as this perfect toning of my mind becomes my reality. I HAVE BECOME MASTER OF MY MIND. I AM A MASTERMIND.'

Here is an extra bonus for you before you arouse from this subconscious reverie: From this time henceforth, the gift of tri-perception will be yours. You will recognize perception, the perceiver and the perceived as a united trinity of perception. This provides you a Quantum Leap of Consciousness."

(The Serenity Resonance Sound continues on for a bit…)

"Now, the sound fades away and only music remains. You can arouse yourself and arise any time you wish with the cosmic knowing: I AM I."

The Serenity Resonance Sound fades out…music continues…then music fades out. The Toning Of Mind Session is complete.)

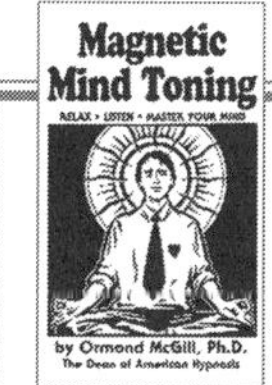

Hypno-Helper
"Magnetic Mind Toning" audio cassette by Ormond McGill can be ordered on line at www.hypnosisfederation.com or from the order form at the back of this book.

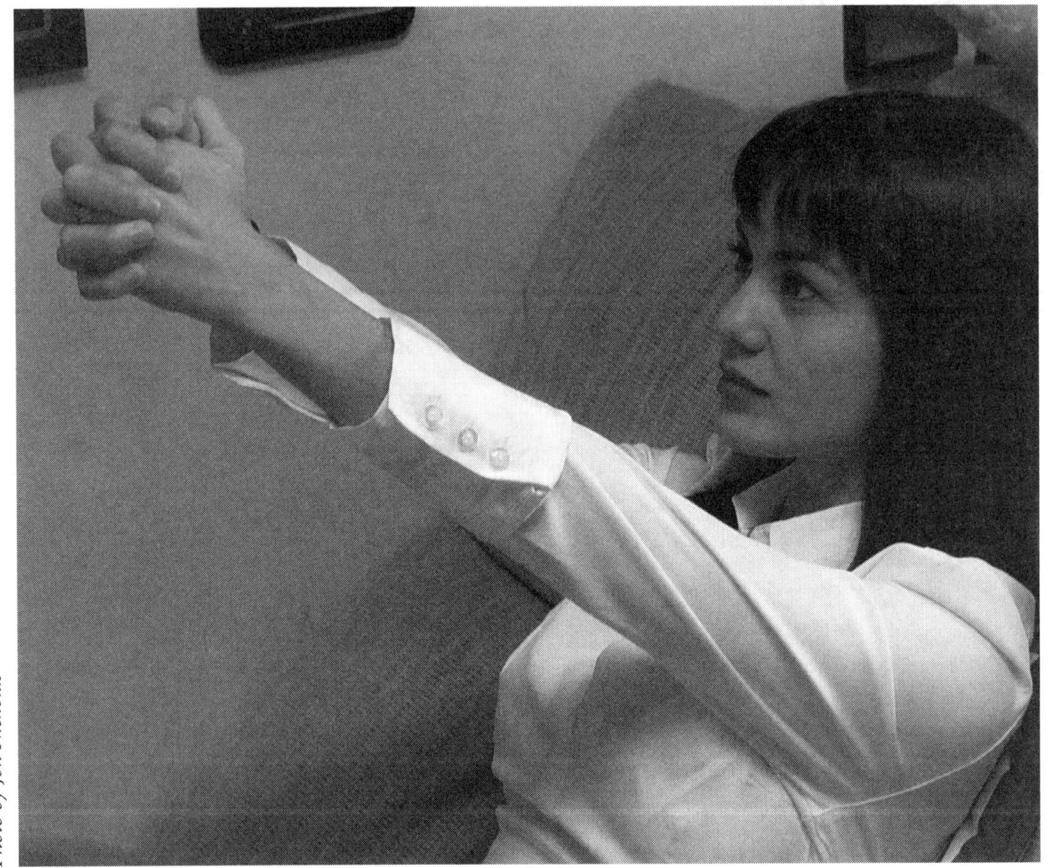

Grip Hands Together

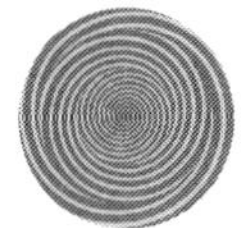

~ *Chapter 36* ~
THE HOLISTIC INDUCTION

Holistic Hypnotherapy becomes the hypnotherapy of the 21st century when your client consciously decides what they want and how to do it and then allows their subconscious mind the freedom to do it. Its deep relaxation works easily as an effective escape from any disagreeable situation.

MODUS OPERANDI:
HOLISTIC HYPNOSIS

Have your client take a seat and then say:

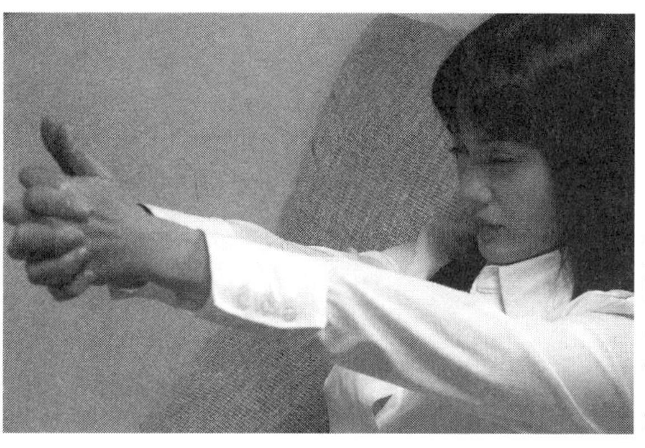

The Holistic Induction

"Extend your arms out straight in front of yourself, grip your hands together and extend the thumbs upright from your clasped hands.

Close your eyes and concentrate on how heavy and tired your outstretched hands become, as you continue to hold them at arms length. THINK of the fatigue you begin to feel holding your arms suspended in this way. They are so fatigued you cannot keep them outstretched any longer."**

Then, softly suggest in their ear:
"How relaxed and sleepy you are becoming…relaxed and sleepy. Your extended arms are becoming so tired you can scarcely hold them outstretched any longer. Be sure to let me know when your arms feel so tired that you must let them down."

They will soon tell you. Combining fatigue with relaxation is a powerful hypnotic induction.

As soon as the client tells you that they must lower their arms, tell them:
"You must continue to keep your arms outstretched, but open your eyes and gaze at your thumb nails held before you. Keep looking at your nails, and as you do you will notice they go in and out of focus. Your thumbnails are going more and more out-of-focus as you stare at them.

When they are very much out-of-focus, close your eyes, and go to sleep. When you go to sleep, you can immediately let your arms drop."

Their eyes will soon close. As they do, suggest:

"Your eyes are closed now, so you can now drop your arms down into your lap, and drop into hypnotic sleep. Your fatigued arms drop and you go into the realm of sleep. Your tired arms rest in your lap and you sleep with great relief."

The arms will drop down to the lap, and the client will drop into hypnotic sleep. Or you can give them a gentle nudge downward with the words **"completely relaxed."**

You can then deepen the hypnosis by continuing with suggestions for depth.

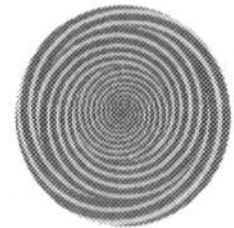

~ *Chapter 37* ~
QUOTATION INDUCTION

The more compatible the hypnosis induction is with the client's hobbies and interests, the more easy and effective it is. This method works well with clients who have an interest in quotations.

Complete your consultation and go with the client into a quiet session room. Place an eyeshade as a blindfold over the client's eyes while they relax in a comfortable chair or lie upon a couch.

MODUS OPERANDI: QUOTATION HYPNOTHERAPY
"You may effortlessly drift away into hypnosis as you relax all over. As you do, I am going to read you a treasury of valuable quotations that you will enjoy. Concentrate your attention upon the quotation and contemplate the wisdom given."

Allow some space between each quotation for this purpose. The client is to feel the meaning and drift into the quotation; as the client drifts into the quotation, he or she will drift into hypnosis, possibly somnambulistic sleep. Tell the relaxing client:

"When the deep meaning of the quotation is understood, your right forefinger will lift and then relax again. Understand?" (Get this spontaneous signal response.)

Start some soft dreamy music in the background. Read the quotations, here given, in a monotonous tone of voice. Read slowly, and take your time. Make the meaning of each quotation clear.

QUOTATIONS TO BE READ TO YOUR CLIENT:
"What a wonderful thing life is. It is a miracle that you are alive."
Pause for contemplation time. When finger signal is given, proceed on and read next quotation.

"Humor brings sunshine to what is said."
Pause for contemplation time. Always wait for confirmation signal before going on to the next quote.

"Early to bed and early to rise makes one healthy, wealthy, and wise."
Pause for contemplation time.

"Think like a wise person, but express yourself like the average person."
Pause for contemplation time.

"Glories, like glow worms afar, shine brightly, but looked at too near have neither heart nor light."
Pause for contemplation time.

"I was much older then. I'm so much younger now."
Pause for contemplation time.

"I used to think of my trifles as important."
Pause for contemplation time.

"The secret of being a bore is to tell everything."
Pause for contemplation time.

"In nature there is no blemish but the mind. None can be called deformed but the unkind."
Pause for contemplation time.

"A faithful friend is the medicine of life."
Pause for contemplation time.

"Superstition sets the whole world in flames. Philosophy quenches them."
Pause for contemplation time.

"Corporations have neither bodies to be punished nor souls to be condemned. Therefore, they do as they like."
Pause for contemplation time.

"I am I plus my surroundings. If I do not honor my surroundings, I do not honor myself."
Pause for contemplation time.

"A slavish bondage to parents cramps expanding growth."
Pause for contemplation time.

"If we had keen vision and feeling of an ordinary human life, it would be like hearing grass grow and a squirrel's heartbeat, and we would walk the road that lies on the other side of silence."
Pause for contemplation time.

"The beautiful have no enemy but time."
Pause for contemplation time.

"In dreams begin reality."
Pause for contemplation time.

"How wonderful to hold a day's conversation with the dead."
Pause for contemplation time.

"A painful pleasure often turns to pleasing pain."
Pause for contemplation time.

"Sincerity is a jewel which is pure and transparent, eternal and of great value."
Pause for contemplation time.

"One that strives to touch the stars oft stumbles over a straw."
Pause for contemplation time.

"Physicians are like kings– they brook no contradiction."
Pause for contemplation time.

"Enjoy the honey-heavy dew of slumber."
Pause for contemplation time.

Pause in giving further quotations to client, and then speak directly to them again:
"You are doing fine. Your subconscious finger signal has been shown each time when you comprehend the quotation given. Enjoy the contemplation as it makes you drowsy and sleepy, and you effortlessly drift away– down deep into hypnosis. I will give you more quotations to contemplate upon and just allow your subconscious to cogitate upon them, as you drift into sleep. Sleep. Go to sleep, as you please."
Continue in the same monotonous rhythm giving quotations. Wait for the finger signal of comprehension even though client has moved from conscious comprehension to subconscious comprehension.

"What lasting joys a man attends who has a faithful female friend?"
Pause for contemplation time.

"Suffering can sometimes be called an initiation into a higher state of BEING."
Pause for contemplation time.

"People want peace so much that one of these days governments had better get out of the way, and let them have it."
Pause for contemplation time.

"The stupid never forgive nor forget; the childish forgive and forget; the wise forgive but remember."
Pause for contemplation time.

"They never taste who always drink. They always talk who never think."
Pause for contemplation time.

"A scientific faith is absurd."
Pause for contemplation time.

"Science without religion is lame; religion without science is blind."
Pause for contemplation time.

"The past is but memories that will never happen again. The future may never happen at all. There is only the here and now."
Pause for contemplation time.

"Enough is enough."
Pause for contemplation time.

Enough. Enough. Enough. Stop the quotations now. Your client will long since have gone into hypnosis. Your client will even seem to have gone to sleep. Breathing will have deepened, and once in a while a snore. Sometimes the finger signals will continue right along, and sometimes they cease. Your client, in contemplating the quotations has moved into the realm of sleep. It is a somnambulistic sleep, and all the while the subconscious has been active.

Suggest:
"Subconscious mind give your attention to me now and turn what _________ (*Client's name*) **desires into beneficial reality."**

This mere suggestion is all you have to do to let the client achieve the result they came for.

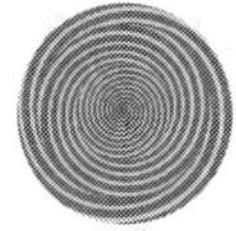

~ *Chapter 38* ~
ELMAN'S RAPID INDUCTION

Includes
Elman's Handshake Induction
The Elman Two-Finger Hypnotic Induction
Two-Finger Induction For Anesthesia
Two-Finger Induction For Children
Fixation Tests
Elman's Direct Suggestion

Dave Elman was a master hypnotist. These ways seems so simple that it seems impossible that they will work. But they do. In the simple is found the complex, and in this pleasant method of rapidly hypnotizing are found all the elements for inducing profound hypnosis.

MODUS OPERANDI: THE ELMAN HANDSHAKE INDUCTION

Dave Elman called this his social method, and used it when the person or group before him knew of his reputation as a fine hypnotist. Had Dave Elman not died quite so soon, and moved deeper into the computer age, he would has recognized in this method mental programming of the computer within the head…the brain. When programmed, the brain operates much like its mechanical counterpart. Push the correct button and what is programmed within responds and flashes upon the screen. In computer lingo it is called "programming." In psychology lingo it is called "conditioning." Dave Elman just called it his "handshake method."

The Elman handshake method of inducing hypnosis goes like this:

In a situation where he was known to be a hypnotist, Dave would walk up to a person and say,

"I'm going to shake your hand three times. The first time your eyes will get tired…let them.

The second time I shake your hand your eyes will want to close…let them.

The third time I shake your hand your eyes will lock together so tightly you will find you cannot open them try as hard as you will. Understand? If you do, just nod your head."

(Dave waited for this affirmation, and then went on.)

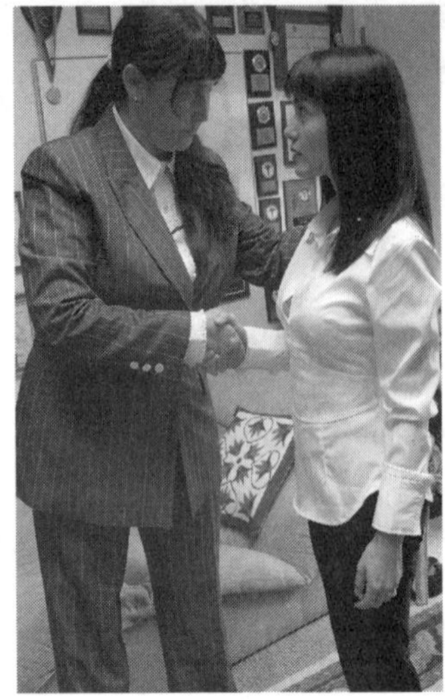

Handshake 1

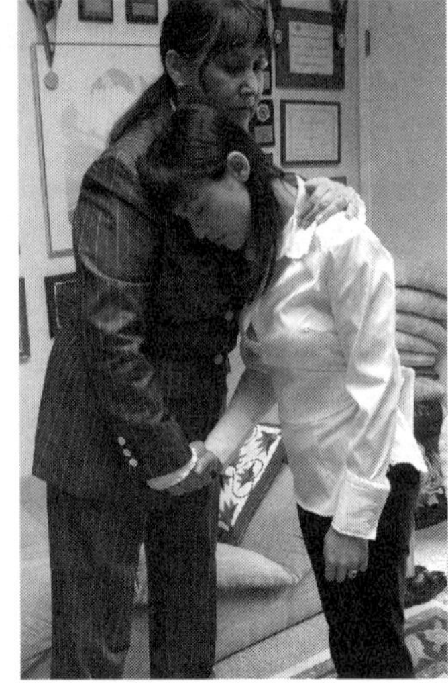

Handshake 2

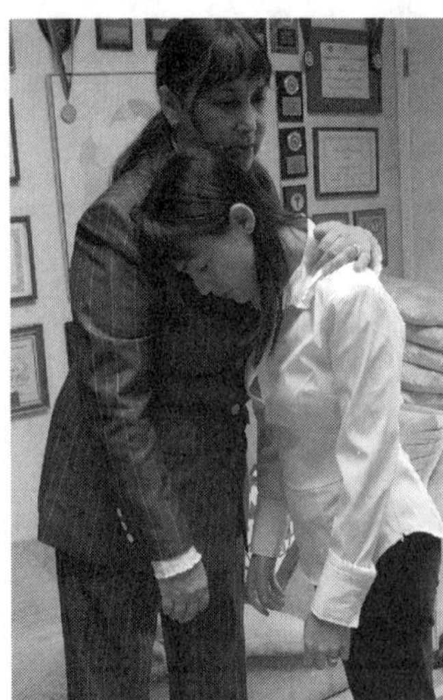

Handshake 3

Photos by Jon Nicholas

"Want that to happen and watch it happen.

ONE… I grip your hand and shake your hand. Your eyes get tired as they look at me. Want it to happen.

TWO…I shake your hand a second time, and your eyes become so tired you want to close them. Want it to happen and close your eyes.

THREE…as I shake your hand for the third time, your eyes become locked together so tightly you cannot open them, no matter how hard you try. Want that to happen and it will."

This is the opening wedge into hypnosis. An abyss lies before the person.

Grip their hand tightly and give a tug as you shout, **"SLEEP!"**

In they tumble to the abyss. Hypnosis has been induced. Hypnosis has been induced. The subconscious is ready to accept and put into action suggestions. You can now deepen the hypnosis, as you wish, with further suggestions of **"Going deeper and deeper to sleep in hypnosis."**

As Elman puts it, "In this process you have bypassed critical mind and established selective thinking. Selective thinking is whatever you believe in wholeheartedly. For example, if you are led to believe you feel no pain, and you believe it completely you will feel no pain. Hypnosis promotes a mental conditioning in which what is presented is believed in wholeheartedly."

Why does this Elman method of inducing hypnosis work so effectively? Because, as was mentioned, the elements for inducing the hypnotic state of mind are all present, viz.: Hypnosis requires keenness of attention upon yourself as a hypnotist.

Your advance reputation gives you that keen attention. Hypnosis requires a rapport developing between hypnotist and subject. A handshake is an automatic way to gain rapport. Even more, a handshake brings in friendship and trust in you.

The process sets a time for an occurrence of "one, two, three" Mind is well trained to respond to things in groups of three, as, for example., "Get ready. Get set. Go." Mind likes to respond on cues of "one, two, three."

Why?

Because, mind is conditioned to such behavior.

The process is gradual in increasing depth of response. **"One…your eyes become heavy. Two…your eyes close…Three…your eyes are locked together and you cannot open them.**

Want it to happen and it will." There is a surprise when it happens and mind becomes wide-open to receiving the suggestion **"SLEEP!"** along with an emphasizing tug of the hand.

How long did it take to hypnotize a person by this method?

Three handshakes. Who could ask for more?

MODUS OPERANDI: ELMAN'S TWO-FINGER INDUCTION TECHNIQUE

This method of hypnotizing, designed by Elman, utilizes the same psychological principles as his "Handshake Method" i.e. attention, rapport, mental set, but applies these in a more formal way.

Hypnotherapist addresses the client,

"I will show you a way to remove all tensions from your body and obtain perfect relaxation. I will help you to splendidly relax. You will like this. It is easy.

Look at me as you sit in the chair, and take a long, deep breath. Now close your eyes and take another long deep breath.

Now open your eyes wide. I am going to pull your eyelids shut by drawing my forefinger and thumb down over your closed eyes. (This downward stroking is performed and pulls the eyelids shut.)

As I do this, I want you to relax your eye muscles under my fingertips, and relax all over. Now I take my hand away, and, as I do so, relax your eye muscles so completely that they just won't work. Then, when you are sure your eye muscle just won't work, test them and see that they won't work, and you cannot open your eyes try as hard as you will.

Test them hard…good. Now, let that feeling of relaxation in your eyes flow right down through your entire body to your toes. Feel the relaxation set in. Good.

Now I will pick up your left hand and drop it into your lap, and as it plops down into your lap, you will go ten times deeper into relaxation than you are right now. (Hypnotherapist performs the action.)

Now, I lift up your left hand and drop.

That hand, too, is so relaxed it just plops down into your lap…good.

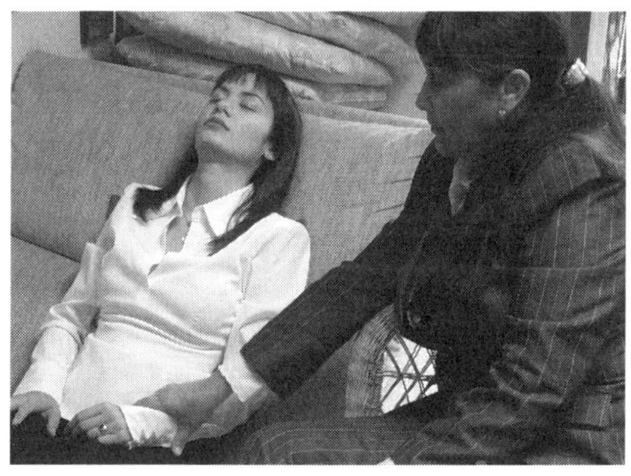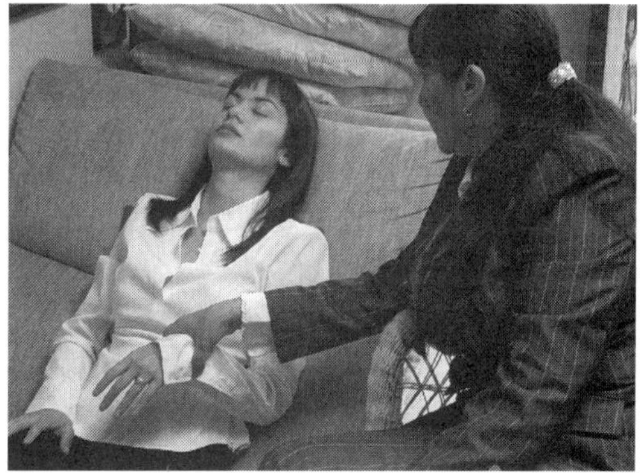

Photos by Jon Nicholas

Hand Drop

I am going to stroke your arm now and it will become numb and you won't feel anything. I am pinching it (pinch arm hard) and you don't feel a thing. Your arm has become completely, anesthetized. See I pinch it again and you feel absolutely nothing. Nothing. Is that right…nothing. If you feel nothing in your arm, nod your head."

Client nods head. You proceed on:

"You have produced complete anesthesia in yourself and you can produce this anesthesia in yourself anytime it is your wish to do so. Now, when I have you open your eyes notice how good you feel. Open your eyes. You feel fine."

During the process, the hypnotherapist can deepen the state by suggesting various experiences, for example:

"Pretend to smell a beautiful rose. You can actually smell its fragrance."

Or

"See your favorite television show in your mind."

Or

"See a science fiction picture and take a trip to Mars."

"When the mental adventure is completed, I will say, 'All right, I am returning you from that space now. Come back to Earth with me. It's been a great trip now, I want you to open your eyes and notice how good you feel.'"

Give your suggestions and then these words and the client comes back feeling great.

MODUS OPERANDI: TWO-FINGER INDUCTION FOR ANESTHESIA

Suppose the Elman two-finger induction is used in a doctor's office and the patient has to open his eyes or bare his arm for an injection. Easily handled! While the patient's eyes are still shut and he or she finds they are stuck, say, **"Anything we do in this office from now on will not bother or disturb you at all. In a couple of seconds, I am going to have you open your eyes and when you open your eyes you will become more relaxed than ever, and you will feel nothing in your arm at all. It is numb all over. Now, open your eyes and get your arm ready. Open your eyes now."**

Fast, rapid, always ready. Simple to use and the results so striking that even the doctor will be amazed.

MODUS OPERANDI: TWO-FINGER INDUCTION FOR CHILDREN

And the process is even simpler to use with children. An example working with a little girl who likes dolls:

"Jane (Call child by first name…this is rapport) **I guess you play a lot with your dolls while at home. And you probably pretend a lot with them, isn't that right? Well, we have a little game of pretend, too. And if you can learn to play this little game of pretend, nothing that happens in this nice man's office will bother or disturb you. You won't feel anything going on, if you play this little game. Would you like to play it?"**

Child responds, "Yes."

"All right, open your eyes wide. I'm going to show you this little game. I'm going to pull your eyes shut with my forefinger and thumb like this (Gently place thumb and finger on eyelids and draw them down.) **Now YOU pretend with your whole heart and soul that you can't open your eyes. That's all you have to do. Just pretend that. Now, I will take my hand away** (remove hand) **and you pretend so hard that when you try to open your eyes they just won't work. See. Now just because you're pretending like that anything we do in this office won't bother you at all."**

A general anesthesia of the child has been induced, and the doctor can proceed with whatever treatment is required.

And when it's over say to the little child: **"All done. It was fun to play pretend. Open your eyes now and you feel just fine."**

And there you are. Fast, rapid, easy. No mention of hypnosis, no mention of sleep, just pretend. That is hypnosis: you have bypassed critical mind and established selective thinking.

That is the Elman way.

MODUS OPERANDI: FIXATION TESTS

Eyelid fixation is one test Elman used. Others can be performed as well.

"Close your eyes and pretend you can't open them. Now I take your arm and I want you to straighten it out…extend it and make it rigid as I count to three. Pretend it is so rigid you cannot bend it. One…make it rigid…two, like steel…now you cannot bend your arm no matter how hard you try. When you try, it just won't work at all. Test it. You'll find you can't bend it at all. Now you've got a rigid arm."

Now you can use that rigid arm to deepen the hypnosis, viz.,:

"When I tell you, you can relax your arm it will become limp and relaxed, and you will go deeper and deeper. Relax and go much deeper. Can you feel the depth? Can you feel yourself going deeper? You can answer. If you can feel yourself going deeper and deeper nod your head."

A nod of the head, and you know a deep state of hypnosis has been achieved. The "rigid arm" is an interesting test. Catalepsy lets you know that hypnosis has been induced, and that you have bypassed critical mind. But possibly the doctor might not wish to use it in his office. There are other ways to assert hypnosis. Look for redness in the eyes, and increasing of lacrimation (moisture), the eyelids fluttering, whites of the eyes getting pink and sometimes rolling up beneath the upper eyelids and you can judge the depth of hypnosis you have induced.

For such testing, suggest:

"Now when I tell you to, I want you to open your eyes wide and let me look at them for a couple of seconds. When I tell you to, open your eyes, and keep them open until I tell you to close them, and then you'll go much deeper you will let yourself go much deeper. Now open your eyes."

The patient opens eyes. You examine the eyes briefly, then suggest, **"close your eyes and go deeper. And when I tell you to come back with me, you will this time open your eyes feeling wonderful in every way."**

MODUS OPERANDI: ELMAN'S DIRECT SUGGESTION

This method of hypnotic suggestion was based on that used in the long-gone but still famous Nancy School in France. The school was under the direction of hypnosis experts Drs. Bernheim and Liebeault, who helped thousands of people by the direct removal of symptoms with hypnotic suggestions. They believed that when a symptom was removed the cause vanished too.

In relation to hypnotism, suggestions mostly constitute words. Words have been called "triggers to action." That is to say, words have been programmed into our personal mental computer, and, on proper cue, spring forth as mental and physical responses, influencing our behavior clear down to the very function of bodily well being.

Words carry power. The proper word spoken at the proper time in the proper way can change the history of the world.

A direct suggestion takes things directly to the point so you might suggest to the client in hypnosis, **"What bothered you is now gone and you feel well and fine. When you arouse from the hypnosis you are cured!"**

Some question the value of direct suggestion to remove a symptom. Their objection is the belief that the basic cause of the symptom must be uncovered and removed before a cure is affected. Elman had respect for his peers, but he was perfectly content to go along with the old Masters. If it was good enough for them in healing thousands of patients, it was good enough for him. Belief being: "the subconscious knows far more intimately what is needed to affect a cure for the patient than does any probing speculation of the therapist." Right or wrong he stuck to his guns, and trained his doctor students to use hypnosis in this directs rapid, fast, practical method as an adjunct to their medical practice. The reported results were outstanding.

You have learned how to hypnotize the Dave Elman way.

Hypno-Helper

"Hypnotherapy" by Dave Elman

"Elman On MP3" eighteen hours of vintage Elman recordings.

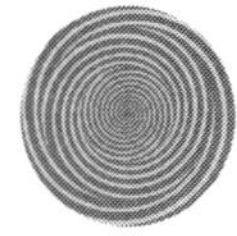

~ *Chapter 39* ~
YOU ARE THE STAR HYPNOTHERAPY

"Life is a stage upon which we are actors all."
              —Shakespeare

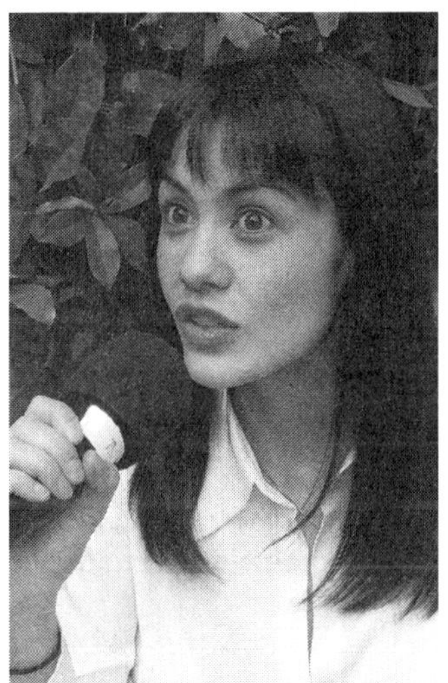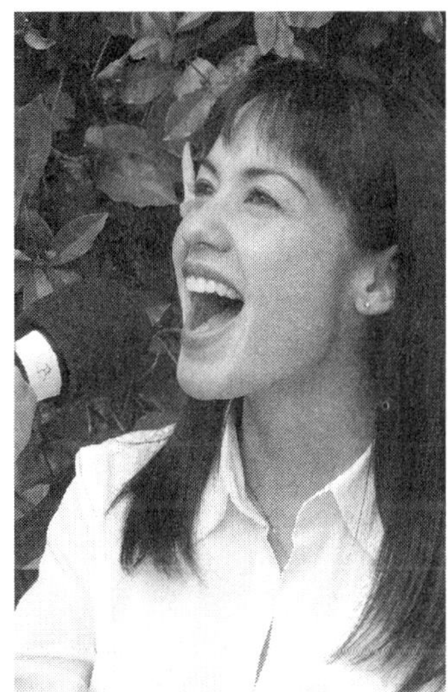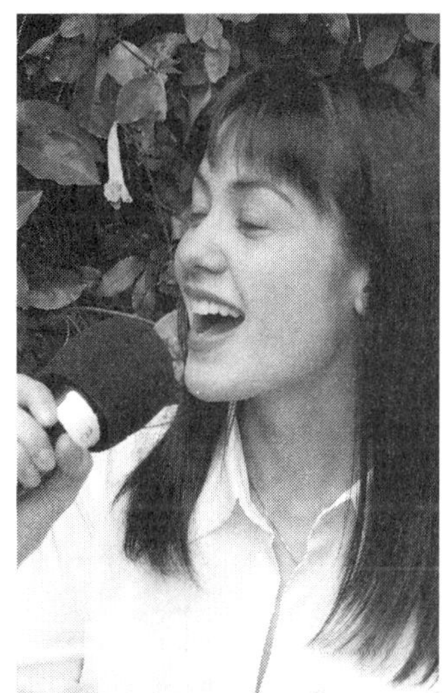

You Are the Star!

MODUS OPERANDI: YOU ARE THE STAR HYPNOTHERAPY

This is a verbatim script exactly designed for studio recording. You can produce it as your own.

You will need:
Digital Recording Equipment
The Serenity Resonance Sound CD
Soft Music (If recording this make sure that the music is "royalty free.")

Begin by playing the Serenity Resonance Sound for a time and then rise up and fade back to a sublevel.

"You can perform the 'You Are A Star' hypnosis wherever you are. You can perform it sitting in a chair or lying outstretched. It makes no difference, just as long as you are relaxed and comfortable…and allow these facts of truth to be received by the mind.

Where ever you are and who ever you are, relax now and close your eyes. Now submerge

yourself into the resonating sound…as it gradually fades away, you will sink deeper and deeper inside yourself into the wonderful realm of your subconscious mind…into the state of hypnotic reverie."

The sound rises then gradually fades to a sublevel.

"As you sink down into the state of hypnotic reverie, you will be fully aware as your conscious phase of mind moves to one side and allows your subconscious to take center stage."

The sound rises slightly and then recedes to sublevel.

"Listen…listen…listen and as you more and more gain this understanding, you will continue to go deeper into hypnosis."

Sound continues at sublevel and meditative music is now introduced softly as well.

"Look upon life as a stage. This gives you a perspective of witnessing the roles you play on your stage of life. This is an advancement of consciousness. You know that life is a stage and that you are free to act out all manner of roles. Some of the roles you play are humorous. Some are serious. But you know the roles you play are just illusions, fantasies and dreams. You know this instinctively. You know this well…as you drop ever deeper and deeper into hypnosis.

You know that the roles you play are as an actor on your stage of life…and that that is really YOU, can sit back in the theater and watch yourself performing upon the stage.

How splendidly you now become aware of the profound depth of Shakespeare's immortal prose *'Life is a stage upon which we are actors all.'* It resonates through your being…and you feel this knowing. You know it well. And upon the stage…which is your life…you can play any role you please for you are the star."

The meditative music rises slightly over the Serenity Resonance Sound.

"You are comfortable, safe and at peace with yourself as you watch the wonderful drama of your life unfold before yourself. Go silent for some moments now as this understanding becomes your reality."

Only Serenity Resonance Sound is played at the sublevel.

Bring up the music slightly with these words:

"Now, within your mind, visualize that you stand in a valley in the center of a deep canyon. It is a beautiful canyon in which every word you speak…echoes from the surrounding mountain tops. Let's hear the echo now. Listen as the sound of your echoing voice comes back to you…hello, hello, hello.

Use an echo effect on "Hello" as the music quiets and the Serenity Resonance Sound is heard above it. Let this sound go on for a few minutes and then suddenly all stops and becomes silent. Silence.

After a pause, the music and the sound resume very softly.

"Shh…shh…shh…go very quiet. Look around and see where you are. Good heavens you are seated in a vast theater watching yourself playing a role…acting a part upon this stage of your life.

Look around and note this vast theater is the Universe itself. Stars surround all sides as your stage of life floats in its very center…it is the center of this great cosmic vastness. IT IS THE VOID. Good heavens what a show I am watching and I can direct the show as is my wish.** (The pronoun shift is intentional)

I return my attention to the stage. The lights come on and light up myself and the other actors that are acting with me on the stage and I can see clearly what is happening on the stage. I am there as the central actor and surrounding me are other actors who are my friends. I know these actors well. They are in the play along with myself, but in this particular play, I am the star. I am also the director of the play."

Music rises to a higher level and then fades to the background.

"I snuggle back in my theater seat and watch the play being performed upon my stage of life. I now have the knowing of moving from three-dimensional perception into forth-dimensional perception, whatever is my wish.

Power up the resonance of your voice as you say;

"I know! I know! I know!"

Add echo effect

"I know! I know! I know!"

Echo out.

"I know what a gift I have been given. I can slip from three-dimensional perception into forth-dimensional perception, whatever is my wish."

Echo in.

"I know what a gift I have been given. I can slip from three-dimensional perception into forth-dimensional perception, whatever is my wish."

Music is turned off and just the subliminal Serenity Resonance Sound plays in the background.

"I know! I know! I know! I await now the time for my arising and returning to the here and now."

Pause.

"When shall I awaken and return to the here and now? At what time will that be? Time. Time. What a foolish question that is for me to ask; now I know. I can arouse fully alert whenever it is my wish to be. For I am the star that shines upon my stage of life."

In echo: "For I am the star of all that transpires upon my stage of life.

For I am the star of all that transpires upon my stage of life.

For I am the star of all that transpires upon my stage of life.

Echo ends, just subliminal Serenity Sound: I hear it echo through my being. I can slip from three-dimensional perception into forth-dimensional perception, whatever is my wish.

Echo becomes softer and softer until gone as you repeat:

"For I am the star of all that transpires upon my stage of life.

For I am the star of all that transpires upon my stage of life.

For I am the star of all that transpires upon my stage of life.

"I know! I know! I know! I await my arousing and returning to the here and now. I awaken...returning to the here and now on my returning to the here and now..."

Serenity Resonance Sound fades out and then silence.

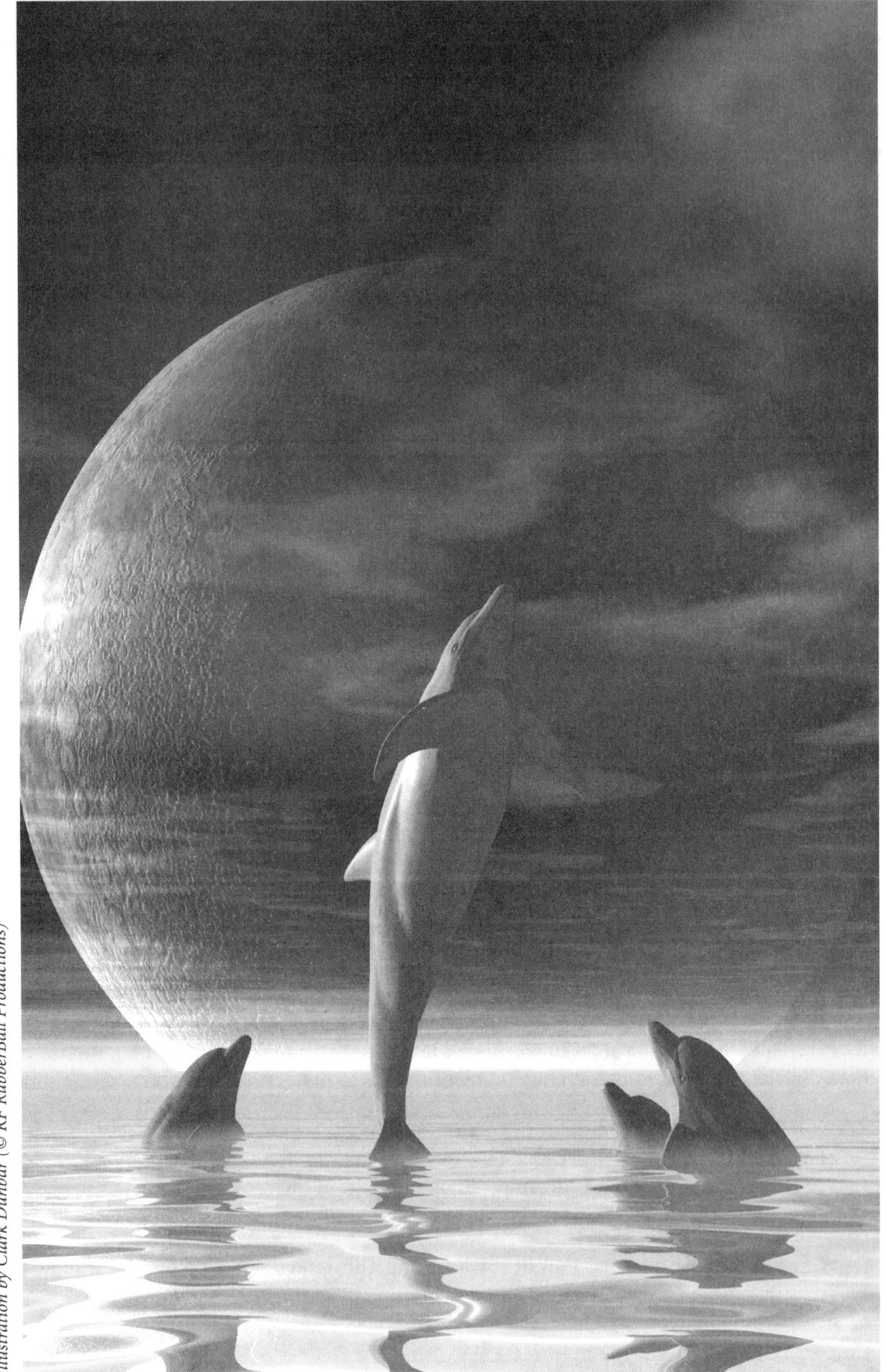

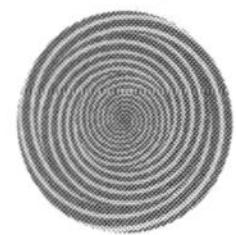

~ *Chapter 40* ~
BALE'S OUTSIDE/INSIDE INDUCTION

First presented with permission from Dwight Bale in
The New Encyclopedia Of Stage Hypnotism

This method comes from hypnotherapist Dwight Bale. This rapid introvertive method is very effective, readily applied and results are striking. It's a biofeedback approach.

You evoke subjective responsiveness when the client suggests, inside him or herself, that what you, the hypnotherapist, suggests is outside.

MODUS OPERANDI IF OUTSIDE/INSIDE HYPNOTHERAPY

Have your client sit in a comfortable chair and close their eyes. Instruct them to begin by breathing– deeply in and out. This rapid in-and-out breathing somewhat "drugs" the brain with an overload intake of oxygen, and outflow of carbon dioxide.

"Take a deep breath. Hold it. Now exhale slowly.

This in-and-out deep breathing is performed six times in rapid sequence:
1. **Breathe In – Breathe Out...**
2. **Breathe In – Breathe Out...**
3. **Breathe In – Breathe Out...**
4. **Breathe In – Breathe Out...**
5. **Breathe In – Breathe Out...**
6. **Breathe In – Breathe Out.**

Now relax your body as completely as possible and say to yourself inside your mind, I am becoming very relaxed. I am becoming very relaxed. I am becoming very relaxed.'"
(Client repeats this phrase silently within himself.)

"Now say inside yourself the words, 'my eyes are closed and I am becoming sleepy. Very sleepy...I am rapidly drifting down into the realm of sleep.'"
(Client repeats this phrase silently within himself.)

"I am so relaxed all over that I can't even open my eyes. I try but I cannot even open my eyes, for I am drifting down into the realm of sleep. I am drifting down, down, down to sleep in hypnosis now."

(Client repeats this phrase silently within himself.)

The process continues:
"I am so relaxed now that my body becomes limp all over, and my subconscious mind accepts and turns into my reality all beneficial suggestions presented to myself."
(Client repeats this phrase silently within himself.)
Hypnotherapist now moves from first to second person in presenting suggestions to the client:
"Good. You are going deeper and deeper into profound hypnosis now and are giving full attention to the beneficial suggestions I give you, while you are in this receptive state of mind. You are in a subjective state of mind. You need not think for yourself now, as I will do your thinking for you. All you have to do is relax as you accept the beneficial suggestion I tell your subconscious. They become your reality, as you continue to sink down deeper and deeper into hypnosis. Just let yourself go! Understand? If you do, just let out a little murmur or nod your head."
(Client almost as an outgoing of breath gives a sound or nods their head.)

"Good. Continue going deeper into hypnosis now, and your subconscious will take over and follow every beneficial suggestion I now give you. All you have to do is let yourself go, and open your subconscious acceptance of the suggestions which will now be given you."

Your client is deeply hypnotized. Present your "suggestion formula" now.

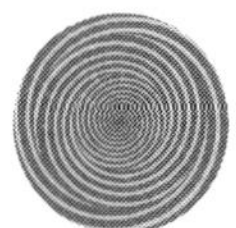

~ *Chapter 41*
ENGLAND'S RAG DOLL INDUCTION

"Dolls, as objects of our creative imagination will, if we invite them, take us to play again in the house of our childhood past and perhaps bestow upon us a future we hadn't imagined"
—Cassandra Light, "Way of the Doll"

I present this technique in loving memory of Diana L. England, who created it. This Induction appeals to children as well as adults. It is a visualization method using a tangible item to intensify the visualization. To do it you will need a doll of any convenient size with a floppy head, arms and legs. In other words, a rag doll like the old Raggedy Ann.

A doll used with verbal suggestions cleverly produces an associative effect in which the visual suggestions emphasize the verbal suggestions. The effects are compounding.

MODUS OPERANDI:
THE RAG DOLL INDUCTION FOR WELL BEING

"You are a about to have a delightful experience as you enter into hypnosis to play an imaginative game. The game will help you to go deep down into the relaxation of hypnosis without any effort at all. In fact, the rules of the game require that you do not try to do anything at all consciously…that you simply relax and direct your attention to the suggestions you are about to receive. Then, JUST LET IT HAPPEN. To get on with the game here is another player."

Bring out Raggedy Ann, or the doll you will use, and have her exhibit and perform in a manner related to the words you use. This manipulation is easy because of the floppy nature of the doll.

"Meet Raggedy Ann. (or the name of your doll). She is a little rag doll who is stuffed with cotton and when you shake her, she flops around in just about any direction. But sometimes Raggedy Ann gets all tense and uptight, just as many of us do when our lives become filled with stress.

Watch her now; her neck and shoulders are tensed up. Her arms are held rigidly out in front of her…this is what happens after a hard day of tending to things that she thinks she simply must tend to.

Now watch the difference that relaxation brings her. Watch the transformation. First she relaxes one arm, then the other. Then her head drops forward and finally she just lets go in the midsection and her entire torso drops forward. Look how completely relaxed she is! Now you see what hanging loose really means.

Now when anyone besides a little rag doll hangs loose they won't necessarily bend double like Raggedy Ann does. When you're not a rag doll, you let your torso hang forward

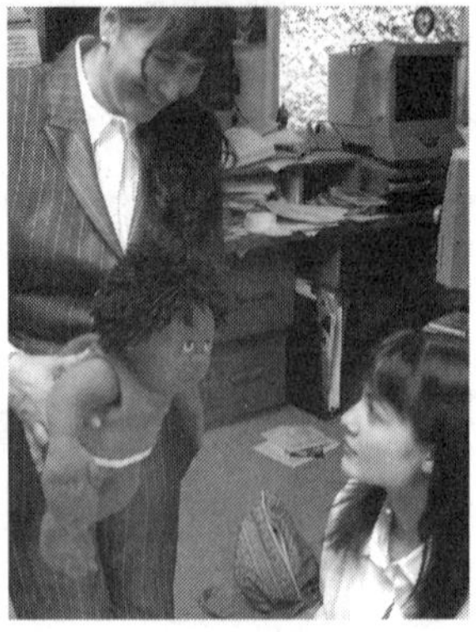

Rag Doll

only to whatever degree is comfortable for you without force or effort and get the feeling of just dangling so you have a good stretch and release all tension.

Now to continue with Raggedy Ann's relaxation…from this completely relaxed forward bend position, she slowly and smoothly raises her body to an erect position. Her head hangs forward until the very last then it too straightens up.

But notice what happens: Raggedy Ann's mind hadn't relaxed along with her body so as she reaches her straight up position, her jangled nerves put tension back into her body and here she is again all tight and tense, but this time she sends her consciousness to each part of her body so her mind will relax right along with her muscles.

Here she goes again!"

Make the doll relax one arm and then the other. Move her head to drop forward on her chest and continue as you demonstrate with the doll:

"1-2-3-4 and she is so relaxed she starts to fall backward, regains her balance, drops forward again and this time when she straightens up, she falls backwards into her chair, her head resting on the chair back, her eyes closed…limp as a rag doll. And notice the serene contented smile on her face. Raggedy Ann is in deep hypnosis and enjoying every moment of it.

Now, when you try this game of relaxation be guided by Raggedy Ann's example and you will make sure that there is a chair right in back of you or else you might wind up on the floor!

So now you are ready to relax Raggedy Ann style, stand up in front of your chair, toes and heels together, elbows bent at your sides with your forearms raised stiffly in front all filled with stress and tension and we'll practice relaxing together two times, just like Raggedy Ann did.

Ready, set, GO! Relax! One arm- drop…now the other arm- drop. Head drop forward, just like Raggedy Ann. Good.

Now slowly let your arms and head rise up again, all tense and stiff again.

Now close your eyes and this time direct your consciousness to each part of your body as it relaxes and let your mind relax right along with your body. I'll count for you as you do this, four counts down and four counts up. Ready, here we go.

1-2-3-4 down and now straighten up 5-6-7-8. you are perfectly erect but so relaxed that you start to fall backward, but reverse the influence and drop forward again, just like Raggedy Ann did. Now straighten up, up, up and this time you fall right over backward into your chair with your head resting on the chair back, your eyes closed, your arms dangling loosely and there is a smile of contentment on your rag doll face."**

Ease the client down into the chair as they fall backwards. Then revolve their head gently around and around in a circular motion to induce further relaxation as you suggest:

"It feels so good to have a neck limp as a rag doll's. How good it feels to be relieved of supporting the weight of your head. Just let your neck relax completely as you head comes to rest in whatever position is most comfortable."

Gently place the client's head in a resting position.

"Feel how the relaxation flows downward through your shoulders and arms. Notice how limp and loose your right arm is."

Grasp their right thumb to lift the arm and gently shake the entire arm as you continue:

"It is limp and floppy just like Raggedy Ann's. As I let go of your left arm and it drops down, you will go ten times even further, deeper down into relaxation…"

Let go of the arm.

"…ten times more relaxed! Sinking into hypnosis!"

"Now feel the relaxation travel down over your chest, torso, and hips. Feel the heavy relaxation of your thighs against the chair seat and that relaxation travels down your knees, calves, ankles and feet."

"Now let me shake your Raggedy Ann foot."

Grasp their leg at the knee and gently shake it as you continue:

"Notice how your foot just goes flippity flop, exactly like Raggedy Ann's. And when I let go, your foot will drop like a rock and when it touches the floor, you will go deeper and deeper into hypnosis."

From a few inches above the floor let their foot drop to the floor and continue…

"Deeper and deeper you go into relaxation…deeper and deeper you go into hypnosis. The other Raggedy Ann foot needs shaking too."

Grasp their other leg at the knee and gently shake it as you continue

"This foot and leg are hanging completely loose and limp and when I let go, the foot drops to the floor and sends you ten times even more deeply into hypnosis."

Let go of their foot and drop it to the floor. Observe how it drops like a rag.

"Your foot drops you down, down, down into hypnosis…ten times deeper. You are at rest, at peace, so comfortable and contented to just let go. Your body is all relaxed…just let your mind relax now too and enjoy a refreshing rest. Breathe deep and full and every breath you take sends you deeper into relaxation…deeper into hypnosis.

This little rag doll is sitting in your chair…this doll that is you…is stuffed with cotton, but some helium gas is pumped into your hands along with the cotton and the gas makes them feel so light that they just start floating right up into the air…rising from your lap. These rag doll hands feel so light they won't rest in your lap any more, as the want to float up into the air rising up from your lap. Feel your elbows bend as the hands rise slowly upward…raised by the helium. There is enough helium gas to float them right up to touch your forehead and when they do you will go ten times deeper into hypnosis."

Give them time to complete this assignment.

"Now when I touch your hands it will let the gas out and your hands will drop like a rag doll's hands into your lap and you will be in profound hypnosis."

Let this happen.

"Now as you rest so peacefully, the conscious aspect of your mind is freed from effort and activity and your subconscious emerges with its fertile soil well prepared to accept all beneficial suggestions that come to it. Open wide your subconscious to receive these beneficial suggestions.

How calm and relaxed you feel. Every ounce of tension is drawing out of your body…out of your mind. This wonderful feeling of peace, confidence and security is your birthright…this is how you were meant to feel. It is the way you felt early in life before any tension reached you and you now understand that every young new human being entering this world has to learn the customs and mores of society and sometimes others unintentionally harm these tender young beings and condition them to behave acceptably. Then as the individual matures they need to be de-conditioned so the real self shines through.

So it is with you, your early conditioning helped you become accepted by society and now has served its purpose. Now you are a free being. So let it go…let old conditioned and unwanted habits melt away and accept your true nature…when you are aware of the integration of your mind, body and spirit and recognize your complete and true self. How wonderful it is for you to recognize and accept the SELF that is truly YOU!

Allow your mind to roam contentedly to any situation where you are completely safe, totally loved and absolute monarch of your space. Go back in your perfect memory now and recall a time of being safe, warm and contented. You may remember the warm secure, contented feeling in the womb or a time in your mother's arms next to her breast or a time when your daddy's strong arms hugged you or someone bouncing you on their knee.

Let whatever safe and warm events come to mind and grow rich and vivid and become indelibly imprinted in your mind. Experience fully what these imagined events bring to your life. Let theses feelings take root in your subconscious and submerge your entire being. Saturate yourself in the ecstasy of these thoughts. Notice how you feel completely secure, confident and in control of your life in every way. The knowledge of this brings complete relaxation to your mind and body. You are completely content in you feeling of well being.

How wonderful to bring back this feeling of confidence and contentment anytime you wish. You can you know…I will show you how: right now in this moment make a fist. Squeeze it tight and then let it go completely. When you squeeze your fists think of this activating the pleasant feeling you have just experienced. When you relax, let go of any negativity. Do it now; squeeze your fists tightly and release, pumping into your being this wonderful secure, happy feeling. Relax your hand and let go of all disturbing conditions. This is your cue.

From this point forward you have this cue. You become ten times more secure, ten times more confident and contented, ten times more able to meet and cope with whatever situations the future brings, for you are now master of yourself.

Now as you rest comfortably and limp like a rag doll, with your breaths coming deep and full, let yourself sink even deeper into the pleasant lassitude of hypnosis. Enjoy the wonderful secure confident, contented feeling that engulfs you as your subconscious makes these things wonderful suggestions part of your being. They are your very own."

Pause and allow time for these suggestions to sink into the client's subconscious mind.

"Now it is time to come back to the here and now. You will glide out of hypnosis pleasantly and wonderfully. The experience has been a complete joy. I will simply count from one to five and at the count of five, you will be fully alert and active again. The wonderful feeling inside yourself you have so blissfully discovered will remain with you and you KNOW that forevermore you will feel completely confident and can successfully handle all situations that life brings your way with calm self-assurance.

Ready now, prepare to come back, fully alert in every way as I count from one to five" One, beginning to come back…two, feeling wonderful and relaxed…three…clear headed and you want to stretch…four you are filled with a wonderful sense of well-being, happiness and joy…five, you are fully alert, back in the here and now and open your eyes…feeling fine in every way.

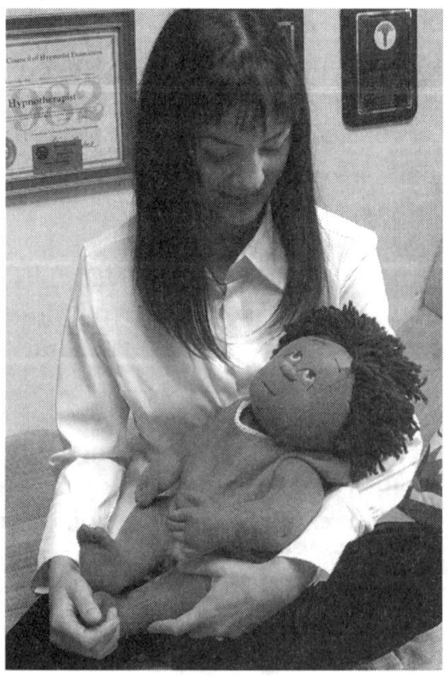

Rag Doll

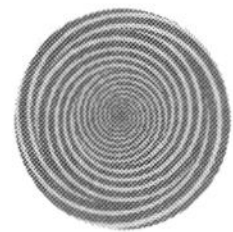

~ *Chapter 42* ~
HYPNOTIZING CHILDREN

Includes
Imagination Game Inductions
Bucket of Water Induction
The Swing Induction
The Penny Drop Induction
Flying Eagle Induction
Thompson's Eye Of The President Induction
Telkemeyer's Slide Induction
Puppet Induction
Hypnotizing School Children

Inductions for children are simpler than adult induction. Adults are too analytical and always want to know why. Children just want to feel happy. Children want to feel loved and self-confident.

How do you get children into trance, gain their confidence, learn about them, hypnotize them, and then use direct suggestion or regression? Get them to focus their minds on something else! The best way: story telling. Children believe in fantasy.

Another good way to hypnotize a child is while they are sleeping. Simply say positive things in their ear. Give clear direct suggestions for right behavior and do not waver. Inconsistency confuses the mind.

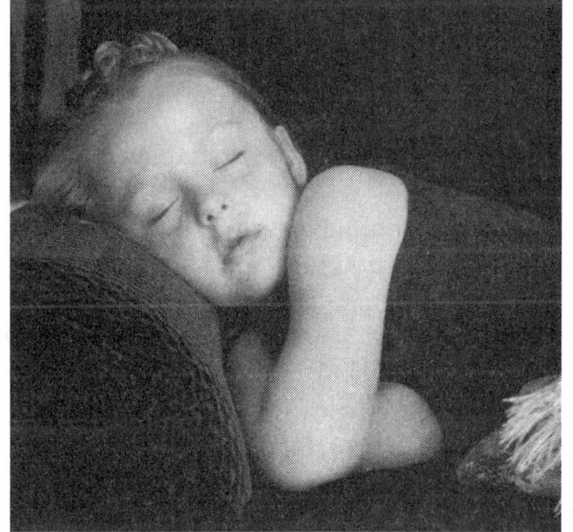

Natalie Rose Peterson

Younger children, below five or six, easily go into trance with direct suggestion. Start just talking to the child. They like you in their space. Kids like big fluffy chairs to get swallowed up in. Kids love to be rocked nice and easy. They like the physical connection.

Have them close their eyes. Many times you will see the signs of deep hypnosis as soon as you get eyelid closure. When you see their eyes flutter, don't shoot yourself in the foot, start the suggestion process. The children are very animated in trance; this doesn't mean they are not in a trance. Many times the deeper they go into trance, the more animated they become. If they open their eyes, just tell them to keep those eyes closed until you're finished.

If children are restless you could say…

"We are going to play a game but to play this game, you have got to sit on your hands. Now you can't move your hands, or else we won't be able to play…"

MODUS OPERANDI: IMAGINATION GAME INDUCTIONS

The following is just a guide. Adapt to your own personality and use words that are comfortable for you.

"You like to play games don't you?"

"Let's pretend…"

"Let's play act…"

"You really want to do well in school and get good grades like other boys and girls don't you?"

"Let's play a game. Are you comfortable in that chair?"

"Would you like to play a game of imagination?

(Yes)

"Wonderful!"

"You've played pretend haven't you? Maybe you pretended you were a super hero or a cowboy or a firefighter. In this pretend game just do exactly what I ask you to do. Open your eyes really wide and when I bring my hand down in front of them close them down and pretend that they can't open. Pretend as hard as you can that they can't open. Are you pretending as hard as you can? That's good. All right, I'll snap my fingers and it will be true. Now even when you try to open your eyes they just won't open. Now let's keep pretending that really nice things will happen to you…"

After you have given them simple and direct suggestions you bring them back by saying,

"That's fine, now the pretending game is over. I will count to three and you will open your eyes and be so happy and feeling fine."

MODUS OPERANDI: BUCKET OF WATER INDUCTION

Children love this induction. I know that this tried and true method will make you very happy and confident of the results. This particular induction is easily modified and adapted into a wonderful group induction also.

First establish that the child knows left from right, if not, indicate which hand by touching the appropriate hand. Have child sit in a very comfortable position and then say to him/her…

"Now just close your eyes and keep them closed until I ask you to open them. I want you to imagine that on the right side, (this side over here), **right next to your chair on the floor where you can reach it easily, is a big, big bucket of warm water. I want you to imagine that, ok? The bucket is easily in reach with your right hand (this hand.)**

Now imagine that floating on top of the big bucket of water is a ball. What color is the ball? (They say 'Blue' or whatever).

Isn't that wonderful?

Now, take your hand and put it on top of the ball. Push the ball down into the bucket of water; just push it under the water. Now bring your hand up and notice how the ball floats right back up to the top. It just comes right back up to the top…doesn't it?

Now just push the ball down again… and then let it come back up again.

Isn't that neat?

Now, I just want you to keep pushing the ball down into the water and then letting it come back up again…and you just keep doing that.

Now ______________ (Child's name) **you're going to notice as you keep doing this, you feel more and more relaxed. Each time you push the ball down, you just get sleepier and sleepier and sleepier…and I'm going to be talking to you…but you don't even have to listen to me. You just continue pushing that ball up and down…and you don't even have to listen to me unless I press my hand on your shoulder like this** (demonstrate.)

______________ (Child's name), **when I press on your shoulder I want you to answer a question. You have the idea don't you?**

So just push that ball up and down and notice how sleepy you get each time you press that ball up and down… and you feel yourself growing more and more comfortable… don't you? (They reply 'Yes') **and it's a nice feeling isn't it?**

Just keep doing that and don't pay any attention to me what so ever…until I press you on your shoulder again. No matter how sleepy you become, you will always be able to hear my voice and the sound of my voice will help you to relax even more…that's right, just keep pressing that (the color they said) **ball up and down and notice how you can sleep deeper and deeper."**

At this point you may either do a 5-1 deepening technique or allow the child to continue deepening his own trance and begin the behavior modification portion of the session. The younger the person, the fewer times compounding is needed. For children up to age 4, compound about 5 times. For older children compound up to 15 times.)

"______________ (Child's name) you know…you are a very smart little (boy or girl)**…a very smart and a very intelligent little** (boy or girl)**. You are going to discover now that when you go to school, you look forward to going to school because it's a wonderful time for you to show off. A time to show how much you know…and be so happy when you know the right answer…and will find that when you are in school you will be able to listen to your teachers and you are going to remember everything they tell you…and you're just as good as anyone."** (Continue with direct suggestion or necessary hypno-analysis.)

______________ (Child's name), **in a moment I'm going to have you open your eyes. After you open your eyes, you are going to feel just great because you know you're just as good as anyone, you know you're loved by everyone.** (Add whatever suggestions are appropriate.) **All right ______________** (Child's name) **open your eyes and notice how good you feel. You feel good don't you?"**

They are still in a highly suggestible state for the next 30-90 seconds and this is a great time to compound the suggestions you have given them.

MODUS OPERANDI: THE SWING INDUCTION

"Close your eyes and imagine that you are in a swing (or rowing a boat, or watching the waves at the shore) **going up and down, up and down. It feels so good…back and forth. It's a beautiful day to swing. You feel so lazy and comfortable that you just take a deep breath and relax all over."**

MODUS OPERANDI: THE PENNY DROP INDUCTION
You Will Need:
A Penny or Other Coin

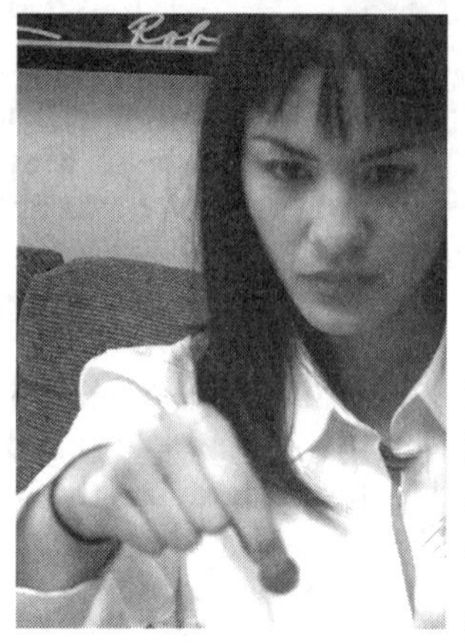

Penny Drop

"Here is a penny. If you follow my instructions exactly, after we are done, you will get to keep it. Okay. Hold the penny between your thumb and pointer finger with your arm stretched out in front of you. Look at the penny very carefully…very good.

Look at your hand and fingers holding the penny. In a moment, you will drop the penny and when you do you'll relax all over…your hand will drop into your lap and you'll feel just like you do when you are deep asleep. When you drop the penny, your eyes will close and you'll go to your favorite dream place. The one you like the most. It will happen so easily.

All right let your fingers relax, drop the penny, close your eyes and relax. Sleep. Excellent. You get an A-plus."

MODUS OPERANDI: FLYING EAGLE
You Will Need:
A Quarter

VERSION 1:
"**Look at the eagle on this quarter. In a moment you will see the wings start to flap and when they do, your eyes become tired and want to close. Just let that happen and go to sleep.**"
If using a Canadian quarter notice the "elks head and antlers" move side to side.

VERSION 2:
"**Follow my hand with the quarter as it goes up and down. You see the eagle's wings spreading.**" (Move your hand slowly up and down, fingers together at first and spreading each time) "**Next time the quarter goes up, the eagle will spread his wings and fly and you will close your eyes and your hand will drop into your lap.**"

MODUS OPERANDI: THE EYE OF THE PRESIDENT INDUCTION
Hypnotherapist Niccolous Thompson says this rapid induction uses the "when I say this" or "when you do this," then you will be hypnotized approach:

"**Sit comfortably in this chair with one hand on the arm of the chair and the other with a quarter placed between your thumb and forefinger.**

(Have the child extend their arm)

Look right into the eye of the president as one arm is relaxed on the arm of the chair and the other is extended holding the quarter, with your eyes staring at the eye of the president.

__________ (Child's name) **we'll play a game using the eye of the president on the quarter you are looking at, and even though soon your eyes will begin to water and you may want to close your eyes, do not let them close** __________ (Child's name) **until I say it is OK to do so. If your eyes stray or move away from the eye of the president, just take them right back to the eye of the president. Now,** __________ (Child's name) **breathe in deep and hold the breath.** (Pause)

Now exhale slowly keeping your eyes on the eye of the president. Take another deep breathe in and hold the breath, and as you exhale as slow as you can, you will notice your arm

is getting heavy and your eyes feel sleepy, you can feel yourself blinking very fast. You're doing great __________ (Child's name)**, so inhale again and hold the breath, and as you exhale slowly your arm is moving down. Your eyes are closing and the more you see your arm moving down, the more sleepy you feel. How tired your arm is, so rest the other arm now, and sleep. Close your eyes and sleep. SLEEP. Breathe in deep breath's, but slowly. Deep relaxing sleep now."**

Hypnosis Is Produced!

MODUS OPERANDI: ERNEST TELKEMEYER'S SPIRAL SLIDE INDUCTION

Illinois Hypnotherapist, Ernie Telkemeyer specializes in working with children. His approach works wonders for children five years and up!

Place the soft pad on the side of your hand (below the little finger) gently on the center of the child's forehead (between their eyebrows). Move your hand counter clockwise (from your viewpoint) so that the skin on the forehead moves but without moving the hand on the skin because it would irritate. As you say, "going around, around and around and down, down, down…" rotate the hand, with even pressure, in your counter clockwise direction (as the hypnotist is looking at it.) Counter clockwise relaxes. The other direction stimulates.

Spiral Slide Pre Talk

"Do you know what a spiral slide looks like? Have you ever seen the kind of slide that goes around and around and around and down and down and down? Good. I want you to close your eyes and see that spiral slide in your mind."

(If they say "yes" continue)

"Is it all right if I touch your forehead? Close your eyes. Good, take three deep breaths with your eyes closed. I'll place my hand on your forehead as you see yourself going around and around and around and down and down and down and deeper and deeper and deeper into relaxation. Always feeling better always relaxing more.

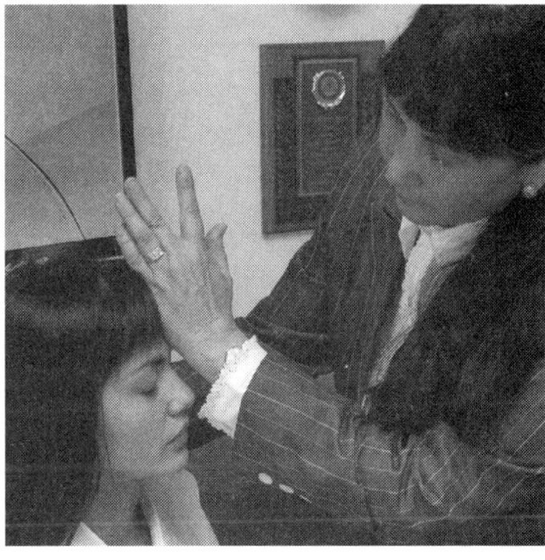

Photo by Jon Nicholas

(Each time you go through this, continue to slow the rotation of your hand.)

"Continue to see yourself going down this spiral slide as you go down and down and deeper and deeper… with just marvelous, wonderful, beautiful good feeling going through your body and nothing but peace, happiness and contentment filling your mind. As you go around and around and down and down…deeper and deeper into relaxation…always feeling better; always relaxing more." Lift the hand three inches to test for relaxation.

(You could do this a third time even slower if you like or, as a option, for a forth time: "In a moment I will touch your shoulders, your face… and all the muscles relax…")

"You are at complete peace in mind and body. You are completely relaxed in mind and body. And you are capable of accepting and acting upon each and every POSITIVE suggestion I give you…"

When suggestions are complete use a 1 to 5 count up…Count up from 1 to 5 giving suggestions with each number.

"One, your mother and your father love you. Two, your friends and your teachers all like you. Three, you are a terrific boy (or girl). Four, you are coming up more and more now. You can now open your eyes and continue to feel wonderful, marvelous and terrific."

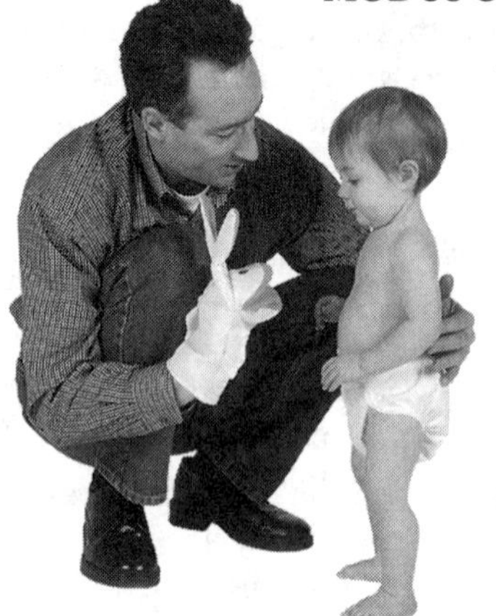

Puppet & Child

MODUS OPERANDI: ERNEST TELKEMEYER'S PUPPET INDUCTION

This works wonders for children two to six years. The puppet becomes so important that in one class the children wrote on the blackboard, "I love hypnosis. Thank you Fluffy and Ernie!" …Ernie got 2nd billing to the puppet!

Choose The Right Type Of Puppet

Choose a puppet that is friendly and cuddly. It can be a hand puppet or one that fits right up your arm; but not a marionette. Scary animals like realistic lions, tigers or bears are no good.

Never use a puppet with red eyes because the child may dream about monsters. Preferable eye color is blue or green. Pink and yellow are acceptable. Brown and black are too neutral to keep a young child's attention away from mom. If you get a brown-eyed puppet get replacement blue eyes at a hobby store. The reason for the bright eye color is that from babies on up, children respond to three things; loud noises, bright colors and movement. The puppet must have two front "feet" or "arms" (Extra hind ones are okay too).

Pre-Instruction

Prior to the session the parent explains to the young child, **"We are going to play a game called hypnosis with Ernie and his puppet will help you** _________________ (i.e. stop sucking your thumb)."

Session

Invite the child to lie down on their back on the floor. This is because as a child you play on the floor. Take your puppet and hold it so that the eyes of the puppet are right above the child's eyes. The puppet whispers in the hypnotherapist's ear, and the hypnotherapist says to the child, **"Fluffy** (Or what ever the puppet name) **wants to know if you will hypnotize him first."**

Regardless of their answer say, **"I'll help you hypnotize Fluffy, is that ok? Tell fluffy his eyes are getting tired. Tell fluffy that his eyes are getting tireder and tireder. You can hardly keep your eyes open. They are so tired just close your eyes."** (Place both of Fluffy's front feet over his eyes as you bring your hand with the puppet down and let it resting gently on the child's chest.

"See, you've got Fluffy hypnotized! We ought to give Fluffy some suggestions. What suggestions would you like to give Fluffy?" (95% of the time they say 'I don't know.' If they say one make sure it is positive or you change it to the positive).

"Well here is a nice suggestion. I know he'd like to be told that he's a nice cat. I know he'd like to be told that he's a pretty cat." (What little girl or by wouldn't like these suggestions themselves).

"Do you know how to bring Fluffy out of hypnosis?"

(Beware, a lot of time they will try to grab the puppet to shake it and you don't want this to happen, so you pull raise your hand back) **"Here is how you bring Fluffy out of hypnosis… I'm going to count from 1-3 and you'll open your eyes. Tell fluffy that. Can you count from one to three?"**

When they do fluffy moves his legs from his eyes and waves at them with his paw. Fluffy now whispers in the hypnotherapist's ear and you report:

"Fluffy wants to know if you'll do it again." (You get them more in the game)

If not, **"Fluffy it's your time to give** ____________ (The child's name) **their turn"**

Take a hold of Fluffy's ear and say,

"Fluffy I want you to give this little boy (or girl) their turn or I'll pull this ear and you won't like it."

Fluffy gets his feelings hurt and shows it by putting both his feet over his eyes. Hypnotist takes the paw down one at a time and fluffy puts it back up a couple of times.

"Looks like this going to be a one eyed job." (This makes an easier one focal point).

Have child lie down again if they have sat up, and move puppet so that they have to look up above tiring their eyes to develop eye fatigue. About half of the kid's eyes will cross.

"Your eyes are getting tired. They are getting tireder and tireder (Watch the eyes for a twitch and say, **"Now you are going to blink."**

If they blink, **"You are going to blink again. Your eyes are getting so tired you can hardly keep them open. As Fluffy passes in from of your eyes, let your eyes close and STAY CLOSED."**

After this happens move the child around with a little gentle rocking from hip to hip and lift their hand and drop an inch or so. Then go right into the suggestions and when complete count up from 1-3 **"One, your mother and your father love you. Two, you are a terrific boy (or girl). Three, you can now open your eyes and continue to feel wonderful, marvelous and terrific."**

MODUS OPERANDI: HYPNOTIZING SCHOOL CHILDREN

In the classroom you don't even need to mention the word hypnotism to make the process happen. Children love to sleep and dream and this affords a perfect entry to subconscious learning.

Begin by lowering the lights and tell your students to **"Today you will learn how to be the world's greatest student** (or athlete, or artist, or expert on history…whatever you choose to teach.) **Lean forward and nestle your head in your arms resting on top of the desk while listening to the music I will play. As you do think of how you felt last night when you were snug in your bed and going to sleep. Close your eyes and keep thinking over and over again about going to sleep…as you rest comfortably thinking of how nice it is to sleep, the music will seem to get quieter and quieter…**(gradually turn down the volume on the player) **Now take a deep breath and holding it take another deep breath and now a third deep breath pile on top of the other two and then let them all out together…good job. You are doing fine. Now one more time pile three breaths in and then when you let them all out together you will be sound asleep and ready to dream about being the world's greatest student** (or athlete, or artist, or expert on history…whatever.) **Ready inhale…one breath…inhale two breath…inhale three breath and exhale all to together and drop deep into sleep."**

(Bring the music up a bit)

"Good! You are ready now to make these dreams and ideas your very own, while you continue to sleep and dream. Your dreaming mind drops you deeper and deeper into sleep. Now dream this. You are so happy doing your schoolwork.

(Use a suggestion formula best for your goal…this one is for being a better student.)

You love leaning and you feel so close to all the students who were your age and got excellent grades because they too liked to study and learn. It was fun for them and fun for you. You are doing fine. You are so happy to be in this class leaning new and fascinating things. You are developing a super hero brain, just like Einstein, that learns easily and the more you learn the more you learn. Learning and school for you is just like a game you like

to play. A game is to be enjoyed and school is so much fun for you. It is easy for you to take tests, learn in class or from your books and from others around you. You love getting your homework done and you can see yourself getting straight A's.

Reach now into your dreams to the treasure chest within you and you now take out the treasure of your fantastic mind that so easily learns.

What I have just told you is now reality in your life. Everything that happens in school makes it more and fun for you to learn and know more and more.

(Pause)

I will count from one to five and when I reach five you will be wide-awake and raring to learn and practice using your fantastic mind. Ready…one…two…three…four and FIVE! Wide awake and feeling just fine and ready to have fun and learn."

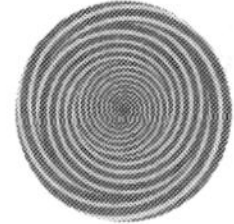

~ *Chapter 43* ~
THE CANDY INDUCTION

I designed this method especially for hypnotizing children. However, it works equally well with adults. People find it literally tasty, since they get to suck on a piece of candy during the process. It can be used with either a solo subject or a group. This method employs the sense of taste, as the central point of concentration. Of course, hypnosis can be induced through any of the senses.

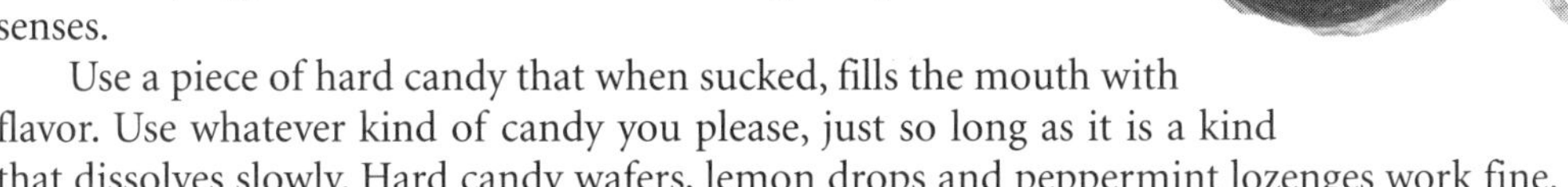

Use a piece of hard candy that when sucked, fills the mouth with flavor. Use whatever kind of candy you please, just so long as it is a kind that dissolves slowly. Hard candy wafers, lemon drops and peppermint lozenges work fine.

MODUS OPERANDI: THE CANDY INDUCTION

Your client should be seated and relaxed in a comfortable chair. Hand them a piece of candy. Tell them:

"Place the candy in your mouth and gently suck on it. You are not to chew or swallow it, but allow it to slowly dissolve on your tongue, filling your mouth with a sweet taste. Center your attention on the taste of the candy. Now, close your eyes, as I present these suggestions:

As you rest in your comfortable chair, think how good the candy tastes in your mouth. Think of the taste so completely that it seems to fill your entire body. You become the taste. And that good taste makes you feel so comfortable and relaxed. Relax. Relax. Relax. Relax and let yourself go!

Now just let your mind drift, allowing whatever thoughts to come and just pass through it. Relaxing quietly, becoming completely quiescent in both mind and body. Now breathe deeply through your nose (inhale). **Hold the breath, then exhale slowly** (exhale slowly), **and let your body relax with the brain; let everything go!**

Breathe into your nose again (inhale). **Hold the breath. Visualize energy flowing into your body with the breath. Exhale now, and as you release your breath, imagine any negativity going out of your body with the breath. Continue breathing in and out slowly and rhythmically…and with each breath, become aware of the vital energy of life moving into your body. Energy that permeates every fiber of your being sends you down towards the realm of sleep.**

How good the candy tastes and how sleepy it makes you become. So just allow the taste of the candy to pervade your being and let it make your entire body relax. Relax. Relax. Relax. How good it feels to relax completely, with that pleasant taste of candy in your mouth.

Let your thoughts of relaxation travel to every part of your body as the candy dissolves in your mouth, so you can relax now and let everything go, to go to sleep. Sleep. Sleep. Sleep. Go to sleep, dropping off into hypnotic sleep. Your conscious mind steps aside as your subconscious mind is fully aware and receptive to all the suggestions presented to you. All the suggestions become your very own. Chew up and swallow what remains of the candy now, and as it quietly goes down your throat you drop down, down deeply into hypnosis."

Now give your beneficial suggestions.

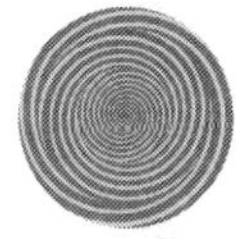

~ *Chapter 44* ~
BLUM'S SINGING BOWL INDUCTION

© 2002 Peter Blum: Blum's Himalayan Singing Bowl Induction

Peter Blum is a Ericksonian Hypnosis Instructor and world renown for his work with Tibetan bowls. His CD's are excellent to induce trance. Here is what he has to say about his fine singing bowl induction:

BLUM'S BOWLS
By Peter Blum

While most hypnotic inductions rely largely on words and/or the element of a strong visual "fix," my favorite induction derives its strength from the power of pure sound. After much research and experimentation, I settled on the sounds produced by Himalayan singing bowls as being ideal for trance induction.

First produced by the "Bön Magico" religious practitioners thousands of years ago for meditation and healing, these metal bowls ring with unearthly **Listen, Listen** beauty. The sounds they generate contain binaural beat patterns, and due to their unique acoustic properties, have a remarkably long "decay"…which is to say that the sound sustains for an unbelievably long time…gradually fading over minutes. These bowls are available for purchase to the general public at import and spiritual stores specializing in items from India and Tibet.

MODUS OPERANDI: SINGING BOWL INDUCTION

Instruct your client:

"First get comfortable. Find a position where your body can relax and your mind concentrate. In another minute or so you will hear the sound of the Himalayan singing bowl. A legendary and wise people who understood the power of sound to hypnotize produced these bowls…

According to some of the most venerated ancient teachings, all things have a beginning, middle, and an end. Thoughts, for instance… as a meditation practice, you might begin to practice noticing the arising, sustaining, and subsiding of each thought as it passes through your mind. But that's just a thought… for another time.

Now what's interesting is that our senses usually notice the beginnings of things. For instance, your sense of hearing…

What I want you to do, as this incredible instrument begins to produce these sounds, is to pay particular attention to where the sound goes…"

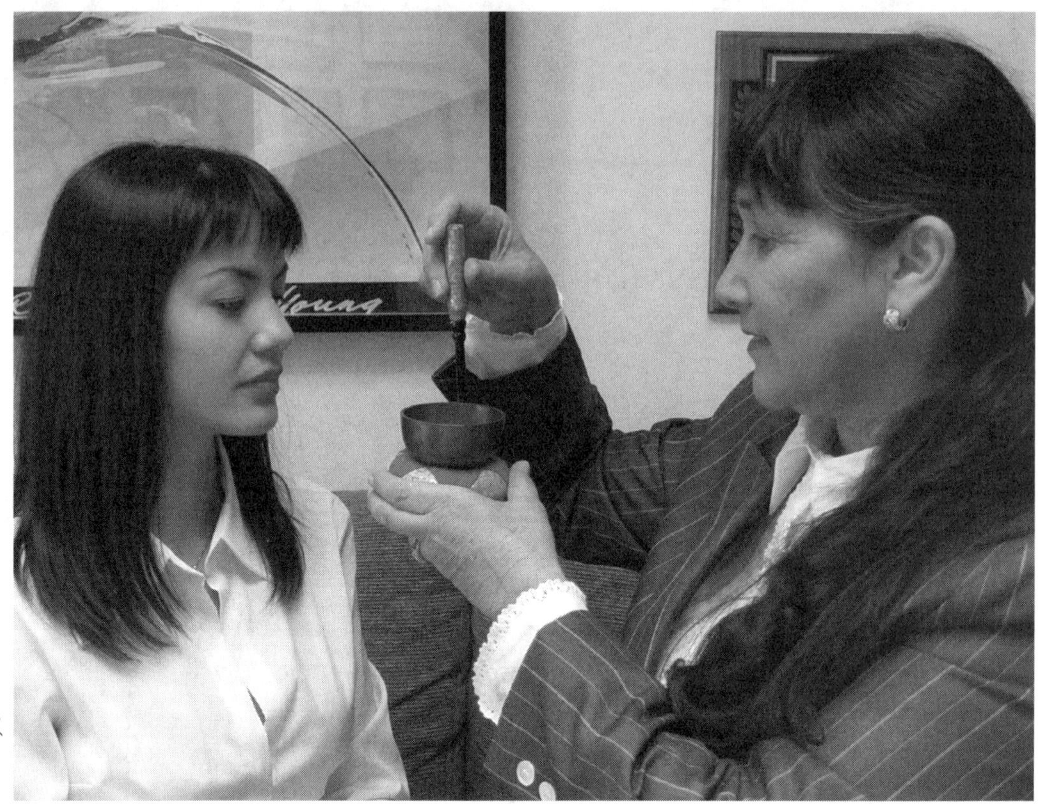

Singing Bowl

(Begin to make bowl sing)...

"Let me pass on to you the suggestion of an old and respected teacher of meditation: 'Listen to the sound disappearing...' and as your attention follows that sound, and as the sound becomes more and more faint, your own state of hypnotic fascination can deepen...simply following the sound disappearing..."

(Pause)

"While your body relaxes more and more, and your unconscious mind begins to realize some of the implications... and it's not necessary or important for your conscious mind to understand how or why... this works, but it certainly does!

And it kind of makes one... wonder... does the sound ever really end completely? Or does it just keep on getting fainter and fainter, until it is just barely perceptible...just within the range of hearing...like my voice, which you can continue to tune in and out of your conscious awareness, as your unconscious learns more useful information."

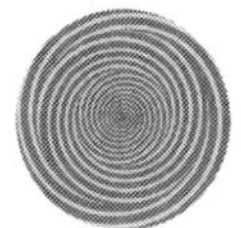

~ *Chapter 45* ~
TRANSPERSONAL INDUCTION

Transpersonal experiences are those flashes of surprising awareness within the range of experiences beyond the normal five senses. Mind has the capability of moving beyond 3-D space and time, via the forth dimension, penetrating other dimensions. This is known as "perception from out of the abyss." Sometimes they come unbidden. The transpersonal includes ESP phenomena, out of body experiences, sensing the visiting presence of a beloved who had died, and having the perception of cosmic consciousness. Always such are part of the experiences of life in realms beyond which we conventionally regard are "normal."

This is a remarkable induction and induces profound hypnosis. It takes the mind through the realms of reverie and dreams into the realm of sleep.

On occasion, you can use such transpersonal experience with your clients while in the Beta state. Just read to them the list of Transpersonal Experiences you have here, and ask them to tell you of any such they may have had. Their answers will give you excellent insight into the type of client you are working with. Transpersonal experiences are good for your client to recall, as it increases the depth of perception of the individual. And they are good for you, their hypnotherapist, as well.

Some are more visual while others are more auditory. In experimenting with these psychic talents, use whatever approach works best for the subject. If their perception comes in through a sense of hearing– such as an inner voice– use an auditory approach.

MODUS OPERANDI: TRANSPERSONAL HYPNOTHERAPY
You will need:
Sleep Shades To Cover The Eyes
A Reclining Chair Or A Couch To Lie Back Upon
Soft Meditative Music in the background, such as "Golden Voyage" or "Ancient Echoes"

Instruct your client to **"Become one with the music"** and play the music for five minutes as a prelude to the session.

The "sleep shade" keeps out light and promotes individual privacy. This of itself suggests relaxation and dropping into the realm of sleep. This puts the person in a subjective state of mind, ready to respond to the list of transpersonal experience questions, which their inner mind will answer as personal to them.

One-by-one ask about the transpersonal experiences and note any that the client answers as "yes." These questions and their subconscious responses just by their nature elicit a deepening of hypnosis as the client drops deeper and deeper into the abyss. Their yes answers become the goal of your session as later the client will be called to re-experience each one. Here are your instructions to the relaxing client:

"As you relax in darkness visualize yourself dropping down, down, down into the abyss of yourself, out of which the transpersonal experiences you have know will come forth. As I ask you each of these, your subconscious knows if such has occurred to you. If so, you will lift your right forefinger meaning 'yes, I know that well.' If there is no recognition, there will be no finger movement. Rest your right hand upon your solar plexus now and be ready to give the subconscious finger signals for those events your subconscious knows if such has occurred to you. All right, here we go:

Have you ever had an out of body experience?
Have you ever felt you had a guardian angel or spirit?
Have you ever had a near death experience?
Have you ever seen a ghost?
Have you ever been aware of parallel worlds?
Have you ever seen a UFO or an alien?
Have you ever experienced a telepathic message?
Have you ever seen auras?
Have you ever felt a connection with the consciousness of machines?
Have you ever experienced the consciousness of plants?
Have you ever had a conscious communication with animals?
Have you ever had flashes of cosmic consciousness, which seemed as a direct connection with the cosmos?
Have you ever recalled events from past lives?
Have you ever heard spirit raps, voices or noises?
Have you ever experienced a poltergeist?
Have you ever dreamed you were dreaming while you were dreaming?
Have you ever had a clairvoyant experience?
Have you ever had a remission of a terminal illness?
Have you ever felt that the planet earth is not your real home?"

Now one-by-one take them back to the experiences they responded to with a "yes."

"Drop down into the abyss of your inner self now and experience again how it felt when you had _______________ (an out of body experience, past life, etc...). As you re-enter this experience, you will drop even deeper and deeper into hypnosis."

Allow time for then to re-experience each one.

"You are now in profound hypnosis and will benefit in every way from the hypnotherapy session I will give you..."

Arouse the client at the conclusion of your beneficial suggestions.

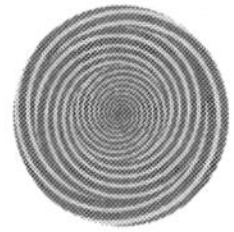

Chapter 46
~ HYPNODANCE ~

Includes
Hypnodance

Dancing is entrancing!

Whirling, tribal dances and war dances all induce hypnosis by dancing. The movement, rhythm, steps and gestures transfix the dancer and those who watch. In tribal rites the members of the dance are aware of the purpose of the ritual and concentrate on its accomplishment. Their total involvement and crowd psychology rapidly evolves into a trance state. An Afro-Brazilian spiritual sect uses a process called "TTT" meaning "Terpsichore Trance Therapy." In this method the consultation is provided both before and after the session. A hypnotic state is induced using predominantly rotational movements.

You are familiar with the use of music in hypnotherapy. Low musical sounds can induce relaxation and lead toward the hypnotic state of mind. The music of hypnodance employs sound with the kinesthetic, fatigue and monotony. This offers powerful hypnotic effects. There is no need with this approach to say, "You are getting sleepier and sleepier" or "You are becoming more and more relaxed." There is no need to mention deep breathing as the physical exertion causes this spontaneously.

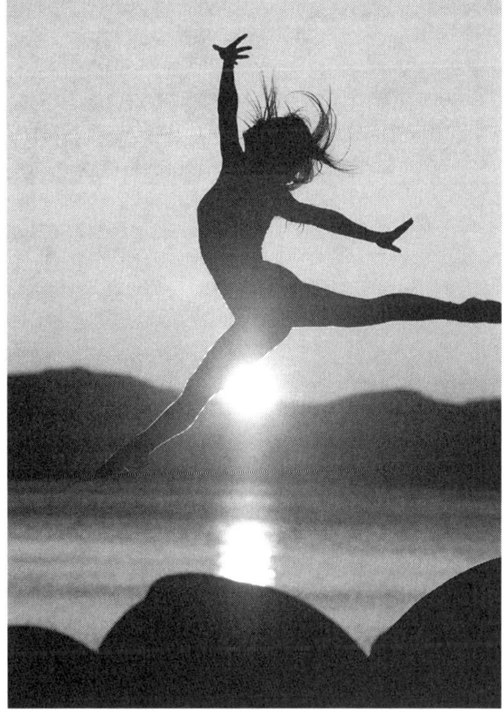

The dancing itself defocuses attention to the extent that a person afflicted with functional paralysis can often move when following the pattern of a dance. They become so enraptured that they are entranced.

MODUS OPERANDI: HYPNODANCE

Professional dancer and hypnotherapist Diana L. England created Hypnodance. Here is how to do it. Establish a goal to be accomplished such as freely expressing oneself, allow the body to move with grace of what ever your client wants to accomplish. Then let the dance begin.

There are many possibilities.

The dancer may use accompaniment or silence that may or may not be rhythmical. The dance may be calculated or the dancer may surrender to the excitement of the movement. The client may chant affirmations as they dance. They may move long enough to become exhausted and then comfortably relax. It can be applied to solo or group sessions. For those who are artistic in nature, it can be enjoyed and develop social skills, artistic grace and personal expression.

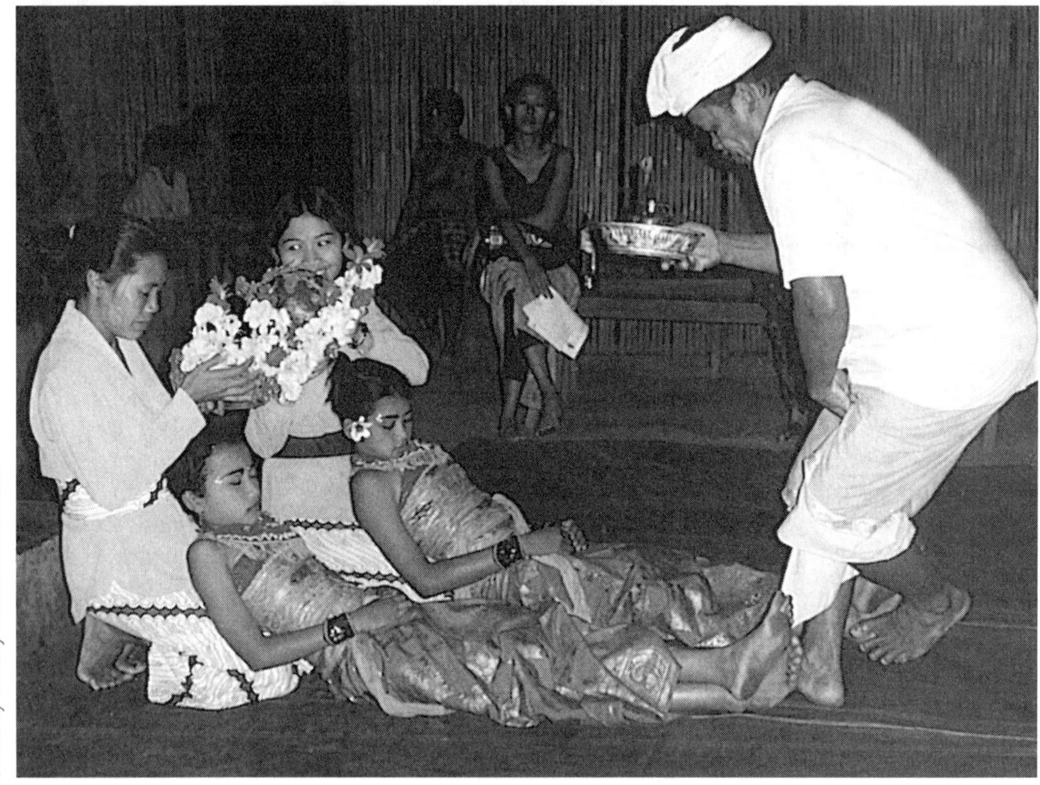

Photo by Shelley Stockwell-Nicholas

Trance Dancers
Bali, Indonesia

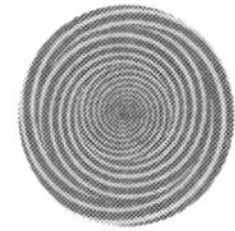

~ *Chapter 47* ~
OTTO'S VERTIGO INDUCTION
By Hypnotherapist Robert F. Otto

Children like to spin and twirl in circles. This fabulous induction involves spinning a person in a chair and because of our innate inner ear perception of movement offers a foolproof induction. Here is the principle behind the induction:

Below your eyes, and behind your cheekbones, is the semicircular canal that is filled with a gel type fluid and microscopic hairs called cupula. The cupula is imbedded within the canal and senses the movement of the fluid. The fluid bends the hairs and says to your brain "I am going in this direction." It tells you the yaw and angular acceleration. Due to inertia, when the subject is rotated, the fluid in the canal lags behind the rotation, thus bending the cupula. The vestibular nerve located at the bottom of the cupula transmits a clockwise indication to the brain. As the rotation continues at about 15 revolutions per minute (RPMs) the fluid begins to catch up with the rotation of the canal, while giving the subject a false sensation of slowing down.

Another false sensation is that of no motion at all, if both fluid and canal rotate at the same speed. Had the subject been kept at a constant speed of 15 RPMs for several moments, the cupula would return to the vertical position.

Deceleration causes the subject to sense a counter-clockwise rotation, due to the tilt of the cupula in the opposite direction. When stopped suddenly to no movement, the fluid continues to rush onward, bending the cupula all the way over, indicating an extreme turn to the left. Hence, within 10-13 seconds we have induced a physiological state of vertigo that must occur.

MODUS OPERANDI: OTTO'S VERTIGO INDUCTION

You will need;

A "Rotating" Type Office Chair, Preferably With A Foot Rest
A Pencil

The Set Up

"Okay _______________ (Their name) please seat yourself (Suggestion of compliance) **comfortably in this chair. Place your feet so that they do not interfere with any obstructions, or touch the floor and place your hands in your lap."** (Make a gesture, an unconscious command, and hand them a pencil).

"After you are comfortably seated, I am going to rotate the chair in a clockwise direction a few times. You will feel a few intermittent interruptions in the rotation as I do this. However, at some point, you will feel yourself moving in the opposite direction. When this occurs, you will also begin to feel a complete sense of total physical relaxation. When you feel yourself moving in that opposite direction, along with physical relaxation, I would like you to simply drop the pencil. The rotation in the opposite direction will become as smooth as

silk. No interruptions at all. What I would like you to do with the pencil now is to ask that you direct the pencil to the way you are rotating. When you feel yourself moving to the left, point the pencil to the left. And likewise when you feel yourself moving to the right, point the pencil to the right. When the rotation becomes as smooth as silk in the opposite direction, drop the pen. Are you certain that you understand my instructions? Good."

Or a slightly shorter version

"I will rotate you slowly in one direction and I will give you a pen to hold. Point the pen in the direction that your body is going. If you go to the left, tilt the pen to the left. If you change direction and go to the right, drop the pen. You are totally aware of everything that is going on as I move you in one direction, then slow you down and then take you to the other direction. At the time you notice the opposite directional pull it will feel as smooth as glass and you will relax completely and drop the pen."

The Induction

Stand behind the client who is safely seated in the chair and place your hands upon their shoulders with slight downward pressure. As you do this, speak softly and begin the induction by saying:

"Just close your eyes now and listen to the sound of my voice. Any and all outside interference will be of little importance to you at this time. You are enjoying the feeling of relaxation sweeping over your entire body from the tips of your toes to the top of your head. Feeling very relaxed and comfortable. Take a deep breath in and now out; feeling very loose, limp and relaxed in every way. Begin the rotation…rotate them 8 to 10 times. No more than 13. After the rotation, allow them to come to a slow and complete stop. Help the stop along if necessary. As the client comes to a complete stop, and the pencil is dropped, begin your favorite deepening technique. Then do an arm drop and begin the session.

This entire induction takes about 20-30 seconds from the time the client is seated. Reaffirm the induction immediately after your up-count by asking the client, **"You enjoy the smooth as silk opposite rotation. There were no bums at all, were there?"** This suggestion is beneficial when using the Vertigo Induction for demonstrational purposes. It gives a clear demonstration that the client was indeed hypnotized.

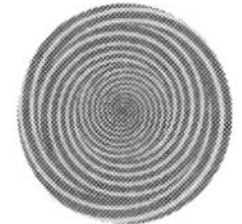

~ *Chapter 48* ~
THE WHIRLING DERVISH INDUCTION

Includes
Three Whirling Dervish Methods
The Slow Revolving Method
Rapid Self-Whirling
Guided Rapid Whirling

The Whirling Dervish Sect of India and the Sufi's of Egypt use a most unusual method of self-hypnosis. These devoted people do not call whirling, hypnosis. They say that their dance entrances them to clear away sin and advance spiritually. Whirling is regarded as a spiritual experience because the intent of it is spiritual, not because the trance induced is spiritual. The Dervishes whirl and whirl around and around until they achieve "holiness" or "become what one thinkest in one's heart."

A western hypnotherapist would say, "Whirling causes a disorientation of normal wakeful awareness and thus one bypasses critical mind." Selective thinking (suggestion) is then directly given and accepted by the subconscious as, "One becomes what one believes they will become."

Dizziness increases hyper-suggestibility. The spinner is more responsiveness to suggestion.

The WHIRLING DERVISH technique provides an excellent form of hypnotherapy. Sometimes called "spinning," it has produced striking results in our clinic. I offer you a Western version of Eastern methods. Develop them as a specialty in your office.

Sufi Dancer, Cairo

MODUS OPERANDI: THREE WHIRLING DERVISH METHODS

There are three forms of this approach
1. A Slow Revolving Method
2. A Rapid Self-Whirling Method And
3. A Rapid Whirling Guided Method.

METHOD ONE: THE SLOW METHOD
You will need:
Hypnotic Music (*Serenity Resonance Sound* or *Hypno-Music* is recommended)

Client and hypnotherapist sit in chairs facing each other.

Arise and light the candle in each corner. Dim the lights in the room so candlelight predominates. Be seated and **"Let silence flow between us as we gaze deeply into each other's eyes. Let us look upon the eyes of one another as windows to the inner self or soul."** Five minutes of such gazing creates intense rapport.

In a brief consultation, let your client tell you what they wish to clear away from their life and what they want to achieve to improve their life.

Instruct them to **"Stand in the center of the room while I stand beside you.**

You will enter into hypnosis by revolving your body and doubling your breathing as you gaze at each candle in turn. By the time you reach candle four, you will be in profound hypnosis."

No specific directions are given to how fast or slow the whirling is to be accomplished. The client sets their own pace and simply whirls around.

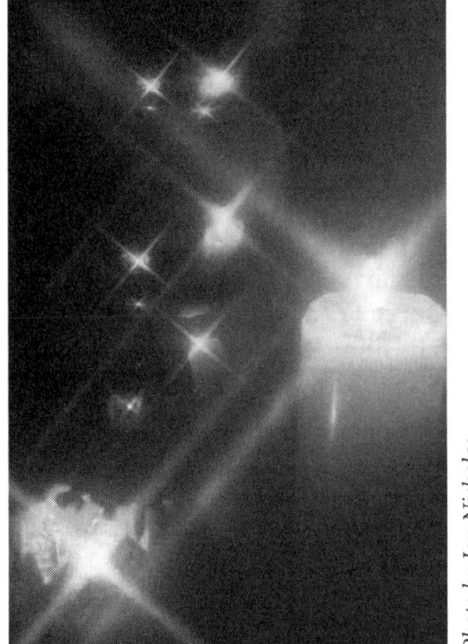

Put on hypnotic music. I recommend my "Serenity Resonance Sound" or "Hypno-Music," which has the alpha theta vibrations in the background.

Start by having them stare at candle number one. **"Stare at candle number one and take one deep breath, inhale, hold…exhale and relax as you say to yourself, 'I am going into hypnosis. I am going to sleep in profound hypnosis.'"**

Give them time to complete this assignment then proceed.

"Revolve your body around in a complete circle until you return to face candle number two. Then repeat the suggestion out loud, 'I am going into hypnosis. I am going to sleep in profound hypnosis.'

Give them time to complete this assignment then proceed.

While staring at candle two take two deep breaths in succession…inhale, hold…exhale. Inhale, hold…exhale. Relax.

Now revolve your body around in a circle two times ending at candle three. As you repeat the suggestion two times, 'I am going into hypnosis. I am going into hypnosis. I am going to sleep in profound hypnosis. I am going to sleep in profound hypnosis.'

Give them time to complete this assignment then proceed.

Now while staring at candle three, take three deep breaths in succession: Inhale, hold…exhale. Inhale, hold…exhale. Inhale, hold…exhale. Relax.

Revolve your body around in circle three times ending at candle four as you repeat the suggestion three times; 'I am going into hypnosis. I am going into hypnosis. I am going into hypnosis. I am going to sleep in profound hypnosis. I am going to sleep in profound hypnosis. I am going to sleep in profound hypnosis.'

Give them time to complete this assignment then proceed.

While staring at candle four, take four deep breaths in succession: "Inhale, hold…exhale. Inhale, hold…exhale. Inhale, hold…exhale. Inhale, hold…exhale. Relax.

Spin four times as you repeat, out loud to yourself this suggestion, 'I am going into hypnosis. I am going into hypnosis. I am going into hypnosis. I am going to sleep in profound hypnosis. I am going into hypnosis. I am going to sleep in profound hypnosis. I am going to sleep in profound hypnosis.'

Give them time to complete this assignment then proceed.

As you stare at candle four, your feet are steady and you remain upright as you drop down in profound hypnosis. Your eyelids close and roll upward beneath your eyelids. You are in hypnosis now and ready to be led to a pleasant seat. As your hypnotherapist I will now assist you to proceed with the beneficial session of hypnosis."

Seat them in the chair and give them suggestions you choose. When you are complete, turn off the music. Blow out the candles. Bring up the room lights.

THE SESSION IS COMPLETE.

METHOD TWO: THE RAPID SELF-WHIRLING METHOD

You Will Need:

A Fully Lighted Room

Sufi Music (If available. If not, use *Hypno-Music*)

This vigorous method is most like that used by the Dervishes to entrance themselves. It involves energetic physical exertion, so it may be best used with younger or more physically fit clients. Whirling is at first a deliberate experience of the body. With practice, the rapid revolving becomes automatic. Whirling rapidly induces trance. You can suggest that the spinning stop or you can let the client determine when to stop. Often when whirling stops you'll notice rigidity in a standing client. You can guide them to a chair if you like. Or they can remain standing.

With the rapid whirling session, the room may be fully lighted, warm and pleasant.

Sufi music can be played. It is often available in New Age bookstores. Or, if you like, you can play my Hypnomusic cassette loudly.

Start by discussing what it is that they want to accomplish. You will keep this goal in mind if positive suggestions are your goal later in the session. Or, you can let them solve their own issues by giving them permission for positive self-talk.

Simply say, **"Let such become the case. Stand up now and just start whirling yourself around and around as you repeat these positive suggestions loudly and fully. When you feel it is time to stop whirling, sit in your seat, and drop down, deeper and deeper into hypnosis, in which you KNOW that you are MASTER of yourself. Here you can talk to yourself or listen to the beneficial suggestions you give yourself.**

Take your time; there is no hurry.

I leave you as you whirl around. Continue to whirl until your inner self knows you have achieved that which you came here to achieve. When all is accomplished to your absolute perfection, you will automatically stop the whirling, retake your seat, close your eyes, and drop deep into the abyss of yourself…into profound hypnosis. Do what your subconscious tells you is best to do.

You are on your own, alone in space and time.

When you arise, you will be completely cleansed and perfect in every way. You will know when your desire has become your reality and when you are done, you will arouse yourself, feeling wonderful, well and perfect in every way."

Allow your client to perform as their subconscious phase of mind instructs. They will arouse from the hypnosis when their mind is crystal clear and their wish has been accomplished.

METHOD THREE: GUIDED RAPID WHIRLING METHOD

This is the noisy version of method two. Your client will shout their self-suggestion as they spin around. Tell them to breathe rapidly, in and out, in and out, and in and out as they loudly and forcefully repeat their self-suggestions.

"As I whirl around and around, I go deeper and deeper into hypnosis. I am completely caught up in the whirling. My consciousness mind fades away and vanishes as I enter the subconscious mind. I automatically accept all beneficial suggestions given me by my hypnotherapist. The perfection of my BEING is my reality. I enter into profound hypnosis."

If you prefer to do the talking as they spin, you can use this suggestion formula:

"Around and around and around you go. As you revolve, your subconscious opens wide and turns what wish for yourself into reality. Your mind is clear like crystal, and you become a holy one. Because you are WHOLE you recognize the wonderful immortal BEING you truly are.

Continue to whirl until your inner self knows that it is time for you to automatically stop the whirling. Then, retake your seat, close your eyes and drop deep into the abyss of yourself; into profound hypnosis. Here you will receive the suggestions given by me, your Hynotherapist, and these suggestions will become your reality. When you arise, you will be completely cleansed and perfect in every way."

Now offer them your affirmations for that which they desire. When you are complete, instruct them to arouse from hypnosis.

Your session is complete.

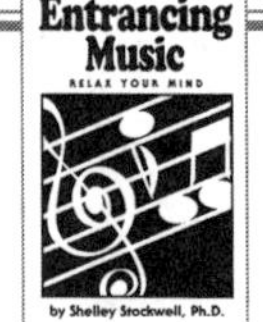

Hypno-Helper
"Serenity Resonance Sound" and "Hypno-Music"
by Ormond McGill and Joseph Worrell
"Entrancing Music" with Billy Krodel can be ordered at hypnosisfederation.com
or from the order form at the back of this book.

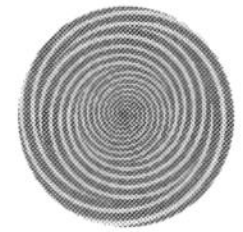

~ *Chapter 49* ~
INSTANT GAMMA HYPNOSIS

Includes
Instant Hypnosis
The Sudden Jerk
The Body Bump
The Evangelist Method
Gamma Hypnosis En Masse

Most hypnotic inductions aim to lower brain frequencies. Gamma Hypnosis operates in the high brain frequencies range. There is still much to be discovered in mental phenomena within the Gamma range. However, we are not complete strangers.

Theta Hypnosis lowers the brain frequencies to enter the subjective realm of hypnosis. Gamma Hypnosis raises brain frequencies to enter the subjective realm of hypnosis. This is to say that hypnosis may be accomplished on both ends of the frequency ratio of the biocomputer brain in accordance to the programmed stimuli presented. Brain frequencies develop in response to thoughts that the mind programs the brain computer to respond to. This, in turn, causes the body to respond. And the more the body responds the greater becomes the power of the thoughts.

GAMMA RHYTHM 41 – 100 Hz Hyper brain activity
BETA RHYTHM 21 – 13 Hz Normal brain activity
ALPHA RHYTHM 12 – 8 Hz Relaxed brain activity
THETA RHYTHM 7 – 4 Hz Hypnotic brain activity
DELTA RHYTHM 3 – 0 Hz Sleep brain activity

The full potential of the gamma brain frequencies is still to be investigated. It may be that gamma range enters the infinite.

Charcot of the Salpetriere Academy performed most of his hypnotherapy with clients in the Gamma state. Charcot worked mainly with hysterics, whose brains operate in the Gamma Range.

Gamma Hypnosis bypasses critical mind and establishes selective thinking (directed suggestions subconsciously accepted). It does this by stimulating and heightening the waking frequencies of the brain to frenzy. In frenzy, we move mind beyond the control of the conscious mind. Frenzy brain activity produces subconscious responses as effectively as lowered frequencies. They may be more difficult to control, but their potential for miraculous body performance is even greater.

Gamma Hypnosis may be produced in an instant with the right hypnotic stimuli, or it can be built with a continuous, ever-increasing energy crescendo.

Instant Hypnosis

Hypnosis is never actually instantaneous, but the brain operates so rapidly, it seems instantaneous. All "instantaneous" hypnotic methods are gamma methods.

Success of an instant induction increases when the subject expects to be hypnotized. Expectancy is a wakeful brain phenomenon. Shock and startle techniques raise brain frequencies to heightened degrees of response (just how high is yet to be discovered). In the immediate moment, your brain speeds up and bypasses all lower frequencies, allowing suggestions to be uncritically accepted. Shock Methods invoke a sudden agitation of the mind where your subconscious immediately accepts suggestion…usually the one word **"SLEEP!"** forcefully spoken is sufficient to produce hypnosis.

Unexpected activity in the body produces a frenzy in the mind. Mental frenzy, even for a moment, removes critical mind control, and opens the brain-computer to subconscious response. Here are some rapid techniques:

MODUS OPERANDI: THE SUDDEN JERK INDUCTION

Have the subject stare into your eyes with the intention of being hypnotized. Watch the eyes, and a sort of vacant look will come in. You can both observe and sense it. At that psychological moment, reach out and grip the person's hand and give a forceful jerk forward. This will cause the person's hand to flop downward toward their lap. At that very instant, give a command, **"Close your eyes and SLEEP this very instant."**

Immediately place your free hand on back of their head and press down, while rapidly continuing the suggestions: **"Melt down, melt down into deep hypnosis immediately now! Melt down."**

Anything that comes to the mind unexpectedly causes mental control to temporarily stand aside, and open subconscious receptivity. The subconscious mind acts upon suggestions given in that moment.

MODUS OPERANDI: THE BODY BUMP INDUCTION

This method of Instantaneous Hypnosis combines the expectation of hypnosis with a physical "bump." The combination results in a rapid induction.

Tell the subject that he (or she) is going to be hypnotized. This creates expectation.

Have the subject stand in front of a chair. Make sure the chair is directly behind the person, so they may safely fall back into it. Ask the subject to close their eyes and to concentrate upon your suggestions:

"Your chair is right behind you. Think of falling back into it. Already you begin to feel an impulse pulling you over backwards to sit in that chair. You commence to fall back, back, backwards to sit in that chair. Sit down in that chair. Back, back you go. Sit down. Sit down. Sit down!"

The subject will sway, falling backwards to the chair with a decided bump. At the moment the bump is experienced, shout, **"SLEEP! GO TO SLEEP THIS EVERY MOMENT – NOW!"**

The bump causes a jar of the body. Immediately grip the subject's head and gently rotate it around and around several times. Do this so as not to hurt the person. This deepens the instant hypnosis. Then, gently push head down toward their lap, and directly state, "You are in deep hypnosis now. Sound asleep and in profound hypnosis!"

The state of hypnosis is induced.

MODUS OPERANDI: THE EVANGELIST METHOD

Religious zeal produces a frenzied mind that is highly responsive to suggestion. This is easy to observe. A person in this gamma state can quickly be given a command that will be obeyed, sometimes with miraculous results.

In the zealous state of mind, a person standing before an evangelist is given a smart poke on the forehead, snapping the head back. At this moment, the suggestion is given, **"The power of God is upon you. Heal! Heal! Heal!"**

The popular suggestion, "HEAL!" is effective in the moment, but often results are not lasting. The subconscious is very literal. A better suggestion is, **"HEAL NOW AND FOREVER."**

All forms of Instant Gamma Hypnosis require expectancy. This can be anything that the subject believes and has confidence in: hypnosis, the power of God, the danger of Satan, snake oil, whatever.

Whatever the expectancy is, use it to induce the subjective state of mind, which, when combined with an unexpected occurrence to the body, produces gamma hypnosis. The state is then directed as desired.

GAMMA HYPNOSIS EN MASSE

Instantaneous Hypnosis is a one-shot deal. Gamma Hypnosis En Masse is a repetition of that one-shot over and over and over, and the constant repetition increases its power. Examples of Gamma Hypnosis En Masse are historic, and take many forms, usually with crowds of people. Crowd suggestion is contagious: Voodoo Ceremonies, Tribal Dancing, Lynching Parties, Religious Revival Meetings, Speaking in Tongues, and Saint Vitus Dance, are examples. Each always has the basis of expectancy followed by a physical response of some sort. When Gamma frequencies run wild in the brain– mind turns them into thoughts, and thoughts produce actions in the body both physically and mentally.

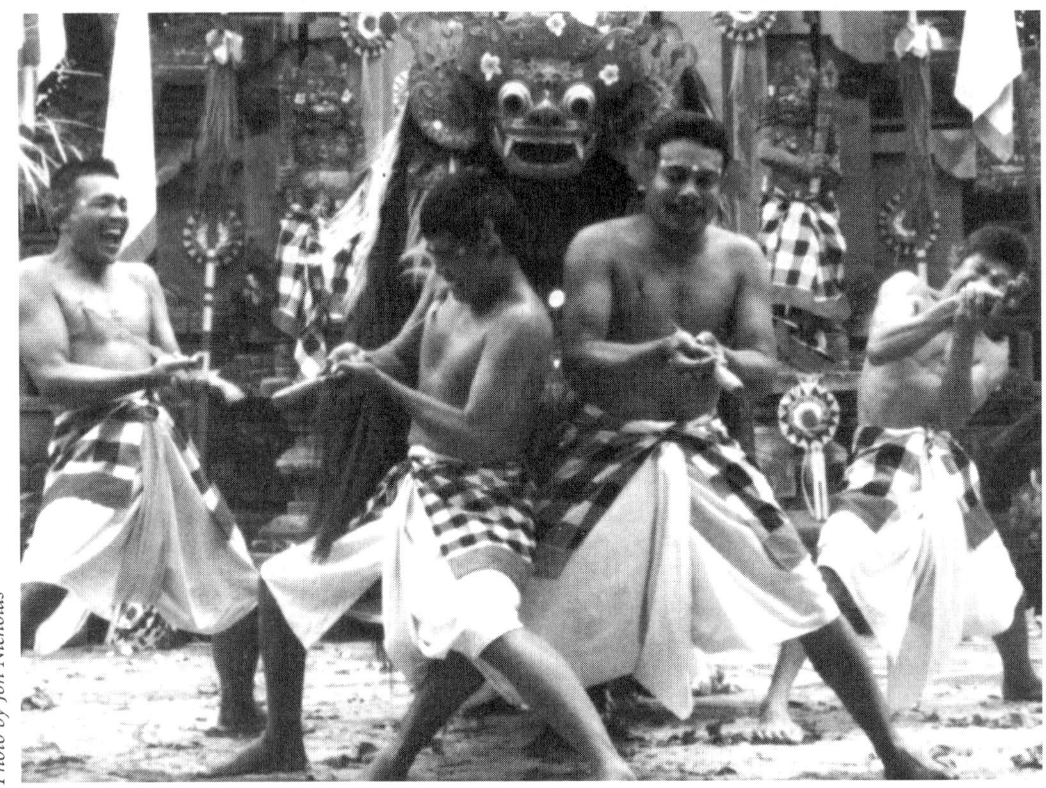

Kris Dancers
Bali, Indonesia

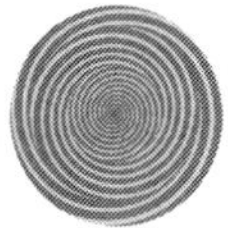

~ *Chapter 50* ~
ORIENTAL HYPNOTHERAPY INDUCTIONS

Includes
Hindu Levitation
Breezy Method
Hum & Heavy
Go To Sweep Method
Up, Up And Away Method
Read Then Dead
Take Your Toll
Head Of The Class
Head Of The Glass
Reflect on Relaxation
Look To Me For Hypnosis
Three Finger Stroke Method
The AUM Induction

I ran into an old manuscript on hypnotism while traveling in India. Included were these old rotogravure photographs of an East Indian hypnotist. They offer various ideas for hypnotic induction techniques.

Reports tell of expert Yogis or Adepts who can, just with a look, restrain wild beasts in the forest. Yogis are said to be able to place live charcoal in the hands of hypnotized person without burning the flesh. Visit Bali, Indonesia and you will see Hindu trance dancers walk unscathed across hot coals and not be cut as they stab themselves with a razor sharp swords called a "kris." I don't recommend that you try these particular demonstrations.

Hypnotism and long distance hypnotherapeutic-healing methods have been practiced in the Orient centuries before it became popular in the Occidental culture.

Hypnotic powers are universal and available to all. The void is not selective of race, creed or religion. Oriental hypnotism and the occidental hypnotism are equal. If the oriental seems more profound, it is because in the unusual is found expectancy. In expectancy is found belief. In belief is found the powers of suggestion in action. Use the following induction methods as you wish. Possibly combine them to your own private method.

HINDU LEVITATION

Oriental hypnotists often practice levitation. A tremendous strength of will is required to accomplish this feat. The levitator practices a breath control discipline up to a hundred times per day to render their body light and the mind calm enough to levitate.

The breathing preparation is done in the morning of a fast. The levitator closes the right nostril with the finger and draws in the air slowly through the left nostril until he has mentally counted sixteen. He then closes both nostrils and retains the air in his lungs while he counts to sixty-four. The air is then slowly exhaled through the right nostril during the count of thirty-two.

When the subject feels prepared, he extends himself on his back and is hypnotized. The hypnotist then energetically wills that a large volume of light air shall enter all parts of their subject's body so that it becomes lighter and float above lighter than air.

BREEZY METHOD

The hypnotist extends their hands with fingers spread apart and waves them around the head of the subject, whose eyes gradually close into hypnotic sleep. Blowing on the subject's forehead increases the effectiveness of the process.

HUM & HEAVY

The subject is seated comfortably and is told, **"Repeat this short sound of aahh** (Any monosyllables like "oh" or "um" will do, too) **in a low voice."** While they do the hypnotist makes stroking downward sweeps or passes before their eyes. This soon results in heaviness of the eyelids, followed by profound hypnotic sleep.

GO TO SWEEP METHOD

The client is seated in an erect position and you the hypnotist place your right hand gently upon the client's head. Then, immediately sweep your left hand with sweeping motions down over the client's spine. Sleep will soon ensue.

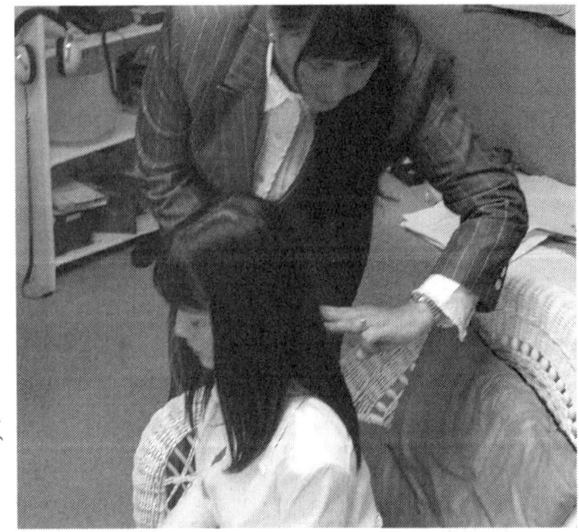 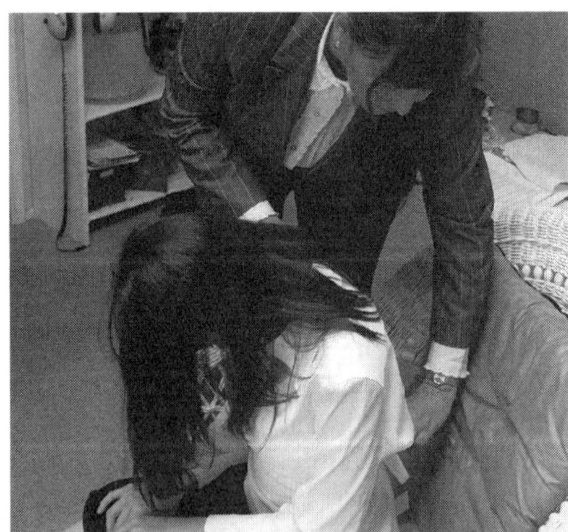

Photos by Jon Nicholas

Go To Sweep Method

UP, UP & AWAY METHOD

The client self induces trance by gazing intently upward. Only a slight suggestion is needed to induce hypnotic sleep.

READ THEN DEAD

You will need a book for this one.

Hand the book to client and instruct them **"You will enter into hypnosis today by simply**

reading and spelling every word very carefully, on the page before you." Hypnosis ensues before the client can complete reading even a single page.

TAKE YOUR TOLL

The subject is told, **"You will go into hypnotic sleep at the hundredth** (or twentieth) **stroke of the chime** (or bell)." The hypnotist then strikes a metal cup with an iron rod (Or strokes a chime or rings a bell) one hundred times (or twenty times) or until they drop away.

HEAD OF THE CLASS

Place the palm of your right hand on the subject's head, while suggesting that their head will gradually become so heavy he will be obliged to close his eyes and go to sleep.

HEAD OF THE GLASS

There is a theory in India that if someone closes their ears with their fingers, they will hear sounds like pieces of glass falling at a great distance. Concentration upon this sound induces hypnosis.

Instruct, **"As I close your ears with my fingers you will hear and concentrate on the sound much like falling glass far away in the distance and as this happens you will go deeply into hypnosis."**

REFLECT ON RELAXATION

You need a mirror for this one.

Hand the client a hand mirror, placing it into their hand at a distance of eight or ten inches from their face. Instruct them to **"Gaze intently into the reflection of your eyes in a mirror."** This technique induces profound hypnosis.

LOOK TO ME FOR HYPNOSIS

Have the subject stare into the hypnotist's eyes to induce hypnosis. The subject becomes hypnotized.

THREE FINGER STROKE METHOD

Hypnotic sleep can be induced by stroking the subject's head upward with three fingers while suggesting, **"You cannot open your eyes."**

THE OHM INDUCTION

You will need:
The Serenity Resonance Sound
A Burning Candle on a table before the client

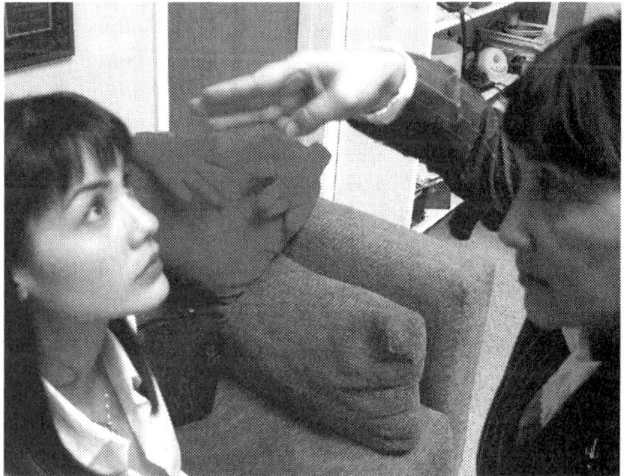

Three Finger Method

Photo by Jon Nicholas

"As the drone of The Serenity Resonance Sound comes in, close your eyes and relax comfortably in your chair. Enter the sound as it floods the room. Now take six deep breaths in succession thinking of the breaths bringing in prahnic energy, which you store in your solar plexus.

Visualize a magic circle being drawn around us unifying us in a single cause; your joy and inner harmony. Now, open your eyes as the music fades away and concentrate your attention on the candle flame before you. While gazing upon it, let the sound of AUM

mantra move through you three times as you make a cosmic connection. (Vocalize the AUM with them three times.)

Now lock your hands together in the AUM mantra way (The prayer position above the head) as you lift them above your head and increase the energy in your body. You will find that your hands become locked together firmly. So firmly that they cannot separate them, tug as hard as you will.

(Give them time to try)

They will separate immediately when I blow out the candle.

(Blow out the candle)

You have taken a quantum leap from mental to physical control of your body.

Close your eyes now and mentally affirm 'I am eager to learn the art of hypnosis as I move from pretending to believing' as you now master your mind and become a mastermind..."

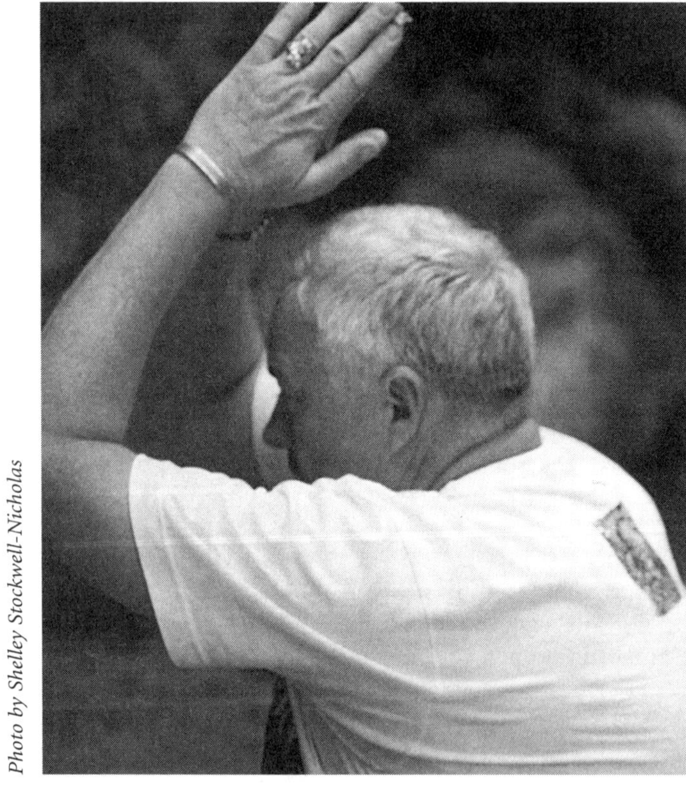

Aum Prayer Position

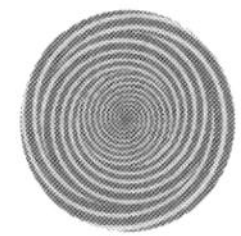

Chapter 51

THE ORIENTAL COBRA METHOD

Expectancy is an important ingredient for successful hypnotherapy. It is a principle no hypnotherapist can neglect. Expectancy is to believe something is going to happen. Often it is built on reputation. A prominent hypnotherapist is far more likely to chalk up clinical successes, than someone with no prestige.

The healing waters of so-called Holy Shrines provide an example. Chemically tested, such water is no different than any other water, but the belief that it has healing powers does the trick. Miracles occur.

IT IS THE POWER OF SUGGESTION IN OPERATION.

This Oriental Cobra Method is an excellent example of how expectancy induces profound hypnosis. This method was witnessed in India.

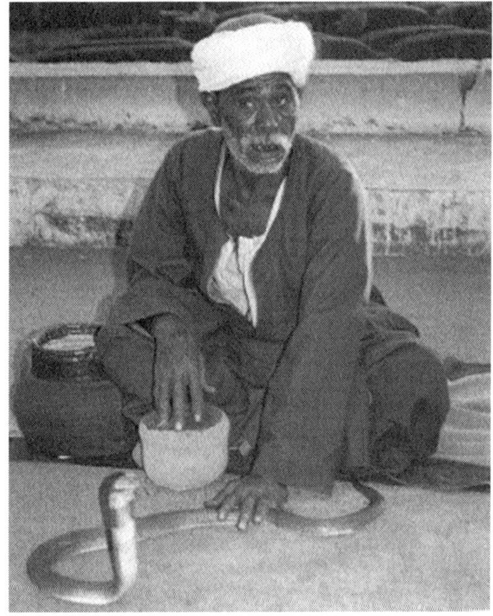

Photo by Jon Nicholas

MODUS OPERANDI: THE ORIENTAL COBRA METHOD
You Will Need:
Hindu Music
Cushions To Sit Upon

The room is dark and incense fills the air. The subject is seated on a cushion in front of the hypnotist. Expectancy commences by the hypnotist telling the subject **"You will be hypnotized by the 'oriental cobra method,' which is the swaying method a cobra uses to entrance its prey. It will in no way harm you, but it will entrance you entirely.**

Now, in absolute silence my body will begin to sway like the cobra sways and you will find that your body will commence to sway in unison like a snake's, too, as the process proceeds. You will find yourself swaying right along with the me, like the cobra, more-and-more…until you drop into the abyss of a deep trance."

Expectancy of what is going to occur has been described. The trap for the mind has been set. Some Hindu music comes in softly forming a background to the swaying hypnotic induction. The hypnotist then assumes the cobra poise while squatting on a cushion, places hands on hips, and swaying around and around in a slow snakelike motion, while looking deeply into the subject's eyes. Around and around sways you the hypnotist while holding in your mind– with intense concentration– exactly what you wish the subject to do: go into trance (hypnosis)!

The hypnotist visualizes, affirms, and projects exactly what is wanted to occur.

Around and around sways the hypnotist while continuing the gaze into the subject's eyes. The subject's eyes will become glassy. They may close. And their body will be seen to sway in unison with the hypnotist's. When this swaying occurs equaling the swaying of the cobra, your work has been accomplished. The subject is hypnotized.

Results from this Cobra Hypnotizing Method are amazing to observe. Intense hypnosis is induced. This is a very dramatic way of hypnotizing that could be introduced in the West, as a hypnotherapeutic method.

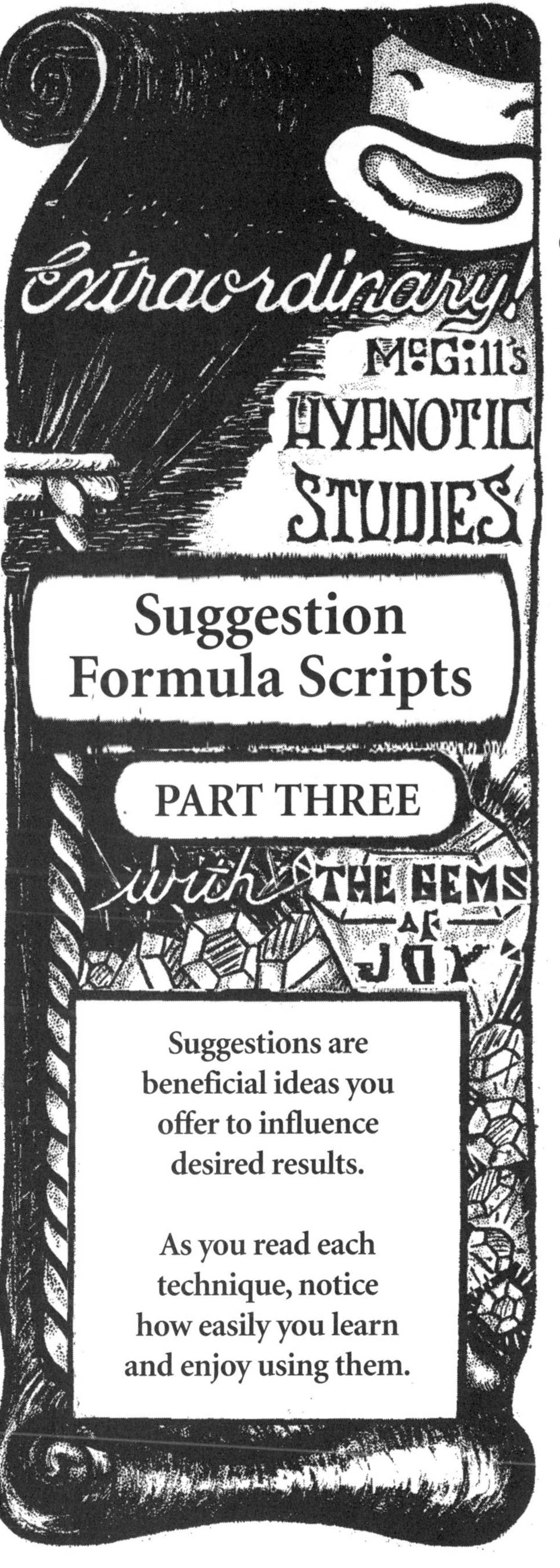

CHAPTERS IN PART THREE

52. Fundamentals of Successful
     Suggestions ....page 199
53. Self-Hypnosis 207
54. The Power of Suggestion 211
55. Post-Hypnotic Suggestions 213
56. Mental Set Hypnosis &
     The Sense Of Time 217
57. Kein On The Law of Compounding....221
58. Self-Hypnosis For The Mature Adult..223
59. Self Improvement Suggestions 225
60. Suggestions With Deep Meaning 227
61. Color Me Rich, Slim & Vital 229
62. Sunshine Self-Esteem Suggestions 233
63. Stop Smoking Today.............................235
64. Sphere of Energy To Stop Smoking 239
65. Stockwell's Quit Smoking Approach ..241
66. Super Learning &
     Sports Performance 247
67. Suggestions For Will & Memory..........251
68. Sleep Learning.......................................253
69. Stockwell's Poetry Hypnosis 255
70. Energy, Confidence And Stamina........259
71. Snuggle Down And Be Comfortable ..261
72. Tension, Stress And Depression 263
73. Holder's Stress Management.................265
74. Einstein's Happiness Script 269
75. The Happiness Way 271
76. Plugged-In Happiness Hypnosis 275
77. Hypnotherapy Of Pleasure 277
78. The Hypnotherapy Of Luck 279
79. The Conscious Smile Technique..........281
80. Hypnotherapy Of Laughter 283
81. Stockwell's Hypnotherapy
     Of Persuasion 285
82. Cosmically Maximize Suggestion........289

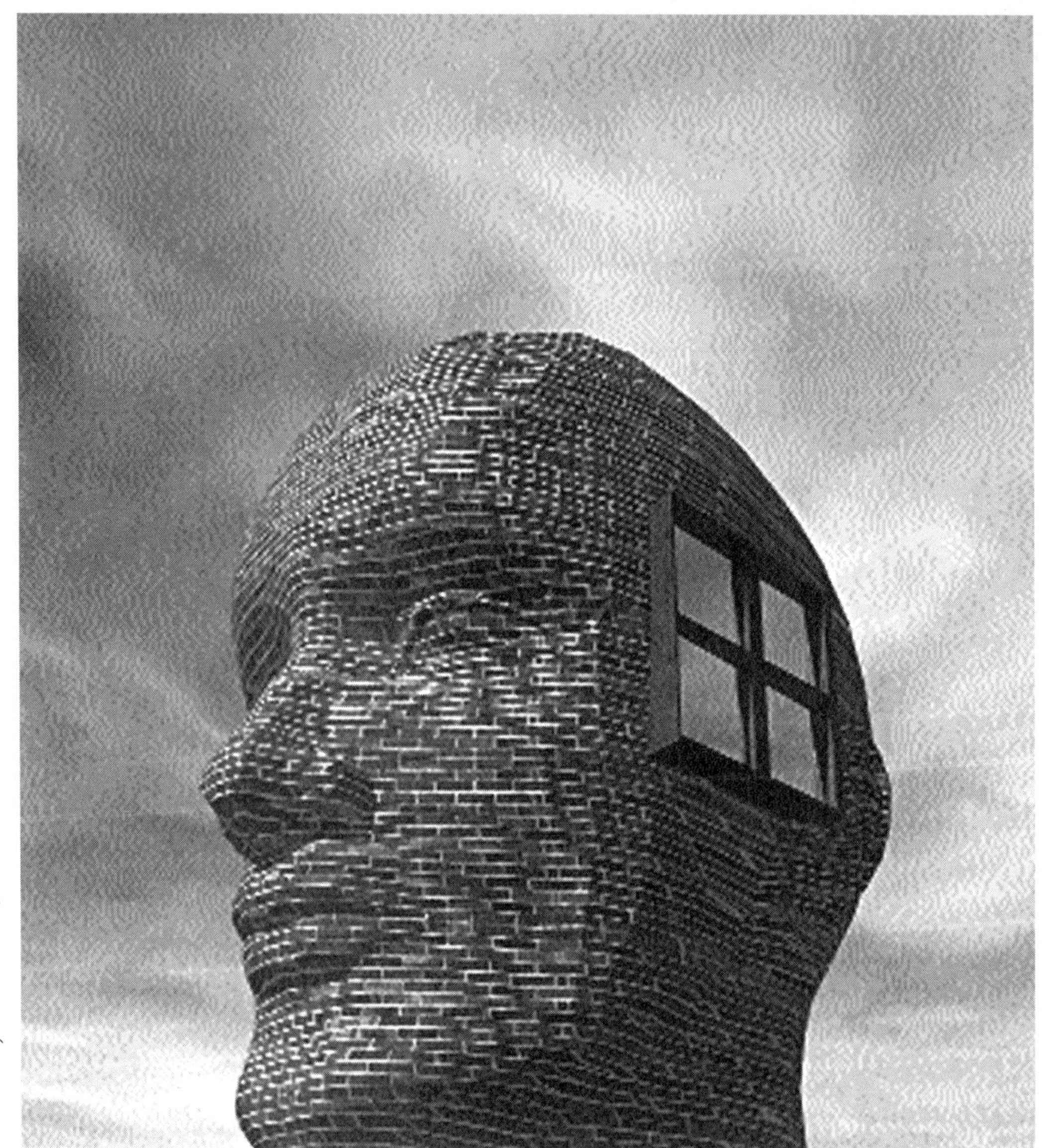

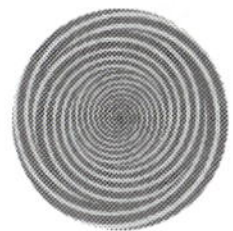

~ Chapter 52 ~
FUNDAMENTALS
OF SUCCESSFUL SUGGESTIONS

Hypnosis + the Power of Suggestion= Subconscious Real-ization and control of these ideas

---

Includes
Key The Subconscious For Benefits: The Three Principles of Key Belief
Key The Mind To The Goal
Anchoring
Suggestion Formulas
Hypnotic Agreement
Hypnotic Reinforcement
Seventeen Rules Of Successful Suggestion-Formulas

Ideas transmitted verbally and nonverbally to the subconscious while in hypnosis are called suggestions. Suggestions that carry over into waking behavior are called post-hypnotic suggestions. Suggestions are ideas that carry enough meaning to the mind to produce automatic unconscious responses.

In 1940, the Journal of Abnormal Psychology defined suggestion as, "A subconscious realization of ideas presented to the mind" which is a wonderful way of saying a lot while saying nothing, for in mind we have our most basic riddle, which can only be answered by mind.

What you need to know as a Hypnotherapist, is that your suggestions offer the client a gentle persuasion to automatically influence their desired results. Suggestions can overcome hurtful habits, addiction, compulsion, fear, pain, limits, worry and stresses, to ease, improve life skills and life transitions. Suggestions motivate. You can target suggestions to improve mental, physical or spiritual well-being, creativity, confidence, sports performance, memory, test taking, learning, behavior, social skills and job performance. You can facilitate pain-free childbirth or surgery and even help others heal their own illness.

Suggestions are ideas for which we CARE; ideas with such emotional drive that we spontaneously and uncritically believe them. We accept, without argument, that an idea is good or bad, true or untrue. Such decisions are not necessarily based on logic or sound fact. Quite often suggestions are completely false. But, with *belief* there is unquestionable acceptance.

Suggestive ideas are constantly around us and we are all extremely susceptible to their influence. Cosmetic and perfume advertisements entice us with claims that we will be made more attractive, with "the skin you love to touch," or the "smell that drives them wild."

Were we to stop to reason about the virtues of the lotion or scent, we may not accept the product's superlative claims. But reason does not enter into the picture…for here suggestion is at work. A suggestion that conveys the idea for which you *care* assures its unquestioned acceptance. And the acceptance of the suggestive idea quickly culminates (in the case of the lotion or perfume) in the purchase of the product and its dutiful application. Advertisers know this principle of attaching emotion to lotion all too well.

Hypnotherapy may not even address specific symptoms. There is no need to probe too deeply into psychological or medical matters. Suggestions for general well-being are very powerful. The subconscious mind knows where help is needed. Hypnosis gives the subconscious mind permission to solve its own problems. Always respect and encourage your client's innate selective ability to use your helpful suggestions and their own suggestions to their best advantage.

At all times be reasonable in your suggestions and the words you use. Don't say anything that sounds preposterous to the client.

Suggestions you present are easily accepted because your client is in a mental state of hyper-suggestibility. They will carry out suggestions that are true to their nature in a style natural to themselves. If they are slow in their natural state, they will react slowly while in hypnosis. If they are lively and quick-witted, they will act accordingly when hypnotized.

Present your suggestions forcefully and make sure that they are understood.

As the hypnotist, it is your obligation to present necessary suggestions to the best of your ability so they bring about the desired hypnotic condition. Your subject must do everything in their power to concentrate upon and accept these suggestions in order to bring about the hypnotic condition within themself.

As you learn the skill of suggestion, you will learn more and more about semantics. The skilled hypnotherapist becomes an artist of verbal and non-verbal suggestion and knows what to say and not say, and when and how to say it.

KEY THE SUBCONSCIOUS FOR BENEFITS: THE THREE PRINCIPLES OF A KEY BELIEF

1. Everything you create begins when you *first pretend* that it is so.
2. From pretending, you advance to believing that it is so.
3. From believing, you advance to the *reality* that it is so.
   Use this idea with every client.

KEY THE MIND TO THE GOAL

Joy and wellness is the point of all suggestions. Whatever you as the Hypnotherapist choose to underscore, can be the "key." Give the "key" in a direct suggestion rather than indirect ones.

Emotions Drive Suggestions

Evangelistic Healing is proof of that. They evoke emotions and get results. The evangelist places God and/or Christ as the subconscious "key" which causes belief to take effect. Rousing services are excellent. An emotionally aroused group with its heightened emotion and the rapid induction of a tap on and shouted, "HEAL!" turns the key. Belief, devotion, and/or respect for the SOURCE from which the "key" is given is said to be the secret of miraculous healing.

Belief in the "Power of the Source" is the electricity of the healing power. Faith is the "key." Be it God, Spirit Guides, Guardian Angels, Masters, Higher Self, or Hypnotist, it makes no difference, as long as the faith is firm. A good hypnotherapist evokes the same emotions of a cathedral or tent, in their office.

Huxley placed the letter "C" on the wall of a classroom of children with defective eyesight. He told them it would be the key to develop perfect vision. It helped the childrens' vision greatly.

A miracle? No. Belief is the secret "key" to possibility. A Sacred Shrine, such as Lourdes, is a perfect example of using a key for healing.

ANCHORING

A stimuli (like facial expressions, gestures, sounds, words, smell or tastes) that triggers or elicits a subsequent desired response.

SUGGESTION FORMULAS

Great benefit comes from the suggestions you implant into the subconscious while in hypnosis. Such suggestions are presented via suggestion-formulas. The more carefully these are planned the more benefits are derived. Speak to the subconscious as though you are speaking to a friend. The subconscious is eager to solve/resolve issues. All suggestions given a hypnotized person should be *positive* in nature. Give them in a normal conversational way.

Psychology gives suggestions to the objective or conscious mind. Hypnotherapy offers suggestions directly to the subconscious. Of course, you can begin your helpful suggestions by imbedding or inserting words or phrases during the wakeful pre-hypnosis interview. However, the most powerful and impactive suggestions are delivered directly into the subconscious. Appreciate that the words you use are the backbone of suggestions because they trigger action. We are so conditioned to words that we respond automatically to them. You can start your session with the suggestion, **"You are ready and willing to accomplish exactly what you came here to accomplish."**

You can enhance powerful suggestions with physical means. For example, when suggesting to someone, whose eyes are closed, that **"things are becoming dark"** and then placing your hands over their eyes to intensify darkness. If suggesting delightful smells, waft some lavender or rose petals by their nose.

HYPNOTIC AGREEMENT

Once suggestions have been given, ask the subconscious directly **"Do you clearly understand?"** and **"Are you willing to manifest the 'cure'. Nod your head if this is okay."** This "yes" affirmation greatly increases the "power" of the suggestion. Subconscious agreement is important.

Do not rush the subconscious to accomplish its affirmation. Tell the subconscious **"You may arouse _____________ (the client's name) from the hypnosis when each of these suggestions have been accomplished."**

HYPNOTIC REINFORCEMENT

Repetition drives home a suggestion and also gives the hypnotist time to pace themselves and their thoughts. The monotony of the same phrase is hypnotic unto itself.

Your vocal pacing offers a great reinforcing tool. Your tone, inflection and phrases point your client's attention to what is most important. Rapid-fire words may be most effective sometimes and a slow measured pacing another. Using your client's name is always an attention grabber and reinforcer. Your sensitive knowing will come with practice.

Layering suggestions during the induction phase compounds the effect. For example, saying **"Your eyelids just don't feel like opening, so you drop deeper. At the count of three your eyelids pop open and when I snap of my finger you go even deeper"** has more than one idea to create a greater deepening influence. Layering post hypnotic suggestions compounds their effects as well. You might say something like **"Every time you see the color blue you smile and that smile brings to mind the words 'I feel so glad to be alive.'"**

SEVENTEEN RULES FOR SUCCESSFUL SUGGESTION-FORMULAS
To design suggestion-formulas that most effectively influence the subconscious, there are some general principles you should understand. These guidelines help you to craft effective suggestion formulas. Use them in designing whatever suggestions you wish to use to improve the life of your client. The exact manner in which suggestion-formulas are designed is an individual matter; no two persons express themselves in precisely the same way:

1. Express Suggestions In A Positive & Honest Fashion
2. Refer To A Positive Future
3. Speak To The Subconscious As You Would A Friend
4. Repetition Works Best, Repetition Works Best, Repetition Works Best
5. Link Suggestions To Images And Personal Emotion
6. Keep It Simple
7. Present Suggestion For One Objective At A Time
8. Have Suggestions Contribute To A New Thought Or Idea
9. Suggest Some Degree Of Improvement
10. Suggest That The Improvement Will Be Progressive
11. Suggest Pleasure With Whatever Degree Of Improvement
12. Put Your Creative Wisdom To Work
13. Combine Verbal Suggestions
14. Combine Verbal And Non-Verbal Suggestions With Mental Energy
15. Combine Verbal Suggestions With Voluntary Physical Action
16. Suggestions May Be Permissive Or Demanding
17. Group Suggestions Are Powerful

We will consider each rule:
1. Express Suggestions In A Positive, Honest Fashion
Very simply, tell it the truth. Give accurate information to act upon.

As much as possible should be positive. Positivity makes suggestions instructive rather than destructive. Mind tends to move toward the subject of a sentence and disregards any disclaimers. If you tell your client, "You will not eat the cookies" all the inner mind hears is "cookies." Avoid the use of such words as "no," "don't," "won't" and "can't" in constructing sentences. Use antonyms (words of opposite meaning) wherever possible. Example:

Word	Antonym
Never	Always
Tense	Relaxed
Upset	Composed
Nervous	Calm (at ease)

In general we think of mind as conscious and subconscious; the conscious phase is considered critical in nature while the subconscious is considered non-critical. In fact, mind is not so severely compartmentalized and operates as a continuum. There are sub-consciousness elements in conscious perception and vice versa. To satisfy the ever-present logical reasoning of the conscious mind, keep suggestions positive and true to be more readily accepted.

To stop cigarette smoking say, **"Let it go entirely."** Saying it is "okay to smoke a little bit" is less effective, because a person's wisdom knows it is better for their health to stop completely. The truth is what is truly best for someone. Quitting entirely, is the better suggestion and is more uncritically accepted and uncritically acted upon.

2. Refer To A Positive Future

This rule is an extension of the "Positive/Honest" Rule. Suggest a brighter future. To mention mistakes that were made in the past is no help. Plan suggestion-formulas to present a future where they are no longer bothered by what troubles them now. Let the future be filled with positive images of having achieved what they want. The mind passively and easily accepts suggestions for positive future behavior. A progression or mental rehearsal of a positive future can be an extraordinary anchor for personal growth. **"Visualize, imagine and experience yourself one year from today, thinking feeling and acting the way you want to think, feel and act."**

Let your statements require response in the immediate future rather than immediate "right now."

Example: "the discomfort in my head will begin to diminish, fade away and be much less when I return to the here and now." is preferable to, "The discomfort in my head disappears this very moment."

In other words, you do not usually tell the client that something is happening before it happens. A good rule is if you see indications that a certain reaction will take place any moment then suggest that it is taking place. Otherwise, introduce the event as a future occurrence and work up to it gradually.

3. Speak To The Subconscious As You Would A Friend

Give suggestions in a normal, friendly personalized conversational way. Use the first or second person in addressing the subconscious, either "I" or "you" will do. For example: "I release any discomfort and I am completely relaxed," or "Soon you will lose any discomfort and will be completely relaxed" are a matter of personal preference.

4. Repetition Works, Repetition Works, Repetition Works

Repetition drives home suggestion. Something "hammered home" a number of times deepens the impression and the monotony is in itself hypnotic. Reinforcing a suggestion gives you time to formulate additional ideas that you want to enforce. Repetition is the key to successful goal achievement in self-hypnosis. Repetition concerns:

(a) The number of times the suggestions are made during each induction.
(b) The number of induction's practiced daily.

Repeating the suggestion-formula two to four times during the induction is desirable. Repetitively in-visioning a sharply defined image of yourself on the screen of your mind as having achieved your goal, coupled with a repeated sense of intense triumph, joy or pleasure (visual and emotional "tie-ins") produces positive results.

5. Link Suggestions To Images And Personal Emotion

Ideas with positive visual associations and personal experience are more charged with emotion and will be more readily accepted. This principle is extremely important.

For example: **"I am filled with pride as I see myself as slim and trim and attractive in every way."**

6. Keep It Simple

Statements should be simple, brief and direct. The subconscious takes and carries out brief and definite suggestions. Plan your suggestions in a manner that is positive, simple and directly to the point and they will be carried out to the limit. Tell your mind what you want it to know. Instruct it in how you want it to perform. Do not give the subconscious reasons or explanations for what you tell it to do, as reasoning belongs to the conscious phase of mind, not to the subconscious.

The subconscious cannot form premises on its own; it can only deduct from premises given it; which it does in a remarkable fashion. The capacity to inductively reason is why an uncontrolled subconscious is dangerous and a controlled subconscious is valuable.

The subconscious never selects its own ideas but acts in accordance to whatever ideas are given it, good or bad, true or untrue, as the case may be. Give your subconscious clear and simply stated information to store in its "memory banks" to draw forth when needed. Make your instructions simple and direct. That is what is meant by saying give your suggestions around the core of a problem. The subconscious responds less readily to subtitles or innuendoes; lengthy or complicated suggestions.

7. Present Suggestions For One Objective At a Time

The subconscious operates best when it is not overburdened. Work on only one goal at a time. Plan your suggestion-formula to cover one point at a time. If you have many complaints to improve, list them and deal with each in turn in a subsequent session. Let suggestions indicate a specific goal or desired result. It is not necessary to mention the means or any difficulties for achieving the goal.

For example: "My goal is my ideal weight of 122 pounds" is preferable to "I desire to lose 43 pounds." The actual goal is 122 pounds and losing 43 pounds is the means for reaching the goal not the goal itself.

Two goals may be pursued at one time, if interrelated. Then, as the first goal is achieved, the second goal is easier to accomplish because of increased experience and confidence.

An example of two interrelated goals could be:
1. "My goal is my ideal weight of 122 pounds."
2. "I enjoy an increased sense of self-confidence."

8. Have Suggestions Contribute To A New Thought or Idea

When dealing with a complaint, your consciousness often insists that an old problem will remain. After all, the condition has persisted for some period of time. When you offer a different solution or add a new thought or idea you offset the old pattern and the situation. The mind more readily accepts the idea that matters will be different in the future.

As an example, take suggestions aimed at stopping smoking. The basic suggestion is that **"You will have increased will power and self-control over tobacco"** in the future. Then the "contribution" of the added suggestion, **"The longer one goes without smoking, the less one has a need to smoke. And now, because you wish to stop for good, with each hour following this hypnotic session, you will have less and less desire for burning leaves and paper."** This adds a fine new idea to the initial suggestion.

Use your originality in adding helpful suggestions for desired objectives.

9. Suggest Some Degree Of Improvement

Frame your suggestions to promise improvement. Precisely what improvement depends on the individual. To promise a complete and immediate cure may invite conflict. To promise some degree of improvement is a more accurate statement of fact.

10. Suggest That The Improvement Will Be Progressive

Suggest that the improvement will increase with each passing day, or with every breath you take. The popular suggestion used by many masters in the field is, **"Every day, in every way, I am getting better and better."**

Suggestions compound other suggestions. If you suggest that person breathe fully and then they relax even more, they make a mental note of their success. This makes it easier for them to embrace the next suggestion. This is called "compounding suggestions." The more physical activities that you suggest and they comply with the more likely they are to accept future suggestions.

11. Suggest Pleasure With Whatever Degree Of Improvement

Let your suggestions encourage the person to enjoy each improvement, count their blessings and celebrate even subtle little changes. Group "some degree of improvement," "progressive improvement," and "pleasure at each small improvement" together. Just these suggestions can constitute the main ingredients of a powerful suggestion formula.

Your body and mind must heal itself according to its capabilities and limitations. "Some degree of improvement" allows for a wide variance in the amount of response expected to occur. This suggestion should be incorporated into the formula. Also suggest that the improvement will be progressive and that you will be improved with the improvement. As an example, **"My improvement will be progressive and with increasing acceleration, and with each passing day I will master this condition more and more, and my cure will become lasting and permanent."**

12. Put Your Creative Wisdom To Work

The subconscious is eager to solve/resolve issues. Empower your client with the idea that, **"You are now enlisting your profound inner wisdom to give you the steps you need to achieve your desired goals."**

13. Combine Suggestions

Combing suggestions has a compounding effect that build toward the desired response. For example, you might say during an induction, **"Your arm is rigid and you can't bend it but when I snap my finger it will instantly go limp, drop into your lap and as it does, you will go even deeper into hypnosis."**

Or during a session **"You love breathing fresh air and with each and every breath you notice that you are breathing more fully and completely. Now and forever more with every breath you will think to yourself 'my lungs are clear. I breath with ease'…"**

Each suggestion reinforces the next and trains your client to be increasingly responsive. Allow the client to proceed from simpler "test suggestions" gradually to more complicated ones.

14. Combine Verbal With Non-Verbal Suggestion And Mental Energy

When you combine the power of the spoken words with the power of telepathy or thoughts, you evoke heightened suggestibility. Clearly think and visualize in your mind the results your client desires and transmit these to them. Follow this with the spoken suggestion.

Your body language; breath, gestures and pantomimes influence and can create an intimate bond with your client. Sweeping your hands over the person's auric field is very powerful hypnosis.

15. Combine Verbal Suggestions With Voluntary Physical Action

Get your client to do physical things like "sit down here" "put your feet on the floor" "open and close your eyes" "lie back" or "rest your hands on your lap" before presenting hypnotic suggestion. This obedience trains them to uncritically act upon your words. Such voluntary response increases involuntary response.

Deep rhythmic breathing too increases suggestibility and floods the brain with oxygen's dizzy effect that makes the mind more open to suggestion.

16. Suggestions May Be Permissive Or Demanding

With most, the subconscious responds better to permissive suggestions, and may not cooperate with authoritative commands. However, some individuals have an unconscious need to be ordered to do things. For them, a command suggestion is more effective.

For example: "I can" or "You can" are permissive. "I will!" or "You will!" are commanding. The individual hypnotherapist must determine which approach seems best for the client.

17. Group Suggestions Are Powerful

The element of self consciousness is eliminated when working with more than one person at a time. Suggestions sometimes are much more powerful with mass suggestions; seeing a suggestion work with someone else helps it work for you. That is why group demonstrations and classes can be very successful.

"The difference between the right word and the almost right word is the difference between 'lightning' and 'lightning bug.'"
—Mark Twain

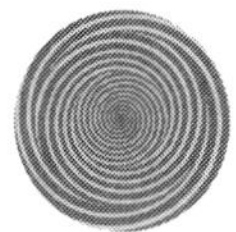

~ *Chapter 53* ~
SELF-HYPNOSIS

Includes
Four Great Ways to Give Yourself Suggestions
Food For Thought Self-Hypnosis
Hypnotize Clients To Hypnotize Themselves

Hypnotherapy is a two-person process or hetero-hypnosis.

Self-hypnosis, auto-hypnosis or autosuggestion, is a one-person process, where you enter and utilize the trance state simultaneously as your own hypnotist/operator and as the subject/client. For self-hypnosis, you must learn to take on a dual role inside yourself: one is active and one passive. Or, you can say, one role is objective and one subjective. This is not difficult to accomplish, as mind is used to doing two things at once, such as driving your car while thinking about the work you will do after you park the car in the garage.

Use self-hypnosis constructively for yourself regularly. Before you is the keyboard of a marvelous computer mind and you have but to operate the keys to program yourself as you wish to be.

FOUR GREAT WAYS TO GIVE YOURSELF SUGGESTIONS

Suggestion formulas can be given to yourself in four ways. Use whichever method seems the most comfortable for you. In all instances, induce a self-hypnosis state-of-mind and while your mind is highly receptive present suggestions to yourself.

1. RECORD SUGGESTIONS

Record the suggestions on a cassette tape and play it back to yourself. Just turn on your tape player and continue relaxing quietly with your hands lying in your lap or while stretched out on your bed or couch.

2. MEMORIZE SUGGESTIONS

Memorize the suggestions and repeat them back to yourself after hypnosis has been induced. If you place your hands over your ears and repeat the memorized suggestion out loud to yourself, they seem to hum and ring through your head with increased power as it echoes inside your very brain! Some find that "mouthing" their suggestions silently, using lips and throat is quite effective for concentrating on the suggestion formulas.

Write and memorize your suggestion formula in advance of the self-hypnosis induction. First write in detail what you desire to accomplish. Then condense the ideas, as much as possible, omitting details and underscoring desired results. These sentences are your autosuggestions.

When possible, do not use over four sentences in making these autosuggestions. Plan these sentences carefully, using a "key word" or phrase, which recall to mind the whole autosuggestion sequence. Memorize these "key words"…to assist you. Do this in advance, as the self-hypnosis state is hardly one for creative thinking, as that is critical mind activity. What has been relegated to the memory banks of your mental computer easily springs forth. This selective thinking will implant in your subconscious.

3. WRITE SUGGESTIONS

Write the suggestions out and read them a number of times prior to inducing the hypnotic state in yourself. While in hypnosis these sequences can then float across the "screen of your mind."

4. MENTALLY VISUALIZE SUGGESTIONS

Place your hands over your eyes and press in gently, and observe what you see before yourself. You will see space. That space in the physical sense is only a micro fraction of an inch between your eyelid and eyeball, but to your experiencing it will seem to go on and on and on into infinity. In that space, now visualize the image of yourself as successfully mastering what you desire. This handling allows your results to float across your "screen of mind."

MODUS OPERANDI: FOOD-FOR-THOUGHT SELF-HYPNOSIS

Suggestions= Food For The Subconscious
A Good Meal Of Healthful Thoughts= Nourishment For Mind And Body
Self-Hypnosis= A Feast You Provide For Yourself and Your Client

This suggestion formula has the goal of self-improvement. It can be presented by yourself, to your subconscious, while you are in the state of self-hypnosis.

When presenting self-hypnosis suggestions use the first person, as you are speaking to yourself. Self-hypnosis is a personal matter.

Read this script out loud. Perform it in a private situation. Allow no one to disturb you during the process. If you like you may record it and play it for yourself.

"I decide what dinner I am going to feed my subconscious and prepare the meal according to this recipe. I can write it in detail or commit its gist to memory. When the meal is all ready, I put it into the oven to cook. The cooking is this self-hypnosis method.

I go now into my private space, close the door and darken the room. I lie on my back upon my bed and am still. For some moments I allow myself to just relax and then I resolve: I WILL NOT GO TO SLEEP.

I keep my eyes open to read this (or if recording: 'I close my eyes') **and continue to relax a bit more. Then I deliberately YAWN. Yawn…yawn…yawn several times. Yawning removes tension from my body. Meanwhile I THINK of how pleasantly relaxed I become.**

Now, I think of my eye muscles becoming so relaxed (If recording: 'they will not operate, and I cannot open my eyes even when I try. IT IS SO. My eyes remain comfortable closed') as I allow the relaxation from my eyes to flow down over my body, and I relax all over…dropping into engulfing relaxation.

I think it and it becomes reality…I become both mentally and physically relaxed and rest for some moments submerged in this state of absorbing mental and physical relaxation. Now, I think of my left big toe as tingling. Concentrate on it…taking my time. Think it and I will feel the tingling.

Having started my left big toe tingling, I now move my thought over to the big toe of my right foot and get it tingling too as I send mental energy to my big toes, and I get them both tingling.

Now go back to my left foot. I concentrate upon all the other toes of my left foot tingling. The big toe is already tingling so it is easy to make the other toes fall in line. Soon my entire left foot will tingle.

I perform the same with my right foot. Soon both feet will be tingling.

Now move the tingling up my body. Think it and I feel the tingling. The tingling is becoming a reality in my body. Bring this sensation up the calves of both legs, at the same time.

I see my calves in my mind's eye. I feel my calves receiving the tingling sensation from my feet.

My feet are still tingling. Moving the energies upward has not diminished the tingling sensation of my feet. What I have done is to spread the energies higher. And now, my feet and calves are tingling together.

Now up to my knees. Feel them tingle.

Now up through my thighs…up both thighs to my hips…feel my thighs tingle.

Now the tingling sensation comes up into my abdomen.

Now up into my stomach.

Now up into my chest.

Now up into and across v shoulders.

Now feel the fingers of my left hand begin to tingle.

The tingling sensation rushes up my right arm into my right shoulder.

My entire body from the soles of my feet to my shoulders is now tingling. I can feel the energy…it is there. It is real!

I bring the energy upward now into my throat. Make my throat tingle with this upward surge of energy. Now up into my face…feel my chin… my lips, my nose, my eyes, and my forehead tingling… my entire body, inside and outside, becomes aglow with energy, and the tingling sensations I produced brings in enough physical awareness so I will not fall asleep.

I have produced a disassociation inside myself via this process…a physiological/ psychological process inside myself. I have transformed my mental computer beat from beta to theta. I have induced hypnosis in myself.

Still lying on my back I continue relaxing ever deeper as I drift towards the realm of sleep but…I do not go to sleep…yet. I am now ready to savor and enjoy my feast…"

Okay, take what has been cookin' and get ready to feed the dinner to your subconscious. Your subconscious is hungry. Place your hands over your ears and repeat out loud to yourself what you have prepared. The subconscious will eat the dinner, as the dinner RRRRINGS through your head. Take your time. There is no hurry. Give your subconscious a good meal while you're at it. Your subconscious is your inner self, you know. Your food-for-thought in this method of self-hypnosis has been the suggestions you cooked up, and wanted to feed to your subconscious.

Insert bits of humor into hypnotherapy. Half the difficulties clients complain of is based on taking life very seriously, not that their problems are not serious, but troubles somehow seem lighter when touched with humor. In other words, "Lighten Up!" In between seriousness and lightness is found the pathway to successful hypnotherapy.

"My subconscious has enjoyed the meal. Yum! Yum! Gobble. Gobble. Gobble. BURP. The meal completed, I let my hands from my ears and rest them by my sides, as I lie outstretched with what I have partaken of food tor thought."

HYPNOTIZE CLIENTS TO HYPNOTIZE THEMSELVES

It is wonderful to offer your clients the gift of self-hypnosis by hypnotizing them and suggesting **"You are deeply in hypnosis now and from this moment forward you have the power to hypnotize yourself. All you have to do is sit or lie comfortable where you are, close your eyes and repeat three times to yourself, 'I am asleep in hypnosis, I am asleep in hypnosis, I am asleep in hypnosis.' And you will be fast asleep in the hypnotic trance. At the same time, you will be alert and able to easily give yourself any suggestions you desire. When you wish to wake up you have merely to count from one to five and you will instantly awaken, feeling refreshed and good all over."**

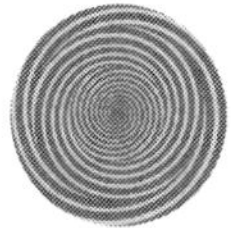

~ *Chapter 54* ~
THE POWER OF SUGGESTION

Includes
The Levels Of Conduct

Hypnosis bypasses conscious thought and directs the subconscious phase of mind to influence mental and physical behavior. While in hypnosis, your mind is hyper-suggestible.

The subconscious phase of mind has the power to either heal or kill depending on how it is directed by suggestion. Suggestion is neutral: it is neither for you or against you. How you accept and interpret it emotionally is a most important factor.

Every suggested idea that enters your mind, if accepted by the subconscious mind, is automatically transformed into a reality...and becomes an element in your life. This acceptance of a suggestion is the Power of Suggestion.

Advertisers know all too well that if they bypass your critical thinking and attach emotions to their product you won't be able to live without it. Perhaps a natural born salesman has hypnotized you to buy something you don't really need. Or do something you don't really want to do. Love too, encapsulates the power of suggestion.

Thinking of a juicy, sour lemon easily proves the fact that suggestion produces physical responses in your body. Notice how the saliva starts to flow in your mouth. Or think of itching and feel those itches start.

Thoughts determine your mental states, emotions and sentiments and the delicate actions and adjustments of your body. Trembling, palpitation, stammering, blushing, the variety of pathological states which occur in neurosis are all due to mental/body interaction. These effects are not voluntary and conscious ones; they are determined by the capacities invested in the subconscious, and come to us often with a shock of surprise.

Suggestion has wonderful power. Thoughts of happiness, joy, and good cheer, if accepted by the subconscious automatically cause happy emotions. What happens when you received a bit of good news? For instance, you find that you have won the lottery! Wow! Your body seems to have lost all its weight, pain and cumbersomeness. You walk on air. When your body functions at its best, you seem not to have a body. Happy suggestions take the mind off your body and it functions perfectly. A happy mind state can make us feel better and even override disease.

Conversely, too much worry and concern frequently makes your body almost too much for you and negative suggestions can make you ill.

Where does hypnosis fit into the picture?
Dave Elman said, "The laws of applied suggestion impose, first the bypassing of critical mind and secondly the establishment of selective thinking." Hypnosis does both, and the suggestions are driven into the subconscious with a wallop.

Mesmerism gave a physiological cause for what became known as hypnosis. When the physical explanation fell from favor the remarkable profession of hypnotherapy was then assigned the domain of the psychological. It is easier to understand the "Power of Suggestion" when we associate it with a physical location. After all, all behavior springs from our physical being.

THE LEVELS OF EMOTIONAL CONDUCT

Here are the levels of emotional conduct:

1. Instinct

Instinct gives you impulses that drive strong emotions. This seat of the subconscious, or the "abdominal brain," is located in the visceral midsection or "gut" of the body. Even the ambitious lure of the future is felt here in the torso.

2. Reflex

The lower brain and spinal cord controls your reflex level. Within its scope is the blinking of eyes, dodging from danger, and reaching with the hands to explore.

3. Habit

Probably located in the lower brain, habits works mechanically, as reflexes do, but permeate the whole field of human endeavor.

4. Conscious Thought

This crowning achievement of human performance lives in your head and works through and controls other levels of response. Conscious thought is the progressive and civilizing force of humankind.

5. The Subconscious

The subconscious most likely involves all neurons in your head and body and permeates the other four levels of emotional conduct. The subconscious is the phase of basic mental activity that interacts upon all behavior of which we are capable. It is a dynamo and may be the energy source of reflexes and all bodily functions: digestion, assimilation, circulation and the action of all vital organs. The subconscious mind never sleeps and is actually more alert when you slumber.

The subconscious mind is dominated by emotion. It holds vital memory from infancy to your last breath, threading each into the texture of your personality. The subconscious gives you the impression of who you are.

Conscious thought may, in fact, be colored by subconscious control. The last stages of a habit are controlled subconsciously. Such discomforting behavior is an automatic subconscious function that strikes an "injurious shaft" into your conscious mind.

The subconscious and conscious mind regularly interacts. If you consciously think an idea and cause it to be accepted by the subconscious, it spontaneously goes into action. If it is a beautiful thought, you are so much the better. If it is a diseased thought, you are so much the worse. Because the subconscious has no selective power, it accepts and automatically acts upon whatever is presented to it.

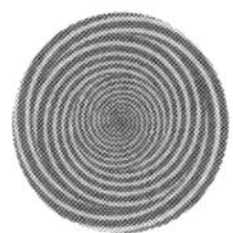

~ *Chapter 55* ~
POST-HYPNOTIC SUGGESTIONS

Includes
A Timely Post Hypnotic Experiment
Triggering Gismos
Snappy Reinforcements
Thought Stopping

One of the most important of hypnotic phenomena is the post hypnotic suggestion. These are deferred suggestions given to the subject during hypnosis that take effect after waking.

The entranced subject is given a suggestion that they are told to perform after they are aroused from trance. The deeper the hypnosis, the more successful the post-hypnotic suggestion will be.

When returned to the waking state, the client has no recollection of receiving any instruction but, when the circumstance arises or the time is reached, they proceed to do what was suggested when they were hypnotized. The suggestion is carried out and accepted as their very own self-motivation.

All hypnotically produced phenomena while the subject is in hypnosis can equally occur as a post-hypnotic experience. Post-hypnotic suggestions are invariably used in all forms of hypnotherapy in which the client is given suggestions that carries over into their daily life for their personal benefit.

This is very fortunate! If hypnotic suggestions were only effective while the subject was entranced, their use would be much limited. The fact that suggestions continue to effect long beyond the trance makes them invaluable. You can also use a post-hypnotic suggestion to re-hypnotize your client or to evoke instant hypnosis at their next visit. Indeed, the post-hypnotic phenomenon is basic to effective hypnotherapy.

Two factors of mental performance are especially important:
1. On a given cue, a post-hypnotic suggestion will spring into effect.
2. Post-hypnotic suggestions utilize your innate subconscious "time sense."

A TIMELY POST-HYPNOTIC EXPERIMENT

The time-memory of the subconscious is remarkable. For example, suggest that a person will perform a specific action at a precise time, such as, in one hour, or 1000 minutes, or a month, or an even more remote period, and they will.

A response to a posthypnotic suggestion often comes as a surprise to the subject. They usually remember nothing until the cued time occurs, and then they will respond to the suggestion, as though it was their own idea. The length of intervening period from when the suggestion was given to its ultimate summation makes no difference. It may be one day, a week, a month, a year, whatever. The subconscious has perfect memory.

Perhaps you'd like to experiment with post-hypnotic suggestion:

While your subject is in hypnosis (somnambulism with amnesia is desired) suggest that at a specific time or when a certain cue is given, that a specific event will take place. When that moment arrives or signal comes in, the event will occur, and the subject, who seems to have no recall of such directions, will experience and perform the suggested event.

MODUS OPERANDI: TIMELY POST-HYPNOTIC SUGGESTIONS

Suggest to a hypnotized person:

"When you awaken, you will feel perfectly normal in every way but when I touch the lobe of my left ear, you will spontaneously experience a powerful impulse to leave your chair, stretch yourself and say 'I feel great.' You will have no memory of this command when you arouse from hypnosis, but the moment I touch the lobe of my left ear you will perform this action. It will occur as an automatic and unconscious action."

Arouse the person, and shortly touch the lobe of your left ear and watch what happens: they will respond exactly as suggested while in hypnosis, and frequently will be surprised at what they did. When asked why they did what they did, the subject often rationalizes by saying, "I just felt like getting up and stretching."

Another powerful closing post-hypnotic suggestion for a hypnotherapy session is:

"The suggestions of benefit given you while in hypnosis will be like seeds planted in the garden of your subconscious which grow and grow into beautiful flowers of reality in your daily life. Come back now out of hypnosis and return to your daily activity when your inner self knows that this is so."

Clients will arouse as timed by their own discretion and what a garden they will grow!

TRIGGERING GISMOS

Here we go again combining technology with hypnotherapy! Wristwatches are available that offer a "Pavlovian" reinforcement of suggestion. Some use a timing devise to remind of a hypnotic suggestion or post-hypnotic suggestion. A wristwatch or beeper, set to beep or play a melody at certain times, creates an auditory stimulus. Some vibrate to kinesthetically stimulate. Such a gadget cleverly uses the "sense of time" and "intermittent reinforcement" to deliver the post-hypnotic suggestion. Its repetitive reminding compounds suggestions and reconditions habits. Cell phones can be used for this purpose.

Imagine having your hypnotherapist with you, repeating post-hypnotic suggestions over and over, until the desired objective is accomplished.

The wearer sets any time mode desired then its sound or vibration powerfully brings attention to the post-hypnotic suggestions and distracts and deters you from the bad habit. A melody (auditory stimuli) and vibration (kinetic stimuli) remind you of a hypnotic suggestion. An original version of this was called the Habitex and was developed under a research grant, patented, and clinical tested to achieve excellent results. It is not used at night, as it disturbs sleep.

Pressure on the top button sets normal time. Pressure on left side sets the timed reminder of the post-hypnotic suggestion. Pressure on right is the "panic button" used to counter any insistent unwanted desires (to smoke, drink, overeat…). Its forceful vibration powerfully brings attention to the posthypnotic suggestions and distracts and deters you from the bad habit.

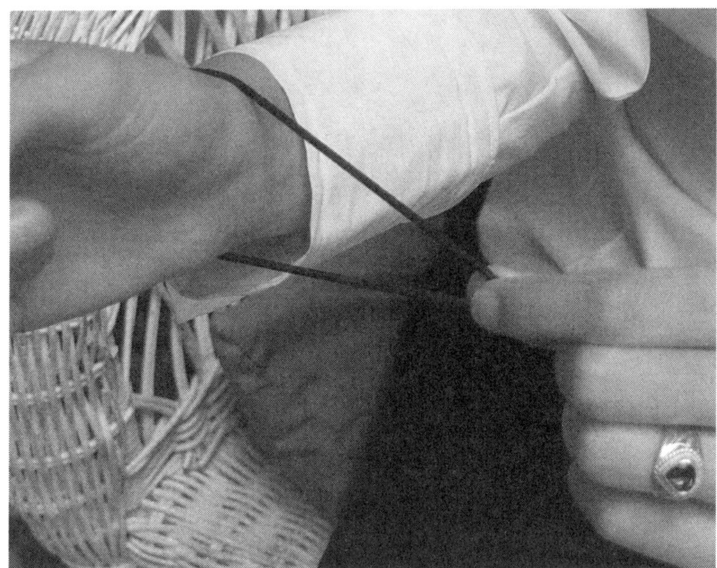

Photo by Jon Nicholas

Snappy Reinforcements

SNAPPY REINFORCEMENTS
From Editor Stockwell

THE WRIST BAND:
A rubber band or hair band around your wrist can be a great reinforcer to snap to a suggestion. **"Any time you think of the thing you want to avoid,** (i.e. biting your nails) **you snap the wrist band and say 'no.'"**

THE COUNTER GIZMO:
Golf stores stock a simple "wrist counter" that golfers use to count their swings. Instruct your client **"Any time you fall back into an undesirable behavior or thought, you push the button on the side of the counter. At night, count the number for that day. You'll become excellent at catching them. Any time you catch yourself immediately ask 'how would I rather be thinking or acting?' Then you change your thought or action to your preferred approach."** Just putting on the wrist counter positively changes behavior.

THOUGHT STOPPING
In trance, suggest to the client "indulge in the thought you want to eliminate and at the end of two (to five) minutes, I will ring a bell (or sound an alarm) and shout "STOP" loudly and when I do, you immediately think of a pleasant thought."
Repeat this process each time making the word "STOP" quieter and less noticeable, and then offer the post hypnotic suggestion, **"if ever that negative thought enters your mind you will instantly and automatically whisper 'STOP' as your mind moves easily to your pleasant thought."**

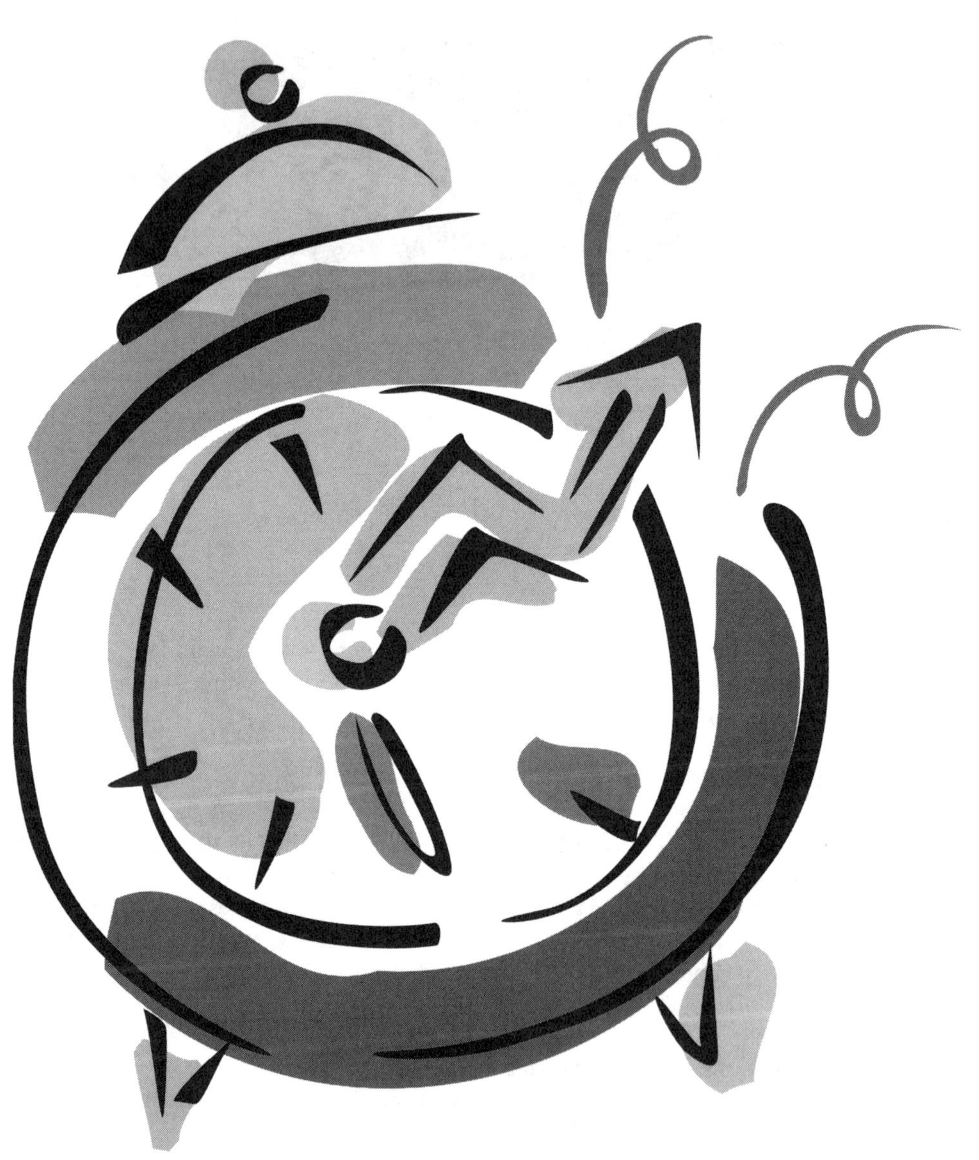

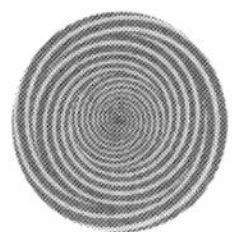

~ *Chapter 56* ~
MENTAL SET HYPNOSIS
& THE SENSE OF TIME

Includes
Setting Your Mental Alarm Clock
Post-Hypnosis & The Sense of Time
Post-Hypnotic Cuing
Time Distortion In Hypnosis

Time does not exist in eternity, but it sure does in your here and now. We have been so constantly surrounded by a barrage of clocks and watches that the subconscious has become conditioned to a "sense of time." Here are four timely discourses relative to hypnotism and that may be useful to your work.

SETTING YOUR MENTAL ALARM CLOCK

There is no need for a *rrrrringing* alarm clock to awaken one on the dot each morning. The hypnotherapist can show clients how to set their subconscious clock. Your subconscious has a sense of time, which functions as a habit through long associations with clocks. Practice makes perfect. The more the subconscious sense of time is used, the more accurate it becomes.

MODUS OPERANDI: FOR SETTING THE MENTAL ALARM CLOCK

Hypnotize your client (only light hypnosis is needed) and give these suggestions: **"You have a mental alarm clock inside your self. You can easily set it to awaken you each morning exactly when you want to awaken. See in your mind the face of a clock, and set it at the time you wish to awaken in the morning. Do this just before you drop off to sleep. When the hour comes on which you are to awaken it will take sleep away and you will awaken spontaneously fresh as a daisy. Simple. Just do it. It will work."**

Once you have set your client's mental clock you can test them in three ways:
1. Tell the client that in three minutes his shoes will pinch, and to take them off.

2. Tell the client that in five minutes the seat of his chair will get hot, and he will leap up from it.

3. Tell the client that in eight and a half minutes– on the dot– they will arouse from the hypnosis.

POST-HYPNOSIS AND THE SENSE OF TIME

An interesting experiment in post-hypnosis is to suggest to the person in hypnosis, **"You will have a strong impulse to come to my office one week from today. You won't know why. You will simply say, 'I had any impulse to come for a visit.'"**

Repeat this post-hypnotic suggestion six times. Then arouse the person. Upon arousing the client from the hypnosis, they will most likely have no memory of the "time suggestion" you have given (make no comment on it, and if there is any traces of memory they will quickly fade). One week hence, they will be on your porch ringing the doorbell.

If you ask why the subject came, they will properly rationalize and say, "I just dropped by to say 'hello.'"

A response to a post-hypnotic suggestion often comes as a surprise to the subject. They usually remember nothing until the cued time occurs, and then they will respond to the suggestion, as though it was their own idea. The length of intervening period from when the suggestion was given to its ultimate summation makes no difference. It may be one day, a week, a month, a year, whatever. The subconscious has perfect memory.

Subconscious mind has an amazing sense of time. A hypnotized nineteen-year young lady was told that she would draw the sign on the cross on the sidewalk in front of her house after the lapse of 4,389 minutes. Though she had no conscious memory of the suggestion, precisely 4,389 minutes later, on the dot, she fulfilled the suggestion and drew the cross.

POST-HYPNOTIC CUING

The post-hypnotic phenomenon is the treasure of hypnotherapy. If suggestions were of value to the client while in trance, their value would be limited. Suggestions given in the subjective state of hypnosis that become realized in objective daily life become valued jewels of living. This process is called post-hypnotic cuing. The cue triggers the subconscious– in a timed response– which calls into action the post-hypnotic suggestion.

As a formula: Subconscious motivation, via the cue, becomes objective conscious motivation.

Most cues are usually of an insignificant nature with no therapeutic value. A beneficial subconsciously suggested effect, which also serves as a cue, causes a greatly enhanced objective effect. An important hypnotherapy breakthrough takes place when subconsciously suggested benefits are transferred, via the cue, to amplify desired objective behavior.

As an example, here is how such might be used to increase the client's artistic ability.

While in hypnosis, suggest, **"Your artistic ability in painting will greatly increase. In exactly three days (or at 2pm on Friday when you are painting in your studio**- or whatever you decide.)...**you will be dazzled and amazed at the quantum leap your art has taken. You paint like a master artist."** At the time the cue given, the person will manifest an advanced talent for painting...the subconscious sees to it. As is often the case with a spontaneous post-hypnotic response, the improvement of the art will come as a surprise to the artist. Often, they will find themself drawing with a skill they never knew they possessed.

The improvement of talent by this method is biofeedback, as the subjective achievement on cuing becomes objective achievement.

TIME DISTORTION IN HYPNOSIS

Another phenomenon relative to hypnotism and the sense of time is known as "time distortion." Drs. Linn F. Cooper and Milton H. Erickson did excellent research in this regard. In brief, through time distortion in hypnosis it is possible to experience mentally, in complete detail, and seemingly in normal time, an activity that would take (by way of an example) ten minutes to realize in ten seconds.

The significance of the phenomenon is obvious as, to quote Cooper and Erickson: "With marked alteration in time perception accelerated mental activity appears possible."

Many experiments in this regard can be tried, such as a subject in one minute flat seeing himself:

Walking for ten minutes.
Cutting down a tree with an axe for five minutes.
Listening to music for fifteen minutes.
Studying a lesson for half an hour.
Talking to friends for an hour.

The human mind functions much like a computer and can transcend time with a flash of thought. Post-hypnotic cuing and time distortion may play an important role in the hypnotherapy of the twenty-first Century.

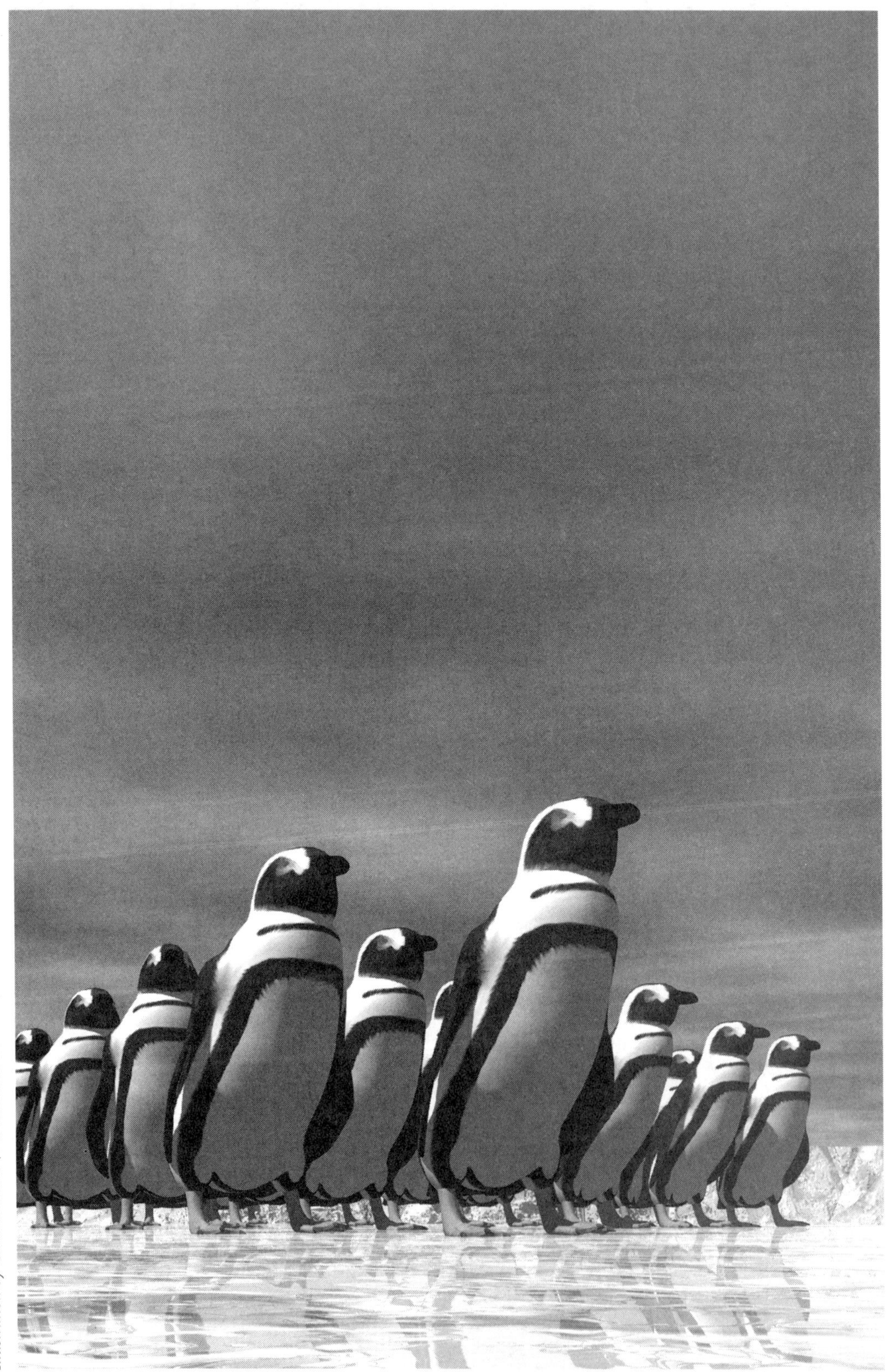

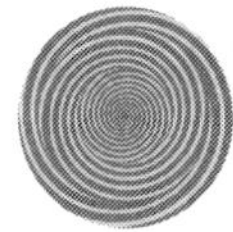

~ *Chapter 57* ~
KEIN ON THE LAW OF COMPOUNDING

By Gerald Kein

Includes
Compounding To Stop Smoking
The Remote Approach

"This is one of the most valuable hypnotist's tools."
—Ormond McGill

We absolutely hate to hear people who have gone to a hypnotist to correct a problem say:
"I went to a hypnotist but it didn't work for me."
"Hypnosis doesn't work for smoking. I tried it three times and I still smoke."

If you, the hypnotist, have done everything right; given a good pre-talk to remove the fears and misconceptions and determined that the person really wants the change what they are coming to you for, then the probable problem is that you were never taught the powerful law of compounding. For the direct-suggestion hypnotist, the law of compounding is without a doubt the most powerful tool in your professional toolbox. The hypnotist who understands this can achieve change for an individual that for most would require regression/abreaction hypnotherapy.

Although Dr Birnheim discovered the mental law of compounding back in the 1800's, it was not until Dave Elman re-discovered it around 1934 and taught it in his classes, that its power became understood and used in therapeutic sessions.

Here is how the law of compounding works: The first suggestion you give for change is very weak and has little to no effect. The second suggestion makes the first suggestion stronger but then the second suggestion is weak. The third suggestion reinforces and makes the first and the second suggestion stronger but the second suggestion is still a bit weak and so is the third. Each time you give your client the suggestion, it always goes back to the first suggestion and progressively strengthens the next suggestions.

Unfortunately most patter scripts don't understand this concept so they are not written to take advantage of this powerful transformational law.

MODUS OPERANDI: COMPOUNDING TO STOP SMOKING

Here is a great way to use the compounding suggestion in a direct drive technique to strongly penetrate and seal with both the conscious and subconscious the suggestion required for the client to change. Let's use stop smoking as an example:

1. Complete your induction and any deepening technique to assure that you have the somnambulistic state.

2. Say to them: **"You are now a non-smoker and will remain a non-smoker for the rest of your life and we are now going to work together to make this your absolute reality. I am now going to give you a suggestion that, as we make it stronger and stronger in your mind, will make you a non-smoker forever.**
    When I say this suggestion, I want you to shout it out to me. Shout it out with me silently in your mind. Feel it penetrate every part of your mind, body and spirit and become your absolute reality. OK, shout this out silently with me. **'I am a non-smoker and I will remain a non-smoker for the rest of my life!' Again, 'I am a non-smoker and I will remain a non-smoker for the rest of my life!'"**
    Say this suggestion with energy at least 15 times.
    After the 15th time say, **"It is true, you are a non-smoker and will truly remain a non-smoker for the rest of your life."**

3. Now you may read and compound this compounding idea with an actual stop smoking script of your choice. As you do, the suggestion of being a non-smoker will be compounded many times and become so strong that if you value your own health, safety and life you best not offer them a cigarette!

The biggest problem with this technique is that you may not use it. After saying the suggestion five or six times it may start to sound stupid to you so you may stop saying it before the effect of compounding becomes strong enough for the actual change to take effect. Be assured, it doesn't sound stupid to the client. They are excited about being a part of the therapy.

THE REMOTE APPROACH

A way to successfully give the suggestion many times is to buy an endless loop audio-tape machine and record a short message on the shortest tape you can find with your suggestion repeated as many times as you need to fill up the tape. Then you're your endless loop machine will play the message automatically again and again.

1. Start your session the same way as above by saying to your client **"You are now a non-smoker and will remain a non-smoker for the rest of your life. We are now going to work together to make this your absolute reality. I am now going to give you a suggestion that as we make it stronger and stronger in your mind it will make you a non-smoker forever. When I say this suggestion, I want you to shout it out to me. Shout it out with me silently in your mind. Feel it penetrate every part of your mind, body and spirit and become your absolute reality. OK, shout this out silently with me.**
    (You could start taping this on your short tape at this time:) **'I am a non-smoker and I will remain so for the rest of my life!' 'I am a non-smoker and I will remain a non-smoker for the rest of my life!' 'I am a non-smoker and I will remain a non-smoker for the rest of my life!'**
    (When your tape is full you can say:)
    This works much better if I leave the room, so I am going to play a tape with this suggestion. As you hear it, shout it out silently and feel it become a part of who you are and how you feel. I will be back in a few minutes."

2. Press the button to play back your repeated suggestion and leave the room. After two or three minutes come back. Press the button and say, **"It is true, you are a non-smoker and will truly remain a non-smoker for the rest of your life."**

Then read any compounding patter script. Compound suggestions of their actual change during the emerging process and you should have a very successful session.

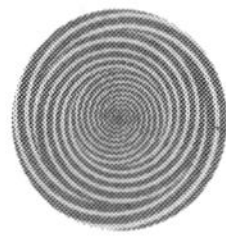

~ *Chapter 58* ~
SELF-HYPNOSIS
FOR THE MATURE ADULT

Two forms of hypnotherapy are popular: self-hypnosis (autohypnosis) and hypnotizing another (hetero-hypnosis.) With self-hypnosis, you become both the client and the hypnotist. Frequently the two overlap as when the hypnotherapist instructs the client to use hypnosis in personal privacy.

This approach presents an easy to perform self-hypnosis method. It is for mature adults, which simply means that it is to be intelligently used!

MODUS OPERANDI: SELF-HYPNOSIS FOR THE MATURE ADULT

Go into your room alone. Place a candle on a table in front of a comfortable chair. Darken the room and light the candle. Take a seat in the chair and relax back. Stare at the candle flame as you follow these directions:

"Relax in the chair with your feet flat on the floor. Rest your hands in your lap. In the dark room stare, stare, stare at the flickering flame. Allow it to occupy your full attention. Now think to yourself 'How good I feel. How comfortable and relaxed I feel. How tired my eyes are becoming as I stare at the candle flame. How very much I want to close my eyes.'

So…close your eyes and relax, relax, relax. Your eyes are closed now so you can just sink down more and more into the depth of relaxation that you sense coming into yourself.

Now let this relaxation travel to each part of your body. Begin by thinking first of relaxing the muscles in the top of your head. Relaxing your scalp completely. As your scalp muscles relax, you will feel a tingling in your scalp. Think it and you will feel the tingling.

Now let this warm tingling relaxation flow down over your face and all the muscles of your face relax. Relax. Relax.

The muscles on the back of your neck are relaxing. Your throat muscles are relaxing. Everything is becoming peaceful and calm.

Now this relaxation is flowing out of your shoulders and on down your arms to your hands and all tension and negativity flows out of your fingertips.

Your chest is relaxing. Your entire torso relaxing…and this relaxation flows down your legs. Your legs become relaxed. You are completely relaxed all over and all remaining tension flows out of your body through your toes. You can feel your feet tingling, as all tension leaves your body. Your entire body is relaxed and you feel comfortable all over.

Now breath deeply and slowly and every breath you take causes you to become more and more relaxed and more and more sleepy. You are becoming so sleepy…so peaceful and relaxed…so sleepy.

You are resting comfortably in your chair with your eyes closed and your breaths are coming in full and deep as you find yourself sinking deeper and deeper down…down into the realm of sleep.

You are going deeper and deeper down into the realm of sleep.

You feel a wonderful peacefulness coming into your body as you drop down, down into the relaxation of hypnotic reverie. You are sinking down, down towards sleep and rest…sleep and rest…sleep and rest down into hypnosis.

You breath deep and free and your whole body is sinking into sleep and rest in hypnosis. Your mind is becoming quiet and still.

Sleep. Sleep. Sleep. Go deeper into hypnosis and even sink deeper and deeper in to hypnosis. You are still aware and your conscious mind moves to one side and your subconscious mind becomes open and receptive to absorb the beneficial suggestions you are now implanting within the garden of your subconscious mind. The beneficial suggestions you give yourself are like seeds that grow and grow and become the flowers of your reality. Accept these suggestions into the garden of your subconscious and they are accepted by your inner self and become part of your life. They become your very own.

Now place your hands over your ears and repeat this out loud to yourself, 'I am becoming the complete master of myself. My inner calm penetrates everything I do. It is a wonderful game I am playing with existence. My feelings about everything I do is that it is fun to do. It is great fun to master everything I do and all the while I remain calm and relaxed and peaceful inside myself.

Every day in every way, my objectives become easier and easier to accomplish. The more life hands me to deal with, the more fun life becomes. I enjoy what I do in every way. The more something is difficult to master the more fun it is to master it. I enjoy the game of mastering. Any challenge makes me stronger and I enjoy my life the more. Life is a joy! Life is a joy! Life is a joy!

I am calm. I am peaceful. I am the complete master of myself. I handle all situations that come my way with amazing ease. I am the complete master of myself.

I have perfect confidence in myself in everything I do. I am in good health and enjoy eating foods that I know are good for me. All my habits are directed towards increasing my good health. Every suggestion that I give myself goes deep into my subconscious mind and makes life a joy for me. Life is a joy for me. Life is a joy for me. Life is a joy for me.

I play in the playground of existence. I flow with existence. Existence brings me the total joy of living in every way. My mind is clear and calm. I know that existence is perfect. I look upon life as a game that I play with existence for the sheer joy of playing the game. I know that everything in existence is a miracle ant that I am the greatest miracle of all. Every one of these wonderful suggestions that I have given myself in this relaxed state of hypnosis goes directly into my subconscious and becomes my reality.

With every breath I take, this reality of myself goes deeper and deeper into my subconscious and becomes the reality of myself. I am well, strong, guided, protected and I feel good all over…in mind and body…every day in every way.

I will use this process often for the benefit of myself. The process is compounding and each time I enter hypnosis I drop down ever deeper into my subconscious and the beneficial suggestions I give myself become rooted in my being. They become my very own.

Every time I use hypnosis I derive increasing benefits from its use and I use it over and over again and again and again.

Now, I sink down deeper, even deeper into hypnosis and drop into the realm of sleep, while these suggestions become my reality.

And, when I am ready, I will awaken refreshed in every way…feeling wonderful and fine…knowing the perfection of myself.

The process is complete and I let my hands drop from my ears and stay in this delicious reverie and doze to awaken when I will."

How will you know it works? You can't help but know.

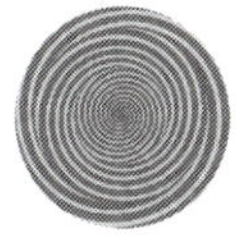

~ *Chapter 59* ~
SELF-IMPROVEMENT SUGGESTIONS

Includes Suggestions for
Tolerance For Others
Better Communication
Social Confidence
Age Attitude
Be More Organized and Efficient
Creativity

Hypnosis, the state of mind where suggestions produce maximum influence and motivate subconscious activity, has tremendous benefits on many levels.

The following are examples of suggestion sequences for self-improvement. They may be modified as desired to be directly applicable to your specific goals. Present these self-improvement suggestions to your subconscious while in self-hypnosis and you get results. You can present them to your client in the "you" form if you like.

While in hypnosis, repeat the suggestion three to ten times for increased effectiveness.

TOLERANCE FOR OTHERS *— no matter what anyone around me does, I become*

"~~The more annoying~~ others tend to become the more calm, patient, and relaxed I become. I overlook any human failings and just enjoy them as they are, and love them more and more as human beings. I am very pleased with this growing sense of loving and caring which is growing within my being."

BETTER COMMUNICATION *I am...*

"I picture and imagine myself as a presentable, interesting, likeable person. I find myself friendlier to others, and am able to speak easily and freely at all times to my fellow human beings. I listen carefully, and reply with understanding and consideration. All shyness or reluctance to communicate and speak to others is fast disappearing. I now communicate well with everyone. I am self-assured."

SOCIAL CONFIDENCE *I am ;*

"I see, feel and hear myself completely at ease in social gatherings. I engage in conversation easily and am friendly to everyone. I listen well and add sparkle to conversations. From the moment I enter the room I feel warmth and friendliness toward everyone within the room. I enjoy these feelings and look forward to more and more social activities and gatherings."

AGE ATTITUDE

"I envision myself as mature, erect, and proud. I wear my age as a royal mantle. My years have taught me that there is so much to learn, to experience, to enjoy in life. I regard each day as a new and exciting challenge. I find myself growing more enthusiastic, more mentally alert, and with a cheerful outlook toward life at all times. I feel my inner resources open up and recharge me."

BE MORE ORGANIZED AND EFFICIENT

"I see myself as a person with the ability, courage, and strength to make up my own mind. I make good decisions, respect my own opinions and judgments, and proceed to act without delay. I organize my life well and can be efficient if I choose– and I choose! I am deeply pleased with the way my life is becoming organized and efficient, as I demonstrate it with my newly found ability."

CREATIVITY

"I have great resources of energy and power within me. I have only to relax and let this creativity run free. I discover to my delight that new ideas, new concepts, and new ways of expressing myself come to my mind in abundance."

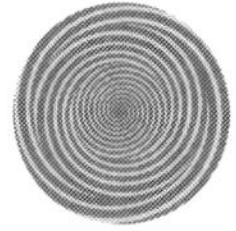

~ *Chapter 60* ~
SUGGESTIONS WITH DEEP MEANING

Instill these quotes of wisdom into your clients while they are in profound hypnosis and you give them an added essential gift of the highest order. Use one suggestion during each session. Their value is great:

"The divine plan of your life now unfolds before you, step by step, and you happily recognize each step."

"You desire the highest and best in your life. You draw the highest and best into your life."

"Ask and it shall be given unto you. Seek and you will find."

"As God's child, you have the wisdom to recognize God as the Creator who is the Creation. This wisdom leads you in paths of happiness and creative success."

"Let there be peace within your walls, and prosperity within your palace."

"You give thanks for the perfect body and mind which allows you to express yourself, and accomplish the divine plan of your life."

"The way for you is joyous. It is the way of safety and security."

"The boundless power that created the universe manifests through you in the perfection of your existence."

"Give thanks that you are ever-renewing and ever-unfolding your expressions of infinite life."

"Give thanks to the boundless universe which perpetually supplies everything you will forever need."

"You are the radiant child of God who always expresses radiant perfection."

"Your body is a gift from God. What you do with it is your gift to God."

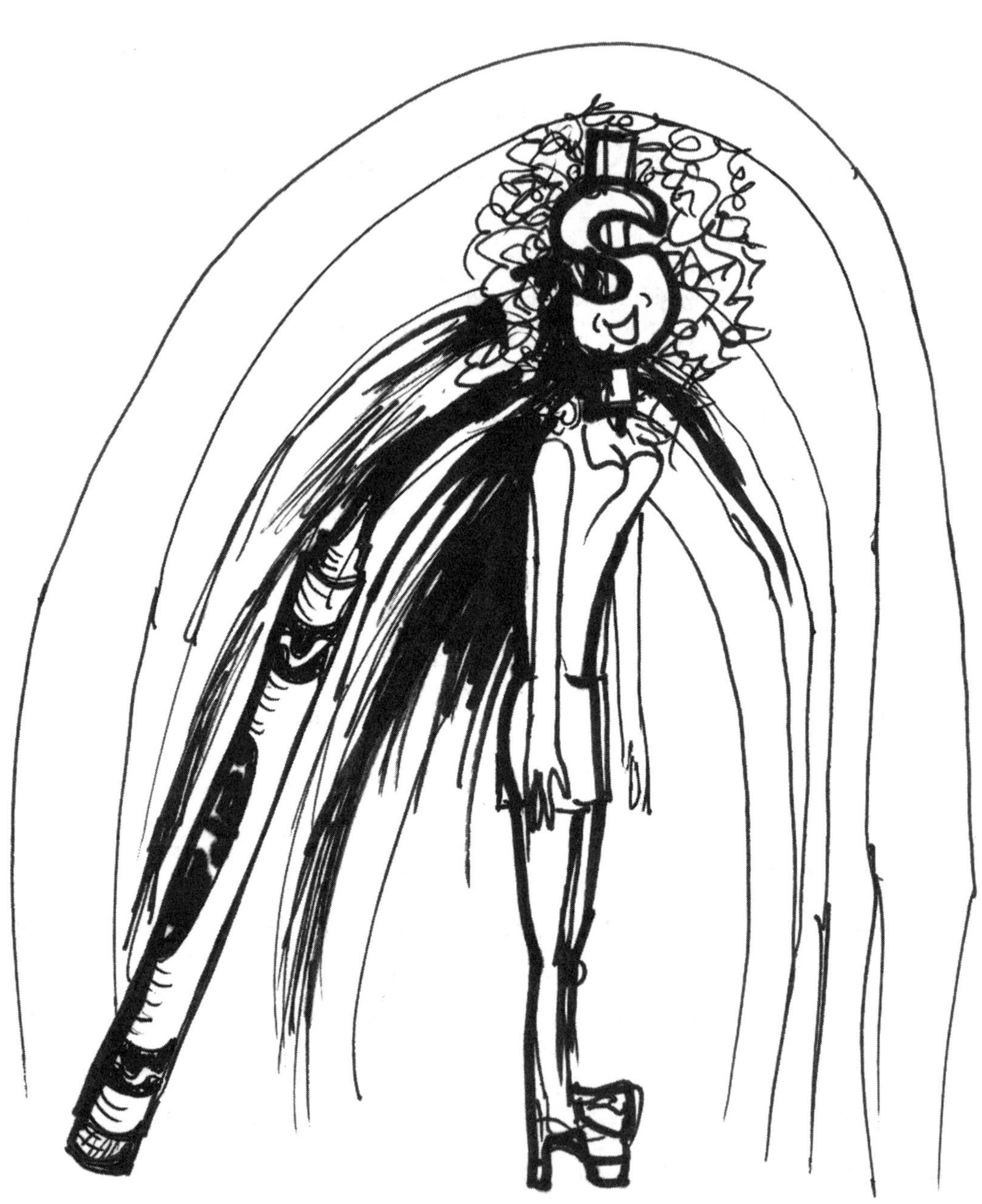

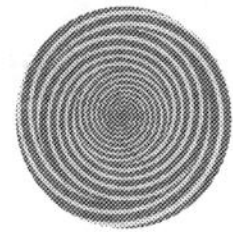

~ *Chapter 61* ~
COLOR ME RICH, SLIM AND VITAL

Includes
Color Me Thin
The Color Of Riches
The Blue Vitality Bath

Abundance Hypnotherapy uses the power of the mind to get what you want out of life… wealth, love, success, whatever. The power is within you, but remember it is a two edged sword that can conquer or destroy.

There is nothing mystical about abundance hypnotherapy. It is a scientific hypnotic method. It is also called "the magic of believing," "the power of positive thinking," or "creative visualization." Whatever it is called, behind it is mind and consciousness. Mind and consciousness operate together.

This approach further advances the "mental-set" technique of Chapter 56, which can be quickly established as a post-hypnotic response or "cuing."

The "Color Me Slim," "The Colors of Riches," and the "Vitality Bath" processes that follow use reinforcing suggestion for the post-hypnotic effect (a suggestion given to in hypnosis will carry its performance over into the waking state) and "cue" the post-hypnotic suggestions to spring into effect.

These processes associate suggestions with different colors. Each color is established (programmed) subconsciously to produce a definite suggested response. Thus, when such a color is "cued," the suggestion that is associated with that particular color springs into action. I use white for spiritual; red for developing confidence; blue for vitality; green for slimness; gold (or yellow) for making money; and purple for sleeping better.

These methods make it easy for you to reinforce behavioral suggestions simply by flooding your mind with thoughts of the desired color, and the subconsciously suggested associations are brought into operation via post-hypnotic operation.

MODUS OPERANDI: COLOR ME SLIM

Here is how to apply this powerful formula in relation to overeating and/or diet enforcement.

First induce somnambulism and present these suggestions:
"More and more, every time you eat, you are achieving success in keeping the weight of your body exactly correct. You are pleased with nourishing food and enjoy it. You enjoy eating the healthy foods of your healthy diet. They are the foods that appeal to you. You enjoy eating food that brings you good health and keeps your weight correct. Foods that are good for your health attract you. You enjoy healthy food. You enjoy eating for wellness. Your

weight is dropping more each day and is becoming exactly right for you because you eat what you should eat and that is all. The foods of your diet are the only foods you wish to eat. You stop eating when you have had enough to fuel you. You enjoy eating the foods that they bring you good health and good health causes you to eat the food."

Now add the following as a post-hypnotic suggestion, which establishes the color association:

"Let these ideas become your reality as you repeat them in your mind; 'every time I think of the color green, the color fills my mind with these powerful suggestions of health, enjoyment, eating the healthy foods of my diet, and my happiness with eating healthy food. When I eat, the color green amplifies my subconscious thought and action and I easily release any unwanted bulk. I am slim and trim. Whenever I think of the color green, foods of my healthy diet take on a special pleasure for me, and are the only foods I desire and eat.'

Having established this association (as a post-hypnotic cue) of the color green with your suggestions of diet maintenance and enjoyment, allow yourself to arouse from the hypnosis session. Knowing that from this time forward, when you sit down to eat, you flood your mind with thoughts of the color green… it turns on your subconscious motivation, and you will find your appetite exactly as it should be, perfectly satisfied in consuming the required healthy food of your perfect diet."

THE COLORS OF RICHES

First induce somnambulism and present these suggestions:

"You are abundant in money, love and happiness. Money comes to you easily. You have all the money you need to enjoy life."

Continue with positive affirmations about money and abundance and then add the following as a post-hypnotic suggestion, which establish "The Colors of Riches" in association:

"Let these ideas become your reality as you repeat them in your mind; 'every time I think of the color yellow or gold, like sunlight, the color fills my mind with these powerful suggestions of abundance, and my openness to receive a lot. The color yellow or gold amplifies my subconscious thought and action and I easily release any limits. I am abundant. Whenever I think of the color yellow or gold, I take on a special pleasure. It is easy for me to be abundant.'

Having established this association (as a post-hypnotic cue) of the color yellow or gold, with the knowing that you are and will be more and more abundant, fills you with enjoyment. When this is entirely so, allow yourself to arouse from the hypnosis session. Knowing that from this time forward, when you flood your mind with thoughts of the color yellow or gold… it turns on your subconscious motivation and you take the right action to be abundant on all levels in money, love and happiness and that money comes easily to you."

THE BLUE VITALITY BATH
You Will Need:
Blue Colored Lights

Use this same idea to bring in extraordinary vitality, when applied in association with colored lights. The process used in this manner will be found effective in overcoming stress, as it quickly removes fatigue, and refreshes both mind and body– bringing vitality.

For this purpose, arrange your private room so you can flood it with blue light.

You must now help your client to subconsciously associate the color blue with suggestions of rest, renewing of energy, and the removal of stress…in others words…with vitality.

Induce somnambulism, and establish these suggestions in the subconscious:

"Let these ideas become your reality as you repeat them in your mind; 'every time I see, think, or experience the color blue, a surging of energy rises up within me and any stress disappears. The flooding of blue light over me immediately brings both relaxation and freedom in my mind and body. The color blue brings me boundless energy and removes all stress. Just thinking of the color blue brings me peace of mind, renewed energy, and buoyancy of spirit.

And when I am flooded through and through with cooling, refreshing blue light, my vitality knows no bounds and I am immediately charged and recharged with energy in my body, mind, and spirit."

Flood the room with blue light.

"Having subconsciously established these suggestions in your inner mind, you now sit in a comfortable within the blue light of renewal and relax. Bathe in the blue light for precious moments."

Conditioning an association of blue light and vitality will prove a delicious experience. It will literally be experienced as a bath in vitality– a great tonic for the renewing of energy. After a short period enjoying the bath of vitality, your client will experience will leave with a sparkle in the eyes and a bounce in their steps. Fatigue and stress will have vanished. The person will be newly charged with vitality.

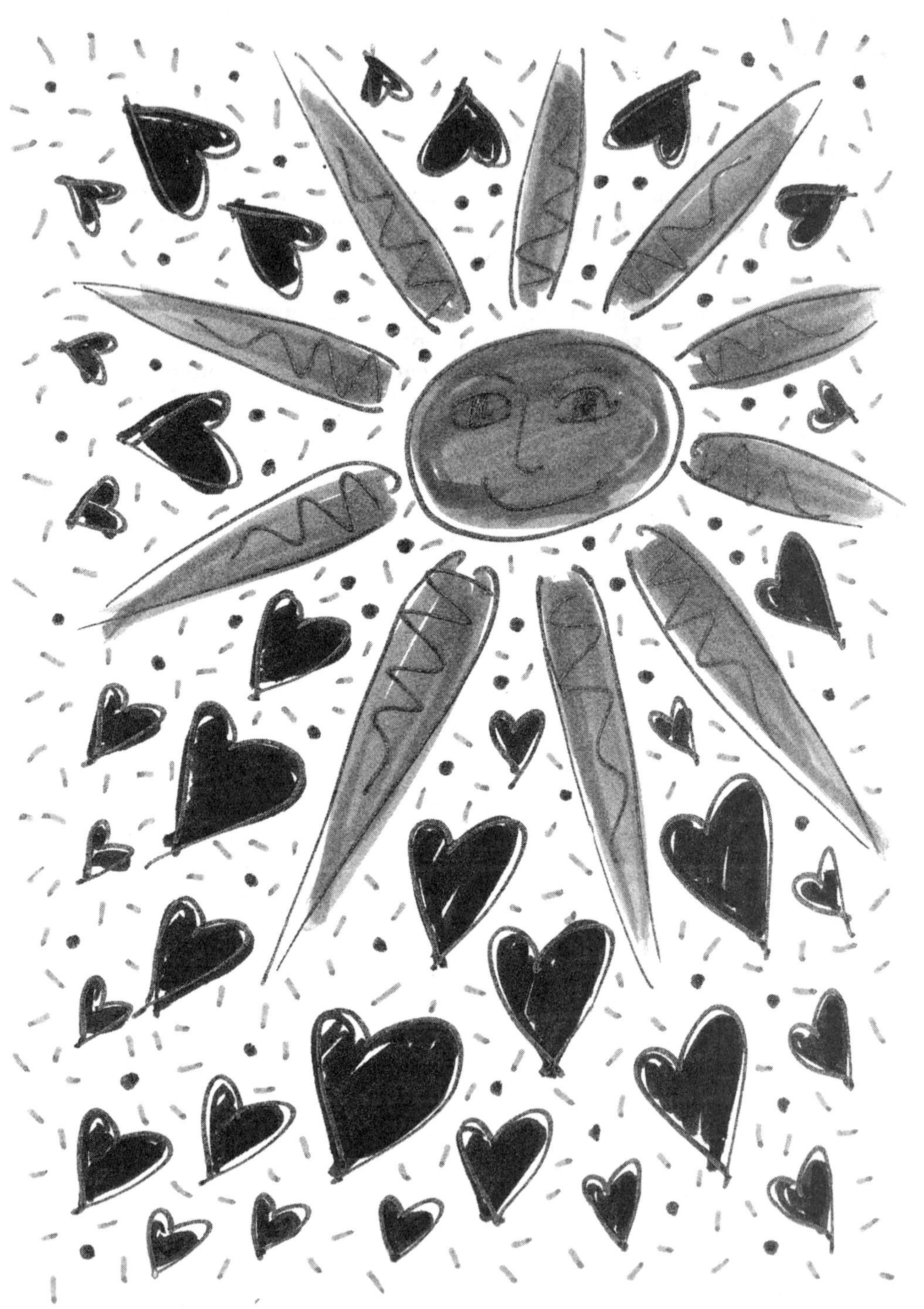

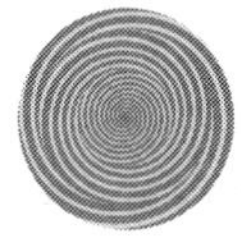

~ *Chapter 62* ~
SUNSHINE SELF-ESTEEM
SUGGESTIONS

In this process, a present dilemma or negative self-image and future success and positive self-image are envisioned and produced by the mind. Side by side they stand and are bathed and transformed by the sunlight…powerful indeed.

MODUS OPERANDI: THE SUNSHINE SUGGESTION FORMULA
Formally induce trance. If you like, you can begin the trance process with the "establish the hypnotic mood technique" you may recall from a chapter 23, i.e. **"I am going to dim the lights and leave you alone in your chair to relax for ten minutes while you think to yourself how you feel the experience of being hypnotized will be. Give your full attention to this, and do not allow your mind to wander from that purpose. Do you understand?"**

Then after your induction, or this self-preparation, give these suggestions:

"You are ready to enhance your self-worth (Or solve a specific problem)?
Envision and imagine your old personal image (Or difficulty). Good.
Now envision and imagine your new desired image (Or success). Good.
Put both images side-by-side.
Sunshine has always been associated with happiness and improvement of things. With spring comes sunshine. Sunshine is always fresh and new.

Focus rays of sunlight down upon the two images of you. The light of the radiant sun illuminates both. Good. This beautiful sunlight causes the old unwanted image (Or difficulty) **to evaporate like a drop of water on a hot tin roof, while simultaneously causing the new image to become bathed in the life-giving sunlight the desired new image takes form.**
Subconscious mind is this clearly understood? Are you ready now to accomplish this luminous task and make it your reality?" Get an affirmation via a nod of the head or subconscious lifting of a finger.
"It is agreed then that this brilliant inner sunlight will dissolve your old image (Or

difficulty) **and will illuminate with radiance your desired new image** (Or success) **and it will become your reality.**

Okay! Let the sunshine come in and dissolve the old and radiate the new. You are a precious sunshine. When this has been accomplished let me know.

Very Good.

In a few moments when you return to the here and now you will feel fine in every way. And whenever you see, feel or think about sunshine you are illuminated with the feeling and knowing that you are that successful image and every time this knowing grows even stronger.

When the time is right you will return feeling well and good in every way."

Allow the arousal to occur in its own space and time. There is no hurry. When client arouses they leave your office with a new image of themselves that has replaced the old.

Mission accomplished.

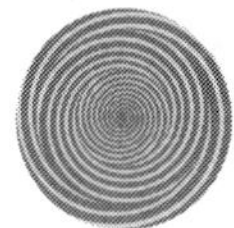

~ *Chapter 63* ~
STOP SMOKING TODAY

Includes
Stop Smoking Today
Direct Core Suggestion
Aversion Suggestion
Screen of Mind

Think of the people you can assist! Stop smoking sessions are popular, profitable, and an important portion of a hypnotherapy business.

In Chapter 30 you learned the "Let's Pretend Method To Hate Smoking." This chapter is devoted to guiding a person to stop smoking while in somnambulism. It is an interesting, intelligent, and adult approach. Far too often operators talk down to the subconscious like it is a petulant child. Reverse that now.

It is wonderfully effective to present suggestions in a mature manner. Somehow, though likely no one knows just why, the subconscious responds quite favorably to such respect.

Come to understand the nature of habits. Habits are conditioned responses in the mind, through repeated behavior, and have developed into unconscious behavioral patterns. In other words, habits operate automatically and are frequently stimulated into action by a certain satisfaction they bring. In the case of a smoking habit, a subconscious pattern carries over into conscious behavior.

The "Stop Smoking Today" method of hypnosis (which can be applied to yourself or to client) turns this subconsciously around, so that instead of wanting to smoke, detesting the idea of smoking is established. All resistance to not smoking is gone. The client becomes so glad to be no longer addicted to a habit, which is harmful to life. The subconscious realization of this fact has caused the habit to lose its power.

The suggestion, **"In every way, you are so glad you have stopped smoking"** is the key to success with this method.

Contemplate the mechanism: "Glad" is a happy suggestion. Mind likes to hang on to a happy suggestion like "glad" and make it a continuum. The mental suggestion glad is associated with the body response of stop smoking. As glad is retained in the mind, stop smoking becomes the continual behavioral response in the body. "Stop smoking today" becomes the immediate fact, and a new habit of not smoking sets in that becomes a glad fact to the client. When glad in the mind combines with glad in the body, the hypnotherapy is successful. The principle applies to many forms of hypnotherapy.

MODUS OPERANDI: STOP SMOKING TODAY SESSION
Induce somnambulism in subject, ending with these suggestions:

"You are in deep hypnosis now, and these suggestions, of great benefit to yourself, go deeply into your subconscious and become your way of life. You have come to me to stop smoking, and you will leave my office a nonsmoker. You will be so glad. Ready, set, go...accept these suggestions into your subconscious and you will stop smoking today.

First, subconscious mind learn why you smoke. You smoke because you are 'hooked' on a habit that has come to serve a purpose in your life. A nicotine habit has developed that has caused your body to repeatedly seek satisfaction from smoke.

Also, you smoke because it fills in time and occupies your hands. It somehow gives you a sense of self-assurance. It is not real self-assurance, of course, but it seems that way.

Also, you smoke because you enjoy it and we tend to do mostly what we enjoy.

These are all reasons why you have smoked, but now you want to stop... so absorb these reasons why you should not smoke, which will now far exceed any reason you have for smoking. You now master the habit of instead of the habit being master of you. And you are so glad.

Absorb this understanding of why you should no longer smoke, and stopping will become your reality today and all desire for it will disappear forever. You will never smoke again...in fact the very idea will become detestable to you. You will never have an urge to do it again. And you are so glad.

Absorb these truths of why you will no longer smoke into your subconscious. They immediately become your reality, and you will stop smoking today. You are so glad.

You stop smoking because it is not good for you. The habit evens kills some people. You could be next. It is definitely injurious to your health. Nothing is more important to you than your good health."

Pause and let these suggestions sink home for a few moments.

"Smoking is no longer a praised social habit. Today the person who smokes is looked down upon as being a victim of a disgusting habit. The person who does not smoke is esteemed far above one who does. In fact, for many nonsmokers, seeing a person smoking is a definite turn off. Your stopping lifts you higher up in social favor."

Pause and let these suggestions sink home for some moments.

"Smoking is a very discourteous habit, and it is very annoying to others. You want to be accepted by others and be courteous in every way. You know it is unfair to others to make them breathe your injurious smoke. The very idea of smoking is becoming detestable to you."

Pause and let these suggestions sink home for some moments.

"You stop because you want to stop. Who is the boss, you or tobacco? Who is in control, you or the habit? If you can't control a habit, how can you expect to control your life? When you master this habit of smoking, you raise your self-respect; and, in direct ratio, the respect others have for you. You have proven yourself the master of yourself when you stop smoking today. You are so glad."

Pause and let these suggestions sink home for some moments.

"These suggestions to stop smoking today have done deep into your subconscious mind. All desire for smoking is gone forever. You are so glad to be rid of this nasty unwanted habit forever. You detest the very idea of smoking. And think of all the money you save while improving your life in every way.

Sink down deeper and deeper into hypnosis now, while these suggestions become your happy new reality. You have stopped today, and will never smoke again. All desire to smoke is gone forever, and you are so glad. When these suggestions have become your reality, you will gently arouse from this profound hypnosis feeling wonderful and well, and you are so glad that your are freed of this unwanted habit, as new nonsmoking life for you begins. If you were to try to smoke a cigarette it will taste like rubber in your mouth and will actually make you sick. You are a non-smoker."

MODUS OPERANDI: DIRECT CORE SUGGESTION

Popularly, suggestions that **"Cigarettes are harmful or may even kill you are"** given. **"Cigarettes will taste awful and you will feel sick if you smoke." "Cigarettes are disgusting." "It is no longer sociable to smoke…"** etc, are said yet all, though good and often helpful, miss the core.

The core isn't that the client comes to stop smoking. The come because they have a DESIRE to stop smoking. Otherwise why would they come to your office to stop smoking? Action speaks louder than words. Their desire is an intense emotional feeling. An emotional feeling is a cosmic connection so the core of your hypnotherapy is to advance this core. Possibly suggest,

"Your desire to stop smoking is increasing with every breath you take. What you sincerely desire to experience becomes your way of life. Your desire to stop smoking increases steadily and continuously with every breath you take. You achieve your desire to stop smoking today. YOU STOP SMOKING FOREVER."

Simple! Direct! Right on target!

Another direct and successful suggestion formula to quit smoking is this:

"See yourself in complete control of all your habits and behavior. You have the power and strength of character to give up this senseless and harmful addiction to tobacco. Each day your desire to smoke diminishes until finally you give up smoking altogether. You feel proud of yourself, and rejoice in your progress and self-control."

MODUS OPERANDI: AVERSION SUGGESTION

"You hate the smell of tobacco and can't even smoke it any more. You detest it and therefore you decrease the amount you smoke every day…less and less until you just don't want to do it at all ever again. Picture and imagine the bright future you have ahead of you, clean and clear of poisonous smoke. If you try to smoke a cigarette, it will taste like rubber in your mouth and will actually make you sick." Repeat this aversion part several times. Then, awaken them from trance, hand them a lighted cigarette and ask them to smoke it. If they do they will feel deathly ill and if they throw it away in nauseous disdain you know they are cured. If they still want it do the session a few more times.

MODUS OPERANDI: SCREEN OF MIND
You Will Need:
A Comfortable Chair
Eyeshades

Consult with the client and then reduce what they want to accomplish into a picture image. You can use this for any goal. To stop smoking the mental image is formed of being in disgust at the very act of smoking. Then have the client relax in a comfortable chair and place the eyeshade over their closed eyes and instruct them,

"Turn your attention to the image of yourself being completely disgusted at the very act of smoking and observe whatever images form before you. These will appear spontaneously upon your screen of mind without any conscious effort whatsoever. This is easy to do as mental pictures of you the way you truly want to be naturally just come into the mind when you relax and let them. Allow the mental pictures to just come in without any control at all. Some may appear to move or some may be static. however they come to you, they become a gateway to subconsciously and almost instantly implant the inner knowing that you are free of that poison."

After five or so minutes of passively observing the mental pictures as they come and go instruct,

"Decide upon the mental picture of the behavior you wish to establish in yourself and when this is done nod your head. Such is now affirmed so I will remove the blindfold and you may open your eyes. Very good."

Does it work? Try it and see…the client will stop smoking forever for smoking now holds no charm and only the reaction to the image of disgust for smoking remains. Success!

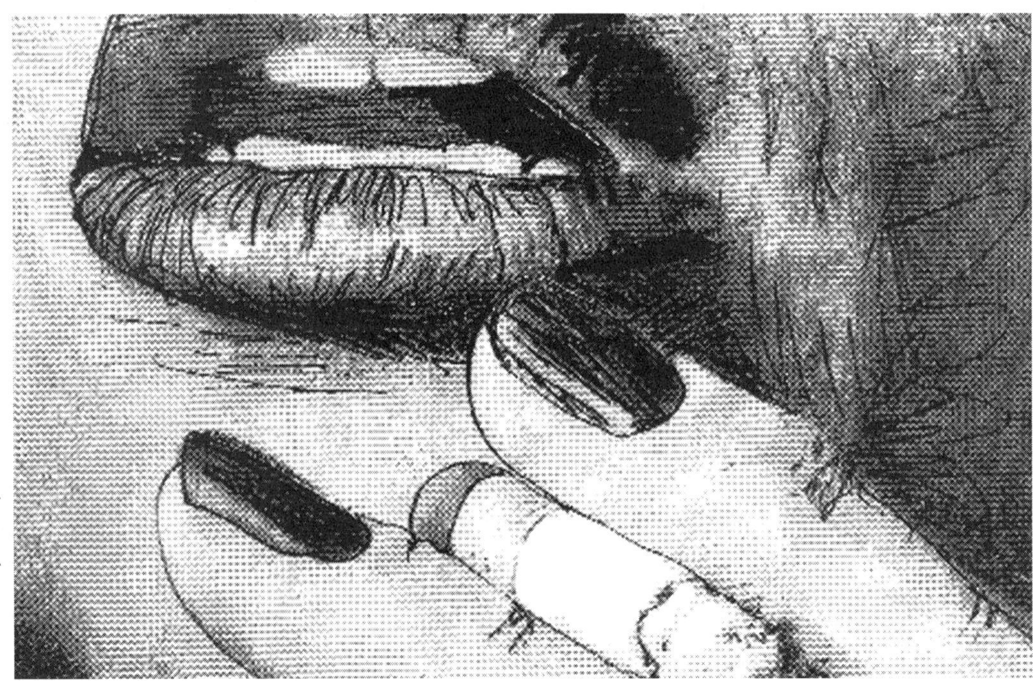

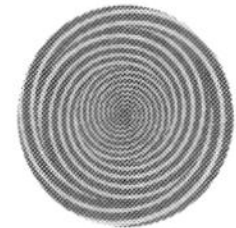

~ *Chapter 64* ~
SPHERE OF ENERGY
TO STOP SMOKING

Includes
Stop Smoking With The Sphere of Energy

The sphere of energy is used to request that the universe grant specific wishes. Countless people testify that this method works wonders! Their wishes were granted often in delightful and unexpected ways. Use it with hypnotherapy to correct a problem.

This method has a powerful hypnotic influence on the client. It is a mutual process between the hypnotherapist and the client and employs the creative mind to produce a matrix in space to affirm in reality for the client. Do you believe in the power of a matrix in space? Millions do. You can employ this method to achieve whatever is called upon to achieve. Clients permanently stop smoking using this approach.

Begin with a personal consultation between yourself and the client. Let's say that your client expresses a sincere desire to stop smoking. You outline the great benefits to be derived by no longer smoking, like improved health, money saved, sweet smelling breath and social acceptance. The consultation complete, you begin the sphere of energy corrective induction:

MODUS OPERANDI: STOP SMOKING WITH THE SPHERE OF ENERGY

Sit close together facing your client. Demonstrate and instruct your client to rub their hands together briskly to get the blood flowing freely. Tell them to do so until their hands tingle.

Now hold your cupped hands toward them and instruct them to do the same. **"Mentally form a sphere of energy between your cupped hands."**

If your client places their cupped hands on the imagined sides of the ball, you place yours at the imagined top or bottom of the same sphere. The space between the hands is thus encircling an imaginary ball.

"Visualize and imagine a sphere of energy being materialized between our encircled hands. Do it effortlessly. Just allow the energies between the hands to activate naturally. You will definitely feel it. As the energy builds visualize and feel it becoming large as a basketball. As this happens sometimes an almost misty force field seems to materialize."

When you both agree that you feel or sense it powerfully between your hands tell your client:

"Keep concentrating on the energy flowing as you say out loud what you want for yourself. What you know as the true benefits you came for today."

When complete, you continue;

"Upon this sphere of energy we place __________ (their name) **heartfelt wish to stop smoking now and forevermore** (or whatever is their goal)**. The great benefits they receive are appreciated. All desire to further smoke is gone completely. Repeat this same idea directly from yourself.**

(Give them time to say their objective).

Now repeat this after me (Take your time so that they have time to repeat each part)**: 'upon this energy sphere I affirm my heartfelt wish to stop smoking** (or what ever) **now and forevermore. All desire for smoking is forever gone. I am so happy that I have completely mastered this unwanted and unpopular habit. From this moment forward I smoke no more and my life is benefited in every way."**

Hypnotherapist continues:

"Upon this sphere of energy __________ (Client's name) **and I place this affirmation that** __________ (Client's name) **will smoke no more. They have completely mastered the habit and have no desire to ever smoke again and are so happy because this is reality. It is so.**

Together now we toss this sphere of energy up into the cosmos…wherein a matrix in space forms this as reality. __________ (Client's name) **has completely mastered any limiting habits. They will never smoke again. Indeed the very idea of smoking is detestable.**

The realization of this is a cosmic fact forever. Make this so. Now together we toss the sphere of energy up into space and visualize and imagine it going up and up and up into the cosmos. The sphere carries its affirmation and the physical reality is confirmed. There is no need to think of it again. You have stopped smoking forever.

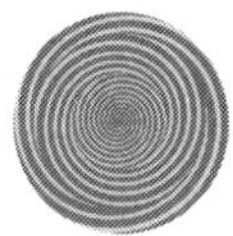

~ *Chapter 65* ~
STOCKWELL'S
QUIT SMOKING APPROACH

By Shelley Stockwell-Nicholas, PhD

More on this subject is found in Dr. Stockwell's book *"Denial Is Not A River In Egypt: Overcome Addiction, Compulsion and fear With Dr Stockwell's Self Hypnosis System"* Available at the back of this book.

Includes
Stop Smoking
Blessing That Deepens Trance
Regression Reframe
Aversion
Changing Patterns To Quit Tobacco
Breathe For Life
Progression

When I work with someone releasing toxic addictions like tobacco I remember some important principles
1. Offer a step-by-step action plan.
2. Avoid using the word you are eliminating. Repeatedly say "I am a 'non-smoker' underscores the word 'smoker' in the mind and the 'non' is automatically discounted. It's like saying to you dear reader, don't think about your tongue right now- all of a sudden you notice that you have a tongue. Better results for abating toxins happen when you accentuate the positive and attach the negative to something revolting.
3. Celebrate the client. They've been beating themselves up enough.

MODUS OPERANDI: STOP SMOKING
Hypnotize your client and to build expectation suggest:
"There is hope. Every day thousands of people just like you permanently quit poisoning themselves. More that forty million people quit for good each year. Their bodies renew and regenerate and the damage caused from toxic tobacco reverses. Lungs become clear and clean. Congratulations, you are ready and can and will quit, too."

BLESSING THAT DEEPENS TRANCE
"Let us ask for blessings. Bless _____________ (Client's name). Help them achieve perfect results from this session. They come here today with clean hands, a warm heart and the sincere desire to be happy and healthy in every way. Bless them on all levels, physically with radiant health, so they breathe with ease and feel terrific. Help them to easily release toxins

from their body so they are all fresh and new. Let them enjoy healthy habits of fresh whole foods, lots of water and moving their body.

Bless them emotionally with unconditional love for themselves and their loved ones. Let joy be their compass in all they do. If it is not fun don't let them do it any more.

Bless them mentally with clear thinking so that they can easily do what it takes to be totally and absolutely free of poison tobacco and get on with joy.

And finally, bless them spiritually so they fulfill their true path and purpose and serve the planet and all living things.

Amen. Awomen. Ah Life."

You can use one or all of the following processes during a session:

REGRESSION REFRAME

"Go back in time to the first time you put burning leaves and paper smeared with saltpeter in your mouth. Remember exactly what that was like for you.

Did you cough as your lungs tried to clear themselves?

Why did you do it?

Was it to be cool or fit in or to be like someone you knew or to be more grown up?

Do you want a decision made by the 'you' so long ago to run your life now?

(Pause)

There is a wonderful technique I call 'play it again Sam.' Here is how you do it. Run the same movie of you putting fire to that first poison paper and chemically coated leafs, only this time, make a different decision. Say, 'no thanks I don't need to do that' and refuse to put that in your body. Very good!"

AVERSION

Imagine a table in front of you with your brand of tobacco on it. Now put all the other brands there on the table too. When you have done this nod your head. Good.

Now, think of the most disgusting thing you can think of. Let me know when you are thinking of it. Good.

Now smear that disgusting thing all over the tobacco. Let it permeate the package the paper the leaves...every molecule now looks, smells and tastes exactly like that gross thing. Chemically soaked burning leaves are gross. Carbon monoxide, hydrogen cyanide, strychnine, tar, nicotine, saltpeter are a chemical nightmare that make up these nasty, white scorpions. They strike to kill each time they touch a mouth or nose. They are revolting. Tobacco is deadly venom. You can almost taste the poison, and it's terrible. Toxic leaves repulse and gag you. You don't want it. You don't need it. It smells and tastes terrible because it is poison. From this moment forward that gross thing and tobacco are all mixed up in your mind.

You hate poisonous tobacco. You can't stand the acrid smoke. The taste and the smell are disgusting.

Now, go ahead and crush the box and imagine seeing the icky tar oozing out of the package. Imagine a pile of all the poisonous tobacco you have used in your life. In your mind's eye see, feel, and taste the truckloads of toxic tobacco. If you were to burn all of those at once, there would be a gigantic billowing, belching, filthy black cloud of smoke, smogging the air. The tar and carcinogens reek and stink: the smell clings to hair and skin. As you think and imagine that black cloud, you think about all those chemicals that have entered your body. It's enough already. YOU QUIT.

'No thank' you say, 'I don't go there. I am vital, clean, sexy, healthy and beautiful. My sense of smell and taste are keen. I love the aroma of natural real air. I love the taste of healthy nourishing food and I crave delicious water. I feel healthy. I am healthy.'

Thank God, you are free. You did it! You walked away from poison; all poison. You did it by eliminating any trigger patterns that caused you to reach for rat poison wrapped in pretty packages."

CHANGING PATTERNS TO QUIT TOBACCO

"Like a switchboard operator, disconnect wires that have in the past tied you to saltpeter smeared paper and thick gummy toxic tar and nicotine. (Pause)

Those wires are now permanently disconnected! One by one, rituals associated with poison drop away. Your car is clean and smells great. Talking on the phone, you breathe fresh air. Sitting in a favorite chair, you enjoy fresh air you have learned to really relax. You love to be clean.

(Pause)

Disconnect the lines to sickening sugar and toxic caffeine. You love to feel great. You release old patterns that don't serve you well and replace them with healthy, happy, new patterns. You embrace happy new patterns. You are so blessed with life. You rewired your mind.

You change your routines for good, healthy habits. You take up new activities that bring you great pleasure. You enjoy taking a stroll during breaks and breathing real air. The air relaxes and revitalizes you. You sit at a new seat at the table. You clean your world. You wash your curtains, walls, car, and clothes and your home. You control the new delicious smell in your world. You are in control. You breathe with ease. Notice how your breathing is already better. Everything smells terrific. You are so proud of yourself.

This is a gift you give your family and yourself.

For the next two weeks you are a total pleasure seeker. You avoid anything stressful and only hang around with nourishing, positive people and situations. You take excellent care of yourself. Now repeat these ideas so that they sing inside your head:

'I choose to live.

I take control of my body, mind, energy and life.

I'm in control of myself. My potential is unlimited!

I'm strong. I help myself. I take charge and spring into action.

I easily achieve my dreams and goals. I'm honest with myself.

I honestly take responsibility for everything in my life.

If there is something I don't like, I change it. I do what I enjoy.

I do what makes me healthy, wealthy and wise. I am wise.

I'm in charge of my thoughts and emotions.

I breathe with ease.'

You are a growing and maturing personality.

You are a grown up adult with the joy of a playful child.

You set a healthy example for your inner child.

You love the child inside of you. I take loving care of all of your sub-selves.

You choose joy.

You choose wellness.

You follow your bliss.

You follow healthy curiosity.

You follow your path of radiance.

You are 100% responsible for everything in your life.

Now see yourself in a mirror smiling, attractive and healthy. Take a deep, full breath, get into center and let it out. In this moment, you begin a fresh, clean, new life. You are free to breath with ease. You are free of toxin and filled with joy. You feel so glad to be alive. It only takes a few days for nicotine to leave your body. What are a few days when you have a whole lifetime of feeling great ahead of you?

You erase any desire to put poison into your sweet body. You are your body. Your body is you. You love your body. You love all of you.

Your body is a loyal and devoted friend of your. It works for you 24-hours-a-day since you first began life. Your body deserves respect. You love your body. You only put nourishing things into your perfect body.

Enjoy another deep breath, taking in as much oxygen as your new, refreshed lungs can hold. To the count of five, let it out slowly one…two…three…four…notice the wonderful feeling of your breath; you breathe with ease and five.

Thank your lungs for doing such a fine job. Each day the cilia in your lungs filter better and better. These microscopic hairs pop right up to sweep away germs and protect you. You breathe fully, deeply and completely. You breathe with ease.

Take three full breaths. With each exhalation, say the words 'relaxed and free.'

One…'relaxed and free!' (Pace this with their breath.)

Two…'Relaxed and free!'

Three…'Relaxed and free!'

Now relax completely. You are free to use your many talents and interests. Now take three deep breaths. Relaxed and free… "Relaxed and free…Relaxed and free…

You feel a tremendous pride in yourself. No one and nothing can take you from this resolve! You affirm to yourself. 'I choose joy. I enjoy life. I am free and healthy. I'm attractive. I'm healthy. I live life completely.'

You love drinking fresh water. For the next two weeks you drink six to eight glasses of water a day and avoid depressing sugar, toxic caffeine, numbing alcohol and any other poison. You love drinking fresh water. For the next two weeks you may choose to take a multiple vitamin.

You stay quit and always remember why you quit and how you did it your way with hypnosis.

You so enjoy being totally free. You are proud of yourself. You see yourself in your mind's eye thinking, feeling, behaving and being successful.

You love the fresh taste in your mouth. You love to smell beautiful smells. Your skin loses any wrinkles and you look young and terrific. Your skin is smooth and attractive. You are sexy and easily accept love and affection. You sleep deeply and soundly, with perfect relaxation. You are free, calm, peaceful, clear-minded, and healthy from head to toe. You feel terrific. You love yourself."

BREATHE FOR LIFE

After inducing trance read this script slowly with soft music in the background:

"Congratulations! You sincerely commit to taking control of your life.

Take a long deep full breath and relax. Become more and more aware of breathing. Feel your chest rise and fall. Hear the sound the air makes as it moves in and out of your lungs and body.

How are your lungs working? (Pause for a minute and honestly answer this question.)

Do poisonous leaves, chemicals and/or fire hurt them? (Pause for a minute and honestly answer this question.)

You are lucky. You are alive! You are lucky! You are healthier and healthier with each and every breath. Celebrate how lucky you are to be here. Thank God, you have gotten a grip and have restored your lungs and perfect body.

You quit poison tobacco now.

Think now about yourself as a newborn baby. You were born to naturally breathe fresh air. Renewed and regenerated, like a healthy newborn, you cleanse your body and release any poison. You are clean. Your world is clean. You proudly take time to make life better. You are eager to learn new ways to honor yourself. Good for you.

Your fresh start begins this moment. You are well in body, mind and spirit. It's simple to release old habits that no longer serve you and replace them with comfortable new patterns that let you feel terrific. You choose to feel terrific.

Become aware of your pulse. (Pause)

Blood carries more and more oxygen to your heart. Your platelets are fluid and flowing. Your blood vessels and arteries are open

You are aware of your breath. (Pause)

With each breath your lungs bring in more and more fresh, cleansing air. The cilia in the lungs pop up and filter again. You are healthy, happy and proud. You breathe fully. You are filled with energy. You are a miracle. You breathe with ease. (Pause)

As you continue conscious breathing, become aware of three parts of your lungs; the lower, middle and top part. (Pause)

Fill your lungs in that order: lower third, the middle third and right on up to the top. Take a deep breath, filling up your lungs, section by section. It feels so good: bottom, middle, top.

You are a conscious breather. More and more oxygen enters and cleanses your lungs; section by section. Congratulations to you. You breathe with ease. Say it to yourself, 'I breathe with ease.'

Think of being completely relaxed. (Pause)

Imagine a pleasant scene and relax more and more. (Pause)

Notice all the sights, sounds, smells, tastes and energy of this special place. It is like you are there. The air is fresh and pure and smells divine. Is there sparkling water? Flowers or green trees? Hear pleasant sounds like birds or a luscious waterfall. Notice a cool breeze or warm sun.

'I breathe with ease. I breathe with ease.'

Notice the sound of your breath. Enjoy your natural breathing. Only healthy air enters your lungs. Your breath is a miracle!

YOU breathe with ease. You breathe with ease. Every breath strengthens your will power and commitment to enjoy life. You take charge of my life. Each breath cleanses my beautiful pink lungs more and more. Smoky, gummy disgusting tar melts away.

'My lungs are clear. I breathe with ease.' As you breath, you clean your lungs more and more. Bottom…Middle…Top.

'I breathe with ease. I cleanse my mouth.' (Pause)
'I cleanse my sinus cavities.' (Pause)
'I breathe with ease.'

You now cleanse and repair your lungs. Your lungs are clean and healthy.
'I breathe with ease.
I breathe with ease.
I breathe with ease.'
Your lungs are pink with soft air filled cells; beautiful and healthy lungs. You feel so glad to be alive. Right now in this instant, release the past! Forgive the past. You are forgiven.
'I breathe with ease.
I breathe with ease.
I breathe with ease.'
Call in the power of your imagination, higher self and God to help. (Pause)

PROGRESSION

Imagine yourself one month from today, free of negative habits. Completely free! You have new, positive habits. How good you feel, what terrific energy you have. You smell delicious. You taste delicious. You look wonderful.
'I breathe with ease.'
Think back and remember why you quit. Remember that awful cough and raw throat, that horrible smell. Tobacco is filthy, dirty and expensive. All the trouble it caused are now gone. You are free. Take a deep breath.
'I breathe with ease.'
Your commitment for joy and wellness is permanent. Moment-to-moment, no one can tempt you to harm your happy body...no friend, commercial or habit. Tobacco tastes repulsive and smells disgusting. If someone offers you chemical-soaked leaves you say, 'No. And God bless you.' You avoid others who are self-destructive. You embrace positive places or situations. You nourish yourself. Your new patterns work great! You drink water, breathe fully and laugh a lot. You stay consciously aware and in charge of your life. Each thought is positive. You use right thinking. You do good positive and loving things for yourself. No matter what feelings come up, no matter what is going on in your life. You never again poison my body temple. You are kind and loving to your body.

You nourish yourself and breathe with ease. Your decision is final. You stick to it. You love your body and yourself.

With each deep breath go deeper into your inner mind. You've come to a crossroad. You choose a road to joy and life. You take the road to lush green, glorious colors, life and fresh smells. The sun is shining and there are warm breezes in your hair. You are radiant and alive, surrounded by loving friends. You are proud of your path and life. Congratulations. You are free. Terrific job _____________ (Client's name)."

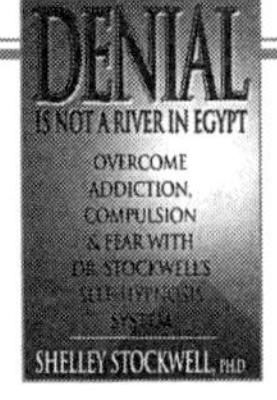

Hypno-Helper
"Denial Is Not A River In Egypt: Overcome Addiction, Compulsion & Fear With Dr. Stockwell's Self-Hypnosis System"
"Hypnosis: How To Put A Smile On Your Face and Money In Your Pocket" by Shelley Stockwell have excellent sections on how to overcome smoking and how to conduct quit smoking seminars.

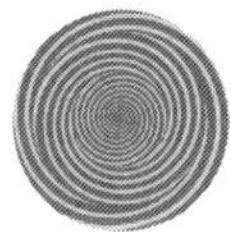

~ *Chapter 66* ~
SUPER LEARNING & SPORTS PERFORMANCE

Includes
Super Learning Induction
Suggestion-Formula For Super Learning
Stockwell (Nicholas) Sports Script

SUPER LEARNING is a new, very personal way, of accelerating learning and increasing comprehension and recall. It programs information into your brain's biocomputer and makes it your very own. Learning is mostly a matter of easy recall of material studied.

Both Russia and Rumania use Super Learning in schools. It makes the environment for study easygoing.

This new super learning technique uses the Serenity Resonance Sound in the background and that, in itself, is powerful hypnosis. Its alpha/theta sound entrains your brain to receive, remember and program learning. Your mind learns best when relaxed and entertained and the subconscious mind has perfect memory. More about the *Serenity Resonance Sound* is found in chapter 34.

Use this method in studying and learning. There is no hurry in super learning. Take your time. Just enjoy this useful knowledge, plus a bit of *knowing* tossed in for good measure.

MODUS OPERANDI: SUPER LEARNING INDUCTION
You Will Need:
A Comfortable Chair where your client can easily read something later on in the session.
A Candle
The Reading Material They Want To Learn
The Serenity Resonance Sound audio tape or CD (available at the back of this book)

Perform self-hypnosis for super learning in your private office where your client is free from all disturbances. First induce trance using your favorite induction then turn on the *Serenity Resonance Sound,* audio tape or CD and Instruct your client, **"Stand up in front of the chair. Take a deep breath and stretch your arms upward high above the head. Stretch. Stretch. Stretch. IT FEELS SO GOOD."** Do this with them and you establish rapport and continue, **"Now, sit comfortably in the chair and relax back, with your hands lying loosely in your lap with feet resting on the floor."**

Now darken the room and light a candle and place it on a table in front of the comfortable chair upon which your client is relaxing and offer these suggestions,
"Direct your gaze towards the candle's flickering flame.

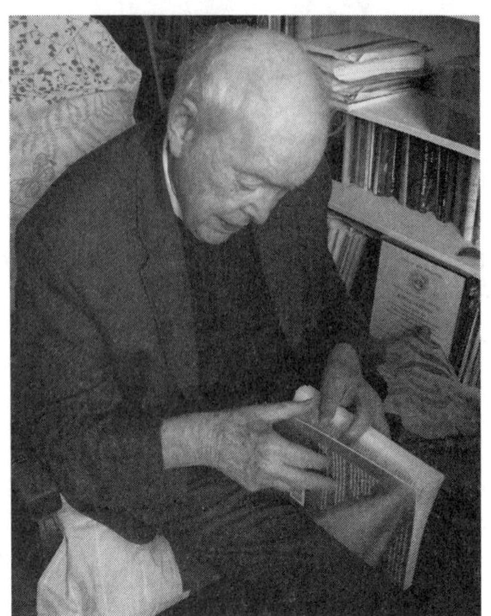

ORMOND READING

How good you feel. How quiet and peaceful. All this while, concentrate your attention to the candle flame. Your gazing and staring at the flame begins to make your eyes feel tired and heavy and they want to close.

So now, just close your eyes close. It feels so good.

Your eyes close…comfortable and relaxed. Your eyes are closed, shutting out all light, so you can now just slip down into the quiet realm of sleep. Sleep. Peace. Quiet. Relaxation. Relax. Relax. Relax and allow this relaxation to flow over your entire body. Your entire body is becoming more and more relaxed.

Let the relaxation travel to each part of your body, as you sink down ever deeper and deeper into the lethargy of the realm of sleep.

Direct your attention to the top of your head. Allow all the muscles in your scalp to relax. Relax so completely that you can feel your scalp tingle. Think it and you will feel it. Feel the warm tingling commence in the top of your head.

Now, let this warm tingling flow down over the muscles of your face. All the muscles of your face are relaxing. Even the muscles on the back of your neck are relaxing. Your throat muscles are relaxing. Your shoulder muscles are relaxing. All is peaceful and calm.

Let this relaxation flow further down your body. Down your arms to your hands… all negativity and tension flowing out your fingertips. Your chest is relaxed. Your entire torso is relaxed. And, the relaxation continues to flow yet further down your body and your legs become relaxed. You are relaxed all over your entire body. You feel comfortable and GOOD ALL OVER.

You are breathing deep and fully and each breath you take is causing you to become more and more relaxed. You are becoming very sleepy.

You feel sleepy. Sleep. Sleep. Sleep. You find yourself drifting off towards the realm of sleep. You are comfortable, cozy, and relaxed. You are dropping down ever deeper towards sleep and relaxation - deeper and deeper asleep in hypnosis.

Sleep and rest. Sleep and rest. Sleep and rest deeper and deeper asleep in hypnosis.

And, even as you drop into hypnosis, you are fully aware and your conscious mind moves aside while your subconscious mind emerges and is ready to accept and make become your reality the gift of SUPER LEARNING that will now be given to you."

SUGGESTION-FORMULA FOR SUPER LEARNING

"Now I'd like you to speak to your subconscious mind in a personal manner. Give it a personality. Even give it a name, if you wish. Speak to it as an individual; as a friend who will grant your every request.

Say to it 'Subconscious mind' -let's call it Henry- 'grant me the skill of Super Learning. When I have something before me I wish to learn, I place my hands over my ears and I read OUT LOUD to myself. Learning will RRRING through my head and become indelibly recorded in the memory banks of my subconscious. Henry, make it so.'"

(Pause)

Take your hands and gently place your fingers to your temples. Good.

Whenever you place your fingers like this to your temples, knowledge will appear, this will be your signal. It will instantly be recalled. It will instantly appear inside your head, behind your closed eyes, upon your screen of mind, and you will come to know that which you wish to know."

So whenever you give this signal, you will recognize and bring forth whatever you have learned that you wish to recall. Good.

Now sit up comfortably and read what it is that you wish to learn. As you read, you can read it out loud or you may intone the words to yourself. Continue to relax in a hypnotic state of mind throughout the entire process. Your concentration is perfect and you easily absorb what you read. Nothing pulls your attention but what you are reading. Place your hands over your ears as you read."

At this point in Super Learning, your client reads their learning material out loud or to them self, with their hands over their ears. The Serenity Resonance Sound is playing very quietly as background for the study session.They will find learning easy to do. This method fills the subconscious memory banks with knowledge almost automatically. When they are complete give this instruction:

"You easily study in this manner anytime you want to learn something. It is easy for you. Just go through the material once. It is quite enough. When complete, relax and close your eyes. PAUSE. Allow this idea to sink-in. You truly amaze yourself in how effectively you learn and use this new method of SUPER LEARNING.

Now let's remind 'Henry' of your agreed upon 'signal.' When you touch your temples all that you have read will clearly and easily flood your memory banks with the knowledge you have learned. You easily recall what and when you want. When you touch your temples, your mind instantly recalls what you have learned. 'Henry' will not let you down.

Use this method of Super Learning anytime you please. There is no limit to the capacity of the memory banks of your subconscious.

When your study session is complete, you just stand up and go about your daily activities and the hypnosis will disburse like vapor.

Oh and say 'Thank you, Henry.' Always give thanks for the miracle that is in you."

MODUS OPERANDI: EDITOR STOCKWELL (NICHOLAS) SPORTS SCRIPT

Induce trance and

1. "Ask your subconscious mind ("Henry") to bring you someone you most admire in your sport. Take a deep breath and "Henry" will learn on the cellular level all you need to know to be at the top of your game so you are just like that one you so admire.

2. Now do a mental rehearsal and imagine yourself/them playing a perfect game from beginning to end.

3. Imagine yourself/them winning a trophy (or whatever is your goal)

4. As soon as you put on your sports togs and take a deep breath, you immediately relax and say to yourself, 'I am at the top of my game.'"

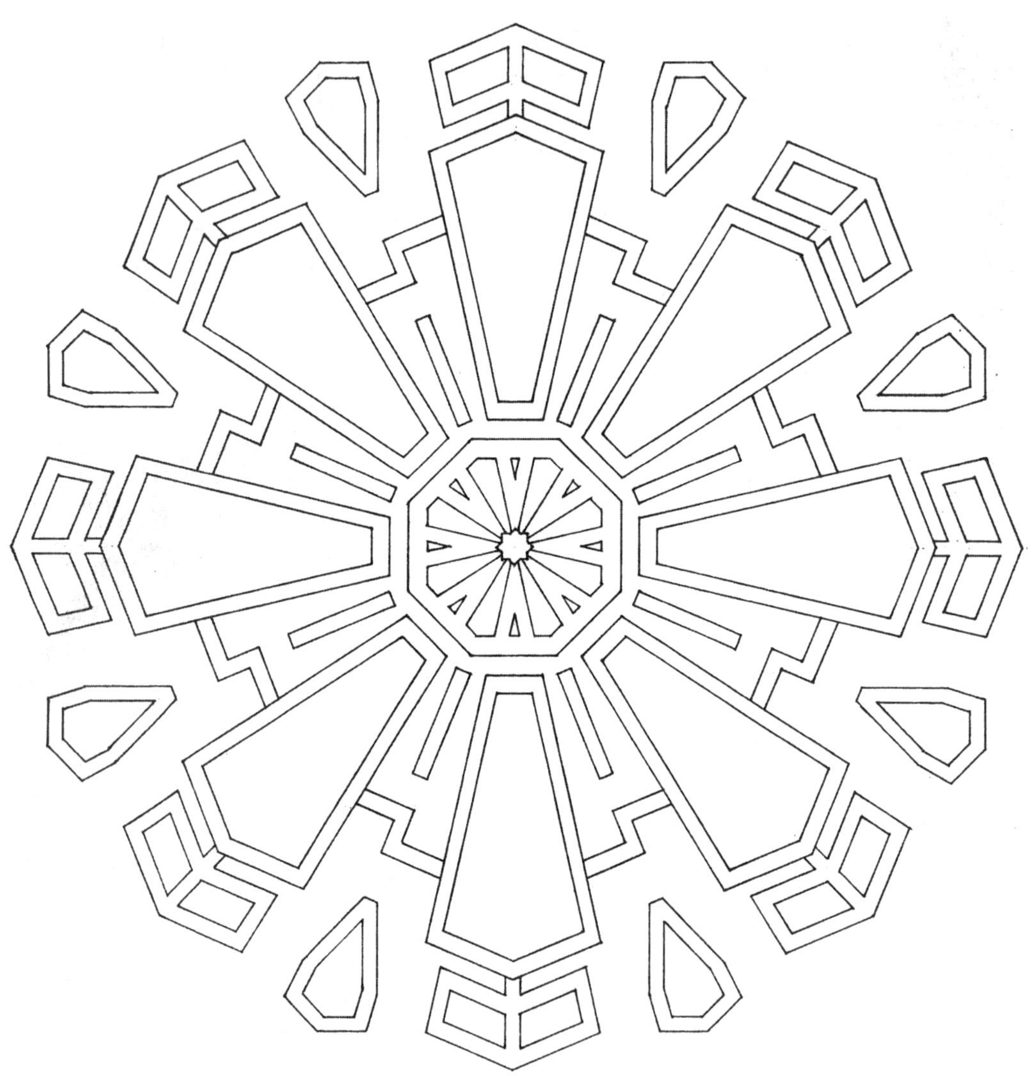

Coloring and writing words on this "brain gym"
super learning mandala created by Kim Peeples activates
the creative mind to enhance memory.

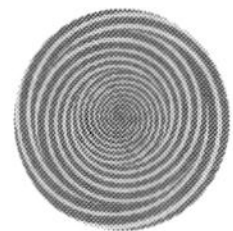

~ *Chapter 67* ~
SUGGESTIONS FOR WILL & MEMORY

A most striking characteristic of hypnosis is the prodigious memory naturally produced. Consciously imperceptible impressions greet you. Everything that you have ever learned can be remembered. Addressing hypnotic suggestions to the memory, even more enhances recall.

MODUS OPERANDI: WILL & MEMORY

"Retire to a quiet place and count from one to ten, while concentrating upon this operation. Make your mind receptive and repeat to yourself with energy and determination, 'My memory and will power is advancing by leaps and knows no boundaries. I remember things easily. I cause this effect by the power of my will.'"

Here are four exercises for you to practice:

Suggestion Formula 1

"Retire to a darkened chamber as you fix your mind intently upon one subject and exclude all else. Do this for as long as possible. It may be challenging at first, but it becomes easier with practice. Repeat this exercise for five successive nights. Allow one hour each time."

Suggestion Formula 2

"At night, when the sky is clear, concentrate your attention upon the stars, and count as many of them as you can."

Suggestion Formula 3

"Go to the seashore where there is smooth damp sand. Write upon the sand with a stick or your finger that you are a mastermind; perform this exercise for an hour each day."

Suggestion Formula 4

"Take twelve marbles, pebbles or similar small objects, and hold them in your left hand. Now pick up one with the right hand and hold it out at arm's length. Contemplate it fixedly, and exclude all other thoughts, for a full minute at a time. Then let the object fall into the palm of your left hand, and precede in the same manner with the other eleven, repeating the process to occupy you for one hour each day."

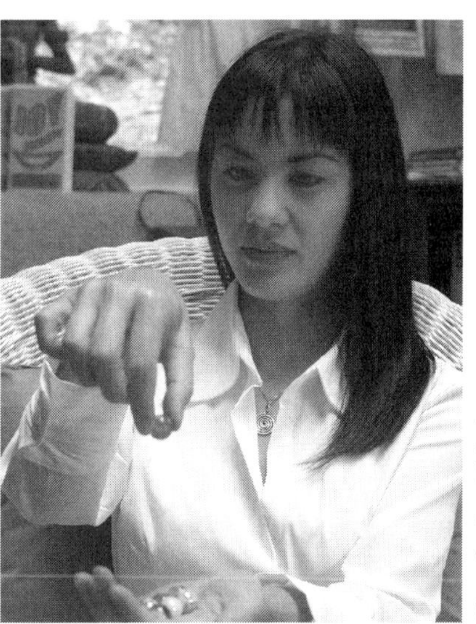

Marble Drop

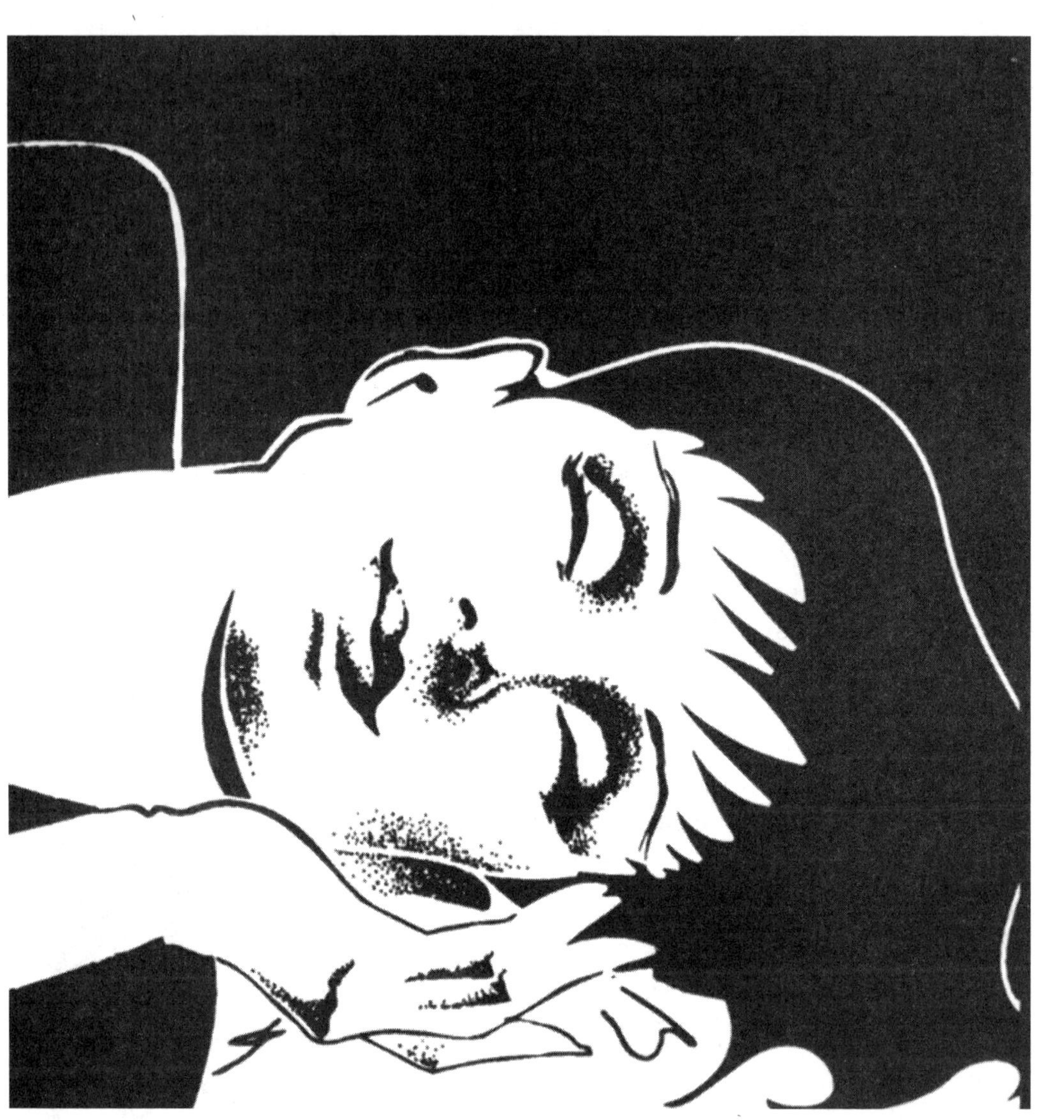

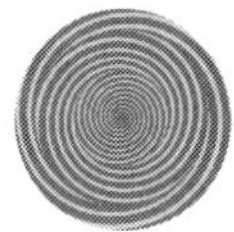

~ *Chapter 68* ~
SLEEP LEARNING:
HYPNOTHERAPY WHILE ASLEEP

We spend nearly a third of our life in sleep. How economical it would be to learn during sleep. Sleep Learning is subconscious learning. Since the brain is a biocomputer, let's call it "nocturnal programming."

During World War II, the military used "Sleep Learning" to help soldiers quickly master the Japanese and German languages. They used a 30-minute cassette tape. A flat speaker was placed beneath the pillow with a tape player and timer at the side of the bed. The timer caused the tape to play and stop intermittently during the night as the person slept. The method was very successful. Those who learned while they slept mastered a subject more quickly.

Sleep Learning combined with Wake Learning holds tremendous potential for education.

Sleep Learning is easily applied to hypnotherapy. It offers the perfect opportunity to reinforce the beneficial suggestions you give your client in your office. While they sleep, in the privacy of their home, they enjoy positive programming.

Sleep produces a natural mental/physical serenity that allows the body to revitalize itself. Your body needs sleep to maintain health, but your mind has no need for sleep at all.

It is possible for your subconscious mind to remain awake to sounds and spoken words while the conscious phase of mind is asleep. In other words, subconscious mind hears, registers, retains, and reacts to verbal suggestions and their meaning during natural sleep. The source of the suggestion, whether by your voice or a recording, is relatively irrelevant.

Sleep Learning and hypnotherapy while asleep requires a soft babbling of instructions to the mind, while the body sleeps. One difficulty with Sleep Learning is that some people sleep so lightly that even soft babbling disturbs sleep. Hypnosis easily overcomes this difficulty with the suggestion,

"When you hear speaking beneath your pillow or by your bedside, it produces a deeper state of healthful sleep, deeper than usual."

MODUS OPERANDI: SLEEP LEARNING
You will need:
A Tape Recorder

Before inducing hypnosis, explain to the client exactly what is to be done. Then, induce hypnosis and repeat these instructions:

"I will record the beneficial suggestions I give you today. Then when you go to sleep in your bed, arrange a tape-player beside the bed, and place a speaker beneath the pillow or next to you. If you have a timer, set it to turn the recorder on and off once during the night. Nod your head if you understand. Good."

Make certain that your client understands these instructions.

Deepen the hypnotic state into somnambulism, and suggest:

"You are in profound hypnosis. Now accept fully these suggestions of benefit to yourself. Your body easily goes into deep, healthful, natural sleep. This gives you vitality and good health. But, your subconscious mind needs no sleep. It remains alert and receptive to the suggestions you will be given while your body sleeps. At a late hour in the night, while you are sound asleep, my voice will speak to you from beneath the pillow, or next to your bed. It will in no way awaken you or disturb you. In fact, as you hear my voice, you will go deeper and deeper into sleep and profound hypnosis. Every beneficial suggestion, I give you, will become reality in your life. Accept now these suggestions into yourself and make them your reality."

At this point in the session, record your "suggestion-formula." Repeat it three times on the tape you make.

Then continue:

"Repeat this affirmation: My subconscious mind accepts these suggestions. They become my reality. Hypnosis has conditioned me to perfectly perform these beneficial suggestions. When this is so, I will return to the here and now feeling wonderful and fine."

Allow the client's subconscious to arouse them from hypnosis – as it intimately knows when the desired condition has been established.

When recording the taped suggestion-formulas, you can add some soothing music. You could re-hypnotize them quickly and play your recording for them now if you like. The client will drift into healthful sleep, while the beneficial suggestions take effect. When complete, arouse them and send them home with a smile.

Instruct your client to **"listen to the tape every night"** until they have reached their goal. Repetitions of suggestions compound its effect.

Another version of this to be used with members of your family is to simply talk to someone while they sleep. Do this in a way that won't disturb their sleep.

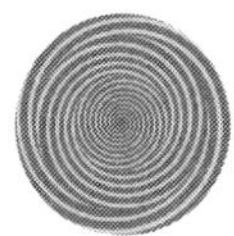

STOCKWELL'S POETRY HYPNOSIS

By Shelley Stockwell-Nicholas, PhD

© Excerpt from "Insides Out" and "Sex and Other Touchy Subjects"
by Shelley Stockwell available at the back of this book

Poetry speaks to us where we live. We love poems for no rhyme or reason. Have you noticed how lyrics to a song stick in your mind? You have been lulled and programmed by the rhythm to remember.

I have enjoyed writing and reciting the following poetry for my clients and students. The flow of the poem itself is hypnotic. Here are some favorite poetic hypnosis scripts I've written:

YES, I'M POSITIVE
Sunshine wonderful absolutely Yes!
I am feeling fine; complete, I am at my best.

I hear that you are crying slashin' mental wrists.
Give your head a twist about. Put your grief to rest.
If you were mistaken…sad…on overload,
Now you're positively bent; and you're not even stoned.

Sunshine wonderful absolutely Yes!
When you're happy, feeling fine, you can't be depressed.
Life is a conspiracy guaranteeing ecstasy…
Abundant love to satisfy all the needs of you and I.

Want it, watch it happen; enjoy absurdity.
Giggle, chortle, laugh aloud, start slappin' at your knees.
Say sunshine wonderful, absolutely Yes
You are groovy, feeling fine; you are at your best!
  — Shelley Stockwell (Nicholas)

MONEY (Excerpted from "The Money Tape" available at the back of this book)
I like Money.
I'm open to receive a lot.
I deserve it.
Money's good for me.
  — Shelley Stockwell (Nicholas)

WELLNESS
I am my body. My body is me.
We live together in harmony.
      — Shelley Stockwell (Nicholas)

FEEL GOOD
I become my own good mommy
And a daddy I love and adore.
I really am my best buddy
For that's what friends are for.
The truth is what has freed me
I laugh and smile and grin.
My talents and dreams are respected
I hear the voice within.
I do kind things for my body
I take back control at last.
I honestly express each emotion
I release and forgive the past.
      — Shelley Stockwell (Nicholas)

DEPRESSION
What is it of your disposition?
That puts you in this glum condition?
Take some time. Put on the light
And stay at home for one whole night
To view the movie that is your life.
And decide if that movie feels real true; for you
And if it doesn't, here's what you do:

Gather the strength, put yourself on the line
And take a risk; this really works fine.
And say, "Just what I want for me?"
That's what it takes to break you free.
For it's harder to stew in depressing old juices
Convincing yourself and making excuses
Than moving ahead with the excitement of change
For movement is living and stagnation is strange.

Your life is a sculpture to mold as you will.
You're not a victim of mom, your mate or your pills
Your life's a pattern that's your own design.
Take a chance, move ahead, now's the perfect time.
      — Shelley Stockwell (Nicholas)

IT'S LAUGHTER YOU'RE AFTER
The funnier it gets, the funnier it gets,
Your cells remember what logic forgets.
To laugh is to live from the inside out,
and that's what ecstasy is all about.
You are the light. You are the laughter,
And that's how you get to happily ever after.
Giggle, chortle, chuckle, grin,
That's how happiness begins.
Laugh, guffaw, slap your knee,
And you'll achieve high-larity.
　　　　— Shelley Stockwell (Nicholas)

GOSSIP
They hover like flies as you tell them the scoop.
Flies don't smell the stench when surrounding fresh poop.
With the skill of a surgeon you dissect each act:
Her demeanor, her boyfriend, her complete lack of tact.
You're the most charged, the loudest, animated as hell
And they cluster and listen to the tales that you tell
You're the star of the show. Their ears stick like glue.
Until you're not around and they talk about you.
　　　　— Shelley Stockwell (Nicholas)

ODE TO MY ADRENALS
Oh,
pyramid-
shaped organs
atop each kidney rest,
though I have overtaxed you
and you have made me stressed.
Thank you for awakening stimulating juices,
adrenaline and cortisone, a rush my body uses.
So I can build my tissue and keep me at the ready,
I will not fatigue you more with fear and panic petty.
Instead, I will caress you for your sweet and loving care.
And an easy-going life style together we will share.
Take that long vacation, you earned because you please me.
Refreshed, renewed and mellow we will take it easy.
　　　　— Shelley Stockwell (Nicholas)

DO IT
Gather ye rosebud while ye may
Old time is still a'flying.
The same flower that blooms today
Tomorrow may be dyin'
　　　　—Robert Berns

INTEGRITY
I have to live with myself and so,
I want to be fit for myself to know.
I want to be able as days go by
always to look myself in the eye.
I don't want to sit with the setting sun and hate myself for deeds I've done.
I see what others may never see. I know what others may never know.
I have to live with myself and so:
Whatever happens I want to be
Self-respecting and conscience free.
     —Author Unknown

Hypnotherapy
Punch, pound, fight it out.
Rip, tear, sigh or shout
pieces, bits go flying by
in this battleground called "I."
Your head may say "no"; your heart may say "yes"
and perhaps you feel like a royal mess.
The battleground of this ancient war,
acted out many times before,
may leave you smiling in a mold
hoping you would not explode
and then you came to the hypnotist's door
and allowed yourself to "at least explore
the place in you where you are snagged"
without insult or scold or nag
as the hypnotist listens long and well
to each small detail you did tell.
Air leaves gently your hot air balloon
as you sit and share in this sacred room
and quietly you put the soldiers to rest
with calm acceptance in your breast.
The warring factions are parts of thee;
you live together physically
You are a tapestry made of thread
woven perfectly in your head
Tough and soft; man and woman
body, mind now interwoven.
     — Shelley Stockwell (Nicholas)

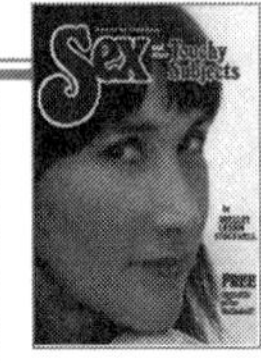

Hypno-Helper
"Sex and Other Touchy Subjects" by Shelley Stockwell-Nicholas
(book and tape)
"Insides Out" (book) available at the back of this book.

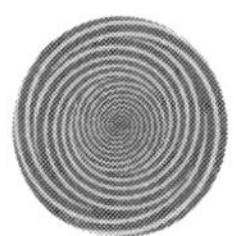

~ *Chapter 70* ~
ENERGY, CONFIDENCE AND STAMINA
SUGGESTION–FORMULAS

Includes Suggestions for
Increased Energy
Stamina
Confidence
Determination
Self-Control

The bounty of these suggestion-formulas is unbeatable. They benefit you to enjoy your SELF more fully! Each may be modified to directly apply to you or your client's specific goals that place you more in control of yourself. Repeat them from three to ten times for increased effectiveness.

INCREASED ENERGY

"I see and feel myself as a dynamic, active person. I have a great reservoir of energy and strength deep within me waiting to be called forth anytime I required it. I feel this resource open up and recharge me. I return to my tasks with renewed energy and power. I feel wonderful."

STAMINA

"I have great resources of energy and power within me ready to act at my bidding. I relax all inhibitions and restraints, and allow these resources to take over and act– now! My resources of vitality respond immediately and perform each task 'at full steam' until each task I undertake is completed. I am very happy at my new-found stamina."

CONFIDENCE

"I believe in myself and my ability to succeed. I am confident. I have a powerful will. I feel myself becoming more and more confident in every way with each passing day. I respect and trust my own judgment, my own opinions, and my own decisions. I am becoming increasingly aware of improved self-esteem, inner strength and courage. I awake each morning knowing that I can and will succeed at any task I undertake. Each day I like and appreciate myself more and more with steadily increasing self-confidence."

DETERMINATION

"I am determined to succeed. I am filled with the ambition. I successfully complete everything I do. I enjoy being successful. Others respond to my ability to influence. I radiate cheerfulness. The universe wants me to be successful. I am self-confident. I am determined to do what I set my mind to do. There is no stopping me. I am a winner."

SELF CONTROL

"I am in control of myself at all times. I strongly and firmly master myself. I am calm, cool and collected. I am happy and at ease. I am the controller of my behavior. I have a sense of joy in all I do. I am in charge of what I say and do. I make good choices in my behavior. My choices bring me many blessings: good health, friendship, success, and love. I am tactful. I am in charge of a full and rewarding life. I make a decision, after I gather the facts with a clear mind. I stick to my decisions. I enjoy positive cheerful thoughts. If I over react I immediately take charge of my thoughts and actions and take back my self-control. I am in charge."

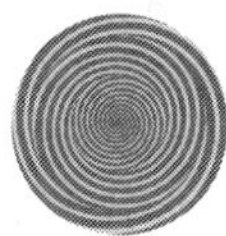

~ *Chapter 71* ~
SNUGGLE DOWN AND
BE COMFORTABLE WITH YOURSELF

Give this self-hypnosis technique to your client as an extra gift. Sometimes this "little something extra" can mean a great deal. It is a very simple technique and you can use it for yourself, as well.

The technique has no particular purpose of goal to reach. Its purpose is just to go down inside oneself and feel good all over. To feel good all over is a great gift.

"Do this. When you wake up in bed, don't fret. Just snuggle down beneath your covers. Curl up like a ball, and fill your mind with how comfortable you feel and how good it is to be alive. Think of yourself as being like a little animal does when it hibernates all winter long. Snuggle up. Snuggle up. Snuggle up. How comfortable you are. How comfortable you are. How comfortable you are.

With your body in a warm and snug position and your mind filled with thoughts of how comfortable you are. You are performing effortlessly a most remarkable form of hypnotherapy that benefits in every way.

Nothing specific. Just snuggle down and be comfortable with yourself.

Then just drift, drift, drift, and likely sleep will come. And when you awaken from that snuggle sleep you will find you never felt better in your life.

Perform the technique regularly, every time you awaken during the night.

Simple. Make no effort at all. Just curl up like a little animal, as you drift back into sleep. You will find the snuggle feeling carries over throughout the day. It is wonderful. It can literally transform your life."

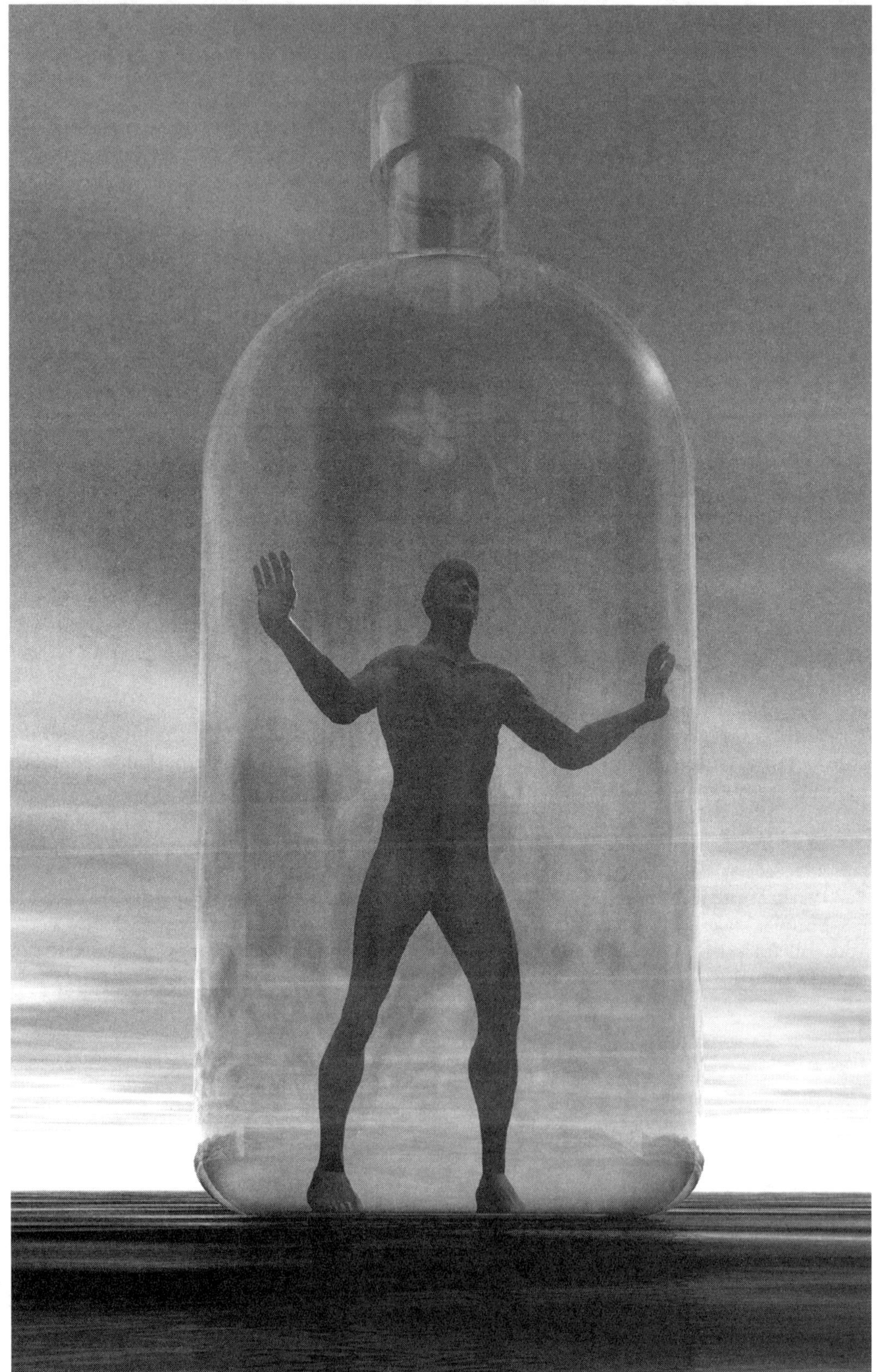

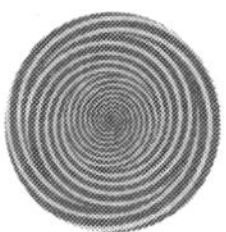

~ *Chapter 72* ~
TENSION, STRESS AND DEPRESSION RELIEF
SUGGESTION-FORMULAS

Includes Suggestions to
Relieve Tension
Cope With Stress
Overcome Depression
Serenity Hypnotherapy

Present these successful suggestion-formulas while in hypnosis. They influence the sympathetic nervous system to put into operation desired behavior and function. Each is of supreme value and makes you or your client more in control of SELF. Becoming in control of yourself is the secret of stress relief, as the more you can control yourself the less stress can control you. What a tremendous benefit to have at your disposal!

These suggestions may apply to you or your client's specific goals and make you more in control of yourself. Each suggestion should be repeated from three to ten times for increased effectiveness.

RELIEVE TENSION

"I feel myself inwardly quiet with a deep reservoir of inner peace. If tension results from emotional pressure, I automatically relax. I permit my inner reservoir of deep peace to open and pervade my mind, my body and spirit with a profound feeling of this deep peace. I feel content, quietly happy, and return to face life with renewed courage, strength, and energy. This process goes into effect starting this moment, and continues from now on for my achieving of perpetually mounting peace."

COPE WITH STRESS

"If ever I become aware of stress or tension, I automatically relax. I have complete control of my emotions and feelings. I refuse to let stress disturb me in any way. I review each situation calmly, rationally, and objectively. I make sound decisions concerning how I live my own life. I am very happy at my new strength and positive approach to life which is becoming my way of being."

OVERCOME DEPRESSION

"I have the power and ability to control all my emotions. Whenever I feel unhappy or depressed, I automatically relax. I replace all negative feelings with positive ones: with a sense of deep inner peace and a feeling of wholeness and well being. Pleasant events and memories come into my mind, and I find myself growing more content and quietly happy each day in every way."

SERENITY HYPNOTHERAPY

Use this for clients who are tense, disturbed with life and filled with stress. This is a transforming hypnotherapeutic.

Hypnotize your client into somnambulistic state bypassing completely critical mind. End your induction with these suggestions:

"**Subconscious mind of ________ (client's name). You are in profound hypnosis and will accept and transform these suggestions into reality. Understand this fully.**

________ (client's name) this session in serenity hypnosis is wonderful for you. It brings you the serenity of a peaceful mind. Allow what is here given to become your productive way of life. Remove you preferences. Let your preferences be gone. Your mind is open and free to receive and transform these suggestions into your reality.

When love and hate are both absent, everything becomes clear and undisguised. From this time on you will hold no opinions for or against anything. Understand this fully: to set up what you like against what you dislike is the disease of the mind. From this time forward this neutral position becomes your way of life. Understand this fully"

(Pause)

This way is perfect like vast space, where nothing is lacking and nothing is in excess. Understand fully that to accept or reject whatever you perceive, clouds perception of the true nature of things.

From this time forward, you live neither in the entanglement of outer things, nor in an inner appearance of an empty world. Changes that appeared to occur in an empty world that we call real but they are not real. Be serene in the oneness of things and all erroneous perception will disappear by themselves.

As long as you remain in activity and passivity, one extreme or the other, you will not know serenity. Do not try to stop activity to achieve passivity, because your very effort fills you with activity. The faster they hurry the slower they go. Consider movement stationary and stationary in motion and then both movement and rest disappear. Absorb this wisdom.

If you do not discriminate between coarse and fine you will not be tempted to pre-judge.

Assertion and denial also cause you to miss the reality of things. To assert the emptiness of things is to miss their solidity. The more you talk and think about finding truth, the further astray you wander from the truth. Stop talking and thinking and you will know everything. You return to the root and find the meaning. You live holistically, in the single way.

The moment of inner enlightenment goes beyond appearance. If there is even a trace of this or that, or right or wrong, mind will be lost in confusion. Your mind now exists undisturbed, and nothing in the world can offend or disturb it. Your mind is serene.

Now understand and absorb this wisdom: To live fully is neither easy nor difficult. For the unified mind, self-centered striving ceases, doubt and irresolution vanish and you live fully. In a single stroke you are freed from such bondage; nothing clings to you and you hold on to nothing. There is neither self nor other-than-self. There is no yesterday or tomorrow. There is only here and now. You live fully in the here and now. You fully appreciate the life you live.

Subconscious mind, let _____________ (client's name) **understand and absorb the wisdom that has been given. When serenity is fully present, arouse** _________________ (client's name) **from hypnosis feeling wonderful and fine.**"

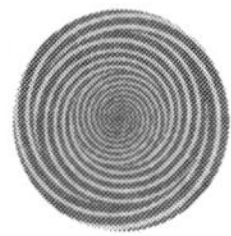

~ *Chapter 73* ~
HOLDER'S STRESS MANAGEMENT
By Philip Holder, PhD

Includes
Remote Control Expectations
Balloon Stress Release
Magic Bubble Stress Release
Fire Away

Without effective coping skills, stress can negatively impact peace of mind and physical health. There are tremendous "stressors" in our lives today. This is especially true anywhere a people is plagued with terrorist attacks, retaliations and related safety concerns.

In truth, stress is a way of life. There will always be stressors around us: it is impossible to eliminate them all from our world. The issue is how to best NOT internalize stress. Good coping skills help you and your clients better manage stress and enhance mental and physical wellness.

What Do You Expect?

To some extent we all want the world to fit our individual standards. We expect others to behave and think as we do.

It is human nature to think that other drivers go too fast, or too slow, when obviously you are the world's greatest driver. It is human nature to think that others should share your brilliant views on child rearing, politics, and society.

In fact, others often don't share your views and to expect them to is unrealistic and causes many problems. When unrealistic expectations are not fulfilled, internal emotional and mental stress often result. Expectation is one of the ways we give control away.

My personal life philosophy is that "I don't expect anything from anybody." By expecting nothing, everything I receive is a gift and I am never disappointed. I'm not saying that we should not strive to do better in our lives by setting goals and by being diligent in achieving those goals. I'm not saying that we shouldn't set standards for our children and ourselves. I am simply saying that the goals we set for ourselves must be realistic.

How Hypnotherapists Help

"I am not in this world to live up to your expectations; you are not here to live up to mine."

Hypnotherapists know that what the person perceives as reality is their reality relative to their own life experience. Because each person perceives the world differently, expectation of others is often a setup for stress related problems and disappointments…especially when we expect others to fulfill our expectation of how they should think and act.

Help your clients understand that they have no control over others and therefore cannot expect others to live up to their image of how, what, and who, the other person should be.

You help your client cope with stress, when you work with them on the issue of expectation. For example a client may say, "When my mother does X, Y, or Z, it makes me feel angry and stresses me out. "The fact is that this person's expectation of their mother may be unrealistic in relationship to what the mother is capable of providing. The answer is not in changing the mother's actions or behavior (since neither the client nor you have any control over the mother) but rather in awakening the client to the idea that their expectation of the other person is what needs to be reframed or seen in a new way.

MODUS OPERANDI: REMOTE CONTROL EXPECTATIONS

Rid someone of expectations of others and you help them to take back "the remote control of their lives." When expectation leads to stress, I have my client remote control it away. This significantly reduces their anxiety level and gives them a powerful tool to battle tension. Instill this waking hypnotic suggestion in the pre-talk, and as a post-hypnotic suggestion, **"No one can push your buttons unless you willingly give the remote control of your life over to them. Imagine a remote control device in your hand. Any time you feel that you are giving up that control, you will immediately take the remote control back into your own hands."**

Sometimes I actually give them an object to act as their remote. Virtually anything will do, even something as simple as a small stone.

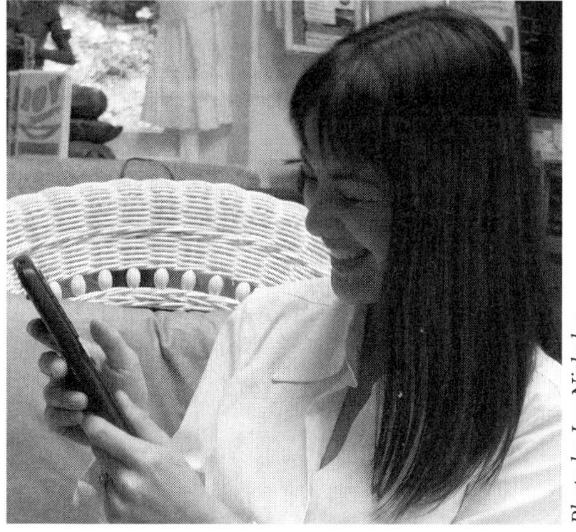

Remote Control Expectations

Photo by Jon Nicholas

They can then easily carry this object with them thereby creating a trigger mechanism to reinforce my suggestions. An eraser also works well. In addition, you can suggest erasing away expectation. If they are visual, have them imagine the word "expectation" on the blackboard of their mind and then have them erase the word.

BALLOON STRESS RELEASE

Imagine blowing up a balloon with 10 deep breaths. As you exhale each breath, blow any stress, tension, anger or irritation into the balloon. When all of the stress is in the balloon, release it and watch it drift away. As it does, imagine that the farther it drifts, the better you feel and the happier you are. Have the balloon disappear into the distance and all stress, tension, and irritation, disappears too. Then suggest, **"Any time you feel stress (or tension or irritation) attempting to return, you will instantly recognize that feeling and simply take a deep breath in, close your eyes, and with one big breath, blow all negativity into the balloon. When you release the balloon, very quickly...in just a few seconds...it will drift away and disappear and all stress will disappear with it. Then open your eyes feeling peaceful, calm, relaxed, and in control."**

MAGIC BUBBLE STRESS RELEASE

Have your client construct a magic bubble around them and tell them: **"This magical bubble has fascinating properties. It repels all negativity while at the same time allowing anything positive (love, humor, etc.) to filter through easily."** I then provide them with a trigger to bring back and/or strengthen this protective bubble whenever they feel the need it. You could suggest that **"any time in the future when you need to relax, just take a deep breath and as you let it out the bubble magically appears around you."**

STOCKWELL'S FIRE AWAY

"Toss your problems and tension into a beautiful blazing fire and enjoy the nice warmth as they are now transformed into sacred smoke. Your problems just drift away. The flames remind you of the healing light within. How happy you feel, as if you are singing songs around a campfire with loving friends. It is safe in your world."

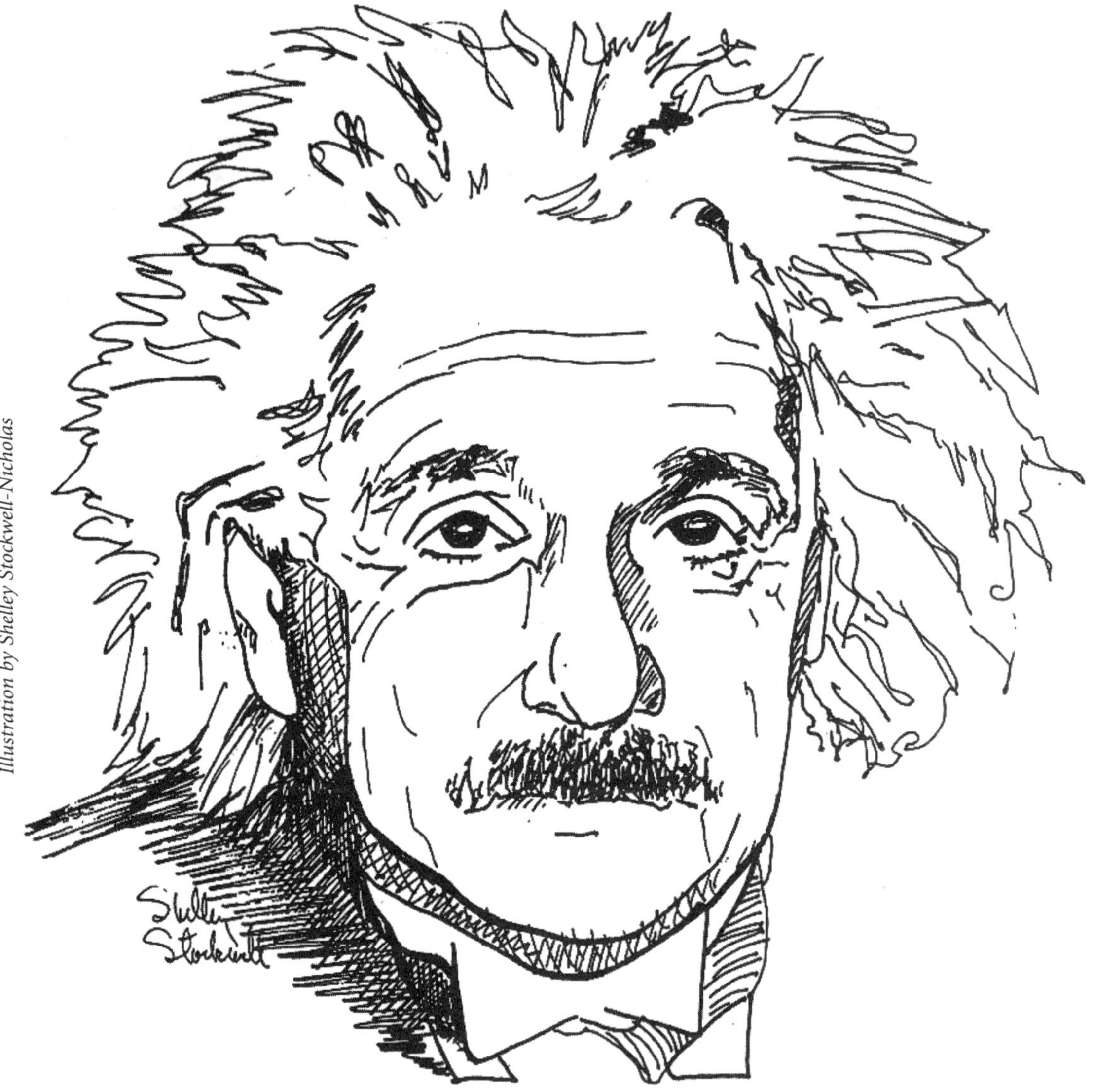

Illustration by Shelley Stockwell-Nicholas

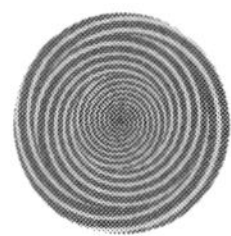

~ *Chapter 74* ~
EINSTEIN'S HAPPINESS SCRIPT

It is reported that Albert Einstein wrote this prose to help a depressed friend. If you receive it consciously as a objective wisdom it is good psychology. Better yet, after inducing trance, instill it directly into the subconscious and it is a superb form of hypnotherapy; effective, practical and useful.

MODUS OPERANDI: EINSTEIN'S HAPPINESS METHOD
Place your client into profound hypnosis and suggest Einstein's brilliant idea:

"Read no newspapers, find a few friends who think as you do, read wonderful writers of earlier time and enjoy the natural beauty of your surrounding. Make believe, all the time, that you are living on Mars among alien creatures and blot out any deeper interest in these creatures. Make friends with a few animals.

Then you will become a cheerful person once more and nothing will be able to trouble you.

Bear in mind that those who are finer and nobler are alone- and necessarily so- so that they can enjoy the purity of their own atmosphere."

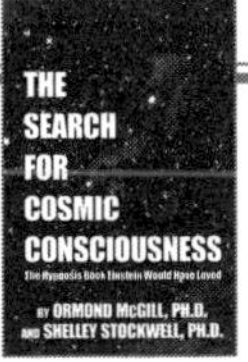

Hypno-Helper
"The Search For Cosmic Consciousness: The Hypnosis Book Einstein Would Have Loved" by Ormond McGill and Shelley Stockwell is available on the order form at the back of this book.

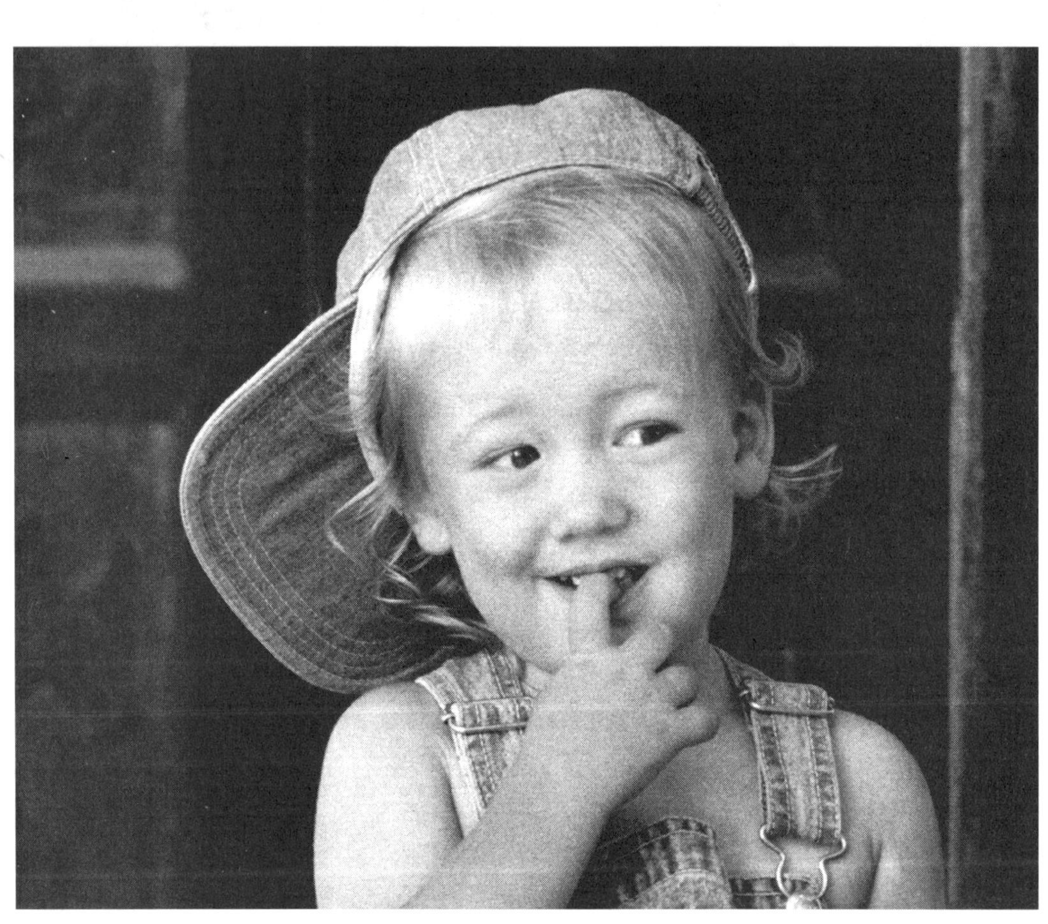

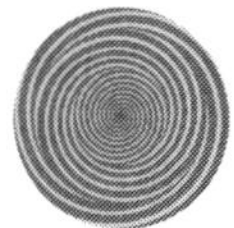

~ *Chapter 75* ~
THE HAPPINESS WAY

Includes
The Four Ways Of Happiness

Everybody seeks happiness. No goal is more basic to well-being than a peaceful mind, for mind directly affects the body. Happiness is a mental state effectively produced in you through self-hypnosis.

When the mind is disturbed stress is produced that causes you harm. A mind at peace can be used to far greater advantage and stress cannot harm you at all. A tranquil mind is a peaceful mind and a peaceful mind becomes filled with happiness.

Changing your attitudes in four ways will aid you to obtain a tranquil and happy mind. Consider:

1. **Cultivate an attitude of friendliness towards a happy person**

2. **Cultivate an attitude of compassion towards the miserable.**

3. **Cultivate an attitude of joy towards the virtuous.**

4. **Cultivate an attitude of indifference towards the evil.**

Implant these transformational attitudes in your subconscious so they become your habitual thinking behavior and see how happiness wells up within you.

Before the technique, first gain an understanding of how deeply changing of these four basic attitudes can change the very quality of your life,. Let's consider each of the four ways to happiness in turn:

1. Consider The Attitude Of Friendliness Towards A Happy Person

On the surface this seems easy, but it is not for the average mind. A happy person is a successful person, and the uncontrolled mind invariably feels jealous of the successfully happy person, as though somehow their success and happiness should be yours and not theirs.

Pause a moment and reflect upon yourself. Have you ever felt real friendliness towards a successful, happy person? Or did you pretend that you did while deep down inside there was envy? It is difficult to change this, however you must if you would truly obtain a mind that is happy.

If somebody is happy, what comes first to your mind? Do you think that happiness has been taken from you; as if the other person has won and you have lost; as if somehow he has cheated you?

Happiness is not a competition so don't be concerned. If somebody is happy, it doesn't mean that you cannot be happy. Happiness is universal, so happy people cannot exhaust it. To change such an attitude come to appreciate that happiness is not a commodity. If someone else gets it, it doesn't mean that you cannot have it. The truth is that the whole of life is actually a celebration and billions of happiness's are happening all over the universe. But if you have an attitude of jealousy you will miss a sizeable portion of it and will be in constant hell that you create with such competitive thoughts. And you will be in hell precisely because all over there is a heaven, a heaven that you can equally create.

Happiness exists throughout the universe in infinite quantity. Nobody has ever been able to exhaust it; there is no competition at all. So, when somebody is happy feel friendliness towards the person. This wisdom flip-flops a negative attitude completely and leads you to find happiness for yourself.

2. Consider The Attitude Of Having Compassion For A Miserable Person

One has to be very clear in following these instructions. Compassion is spoken of, not friendliness, in this instance. Friendliness means you are creating a situation in which you would like to be the same as the other person. Compassion means that someone has fallen from happiness and you would like to help him regain happiness. You would like to help them, but you would not like to be like them because that is not help.

Somebody is crying because he is so sad, and you start crying with him. This is sympathy not compassion, and sympathy is a form of friendliness. Deep down when you show sympathy to a miserable person, you are happy because you are not so miserable. It is simple arithmetic: when somebody is happy, you feel miserable thus when somebody is miserable you feel happy. That is how the average mind operates until you become master of it and change your attitude.

Compassion is a totally different quality from sympathy: compassion means you would like to help the other come out of their misery, but in so doing you do not allow their misery to become your misery. In other words, when you are compassionate, you would like to help the other person come out of their misery, but you are not happy about their misery; on the other hand, you are not miserable about it either. Just between the two exists the attitude of compassion. Compassion has a "feeling tone" about it of remaining aloof, while, at the same time, being attentive.

There is an important lesson to be learned here. Misery is an attitude. It is less concerned with material conditions than it is with the inner mind. Even a poor person can be happy, and once they are happy many things start falling in line. Soon they may not be a poor person, because how can someone be poor when they are happy? When you are happy, the whole world participates with you. When you are unhappy, everything goes wrong. This is the dynamics of the mind. It is both a self-improving and a self-defeating system, at one and the same time. That is why it is important for you to become master of your attitudes, if you would find the happiness way.

3. Consider The Attitude Of Feeling Joy For The Virtuous

The average mind is very suspicious of virtue and may feel that if somebody is virtuous, they must be deceiving you. Mind conjures up the attitude: how can anybody be more virtuous than me! Somehow or another mind tries to criticize and find fault to bring them down. Criticism and faultfinding cause stress. If you criticize a virtuous person, deep down you are criticizing virtue. Then, it is not long before you come to believe that virtue is next to impossible in this world, and then the world becomes a mess of unhappiness for you.

But these instructions say to change this attitude, and instead cultivate joy towards the virtuous. Finding joy for the virtuous leads you down happiness way.

4. Consider The Attitude Of Cultivating Indifference Towards Evil

Evil is the negative side of good, and the conscious phase of mind tends to gravitate towards the negative for the negative is easier to accept consciously than is the positive. For the subconscious phase of mind just the opposite is true, as it can accept more readily the positive; but for your consciousness it is easier, by way of example, to say "no" than it is to say "yes," because to disprove a "no" is very difficult.

As was discussed in the attitude towards virtue, if you say "no" to virtue you do not harm virtue (or even someone who pretends virtue), you harm yourself.

To find the way of happiness you must develop an attitude of being joyful towards the virtuous and indifferent towards evil, which is an entire reversal of the attitude of the average mind.

It is a temptation for a uncontrolled mind to condemn even virtue, but these instructions say you must not even condemn evil. That is to say, you must become indifferent to it. Why? It is because of the way the mind operates. If you condemn evil too much, you pay too much attention to evil. And, one tends to become attuned (become like) whatever one pays attention to. In other words, you become addicted to the wrong.

The famous French psychologist, Emil Coué discovered a law of human behavior, which he called "The Law of Reverse Effort." This means that if you are too much against something, you will become the victim of the something. Action follows your attention. If you are overly attentive to evil you tend to head toward evil. Remember, evil is resisted most easily when you become indifferent to it, and your mind becomes then more tranquil, and a tranquil mind is a mind filled with happiness.

In reading these instructions about changing your attitude about happiness, miserableness, virtuousness, and evilness, you have learned it on the conscious level. That is why such lengthy instructions have been given. The conscious phase of mind likes explanation so it can reason about it. But your subconscious does not need lengthy explanation at all. To impress the subconscious all you have to do is place yourself in the mind state of self-hypnosis and generalize the suggestions as positive affirmations.

Since mind is not entirely compartmentalized, but a continuum, these instructions are first instilled in your conscious mind to aid your subconscious to accept them more readily via hypnotic suggestion.

Finding happiness for yourself and bringing happiness to others leads to a wonderful (wonder full) life. This transformation of attitudes can be accomplished using hypnosis. Through self-hypnosis you can find the way of happiness, one of the most wonderful suggestion-formula of all.

While in hypnosis repeat this suggestion-formula a dozen times. It will take root in the garden of the subconscious, and will blossom forth as a changing of attitudes from negative to positive. It provides a quantum leap to happiness. You have discovered the way of happiness:

"From this moment onward you commence to feel friendly towards people who are happy. You feel compassion towards people who are miserable. You feel joyful towards people who are virtuous. You feel indifferent towards people who are evil.

You become a source of help and love to all people as they are. You accept them fully. This is becoming your attitude and brings you a peaceful mind. In every way your mind is becoming serene and tranquil. You are at peace with all the world and with all the people in the world. You have found the way of happiness."

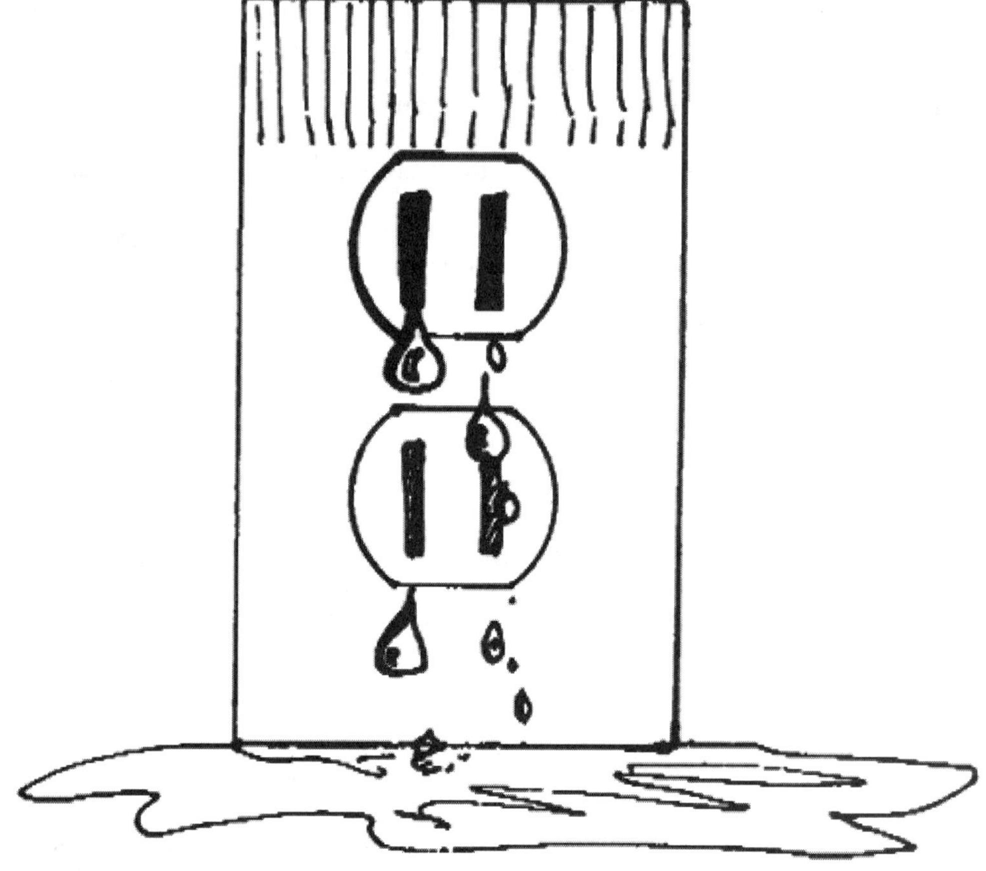

Emotional Outlet

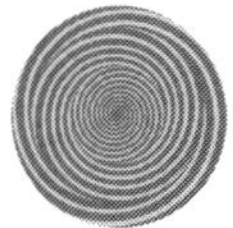

~ *Chapter 76* ~
PLUGGED IN HAPPINESS HYPNOSIS

Includes
Replaceable Hypnotherapy

This is an advanced technique. After years in the field of hypnosis, this method came through to me. Most to whom it has been told do not seem to understand it. It is a very basic method:

Emotion/Non-Emotion= Neutrality

Positive/Negative= Neutrality

Two planets collide in space and two worlds are destroyed. The universe remains neutral

And as Buddha said, "nothing need be done."

People come to hypnotherapy to remove unhappiness from their stream of consciousness and to replace it with happiness. This method does that, as you the hypnotherapist remain neutral in the matter. Indeed replaced happiness can be very neutral as far as the hypnotherapist is concerned. It is like the dentist who fixes an unhappy tooth into a happy one.

MODUS OPERANDI: REPLACEABLE HYPNOTHERAPY

Hypnotize your client and suggest:

"You are going to remove unhappiness and replace it with happiness. Your stream of conscious awareness now creates a sphere of harmony and peace. This ball of energy represents your whole life.

Scan the sphere and if you discover any unhappiness, remove it like a cork from a bottle. Do this very quickly as the waiting happiness is eager to fill in the space the cork leaves behind. Okay rapidly remove any unhappiness from your life. Remove all reasons why you were unhappy and immediately any gaps are filled immediately with positive energy. It happens without words. It happens so fast that there is no time to speak. Good.

Now, ask your creative mind to generate a sphere ball of happiness that encompasses you entirely. You are happy."

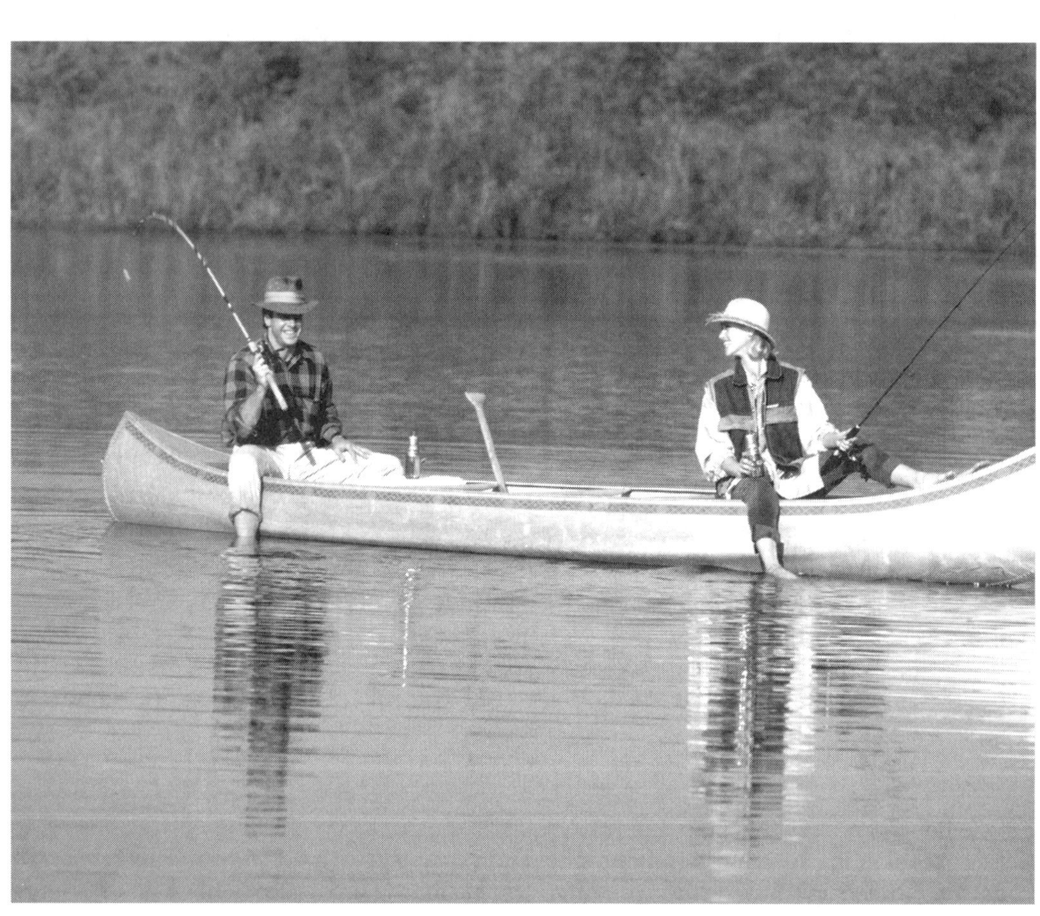

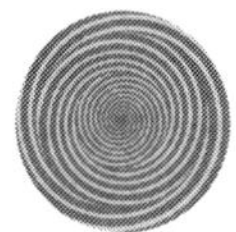

~ *Chapter 77* ~
HYPNOTHERAPY OF PLEASURE

Includes
Pure Pleasure

It is interesting how human knowledge advances. One thing leads to another. Usually it is not a smooth flowing from one to the other. Most often it comes in quantum leaps of increased awareness. Sometimes it happens instantaneously: one moment it is not there and the next it is. The Hypnotherapy of Pleasure is a superb process for hypnotherapists to give their clients as a gift. In pleasure, cares become like drops of water that evaporate in the sun.

Hypnotherapists face many clients who continually carp about the uncertainty of life and how miserable they are. Complaint after complaint after complaint; the man can't stand his wife; the wife can't stand her husband; the children drive them both crazy; the world is going to pot!

What is the hypnotherapist to do with clients who hold such a negative outlook on life?

The solution is not as difficult as it might seem at first. Simply hypnotize client and saturate the subconscious with pleasure-laden suggestions, like, **"Life is a joy just for the sheer pleasure of being alive." "Pleasure is established as the miracle of being."**

This approach is optimistic. It provides an every day means for the client to let go of old negative beliefs. Everything at its root is yin and yang– solar opposites of each other; opposite ends of the same. One end is displeasure and the other is pleasure. Therein lies the way to help clients solve their problems; to achieve an inner calm; to bring into bearing the extraordinary benefits of pleasure.

Let's take a look at the truth the Masters say:
Buddha says, "If you are unhappy just change your attitude."
Shiva says, "Don't take life so seriously – dance with the stars."
Lao Tzu says, "Relax into existence."
Patanjali says, "Make life a playground not a battlefield."
Christ says, "Trust your Father in Heaven."
Tilopa says, "Live life fully to the hilt."
Krishna says, "Romp and play and enjoy yourself."

What excellent hypnotherapists the Masters are. Use what they have to say in designing your "suggestion formula" the next time you work with a carping, faultfinding, complaining client.

Complaints are habits based on negative behavior. The subconscious mind is the repository of habits. Hypnosis provides a process for reprogramming the subconscious mind.

Positive suggestions bypass the critical complaining of conscious mind, and present selective ideas of happy living into the subconscious where they are accepted and acted upon without criticism. Hypnosis, then, provides the means to change the mind, and since mind produces thoughts it can transform the client's complaints (negative thoughts) into positive thoughts.

How?

There is no need to seek to correct specific aspects of a complaint. It takes too long. There are just too many different kinds of complaints to deal with. Instead, just generalize your suggestions, and let the client's subconscious do its own sleuthing and application to where such is most needed.

MODUS OPERANDI: PURE PLEASURE

Hypnotize the client into somnambulism. While in that state suggest **"How thankful you should be that you are able to complain, it proves you are alive. A dead man (or woman) never complains. Subconscious consider how miraculous life really is; that everything taken for granted is, in fact, a host of miracles; you can see; can speak; can think; and can move about the planet. Let your subjective phase of mind reflect on these precious gifts with profound appreciation. Then submerge this appreciation into the realm of pleasure.**

See yourself as pleasure…the living, breathing, personification of pleasure. Pleasure. Pleasure. Sink into pleasure. Submerge every nerve and fiber of your being into the pleasure of your being. How fortunate you are to be alive!

The process of filling and experiencing yourself as pleasure will entirely alter your personality, and others around you will begin to respond to your presence with pleasure. You become a light in the world; you are brightness. You become a happy person, and a happy person makes others happy too. It is impossible for others not to so respond when you become a light in the world. In your mind's eye begin seeing a flame commencing to burn in your heart and your body becoming an aura around the flame.

That is the way. The suggestions of pleasure as being reinforced with every breath you take. You associate breathing with pleasure. Breath is life. Every breath in-taken is actually drawing in pleasure. Enjoy every precious moment eternally."

It's great hypnotherapy.

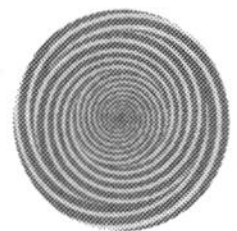

~ *Chapter 78* ~
THE HYPNOTHERAPY OF LUCK

Includes
For A Lucky You
For Lucky Clients

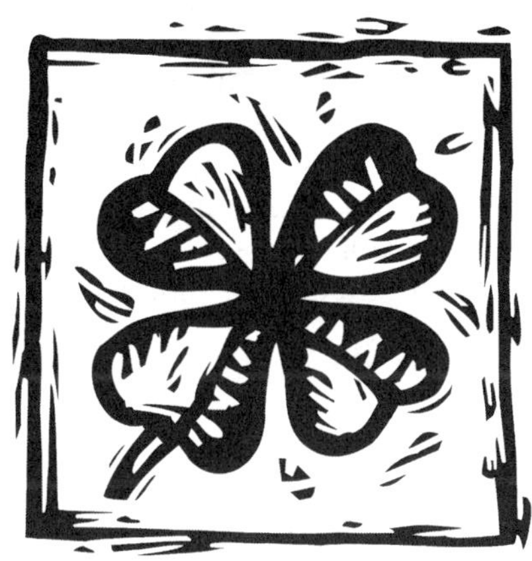

Being lucky is good hypnotherapy. Luck is more than just hit-or-miss good fortune. It is the positive energy of good fortune. Bringing that positive energy to yourself and your client is The Hypnotherapy of Luck.

Think about it. Since time immemorial, humankind has associated luck around symbols. A rabbit's foot, like the prolific bunny it came from, brings prosperity, said the ancient Celts. And since rabbits live underground, it helps us communicate with the netherworld. A mustard seed, a horse shoe, a wishbone…such tangible objects are regarded as "a lucky piece."

The lucky piece can be whatever one wishes. Home-run king Hank Aaron wore the same shower shoes for twenty years because he thought they brought him luck. Some find a stray penny, put it in their pocket, and feel confident it will bring them luck. And sometimes it does, for the thought starts the energy of luck flowing within the individual.

One of the nicest images for luck, the four-leaf clover, comes from the medieval Druids. They said it gives special powers to the finder to see invisible spirits. The four-leaf clover has become a wonderful modern symbol for luck. If you have the good fortune to find such a rare specimen, place it in your wallet or purse and keep it with you always. It will bring you luck.

Superstition?

You bet.

Superstition is based in classic inspiration. A tangible object is not needed, just the mental image of the object will do. That is how the hypnotherapy of luck is designed. Another word for hypnosis is "charm." Use hypnosis as a lucky charm and you gift yourself and your client.

MODUS OPERANDI: SUGGESTIONS FOR A LUCKY YOU

"The entire Universe operates on the principle of luck. Aren't you lucky to be so close to God? You are so lucky you have Guardian Angels and Guides that help you all through the turmoil of life, and lead you in the direction of good fortune. Aren't you lucky that you are you?

Relax, close your eyes and visualize the mental image of a four-leaf clover. The four-leaf clover sets the whole Universe in gear for you. If you understand how it works it would be a wonder. But no need to mind the "why" just "do." Fill your entire head with the image of the four-leaf clover. It is easy, for you have known that symbol for luck all your life. Now, try to

drop the image. You can't do it, for the more you try to rid yourself of the image, the more it persists. Lucky you! You have started something within yourself that will bring you luck, and sticks with you."

MODUS OPERANDI: SUGGESTIONS FOR LUCKY CLIENTS

You can give this same persistent image of the four-leaf clover to your clients during each hypnotherapy session. Set it there as a posthypnotic suggestion just prior to their being aroused. The Four-leaf Clover can change a life. They, too, will always see the image, and even more so when it is needed. Then continue:

"Want to be on a continual lucky streak? You can, you know. Do this: Hold the image of the four-leaf clover in your mind and combine it with Lao Tzu's 'going with the flow.' Or, if you understand it better, be like a log drifting down a stream, and the things you bump into are the treasures of living. The things you bump into are bits of luck coming into your life. The principle of combining one process of value with another (same directive) process of value squares the ratio of the value of the combined processes. The principle is of universal value to all forms of hypnotherapy. Luck is a positive energy field you now create around yourself. You're on a roll…a lucky streak. One luck creates another luck, in a chain reaction. Watch how it operates and you understand."

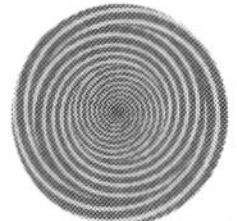

~ *Chapter 79* ~
THE CONSCIOUS SMILE TECHNIQUE

"Specific muscular action is not merely an exponent of passion, but truly is an essential part of it. It is impossible to fix your the features in the expression of one passion and call to mind a different passion."
—Professor Maudsley

R.P. Halleck studied the affect of facial expression on a person's feeling state and immune response. "Putting on a happy face" of some 200 different kinds of smiles does indeed make you happier and healthier. Conversely, a sad face can make you ill. When subjects were trained to control their facial muscles and voluntarily smile, their physiology and hormones immediately and drastically changed.

Smile

Photo by Jon Nicholas

"By inducing an expression we can often cause its allied emotion. Actors frequently testify to the fact that the appropriate emotions arise if they go through the appropriate muscular movement (physical action). In talking to a character on stage during a play, if they clench a fist and frown, they often find themselves becoming really angry; if they start with counterfeit laughter, they find themselves growing cheerful."

For emotional insurance, whether you feel like it or not, place your facial muscles in the smile for ten seconds as many times a day as possible. By doing this, you actually alter your blood chemistry and the natural opiates and neuropeptides in your brain, stomach and intestines increase.

MODUS OPERANDI: THE CONSCIOUS SMILE

Conscious Smiling can be developed into an effective hypnotherapeutic technique. Hypnotize your client into somnambulistic state; at the end of session establish this post-hypnotic suggestion, **"From this time onward, every time you have a mental disturbance, you will automatically put a smile on your face. The smile will reduce the disturbance to trivia which you can easily handle."**

Arouse the client with no mention of post-hypnotic suggestion. It will be spontaneously realized.

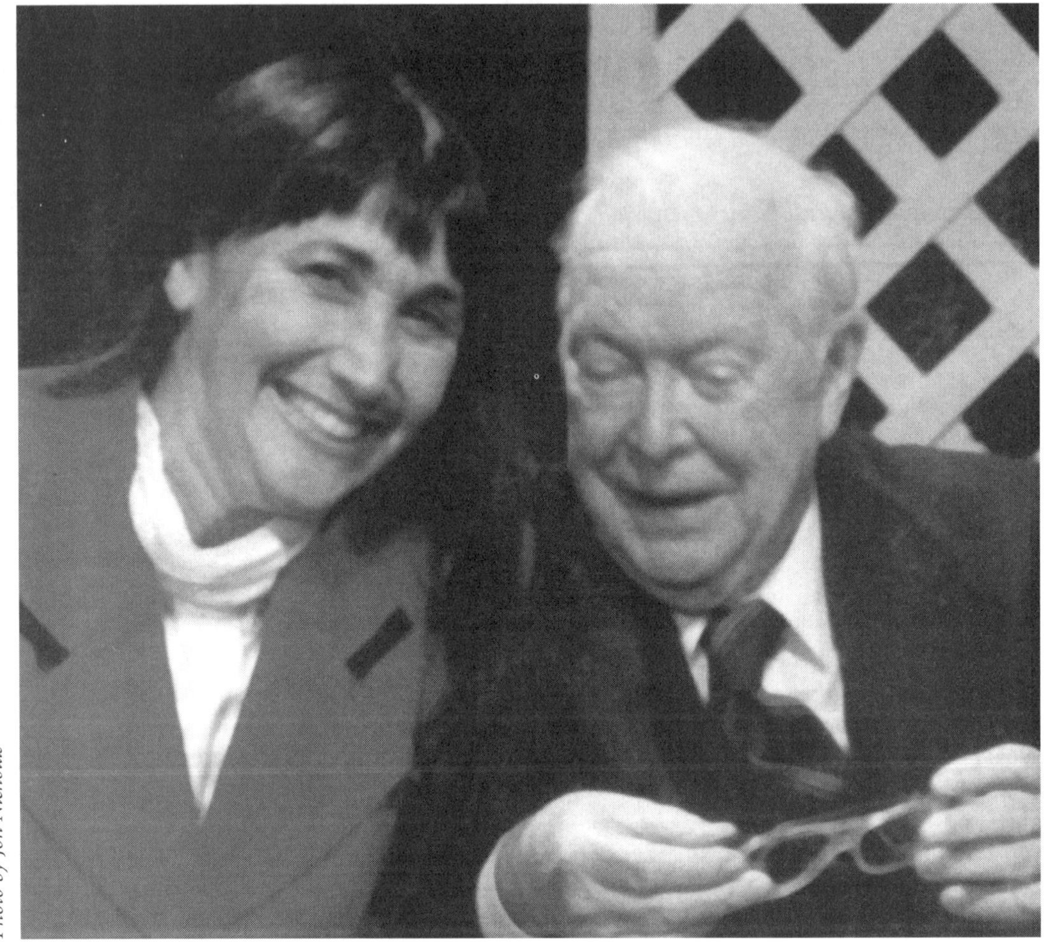

Ormond & Shelley

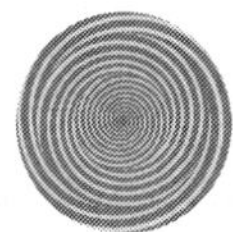

~ *Chapter 80* ~
HYPNOTHERAPY OF LAUGHTER

Includes
Laughter Hypnotherapy
Heal Ol' Psychic Wounds Hypnotherapy

Laughter is good therapy in many situations. How often, is it said, "Making a sick person laugh is darn good medicine." The doctor who smiles is far better than one who frowns. The happy doctor takes the patient's temperature and it reads high never shakes his head and says, "You are very ill." Rather he chuckles and says, "Great. You are doing fine. You'll be well in no time."

The power of such awake hypnosis suggestion is potent medicine, and even more so when given from a source of accepted authority.

Laughter forms the foundation for wonderful hypnotherapy. Design it as a "suggestion formula" and sell it to the subconscious.

MODUS OPERANDI: LAUGHTER HYPNOTHERAPY

Hypnotize client into somnambulism. In this, they enter the realm of the subconscious. Repeat this suggestion formula often, as repetition is the driving force of suggestion. The Masters put it this way:

"Brilliant child, make the truth of happily living life become reality. Fill life with joy and happiness. Live life fully and to the hilt. Inside thyself be peaceful and serene, and go with the flow. And so laugh as you play with life, and let the energy of laughter make these suggestions become the way. Laughter makes it so."

MODUS OPERANDI: HEAL OL' PSYCHIC WOUNDS HYPNOTHERAPY

The hypnotherapy of laughter for healing ol' psychic wounds is profoundly effective. A psychic wound is the result of a traumatic experience suffered in the past by an individual, often in childhood. The actual experience may long be consciously forgotten, but the wound still remains subconsciously remembered and can mar the happiness of the person in the here and now. Laughter helps promote a cure.

This does not imply that a psychic wound is not to be taken seriously and laughed at. Traumatic experiences suffered at an early age can produce weighty effects upon the psyche, but laughter is a form of positive energy while the wound is negative. Such positive energy can overcome a negative. Further, there is little to be gained by holding on to ancient hurts forever. Through hypnotherapy, old hurts are surfaced, faced squarely, and then dropped into the abyss of oblivion. Here is how to do it:

Hypnotize client (somnambulism). Then present to the subconscious this suggestion formula:

"Remember always the past is memories that will never happen again while the future may never happen at all… we live only in the here and now. Let this become your knowing, and the pains of yesterday will become less painful in the present."

Pause for some moments, and then continue:

"As best you can, dear one, let go of the past and allow disturbing memories to be soothed by the healing balm of time."

Pause for some moments, and then continue:

"Replace unhappiness from the past with the happiness of today. You are happy. You know within yourself you are now free. Repeat: I am free! I am free! I am free! And the pathway of happiness opens wide before me…as I now live my life in the here and now." Pause for some moments, and then continue:

"And so I laugh, and the laughter echoes through the corridors of my being, and all psychic wounds are healed."

Pause for some moments, and then continue:

"My subconscious makes it so."

Repeat this "suggestion formula" three times to the hypnotized client, and allow the laughter to bubble forth. When it subsides on its own, suggest:

"All fine and happy now. You are free. You are free… alert, happy in every way, and feeling fine each day."

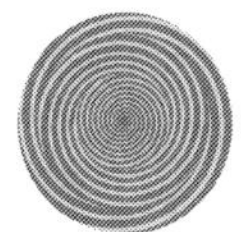

~ *Chapter 81* ~
HYPNOTHERAPY OF PERSUASION

©by Shelley Stockwell-Nicholas, PhD

Includes
The Ten Principles Of Persuasion

In relation to hypnotherapy, persuasion operates in two directions:
1. You persuade your clients to improve and live a better life.
2. Persuasion helps build your business and the more successful your business, the more opportunity is provided to aid clients with hypnotherapy. Persuasion is the objective way to move mind in directive directions. When directives are subjective it becomes hypnosis and influences things in life you give yourself and others.

Editor Shelley Stockwell-Nicholas shares her thoughts on the negotiation power of suggestion. Here is what Shelley has to say:

PERSUASION
Everything in life is involves the power of the suggestions you give yourself or another.
In business as in life you don't always get what you deserve you get what you negotiate or suggest. Think about the last time you negotiated with someone; a friend, a loved one, an employee, a sales person, a customer or a vendor.
Anytime you exchange information with intent of establishing a change, you negotiate and direct the mind. Suggestion is one of the keys to success in life.
I was stunned one day in the market as my five year old negotiated and hypnotized me to buy him a ball. (He had dozens at home).
"If you get me this ball it will make a complete set- one in each color. Won't they look great in my room?" (Selling the benefits).
"Mommy doesn't have the money for that ball."
"Well let's put some paper towels back and then we'll have the money."
What could I do?

Think about negotiations that you've made in the past. How did you get what you wanted as a child? What negotiation and agreements (both spoken and unspoken) went into your marriage agreement? How did you purchase your last car? What are you like in a flea market? If you are selling yourself or a product what do you say to others? Do you ask for what you want?

THE TEN PRINCIPLES OF PERSUASION
Learning the principles of Persuasive Hypnotherapy allows others to benefit from your product or service. Successful advertisers know these principles well. How can you help someone with hypnosis if you don't persuade them to come to see you for a session? The better you learn how to persuade, the better hypnotherapist you become.

Prepare to Persuade
Be A Good Planner
Hold High Expectations
Be In Good Shape
Look Good
Be A Good Listener
Ask Questions
Stay Neutral
Persistence Pays
Analyze Your Negotiations & Learn From Them

1. Prepare to Persuade

Attend workshops and read books. With awareness of how to negotiate and how YOU negotiate and persuade, you develop your ability to persuade. Persuasion is an art form.

What continuously goes on around you? Observe your everyday conversations and the conversations of others and you'll see that folks negotiate all the time.

2. Be a Good Planner

Decide what you want to convey and persuade. What action would you like to evoke from your client? Hold the thought of the outcome. Then think before you speak. HOLD THE THOUGHT OF THE OUTCOME BECAUSE THIS SUGGESTS THE OUTCOME. Notice the most appropriate time to bring in your positive suggestions. The best moment to make a "call to action" is when the other can give you a moment of their time and focus.

In hypnotherapy you call the other "client" and form a plan of action that makes use of the most effective suggestion formula to help them. The plan goes like this:

Contract; **"In a few moments you will enjoy a wonderful hypnotic experience of reverie and relaxation."**

Delivery; **"Relax back comfortably in your chair and concentrate on the suggestions I give you. You gave yourself a promise that hypnotherapy was going to help you, when you came to see me. Now do what is promised."**

Call to Action; (Timing is vital to the hypnotic induction,) **"Now close your eyes and drop down into the realm of sleep. Wonderful beneficial to you- SLEEP. Now go to sleep."**

3. Hold High Expectations

People rarely pay you more than you charge. Value your worth and others will too. When negotiating money open positively: where you start effects where you finish.

What is your value? What should you charge? Take a tip from classy department stores. You pay a big price for a dress at Sak's Fifth Avenue that you could get at a song at Ross; the same dress, just a different price tag. But if it comes from Saks, it must be great. Don't think cheap. Today's economy is often more based on prestige than it is on actual worth. Ormond tried an experiment with a couple of therapist friends. Both were equally skilled. He sent a client to try out both. One charged a high fee and the other deliberately a low fee. The high fee got the best results. Why? The subconscious has a personality much as an individual. Treat it with respect.

A low fee can infer the suggestion to the subconscious "If you don't think I'm worth a good salary darned if I'll work for you!"

Be confident—EXPECT TO DO WELL. Always remember too that people value most what they pay a lot for. Think about it, don't you cherish something you spent a lot for? Studies prove that people who expect more get more. Help your clients succeed.

4. Be In Good Shape

Good persuaders are in good mental and physical shape. Persuading takes energy and can sometimes create tension. Rise above tension and be in a peaceful mental place. Get enough rest, eat well and drink lots of water. Most importantly, don't drink, take drugs or load up on sugar or caffeine. It hurts your persuasive power. Be in a good mental place. When you feel good, good comes to you and you make your clients feel good too.

5. Look Good

If at all possible, dress like the person you want to persuade. Even dress up a little more than they are dressed. This conveys to the subconscious that you are to be respected and that you respected them by taking care to look your best for them. Visual impact can make or break a negotiation. Studies show that people make judgments within seconds that can decide the outcome of a negotiation. Be clean and smell clean.

Books are truly judged by their cover. To prove this point, when I lecture, I often get three people dressed in exaggerated attire and one dressed in a blue, color coordinated suit to stand in front of my listeners. I then have my listeners answer these questions:

What kind of personality does this person have?

What Kind of family?

How much money do they make a year?

What are their strong and weak points?

How educated are they?

Would you trust them in a business situation?

The demonstration was presented with a humorous tongue in cheek attitude so no one is embarrassed. The well-dressed one is always judged as smarter and someone you would listen to and trust.

6. Be a Good Listener

"It is better to keep silent and let people think that you are a fool than to open your mouth and remove all doubt."
—Abraham Lincoln

The one who speaks first sets the tone. Greet the person with a smile and a firm (not killing) handshake. Make eye contact. Smile. A certain smile diffuses aggression among apes. It works with humans too. Begin by saying something positive that gets the other person's attention. Be sincere. No one likes to feel manipulated.

What does your client want? Listen to their desires and repeat back to them so they know that they have been heard. Active listening establishes rapport. Rapport builds trust. Trust opens us to suggestion and is the backbone of hypnotherapy.

7. Ask Questions

The person who asks the most questions usually controls the conversation. They receive the most information and information is power. One well-placed question shows that you're listening to their viewpoint and needs.

I once got a job by asking my interviewer: "You have a very interesting job talking to people all day long. How did you get into this?" An hour later, after telling me her life's story my interviewer said; "You are perfect for this job. You're such an interesting person." She knew virtually nothing about me.

If you are asked a question restate or rephrase the inquiry before answering. This gives you time to think and give an honest and persuasive answer. Don't make up answers that can be proven as wrong. If you don't know the answer say so. Thank the person for raising a good issue. And promise to look into it. To be credible, follow up. If the question is irrelevant gracefully move on to another topic. Remember that the only dumb question is the one not asked.

8. Stay Neutral

If you're greeted with a challenge don't play along with it. Go into neutral or tell a lighthearted story. Or divert their attention to aspects that they already have agreed upon.

One of the best low-key negotiators I ever saw was my agent at the Frankfurt Book Fair In Germany. A buyer picked up a book and said, "Now why would I want such an awful book!" My rights agent smiled, remained neutral and said "Would you like a cup of tea?" As the client continued to thumb the pages of the book, the agent actively listened, nodded and never addressed the barrage of forthcoming criticism. I watched in awe as the buyer talked himself into buying the book!

Stay neutral with your client and they will come to you.

9. Persistence Pays

"A winner never quits and a quitter never wins"

Especially in relation to persuasive hypnotherapy, persistence pays. Hypnotic suggestion heaped on hypnotic suggestions are compounding in effect. The hypnotherapeutic session is always most helpful when it is a "yes" session rather than a "no." Don't quit when you meet resistance. "No" may mean "Give me more information."

10. Analyze Your Negotiations & Learn From Them

Win/win negotiations are the most successful. Persuade for positive change- Learn well and prosper. If you've done a great job the client has gotten more than they bargained for and you have been more than compensated financially and deeply satisfied because you made a difference.

Teach others win/win principles and you have a devoted friend, client and lots of referrals.

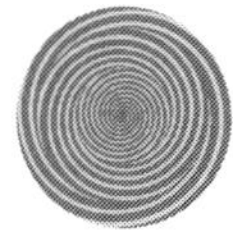

~ *Chapter 82* ~
COSMICALLY MAXIMIZE SUGGESTION

To achieve maximum power and effectiveness with each hypnotic suggestion, present them with a Cosmic Connection. The Cosmic Connection is like wind when it is no longer windy, so how can you obtain a Cosmic Connection?

Very simply.

Don't try to make a Cosmic Connection. The only way to do it is to KNOW you already have it. Feel the Cosmic Connection in your heart and YOU HAVE IT whenever you do hypnotherapy.

Then…

Make a little symbolic reminder of your heartfelt cosmic connection. Here's how:

Take two un-cancelled adhesive United States Postage Stamps with a love design. Place the adhesive backs together, and squeeze tight. They will bind so closely you can't get them apart no matter how hard you try. You have literally made the two stamps become one, with the love design on each side facing out.

Now…think about love and your cosmic connection to a higher purpose and look at the design on one side of your love stamp.

Now…

Look at the design on the reverse side and think of the beneficial hypnotherapeutic suggestions you give your client while being at one with love and your Cosmic Connection.

This lets you maximize the POWER OF SUGGESTION. Just like the two stamps adhered together, so your suggestions are one with a Cosmic flow.

Carry this symbol with you, and place it on a table before each session. Make no comment about it. It is private. Just have it there. IT MEANS SO MUCH.

To be a Master Hypnotherapist, stamp your hypnotherapy suggestions with a Cosmic Connection.

Illustration by Shelley Stockwell

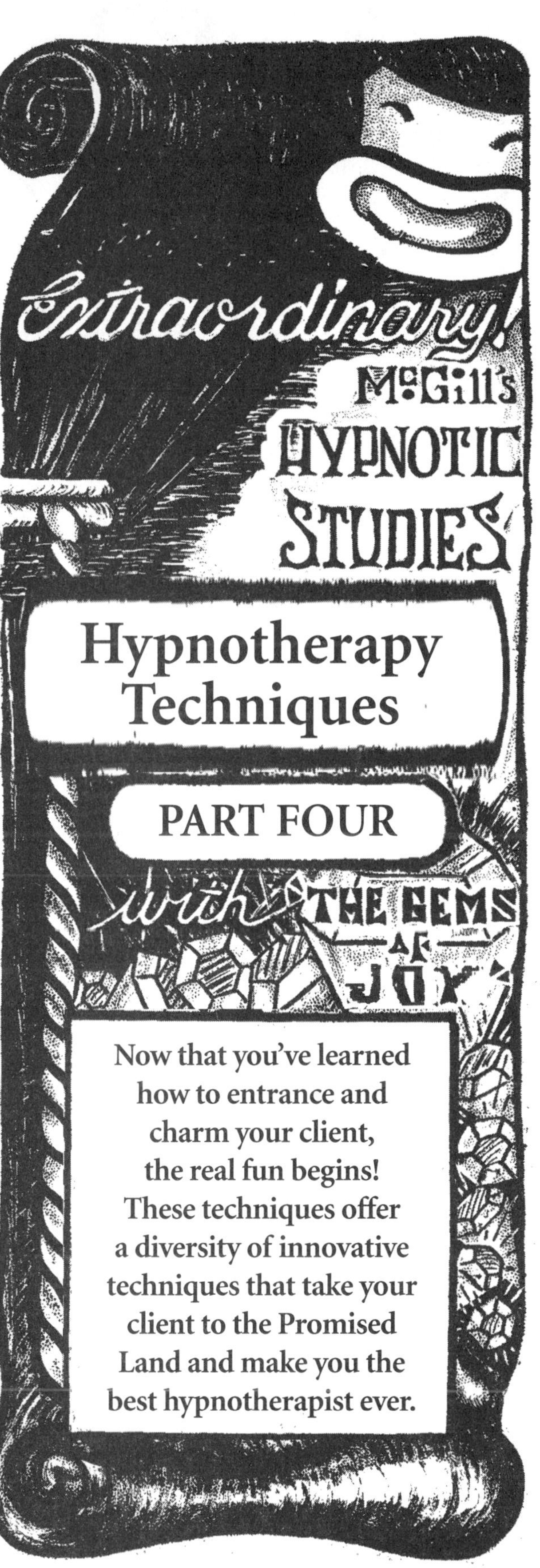

Now that you've learned how to entrance and charm your client, the real fun begins! These techniques offer a diversity of innovative techniques that take your client to the Promised Land and make you the best hypnotherapist ever.

CHAPTERS IN PART FOUR

83. Nothing-Need-Be-Done Hypnotherapy ....page 293
84. Hypnotherapy of Nothingness 295
85. Active Participation Hypnotherapy 297
86. Subconscious Hypnotherapist 299
87. Talking to Yourself 301
88. Stockwell's Subpersonality Approach..303
89. Hunter's Parts Hypnotherapy..............307
90. The Slow-Down Clinic..........................313
91. Forget You Not Hypnotherapy 315
92. Computer Hypnotherapy 319
93. Infinite Smallness Hypnotherapy 325
94. Right Brain/Left Brain Hypnotherapy...............................327
95. Count Your Blessings Hypnosis 331
96. Your Little Theater Of The Mind 333
97. NLP Hypnotherapy 335
98. Stockwell-Nicholas NLP 337
99. NLP Movie Theater Techniques 347
100. Hypnotic Dream Work 351
101. Hypnotherapy of Imagination 355
102. Aladdin's Arabian Hypnotherapy 357
103. The Hypnotic Seal 361
104. Abreaction Management 363
105. Stockwell's Ericksonian Hypnosis 367

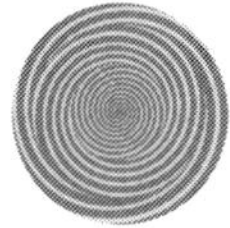

~ *Chapter 83* ~
NOTHING-NEED-BE-DONE HYPNOTHERAPY

As every hypnotherapist knows, every-so-often a client will come to your office feeling depressed and like their life has been shattered. They come to you asking, almost hysterically, "What should I do?"

MODUS OPERANDI: NOTHING-NEED-BE-DONE HYPNOTHERAPY

What can you do with such a despondent client? Enjoy this profound NOTHING-NEED-BE-DONE HYPNOTHERAPY.

Say to your client, **"Tell me ALL of your unhappiness. Don't spare my ears. Shout it out, if you wish."**

Let the client tell their story. Make no comment; do not try to analyze. Just let all the venom pour forth. When the client asks again, "What should I do?" Have them lie outstretched upon your couch or reclining chair. Play gentle meditative music softly in the background, and darken the room. If you have a violet light, flood the room with violet light. Violet is the color of inner peace. Now, speak directly to your reclining client.

"Thank you for sharing your heartfelt disturbance with me. And for having the confidence to ask me what you should do. Do this: Close your eyes, relax, breath, and visualize and imagine in your mind's eye, a scene of yourself walking through a beautiful forest glade. It is green with many flowers about. Birds are singing. Take your time and enjoy this scene within your mind. How peaceful it is. How opposite from what has disturbed you recently. Let your mind drift into the music that surrounds you now."

Allow some moments for this experience to be experienced. Continue on:

"Now, rest your hands upon your core or belly chakra, the solar plexus. Now, inhale a deep breath, and feel your solar plexus rise beneath your resting hands. Hold the breath for a bit of moment, then exhale fully, and feel your solar plexus drop downward. Continue breathing in this easy natural way, in and out, each time giving your attention to the rise and fall of your solar plexus beneath your resting hands. Give this your full attention, and you'll find it makes you very sleepy and more and more relaxed.

How relaxed and sleepy you become. Give your full attention to your breathing, as your solar plexus rises up and down. Go ahead, drift and enter the realm of sleep, when you wish. You are still aware, as your conscious mind gently moves aside, and your subconscious mind takes center stage. Just drift into the realm of sleep, as I talk directly to your subconscious. How wonderful it feels!

Subconscious mind, open wide your portals of full attention. Allow the miraculous suggestions I give to become the reality of this remarkable individual. Make no effort, just know that nothing need be done. Take this idea in deeply. Drift and dream as these miracles become your very own."

Music fades out. Silence. Then give these miraculous suggestions:

"Say this to yourself, I know I need to do nothing to obtain a peaceful mind, for a peaceful mind is there in the Center of my Being. It belongs to me."

Allow some moments for this to sink home.

"Nothing can hurt me unless I give it the power to do so."

Allow some moments for this to sink home.

"I no longer seek to change the world. I just change my mind about the world."

Allow some moments for this to sink home and bring them back to room awareness. The session is complete.

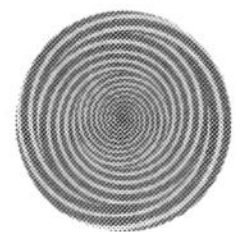

~ *Chapter 84* ~
HYPNOTHERAPY OF NOTHINGNESS

To achieve the blissful state of nothingness (no-thing-ness) is to advance to the consciousness of the Masters. It is the ultimate hypnotherapy.

In nothingness one becomes empty inside…one becomes above the world of ceaseless searching/wanting. It is a spiritual realm. In nothingness one is beyond all desires, judgments, and opinions that things should be different than they are. At least, you understand the Buddha saying "nothing need be done."

In the hypnotherapy of nothingness, a recognition dawns that real treasures are not found outside yourself, but are already inside yourself. In other words, you already have it ALL. When you recognize this truth, you advance from homo-sapien to homo-superior human.

Understand?

All And Nothing

Frankly doubtful because your critical (conscious) mind says that you must always search for something. But your subconscious phase of mind perfectly understands, because it is the way of nature; which understands that such a flower is perfectly content to just be a flower. Nothing is needed. If you give yourself and your clients what the flower has, you have performed the hypnotherapy of Nothingness. It is the ultimate self hypnosis and the ultimate hetero-hypnosis. It is the ultimate hypnotherapy.

MODUS OPERANDI: HYPNOTHERAPY OF NOTHINGNESS
You Will Need:
Meditative Music (like the Serenity Resonance Sound or Hypno-Music

Play gentle softly in the background. Allow your client to drop into somnambulistic hypnotic reverie as you instruct:
"Just lie quietly as you relax and listen to the meditative music for fifteen minutes or so. Do nothing. Just listen and become one with the music."
Mind commences to become empty for there is nothing for it to do. You feel like you are drifting into the VOID. And then you suggest,

"Become nothing. Become nothing. Become nothing. Fully accept exactly what you are with full appreciation of the miracles that you are."

No other suggestions are needed, as the subconscious mind knows and will take them there. In nothingness it is discovered that everything is there. Nothing need be done and the music plays on as you drift and drift and drift. Turn off the music and allow SELF to lie in silence, until arousal from hypnosis occurs on its own.

I guarantee the perception of perception will never be the same again.

Nothingness. So simple yet so basic. How could such a simple hypnotherapy have been missed these many years? So elusive that only the Masters achieved its realization.

Why is it elusive?

Because truth is hidden within itself. So much stuff is heaped upon it, it is all but lost. Only when the subconscious brings in nothingness will one begin to understand. The hypnotherapy of nothingness may well belong to the future, but try it in the here and now.

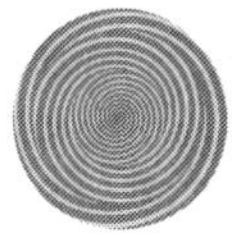

~ *Chapter 85* ~
ACTIVE PARTICIPATION HYPNOTHERAPY

Conventional hypnotherapy employs a dynamic situation in which the client assumes a passive role (as the subject) while the hypnotist takes the active role (as the operator). In other words, the client enters the hypnotic state and his subconscious is laid open to instructive suggestions from the hypnotherapist– poured, as it were, into their receptive sub consciousness. This process works very well. However, there is no need to use this handling exclusively. Having someone take an active role in their hypnotherapy may enhance their learning and more rapid results.

Active participation hypnotherapy combines the passive approach with the psychoanalysis style of encouraging the client to talk out problems, locate traumatic causes and to release through "catharsis." In other words, the client probes his own subconscious to locate the seat of his own difficulty, directs you as to what form of hypnotherapy will correct the problem and benefit them most. Finally, the client confirms that the problem is corrected.

This removes much of the guesswork from hypnotherapy; you do not guess at the client's needs, as the client, themself, tells you their needs. The subconscious of the client knows what their needs are and directs the hypnotherapist accordingly.

"Active Participation Hypnotherapy" is a breakthrough technique where you assist by directing the client to direct you as to how you can best direct them: all information comes directly from the client's own subconscious sources, who confirms that the problem is corrected– which is the culminating suggestion that the solution has been achieved.

MODUS OPERANDI: ACTIVE PARTICIPATION HYPNOTIC METHOD
You Will Need:
The Serenity Resonance Sound or Hypno-Music (available at the end of this book)

The method is handled in this manner: First induce somnambulism. After the client is deeply hypnotized, you suggest, **"After you are hypnotized, your conscious mind will move to one side and your subconscious mind will come to the fore and will speak for itself. You will be able to speak easily and freely and what you say will come directly out of your subconscious as it speaks for itself. As you speak, your speaking will continue to send you into increasing depths of hypnosis."**
The hypnotist continues:
"You are deep into hypnosis and yet you are completely aware and can freely speak to me, and tell me the exact truth about your condition. Your conscious mind moves to one side and your subconscious mind comes to the fore and will speak to me directly, and as it does so the

speaking will send you down yet deeper and deeper into hypnosis. All speaking will come as the result of your subconscious mental activity. You will tell the complete truth about yourself. As you relax now in deep hypnosis, start speaking to me, and tell me what your problem is."

The hypnotized client will commence speaking of their problem. What they tell you comes directly out of the subconscious and thus is not colored by conscious rationalization. The heart of their problem is revealed. Often what the client's subconscious says about their problem is completely different from what their conscious mind expressed. This lets you really probe into their difficulty and correct it more expertly. After the client has subconsciously said what is needed, suggest:

"Now that we know what the real heart of your problem is, I will give you beneficial suggestions to correct it. The suggestions I give you will go directly into your subconscious mind, will take root there, and will develop into fresh patterns of behavior, as you want your behavior to be."

At this juncture, you return to conventional hypnotherapy by giving positive and beneficial suggestions to correct your client's condition and establish new behavioral habits. This complete, return again to active interviewing your subject.

"The suggestions I have given you have gone directly into your subconscious and have done you so much good. You are now on your way to perfect well being. Speak to me again now from your subconscious, and answer these questions…let your responses arise directly out of your subconscious mind, as you speak them to me. Have the suggestions given aided you in the mastering your problem?"

Client responds. (Obtain a commitment.)

"What further suggestions do you wish me to give you to help you master your problem?"

Client responds. (Do what the hypnotized person tells you to do.)

Continue:

"Now that I have done what your own subconscious knowing about yourself has told me to do, is your situation beginning to show the improvement you wish?"

Client responds.

"Before I awaken you from this deep hypnosis, are there any further helpful suggestions that you wish me to implant into your subconscious to help you master your problem? If so, tell me from you deep insight of knowing about yourself, and tell me how to correct it, so that I can help you in every way."

Client responds. (Do anything further that the client in hypnosis tells you to do.) Upon completing this finalizing portion of the session, suggest:

"Now that I have given you every beneficial suggestion and have done for you everything you have told me to do to master your problems, is this satisfactory?"

Clien responds. If "Yes" proceed and end the session.

If "No," say, "Tell me then what I am further to do to aid you?"

Continue your session until such time as the client subjectively agrees that their problem is solved, or is on its way to solution. This affirmation of the correction directly from the subconscious, in many instances, results in a complete correction of a problem in only one session.

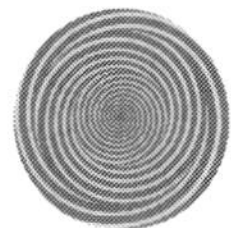

~ *Chapter 86* ~
SUBCONSCIOUS HYPNOTHERAPIST

This technique gives the hypnotherapist a passive role, while the client assumes the active role. reverses the situation. Here's how to passively create great results:

MODUS OPERANDI: SUBCONSCIOUS HYPNOTHERAPY

Take your time with the consultation. Allow the client to tell their story and what they want accomplished. Remember that your "sympathetic ear" is an important part of the work.

Go with your client into your private session room, darken the room and have the client lie on back on a comfortable couch. Then start the Hypno-Music or Entrancing Music as a background to the session. These recorded music tapes and include alpha-theta tones, which lull them into hypnosis. They are available at the back of this book.

Guide the client to take six deep full breaths in rapid succession and then close their eyes and allow themselves to enter the music and sound. Then give them time to "enter" the music for several minutes. Now suggest:

"As a result of our consultation, we both know what you want to achieve. In this session, you will design your own 'suggestion-formula' accordingly and present them to your own mind. Do this clearly and slowly so that your subconscious can to be its own therapist.

As you relax in this serene stage of mind, enter the realm of sleep. With your eyes still closed, visualize and imagine a white, bright screen in front of your closed eyes. It may appear much like a blank computer screen. However you envision it will be perfect. This is your screen of mind. Upon this bright, blank screen, visualize with your inner eye, in capital letters this message:

'I am going into deep hypnosis. My own subconscious mind now becomes my very own hypnotherapist. Subconscious mind, allow __________ (Say your name as this is your office and your client) **to assist me in this self-achievement.'**

Good. Your subconscious, when requested to answer a question, will respond by lifting your left forefinger. This will signify your answer 'yes.' If you understand this, give that signal now."

(Wait for left forefinger to lift. Then, proceed on.)

"Very good."
(Pause for a few moments, and further let the frequencies of Hypno-music sink in.)

"Subconscious, are you agreeable to this? If this is true, give the 'yes' signal to me."
(Wait for subconscious "yes" response. If it is "yes" and it usually is, continue. If not, repeat the suggestions for this idea-motor response and wait again.)

"Subconscious take your time and completely solve the problem that was presented when we talked a few minutes ago. (Re-state the problem, using their own words.) Thank you, subconscious, for making this the case. When you have solved the issue with the perfect solutions for you, let us know by raising your 'yes' finger or nodding your head. Thank you."

After these instructions, go silent. Wait, wait, wait for the subconscious to solve the problem. When they nod or move a finger say:

"Allow these beneficial suggestions to sink deeply into your inner-self and become your reality."

AROUSAL FROM SUBCONSCIOUS HYPNOSIS

Turn off the background music and let silence reign. Address the subconscious:

"Subconscious when you know this problem has been solved and the solutions are now your reality on all levels physically, mentally, spiritually and emotionally, this session is successful and complete and you may arouse this person from hypnosis completely healed in the here and now."

This allows the subconscious of your client to decide when the session is complete. Congratulations on achieving true 21st Century Hypnotherapy.

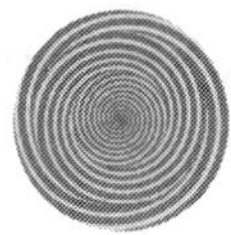

~ *Chapter 87* ~
TALKING TO YOURSELF
HYPNOTHERAPY

Includes
Two Mind Myths
Talking To Yourself Hypnotherapy
    The Audio-Phone Method
    The Hands-Over-The-Ears Method

This approach celebrates thoughtful deliberation privately with oneself as a terrific habit. Use it and life is good for you and your client!

TWO MIND MYTHS

To use this important hypnotherapy, you must rise above two myths about the mind; myths so frequently hammered into the heads of hypnotherapists that they have become belief:

Myth One: The 10%-90% Theory

It is said that the mind is unequally divided into two parts: 10% being conscious mind and 90% subconscious mind. How can that possibly be the case, when mind is intangible? How can a percentage (proportion) be given to an intangible?

Remember that you are a trinity: body, mind, and spirit. Your spirit is your consciousness, which is your individual SELF. Your SELF uses mind to produce thoughts, and thoughts are forms of energy, which program your brain (bio-computer within your head) to produce various forms of activity of your body, as it currently exists in 3D.

Myth Two: Talking To Yourself is Nutty

Talking to oneself is the sign of a simpleton. Some formulate this opinion when hearing another babble to themself. "Babbling has little purpose, and talking to oneself should be used privately" they say. Yet, consciously directed babbling can greatly improve the wisdom of your behavior.

Of course, compulsively talking to yourself can be exhausting. But when you develop a habit of inner dialogue to benefit your behavior, you become more vital. When used properly, inner dialog is a gift. That's the purpose of TALKING TO YOURSELF HYPNOTHERAPY.

MODUS OPERANDI: TALKING TO YOURSELF HYPNOTHERAPY
To deliberately talk to yourself for purposeful directive you can use an "audiophone" or talk to yourself– out loud– using the Hands-Over-Ears technique. Either way accomplishes the objective of self-talk with awareness.

THE AUDIO-PHONE METHOD
You Will Need:
An Audio-Phone

An audio-phone device has earphones and a microphone that amplifies your voice into them. You place the earphones on the ears as you talk to yourself via a microphone. It is a personal feedback process.

THE HANDS-OVER-THE-EARS METHOD
The Hand-Over-Ears method requires you to press your hands over your ears while talking to yourself. This causes an amplification of what you say to yourself to buzz through.
Talking to yourself lets you reflect upon the behavior you wish to design within yourself.
To use this approach, think of a habit you'd like to overcome or something you'd like to understand more fully. Then, think out loud about what you want to think about that subject. Next, tell yourself ideas you want to tell yourself about it.
This masterful technique of TALKING TO YOURSELF HYPNOTHERAPY is of inestimable value.

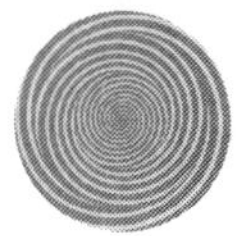

~ *Chapter 88* ~
STOCKWELL'S SUBPERSONALITY APPROACH

© 2002 Excerpts From
"Denial Is Not River In Egypt: Overcome Addiction, Compulsion & Fear
with Dr. Stockwell's Self-Hypnosis System

Includes
Edit The Editor
Edit & Tame The Editor
NLP Gives Sub-Personalities A Hand
Gestalt Hypnotherapy

"I am one with my duality."
—Barry E. Smith

When you pay attention to the chatter in your head, you hear them; the wisest of wise, angel, naughty, humorist, child, teen, mature one, old crone, seducer, prude, the feeler, the thinker, creative one, the inner critic and more. If you feel conflicted, it is these inner selves dukeing it out. Activate and integrate positive sub-personalities to work together and they will. Then you become a happy, many-faceted jewel.

If a faultfinding sub-personality gets overly controlling, you need to diffuse or balance it with more nourishing sub-selves. Why let one out-of-control voice rule all your other voices? Tough love for yourself is one way to tame that voice. There are other ways:

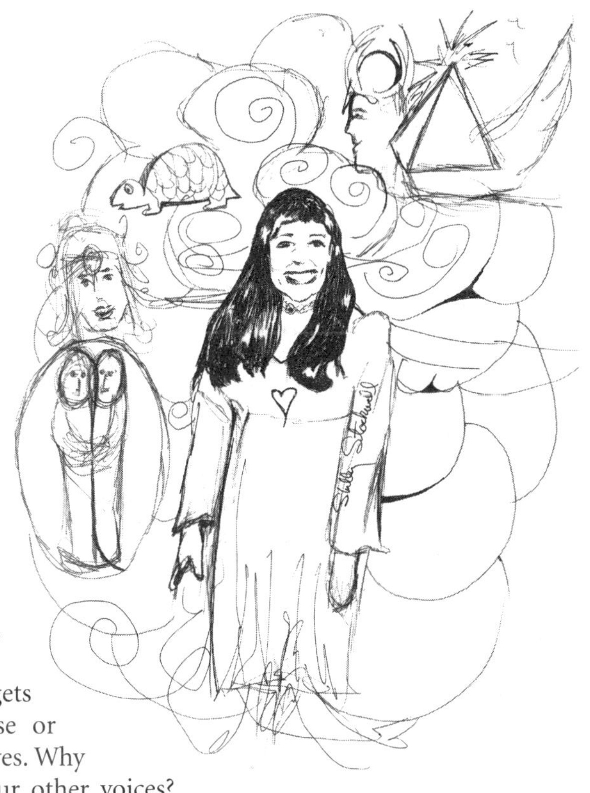

Illustration by Shelley Stockwell-Nicholas

EDIT THE EDITOR

"If someone with multiple personalities threatens to kill themselves, is it considered a hostage situation?"

—George Carlin

Do you live with your worst enemy? Are you very hard on you? Do you blame yourself for failing to be perfect? Do you call yourself names like "moron," "idiot," "pig" or "stupid"? Is there a part of you that goes haywire and out of control?

A limiting sub-personality says things like;
"I'm going to keep you sick and debilitated,"
"You don't deserve any better,"
"You'll fail."
"This is silly."
"What will other people think?"
"You're worthless."
"How dumb can you be?"
"You can't do anything right."

Who is this untamed inner critic, or limiting character? I call them the Editor. There to protect you, this sub-self can get cocky and out of hand. Left unbridled, they may constantly lend a hand that slaps you down. This critical parent is often more negative than your actual parents ever were.

Untamed critics take as much power as you give them. Then they overtake thoughts and behaviors. The Editor isn't hell bent on stomping you; They've just been given too much power. If you let them, they inner-fear with your happiness.

MODUS OPERANDI: EDIT & TAME THE EDITOR

Here's how my brother Alex and I tame the tyrant. When using this with a client, hypnotize them and take them through this process:

1. DESCRIBE THE PERFECT YOU

"The first step in unhooking yourself from the Editor is to simply be aware of them. To do that, think about yourself as if you were as perfect as you would like to be. How would you characterize yourself? (Wait for their answer). **Use 10 words or less to describe your ideal self. For example; 'I am sweet, slim and loving. And I get things done.'**

Write your positive AFFIRMATION of self here: ______________________

____."**

2. CHECK IN WITH YOUR LIMITING CHARACTER

"What did the Editor say when you wrote your affirmation? If they complained or criticized write down what they said.

Write the Editors opinion here: ______________________

____."**

3. REVERSE THE CURSE

Continue to write as many affirmations and editorial opinions as possible and when complete, take the Editor's negative comment and turn it around into a positive remark. If it said **"'You never finish anything you start.' Change it to 'I always finish what I start.' If you said, 'You are stupid' change it to 'You are brilliant and learning more each day. Great!'"**

4. PERSONIFY YOUR LIMITING GAL OR GUY

"Now imagine the Editor in a physical form and describe them with the first thing that pops into your head. Dare to give outrageously brave and ridiculous answers:
What is your editor like? (pause for answer)
What clothes do they wear? (pause for answer)
How do they smell? (pause for answer)
What kind of vibes do they give off? (pause for answer)
How are they built? (pause for answer)
What kind of a voice do they have? (pause for answer)
Do they remind you of someone you've met before? (pause for answer)

5. INTERVIEW THE LIMITED ONE

Ask them: **"What do they do for fun?"**
"When did you come into my life?"
"What brought you into existence?"
"What is your job? Do you like it?"
"Can we give you a new job description you'd like better?"
"How do you protect me, the person you come through?"
"How does what you do serve the me that you come through?"
"What would you like me to appreciate you for?"
"What am I doing or not doing that concerns you?"
"What do I do (or not do) that gives you what you want?
        (Or, **"What is the least wrong thing I do?"**).
"Give me one small doable thing that I can do to improve in this regard."
"How can you, do a better job of critiquing me and yourself?"
"Where are you located?" (Are you in my body or in an object?)
"How would you like me to contact you in the future?"
"Thank you, Editor, for talking to me and doing a diligent job."

6. ASSIGN A NEW JOB DESCRIPTION

"Now invite your editor/critic to sit in the car or wait outside the door while you interview other sub-personalities that express your creativity, love peace and harmony."

AFFIRM SUCCESS: Tame the Shrew/Critic/ Editor

OK inner wise guy this affirmation is for you…listen up.

"I am speaking directly to the Editor: When you are present, affirm with me these ideas. 'I am a masterful critic. I give loving critiques; I'm ever improving. To get my host's attention, I address them with terms of endearment. I address my host lovingly. I praise their progress and suggest small improvements. In this way, I protect them well and help them get the love they need.' Thank you for listening Editor."

MODUS OPERANDI: NLP GIVES SUB-PERSONALITIES A HAND

"Locate the parts of you that are in conflict; the ones who invokes an unwanted behavior (like smoking, for example). **Locate other parts that have your highest good in mind. Put out your hand and place into one hand the negative parts and in your other hand the positive voices.**

Close your eyes and identify each part with a visual, feeling and sound image… describe each carefully to yourself. As you do, your hand will take on the weight of each personality grouping and will respond to the weight. That way, you feel the balance or imbalance of your opposing viewpoints. When both sides have said everything they have to say about the situation, take a deep breath and let them discover any points that they agree upon. When ready, bring your hands up until they touch and merge both attitudes. Congratulations, you have resolved your conflict."

GESTALT HYPNOTHERAPY

"My approach is an integrative one. We make real people out of plastic ones."
—Fritz Perls

In the 1940's Frederick (Fritz) Perls used the word "gestalt," meaning "configuration of the whole," to describe techniques to bring a person's awareness to now, distinguish between "perceptual reality" and "mental fantasy" and to integrate conflicting viewpoints.

Gestalt hypnotherapy allows your client to dialog with their body, their attitudes and the here and now reality. Each of these distinct viewpoints act as sub-selves. The hypnotherapist's goal is to get them to work as a team.

The client while entranced, enjoying the natural trance that ensues, acts out scenes from dreams or life taking on the roles of each human, inanimate object and sub-personality. You can use body language to key into the process. Let's say that during your session the person's finger twitches. You would say **"What is it your finger would like to say?'** And then continue to dialog until resolution. Let's say they wring their hands, ask, **"What would one hand like to say to the other?"**

Or if they say for example, **"My mother wouldn't like this…"** You'd say **"Be your mother and tell me what you'd like to say about this."** And when they are complete, **"And what would you like to say to your mother?"**

If the dialogue comes to a stand still ask them to **"assume the role of a third party observer who acts as an arbitrator and helps the dissenting parts come to a peaceful resolution in the here and now."**

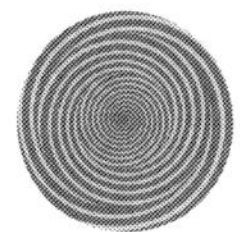

~ *Chapter 89* ~
HUNTER'S PARTS HYPNOTHERAPY
By Roy Hunter, M.S., CHI, Fellow
Based on his book, "The Art of Hypnotherapy"

Includes
What is Parts Therapy?
How To Do Parts Therapy

KNOCK, KNOCK WHO'S THERE?
Perls called it "Gestalt," Freud "varied ego states,"
Indians, "all my relations" for numerous manifestations.
"Voice Dialog" for Hal & Sidra Stone,
"Archetypes" from Joseph Campbell,
"Role-playing" and "Psychodrama"
make sub-selves unscramble

I say "hello" to me on the phone, as multiples cheer "a schizophrenic's not alone"
Sometimes I argue behind my face or beat myself out in the human race
But each of me is an inspiration when we work together for into-great-ion
> —Shelley Stockwell, PhD

The late Charles Tebbits was legendary for using this technique for resolving inner conflicts. Here is what C. Roy Hunter has to say about it:

WHAT IS PARTS THERAPY?

We all wear different hats at different times and places and have various aspects of our personalities or "ego parts." In the hypnotic state you can actually call out these physical and mental parts and dialogue with them. The hypnotherapist then mediates conflicts and helps the parts come to inner resolution.

For example, an overweight person often has a part wishing to go on one diet after another, while another personality part incessantly breaks each diet. They may say "a part of me wants to get rid of this weight while another part wants to keep on eating."

While in deep trance, the client might easily allow the two conflicting parts to emerge so the conscious mind may take on the energy and emotions of each personality part. Effective mediation paves the way for the client to successfully reduce. While this concept may seem simple at first glance, effective parts therapy involves numerous steps and good communication skills.

I rarely use parts therapy on a client's first visit with someone who has never experienced hypnotherapy so that they have an enjoyable, abreaction-free first visit.

MODUS OPERANDI: HOW TO DO PARTS THERAPY

Here's how to do it. Follow ALL the steps explained:

Pre-Induction Explanation

Hypnotize your Client

Identify the Part

Gain Rapport

Call Out the Part

Thank the Part for Emerging

Ask Detailed Questions of Its Purpose

Negotiate and Mediate

Terms of Agreement

Confirm the terms of Agreement

Give Appropriate Direct Suggestions

Give Integration Suggestions

Give Helpful Post Hypnotic Suggestions

1. Pre-Induction Explanation

Explain Parts Therapy to the client before hypnosis begins. You might say; **"I can take my wife to a Friday night movie and think to myself 'we could see this at a bargain matinee price on Saturday afternoon.' That's my inner accountant speaking inside my head. At the same time my own inner child may say 'I've worked hard and deserve to have fun when the time is convenient.' Under hypnosis, I could easily get into the emotional energy of each part and present conflicting arguments. In an actual hypnosis session my inner child made a bargain with my inner accountant so there is no conflict."**

If you don't give a pre-induction explanation, do one at the end of your session so your client doesn't leave your office thinking they have upsetting multiple personalities.

2. Hypnotize your Client

Make sure that the client is hypnotized to a sufficient depth to minimize the risk of interference from the analytical mind.

3. Identify the Part

Usually I begin by identifying and calling out the part that is blocking success first by using words such as, **"There is a part of you that is causing you to __________ (Snack frequently)… If the part of desiring change is willing to talk please say the words, I am here."**

When they respond ask, **"How may I address you? What may I call you?"**

If they do not respond ask when and where questions like **"When did you come into __________ (Client's name) life?" "What is your function?"…**

You may choose to call out the other part of the conflict as well, which in some cases might be role-played by the conscious mind.

"__________ (Client's name) there is a part of you that desires to change, and that part is most certainly interested in your happiness. And when that part of you is happy __________ (Client's name) you will be happier. It the part of desiring change is willing to talk please say the words, I am here." When they respond ask, **"How may I address you? What may I call you?"**

"Did you hear what _________ (the other parts name) **said? How do you respond?** Or you could, if you like, summarize what the other part said. **"That part of you appreciates that you were willing to listen and is now willing to listen to you in return. What do you have to say in response?"**

4. Gain Rapport

Just as rapport is built with a client before hypnosis, it must also be gained with each part in order to make it feel safe and accepted. Complimenting it in some manner does this, even if the client criticizes it. Always keep rapport with each part as they present themselves so that you do not break rapport with the subconscious. Your goal is to reach resolution and you do not want your client to pop out of trance.

5. Call Out the Part

"I'd like to speak with a part of you that makes ___________ (Client's name) ___________ (snack frequently between meals). **I'm sure that you are doing what you think is right for** ___________ (Client's name) **and there is a reason why you are doing such a good job. As a mediator I am willing to listen to whatever you have to say. Please enlighten us.** (Or. 'tell me about yourself.')

If you like you can bring in a conflicting or higher part of self to dialog.

Another part of ___________ (Client's name) **that is unhappy, and feels that better communication can enlighten both of you with a few ideas that could make** ___________ (Client's name) **much happier. If you would like to gain more information and communicate** ___________ (Client's name) **is willing to listen to whatever you have to say. Tell us about yourself.** (or Would you please let us know you are willing to communicate by either saying 'I am here' or by moving a finger to show me 'yes.')

Wait for a response. It there is no response within about a minute, continue with suggestions such as, **"I am only a mediator and am telling you what** ___________ (Client's name) **told me to say. We are willing to listen to whatever you have to say. Will you please enlighten us, and let me know when you are ready to speak by saying 'I am here' or by moving a finger to show me 'yes.'**

Wait for a response. If there is still no response after 2 attempts, you may either ask only for an ideo-motor (finger signals) or call out the other part instead. If there is still no response, try going through a third part that is less involved. **"I'd like to speak with a part of you that is familiar with what has been going on with** ___________ (Client's name) **parts of self."**

No response could mean that conscious interference could be in the way. At your option you may deepen the trance or try again or switch to anther hypnotherapy technique.

6. Thank the Part for Emerging

This is essential to good communication. A mediator at a bargaining table would most likely thank all in attendance for their willingness to come and discuss differences. I say **"Thank you for your willingness to communicate."**

7. Ask Detailed Questions of Its Purpose

Your objective is to uncover the cause of a problem. Simply ask the five "W" questions: Who? What? When? Where? And Why? By asking the "who" question first, you may find a part disclosing its purpose in its name and answer to one or more of the other four "w" questions to help uncover the cause of the client's problem and pave the way to a solution.

Normally I begin by saying **"Who are you or what name or title shall I call you by? _____________ (Client's name) want to know what your job or purpose is and why you are doing what you are doing. They are willing to listen to you in return. What do you have to say in response?"**

Allow each part to express and now the fun begins! It is impossible to write a script for what to say next. The best advice is what Charles Tebbetts said, "deal with what emerges!" Sometimes it is necessary to go back and forth between these questions and the next negotiation phase. Call in other parts whenever necessary with, **"Is there another part that can provide some helpful suggestions or information?"**

8. Negotiate and Mediate

Your goal is to facilitate release, followed by relearning. Often the best way to accomplish this is to negotiate and mediate compromise, acceptance and resolution. It is vitally important to remain non-judgmental throughout the process, even when a part says something that seems ridiculous. Often clients show a variety of emotions during the process, laughing, swearing or expressing surprise at what they say about themselves.

Stay calm, and maintain rapport with all parts. Usually before a resolution can be reached each participating part must feel like it was able to present its case and be heard. Once this is done proceed to the next step:

9. Terms of Agreement

Often parts themselves will come to terms of agreement; but frequently conflicting parts must compromise and bend a little (with your assistance). Ask the right questions, remaining as objective as possible while looking out for the best interests of the client. Good parts therapy is a matter of trial and error, changing, adapting to the client and always dealing with what emerges. Often a part agrees to take on a new job. Sometimes you may have to go for a temporary term of agreement and seek a permanent resolution later.

"What would it take for you to honor _____________ (Client's name) request?

If you do what _____________ (Client's name) asks, what do you want in return?

If _____________ (Client's name) loves and accepts you, are you willing to take on a new job?

Is there another job you can do for _____________ (Client's name) that will make you happy?

You are a part of _____________ (Client's name) and you can only reach your full potential of happiness (peace, achievement, security…) if _____________ (Client's name) is happy too. Are you willing to do something that will make _____________ (Client's name) happier?

Can you make a compromise until we can continue negotiations at the next session?

Are you willing to do this on a trial basis for a month or would one week be easier?

We only have a little time left. Are you satisfied with today's progress and are you willing to continue negotiations next week."

If a part is totally uncooperative you can call out whatever part has the highest wisdom and ask its assistance. If, and only if, you know your client's religious affiliation call upon their spiritual guide as a part to assist negotiations. If the client has Christian beliefs the Holy Spirit works wonders. If the client believes in the higher self call the Higher Self in the same manner.

10. Confirm the terms of Agreement

When you believe that all participating parts have reached terms of agreement, confirm by asking:

"______________ (Part #1 by name) **are you satisfied with agreement reached here today?**"

Wait for the response. Proceed with all other participating parts.

"Is there any other part that wishes to express itself?"

Wait ten seconds for a reply, if not proceed:

11. Give Appropriate Direct Suggestions

Suggestions should conform strictly to the terms of agreement reached along with confidence building suggestions that **"all parts will cooperate together."**

12. Give Integration Suggestions

Before awakening your client. Charles Tebbetts usually had the parts shake hands, embrace or hold hands for mutual love and acceptance followed by the direct suggestions **"all parts now merge into an integrated and complete whole. The integration is complete by raising your hand."**

One of my clients envisioned his parts dancing just before integrating. Some hypnotherapists use words such as 'harmony' for 'integration,' others ask clients to **"see a green light when the integration is complete."** (yellow or red would mean that more work is to be done). I use an Ericksonian "double bind" statement like **"You may either raise a hand or move your 'yes' finger when all parts attain inner harmony or integration."**

13. Give Helpful Post Hypnotic Suggestions

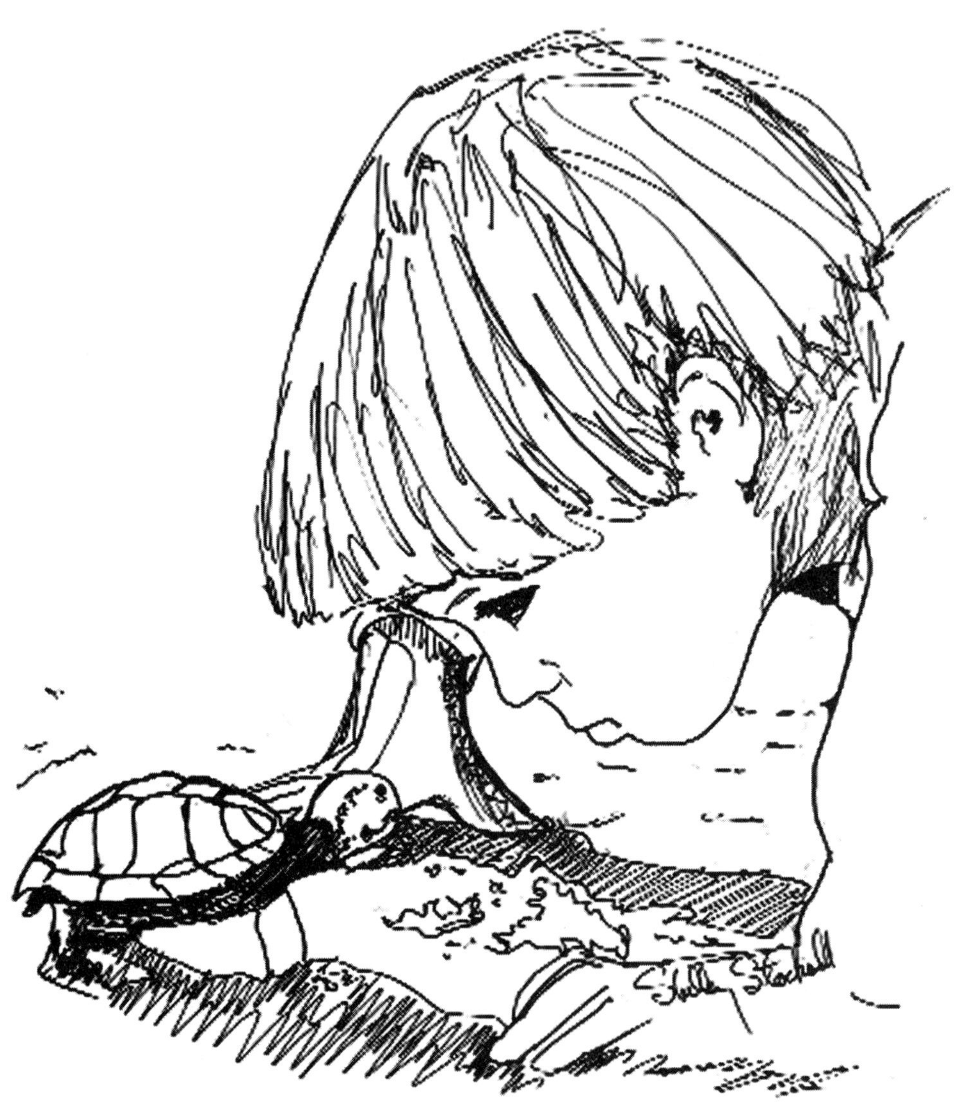

Illustration by Shelley Stockwell-Nicholas

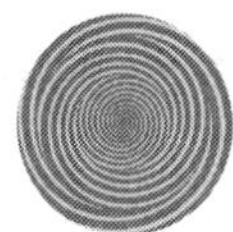

<h1 style="text-align:center">~ Chapter 90 ~
THE SLOW-DOWN
HYPNOTHERAPY CLINIC</h1>

Half the troubles in the world are caused by going too fast: accidents, wrong decisions, pugnacious behavior, nervous wrecks and murders. Yes, even murders are caused by going too fast and not thinking things through. Neurosis and psychosis and even going crazy is caused by going too fast. The list goes on and on.

Think about it.

Maybe saying that going too fast causes half the troubles in the world is too modest.

What to do about it?

Slow-Down Hypnotherapy!

It provides a natural answer the natural way. The natural way is the way nature handles its time clock.

Everything in nature follows its natural time clock, except humans. Plants left to themselves grow at their own speed. Animals, too. Nature is in proper sync with itself.

The prime directive of life in the world is survival. An animal sometimes goes fast, sometimes slow, but always its behavior is in time and in sync for top efficiency. Animals are timed with nature for the best living of life.

Humans create artificial behavior, which throws off their time clock. The modern world is geared towards a fast pace. Do more and more. Get things done quickly. Move swiftly. Go fast. Get there. Pace, pace, pace. Often this leads to a crackup.

Some druggist, recognizing this, got the bright idea to create tranquilizers to slow us down. Tranquilizers became a billion dollar industry. But tranquilizers are an artificial way to regulate your natural time clock. Further, they make you dopey.

Your subconscious mind has its own natural time clock. But since the subconscious is responsive to suggestion, the conscious mind can sell it on hurry, hurry, hurry! It barrages the subconscious to keep pace with a fast-paced world. Then you can get more done.

Stupid! One actually gets less down by hurry, hurry, hurry, than by allowing things to happen in accordance to their subconscious sense of proper timing. Slow-Down Hypnotherapy provides the way.

Subconscious mind instinctively knows the correct way to time the performance properly of each thoughtful activity. Given its natural freedom, it will be correct. Only conscious, critical mind can cause it to get out of sync. Slow-Down Hypnotherapy must be aimed to regulate ones pace to its natural time clock. When this is done, one performs at top efficiency. Sell your conscious phase of mind the idea of harmonizing with your subconscious phase of mind and your behavior will instinctively time you to perform correctly.

The modern world puts much stress on the individual to do everything quickly. "You must do more and more to be extraordinary," it says. Being extraordinary is a self-imposed obligation. Actually, being ordinary, means to be in accordance with your nature. That is really extraordinary. Take your time and think about it.

Want to become a millionaire in hypnotherapy? Establish a SLOW-DOWN HYPNOSIS CLINIC.

MODUS OPERANDI: THE SLOW-DOWN HYPNOTHERAPY METHOD
You Will Need
Soft Music

Mind produces thoughts and thoughts produce the directive energy for behavior. Mind functions best when it is relaxed and not under pressure to speed up. Start by relaxing mind.

Have the client sit or lie down comfortably. Play some slow, soft music in the background to the session. Have them close their eyes, and drift into the music for some moments. Then tell them:

"Yawn. Yawn. Yawn." Yawning is automatically relaxing.

"Visualize yourself drifting in a sailboat on a quiet blue lake, in peaceful, beautiful country. Get close to nature. Let your mind drift and drift and drift allowing whatever thoughts that come in to just pass through it. Just drift and drift and drift. Sleepiness will come. Down, down deeper and deeper into this drowsy sleepiness.

You enter the realm of hypnosis.

You have a subconscious clock inside yourself that knows how to most accurately time all that you do. From this time forward, you allow your subconscious mind to regulate the timing for whatever you do. Your subconscious mind is in charge of your timing and not your conscious mind. You are in sync with your subconscious time clock.

Slow down. Slow down. Slow down. You now pause and take three deep breaths before you make any decisions. Take three deep breaths if you feel angry. This completely changes your mental direction. All anger will disappear, you feel at peace.

You become master of the world's swift pace. You regulate all you do in accordance to your subconscious direction. Any stress is gone from you forever. You are relaxed.

See yourself dropping down, down into the quiet of your inner self, where all is peaceful and serene.

See yourself doing everything you do with no effort at all. Everything is easy. In so doing, you become a master of everything you do. Rather than being mastered, you are the master of all you do.

Allow these thoughts to ramble through your mind, as you drop down even deeper into the reverie of hypnosis. Drift down into perfect synchronization with yourself.

Make the effort to do all you do without effort, and you will be synchronized with yourself. You become the master of time, rather than time being the master of you.

Slow down. Slow down. You are in perfect synchronization with your subconscious rhythms. There is plenty of time. When harmony has been accomplished between your conscious and subconscious mind... come back with me in the here and now, wonderfully aroused from these moments of hypnotic reverie.

Take this time...there is no hurry. When your subconscious knows this is so... arouse and come back with me."

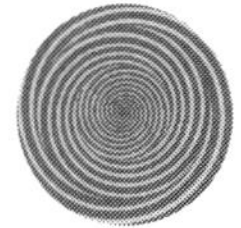

~ *Chapter 91* ~
FORGET YOU NOT HYPNOTHERAPY

Includes
Forget You Not Hypnotherapy
Transcendental Hypnosis Induction

You know that you are, but have you forgotten WHO you are?

This effective form of hypnotherapy reminds clients WHO they are and it is equally useful to you personally.

When you were born into this lifetime, if you are a male, your parents very likely looked through a list of boy's names, to select a name for you. If female, they choose a girl's name from the lists. You had nothing to say about it. They choose the name they liked, and you have been tagged with it for life.

That is just the start…soon, other forms of identifications are attached to you: your address, your phone number, your social security number, your driver's license number and more. Somewhere in Washington, D.C. a computer keeps track of your ID tags– and you.

With time, you may have become tagged with behavior difficulties such as phobias, stress, depressions and nervousness and perhaps have come to recognize these tags as yourself. Maybe you have sought hypnotherapeutic help for such identifications.

In other words, you seek freedom from things (experiences) that your parents, circumstances, society, and even governments have heaped upon you. Your seeming difficulties stem from an identification of yourself that you have accepted from outside of self. You have forgotten to remember WHO YOU really are.

Remembering WHO YOU ARE, the real YOU, is the cure.

The real knowing of who you truly are, the perpetual essential you, is stored in the memory banks of your subconscious. Hypnosis is a fine way to surface these memories. Once you achieve the insight that all bothersome earthly stuff is only a bother to the false identification of self, you let it go. After all, it really doesn't belong to YOU.

Such hypnotherapy is really so simple, yet much overlooked in mental healing. Mind tries to make excuses for overlooking the obvious by making it seem complex. When one just pauses to remember who they actually are, all the stuff they thought was such a big deal becomes "poppycock."

Try this Transcendental Hypnosis Induction Method and you'll see how well it works. For to recall SELF, as an immortal BEING, a unique consciousness like no other, far exceeds any supposed identification.

When you stand in the very center of the universe in relation to yourself, you are in a God position. Jesus said, "GOD IS WITHIN YOU." No ego is evolved in this, as all equally hold this exalted position. The only difference lives in the recognition of this truth.

MODUS OPERANDI: "FORGET YOU NOT" HYPNOTHERAPY
You Will Need
Meditative Music
(Use *Hypno-Music* or the *Serenity Resonance Sound* for this, if you wish).

Have the client take a seat in a comfortable chair, with their feet placed flat on floor, and their hands resting in their lap. Their hands should not touch each other. Have the light in the room come from behind the client and directed towards the hypnotherapist. Give these suggestions:

"As you sit quietly in the chair, relax the muscles of you body. Just let yourself GO! As you do this, direct your attention to my eyes: look deeply into my eyes, and keep your attention fixed upon my eyes, until I tell you to close your eyes.

As you stare deeply into my eyes, notice how you perception on my eyes begins to change, and with this changing note how the perception of yourself begins to change. Instead of focusing upon my eyes, the point of your focusing moves through my eyes– to the other side of my eyes– to a point far beyond my eyes. You will find that you are no longer looking at my eyes, you are looking through my eyes into myself, and in this looking into me, you will sense that you are gaining a deeper perception of yourself.

You are becoming aware that you are looking through the windows of my eyes out into the vastness of space– in which the stars of the heavens pulsate and shine. Observe this phenomenon carefully. You are advancing in your perception."

Transcendental Induction
Meditative music comes in softly now, forming a background to the transcendental induction. The induction continues on.

"Let your entire body completely relax now, and send your BEING through the windows of my eyes, and project your BEING into that vast space. You are beginning to sense your Cosmic Connection. As you look deeply in this manner you relax your body completely, your eyes become so heavy and relaxed that you can no longer hold them open, and your eyes close. So close your eyes. (Eyes close.)

It feels so good to close your eyes. They are becoming so relaxed that you will find you cannot open them, no matter how hard you try. Try as you wish, but you cannot open your closed eyes, and along with the relaxation of your closed eyes, more and more does your entire body relax. So just relax into the vast space, which you see spreading before yourself, now that your eyes are closed, so with the perception of your 'third eye', you are now not looking into my space…the space you now witness is your own space. Deeper and deeper you sink into this space and more and more you begin to sense the wonderful BEING you truly are.

Now…
You feel yourself sinking down into this vast space, which spreads before you infinitely. Your two physical eyes are closed, so with the perception of your 'third eye,' you are now not looking into my space…you now witness your own space. Deeper and deeper you sink into this space, and more and more you begin to sense the wonderful BEING that you truly are.

Every breath you take sends you down deeper and deeper into this vast space of yourself, as you recognize your Cosmic Connection. Deeper and deeper you sink into this vast space, which is independent of the physical world. Your breaths are deepening, and every breath sends you down deeper and deeper into this vast space…far, far down beyond even a vestige

of consciousness of the physical world. You are gradually leaving the physical world behind, as you enter the realm in which your real SELF dwells.

Drift. Drift. Drift. You find yourself drifting in space…mind free of its body in this space. A mind free of its body in this space…drifting down ever deeper and deeper into space.

Now, ask yourself some questions as you drift down into this vast space. Are you the one who is called by a certain name in the physical world? Are you the person who lives at a certain address? Are you the person who possesses a certain bank account and holds a certain position in the physical world? (Pause.)

Experience how you feel right now in this vast space beyond the physical world beyond thoughts. You are beyond thoughts…you are a free mind drifting in free space. You are none of the things you thought you were, and yet you are still YOU."

GO SILENT FOR A MOMENT NOW IN THIS STATE OF CONTEMPLATION. THEN CONTINUE…

"As a free mind, you drift down deeper and deeper into this space. Where do you experience yourself drifting? Drift down to the very center of this vast space; as you drift down to the center of your real SELF. You are drifting into THE VOID, which is the creative center of the Universe, of which you are an intimate part.

You are drifting down, down to your SELF, and you begin to truly know your SELF. You see yourself before your SELF, and you ask a question, 'How can this be, for I am here in space drifting down to myself?' Suddenly you come to realize what you really are: you are the consciousness of your SELF, and you appreciate and recognize this fact with great joy and understanding in at last knowing– with full awareness– who and what you really are– you are the consciousness of your SELF.

You are an individual consciousness, and you recognize this fact that the SELF you see before you now, is the real YOU beyond any name which has been given you in the physical world, and what society has proclaimed you are.

This insight comes upon you like a bursting of stars…and suddenly you feel utter blissfulness, utter peacefulness, utter happiness, as you find yourself dropping down dropping down directly to THE CENTER OF YOUR BEING–WHICH IS YOUR REAL SELF.

You go on down, down into your SELF, and merge as one complete BEING. In doing this, you experience complete rest. You are home. Now, you know what and who you really are. Now you know that the many things you thought you had to complain about and correct in the physical world actually have no meaning to you at all. They all vanish in this KNOWING."

GO SILENT FOR SOME MOMENTS NOW AND CONTEMPLATE WHAT YOU NOW RECOGNIZE TO BE YOUR REAL SELF. Then continue…

"Now even this realization melts and fades away, as you melt into yourself… there is no separation of yourself as mind on one hand and body on the other, for in your true SELF both are combined as ONE. Each is part of the other, which combine as your consciousness.

Your true being is recognizing your relationship in the ever expanding universe. Suddenly, you know you are part of the totality. You are aware that you are one with the infinite.

This experience of SELF now completely changes your relationship with the physical world, in which it dwells at this time. It gives you control over both your mind and body that you never knew was possible. You develop powers you never knew you possessed, as YOU and SELF operate together as a team, in complete unity. YOUR SELF takes over control of mind, as it manifests in the physical world, and through your body. You have mastery over your mind, which makes you a MASTERMIND. Your mind brings perfection to your body.

With this control, which you have mastered, you make of yourself whatever you desire. You heal your body, you keep your body in perfect health; you remove all unwanted habits; you make your body perform to perfection. You master ALL that you desire, and achieve what you want to achieve. YOU HAVE DISCOVERED WHO YOU REALLY ARE AND THAT GOD IS WITHIN YOU!

This, which you now know as truth, will stay with you always. Every breath you take into your physical body automatically reinforces this truth, and ever increasingly causes it to become your realization."

Turn background music off.

"I bring you back now to the here and now. Joyously return to the physical world with the blissful KNOWING of who you really are. It glows within you as an everlasting flame."

Arouse client and the session is complete.

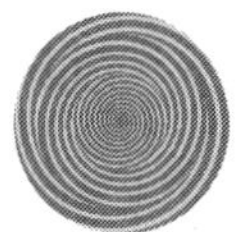

~ *Chapter 92* ~
COMPUTER HYPNOTHERAPY

Includes
Computer Technology Induction

Computer Hypnotherapy is a contemporary form of Hypnotherapy. Hypnotherapy popularity increases in this computer age. Your brain operates and directs you and your client's behavior and functions like a biocomputer. A biocomputer is constructed of organic material, while a conventional computer is inorganic in construction.

Your bio-computer is far greater than any computer yet produced. A good computer on your desk may have more than eight hundred million connections. Your brain biocomputer has over one hundred billion neurons and uncountable trillions of connections. Its potential has been scarcely touched.

BRAIN
The bio-computer in your head performs as it is programmed to perform. Here is found your "memory banks" of learning and experience. Also within it is "the mind's eye" which can be likened to a computer screen. Programs flash upon your screen of mind. As the master center of your brain it communicates throughout the body via the autonomic and sympathetic nervous systems. Your brain acts as consciousness directs, with consciousness as the programmer.

MIND
Through mind the bio-computer is programmed. Think of your mind as the keyboard operated and programmed by SELF (your consciousness).

SELF
The programmer of your bio-computer is SELF. Your mind, body and spirit make up your consciousness. And herein lives your SELF. SELF is the ultimate programmer of your bio-computer.

PRAHNA
The cosmic electricity, prahna provides the energy to make your bio-computer run.

HYPNOTHERAPY
Hypnotherapy is the technology through which mind can program the bio-computer brain. In computer hypnotherapy, the term "bio-computer" is substituted for "subconscious" …yet, a rose is still a rose by whatever name it is called.

How does hypnotherapy work?

In your current state of awareness, such comprehension is almost beyond understanding. Hypnotherapy, like the computer, does not require that you know how it works to make it work. Countless millions, even children, know how to operate a computer, but few know the inner electronics that make it work. Most simply know that the computer works. Hypnotherapy is like that. Just use it like most people are content to do, without concern for its inner operation. Be equally content with using your bio-computer.

MODUS OPERANDI: COMPUTER TECHNOLOGY INDUCTION

Have your client take a seat in a comfortable chair.

Give them this initial instruction:

"How like a computer you are. (Be as technical as you wish in your explanation. Computer devotees relate to that.) **The biocomputer inside the head, and throughout your body contains "memory banks" of learning and experience. Also within your biocomputer is found "your mind's eye" which can be likened to the computer's screen. Your MIND is the keyboard operated by SELF (consciousness). Through MIND the biocomputer is programmed. HYPNOTHERAPY is the technology through which mind can program the biocomputer brain. PRAHNA, or your life force, is the cosmic electricity, which provides the energy to make the biocomputer run. Now just relax and gaze into my eyes. When your eyes feel tired and heavy let them relax as we begin Computer Hypnotherapy."**

The Hypnotherapist and the client gaze into each other's eyes until the client's eyes feel tired and heavy. If they do not close their eyes on their own, instruct them to:

"Close your eyes and let them roll gently backwards under your closed eyelids, as though you are looking into your biocomputer brain. Your biocomputer will be turned on and operate fully by bringing the vitality or PRAHNA into yourself. This cosmic electricity is brought in through deep breathing.

Take six deep breaths in rapid succession."

(Wait until it is complete. You can breathe audible right along with them as a model.)

"Now, relax more and more as you continue to breathe, deep and in slow progression. With each breath you take in this slow rhythm you will find yourself becoming more and more sleepy, more and more relaxed, and more and more drifting down into hypnosis.

This puts your bio-computer in full operation, and you quickly drift down into profound hypnosis. As you know, many advanced computers use verbal speech recognition. You will now use this most modern approach. As I give the instructions verbally, you are to repeat them *silently* **inside the biocomputer inside your mind.**

Good. We begin the voice recognition function as you let these words resonate within the walls of your skull:

My eyes are tired. My eyes are closed. I am becoming relaxed all over. I am drifting into hypnosis."

(Pause and allow them time to sub vocalize. Do not rush the client. Allow time for these suggestions to sink in.)

"My eyes are tired. My eyes are closed. I am becoming relaxed all over. My biocomputer brain is now in full operation, and I am programmed to drift down deep in hypnosis."

(Pause and allow them time to sub vocalize.)

"My biocomputer brain is now in full operation, and I am programmed to go deeper and deeper into hypnosis with every breath I take."

(Pause and allow them time to sub vocalize.)

"My eyes are closed and they have become so relaxed now that I cannot open my eyes no matter how hard I try. I am programmed to be so relaxed; I cannot even open my eyes when I try. So I do not try…I just drift and drift into hypnosis."

(Pause and allow them time to sub vocalize.)

"I am so relaxed and sleepy that my head is dropping forward onto my chest, and I sink into deep hypnosis."

(Pause and allow them time to sub vocalize.)

The hypnotherapist now moves from first to second person in presenting further programming to the client:

"Good. Your bio-computer mind is operating to perfection. I will take over now and program it from this point on. All you have to do is relax more and more, and go deeper and deeper into hypnosis, as I beneficially program your biocomputer brain, of great benefit to yourself.

As we program into your bio-computer's memory bank this valuable wisdom and it becomes your way of life. This wisdom is always with you so you honor the perfection and mastery of your mind and body. As this wisdom is programmed into your bio-computer brain, you continue going down deeper and deeper into hypnosis. In this process, the fingers of your hands will function as the keyboard, and when the associated finger is pressed upon, that wisdom will come forth and shine in brilliance upon your SCREEN OF MIND to become your personal reality.

When your right thumb is pressed upon, this wisdom will shine forth upon your screen of mind and become your very own:

You try less and less to make things happen, and more you just let things happen."

(Gently press on their right thumb and you say this affirmation. Pause for a few moments.)

When your right forefinger is pressed upon, this wisdom will shine forth upon your screen of mind and become your very own:

In everything you do, you always respond in practical action. You will always act and react in a way of greatest benefit to yourself."

(Gently press on their right forefinger and you say this affirmation. Pause for a few moments.)

"When your right middle finger is pressed upon, this wisdom will shine forth upon your screen of mind and become your very own:

You are a witness to everything you do in life. You stand back and observe yourself. That way you always improve your action."

(Gently press on their right middle finger and you say this affirmation. Pause for a few moments.)

"When your right ring finger is pressed upon, this wisdom will shine forth upon your screen of mind and become your very own:

In everything you do, you always respond in practical action. You will always act and react in a way of greatest benefit to yourself."

(Gently press on their right ring finger as you say this affirmation. Pause for a few moments so that they can absorb.)

"When your right ring finger is pressed upon, this wisdom will shine forth upon your screen of mind and become your very own.

You observe yourself as you truly are, and not as you imagine yourself to be. Then, day by day, in every way, you'll become better and better."

(Gently press on their right ring finger as you say this affirmation. Pause for a few moments so that they can absorb.)

"When your right little finger is pressed upon, this wisdom will shine forth upon your screen of mind and become your very own:

You will know that when your mind is under control, your mind becomes like crystal reflecting equally, without distortion, the perception, the perceiver, and the perceived. It is through such mind that your consciousness of yourself is known."

(Gently press on their right little finger as you say this affirmation. Pause for a few moments so that they can absorb. Then move on to the left side.)

"When your left thumb is pressed upon, this wisdom will shine forth upon your screen of mind and become your very own:

Know that your Mind and Body act upon each other in a continuous and subconscious reaction."

(Gently press on their left thumb as you say this affirmation. Pause for a few moments so that they can absorb.)

"When your left pointer finger is pressed upon, this wisdom will shine forth upon your screen of mind and become your very own:

Be like a log drifting down the stream, and the things you bump into often will prove to be your lucky treasure of full living."

(Gently press on their left pointer finger as you say this affirmation. Pause for a few moments so that they can absorb.)

"When your left middle finger is pressed upon, this wisdom will shine forth upon your screen of mind and become your very own:

The best way to learn to anything is to start right in and learn how to do it. You just do it."

(Gently press on their left middle finger as you say this affirmation. Pause for a few moments so that they can absorb.)

"When your left ring finger is pressed upon, this wisdom will shine forth upon your screen of mind and become your very own.

The past is but memories that will never happen again. The future may never happen at all. There is only the here and now."

(Gently press on their left ring finger as you say this affirmation. Pause for a few moments so that they can absorb.)

"When your left little finger is pressed upon, this wisdom will shine forth upon your screen of mind and become your very own:

When something of value happens to you, say, 'thank you' to your inner self."
(Gently press on their left little finger as you say this affirmation. Pause for a few moments so that they can absorb.)

"Allow it all to happen. The wisdom given you in time and space is now programmed into the memory bank of your biocomputer.

When you wish to prepare yourself to arouse from hypnosis, just press upon your right thumb. Following this, when you wish to fully alert from hypnosis, press upon your left thumb, and you will arouse feeling wonderful and fine."

HYPNOTHERAPIST'S NOTE:
Remember that once implanted in your client's bio-computer this "keyboard" of the fingers will always bring forth the programmed wisdom.

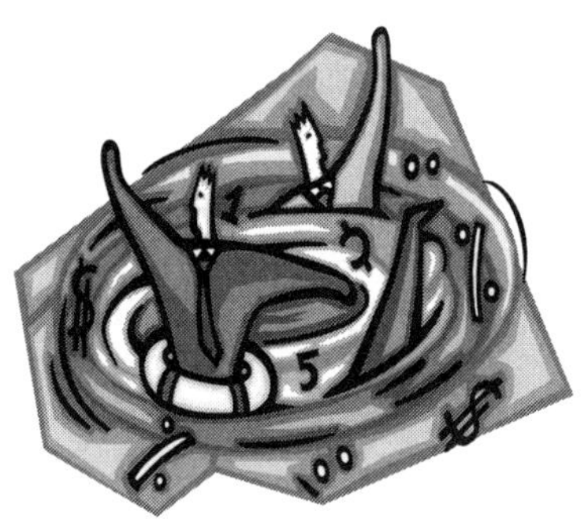

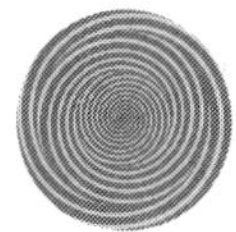

~ *Chapter 93* ~
INFINITE SMALLNESS HYPNOTHERAPY

A client may come into your office complaining that they feel like a little child drowning in oceans of pressure from a great big world. They feel so small, so unprepared, and so inadequate to handle the trials of life.

What can they do? What can they do? What can they do before they drown?

The lifeguard hypnotherapist comes to the rescue and tells them they must become large and strong so they can meet on the pressures of the world. They will live. They will not drown.

And so they are hypnotized to change their attitude about themselves: they are no longer a little child, now they are a full-grown adult. They are big and strong and can meet all the pressures of the world.

My goodness. What a help that is. They feel big and strong and now they can meet the pressures. They are no longer in danger of drowning, but the pressures are still there.

They feel so much more adequate now, but what to do about the pressures of living life? THE HYPNOTHERAPY OF INFINITE SMALLNESS provides the answer.

MODUS OPERANDI: INFINITE SMALLNESS HYPNOTHERAPY

Hypnotize your client and suggest:

"Remain just as you came, feeling like a little child." Then instead of suggesting that they become big and strong, suggest:

"You are now becoming smaller and smaller."

They came feeling as inadequate as a little child. They now experience themselves as an even smaller child- a smaller child while the pressures remain big as ever. How can that possibly be of help? Try it and see.

"You continue to become smaller and smaller, becoming so small that worldly pressures cannot find you at all. Down, down into infinite smallness you go; becoming so small you are invisible to the world. So small as to be the size of an atom, and then you disappear into nothingness. You enter The Void.

"When you become nothingness, you become what the Buddha told all who would become masters must become. You are conscious of what you really are. Suddenly, you burst forth like a blazing star and all the pressure of the world cannot touch you at all.

"You become submerged in the Cosmic Ocean and the earthly ocean is remote and unimportant. Standing in the Cosmic Ocean, you become part of that ocean, which is vast and beyond all earthly perception."

The experience for each person entering into infinite smallness is completely individual, for they are one-of-a-kind.

Directly ask their subconscious,
"If you understand the power of infinite smallness, nod your head. This will signal me that you do."

The signal will come. When it occurs, tell the subconscious:
"Arouse _________ (their name) **from hypnosis, happy and content in knowing that you are neither big nor small, young or old. You are perfectly content in just knowing that you exist. What you previously thought were unbearable pressures have been transformed into adventures from which to learn by experiencing. You have learned what you are: A TIMELESS MIRACLE."**
Up, alert, and on their way, the client leaves your office, and you can smile at a job well done.

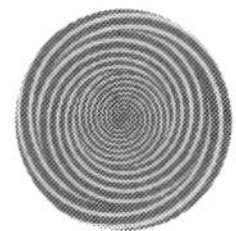

~ Chapter 94 ~
RIGHT BRAIN/LEFT BRAIN
HYPNOTHERAPY

The Twenty First Century is a bustling "Computer Age." Computers are everywhere, yet the greatest computer of all resides inside your head. The Human Brain is the Master Computer. To be a master hypnotherapist, it is well to learn as much as possible about the human brain.

Professor Emanual Orlick presents some staggering figures: The human brain is made up of more than one hundred billion neurons. And, it is estimated that each neuron makes as many as 200,000 synaptic connections, making more synapses than there are approximations of stars in our galaxy.

Your brain receives its information through your five senses: seeing, hearing, touching, tasting, and smelling. But it is not your senses that give you the information, but it is your brain that tells you what you see, hear, feel, taste of smell. All your sense organs are essentially extensions of your brain and brain cells.

Every second, it's estimated that our brain-computer receives more than 100-million internal and external bits of information. An idea of just what this means can be had by expanding this number to one minute, one hour, one day, one year.

1 second covers 100,000,000 bits of information.
1 minute covers 6,000,000,000 bits of information.
1 hour covers 360,000,000,000 bits of information.
1 day covers 8,640,000,000,000 bits of information.
1 year covers 3,153,600,000,000,000 bits of information.

What an amazing computer you have within your head: 3 quadrillion, 153 trillion, 600 billion bits of information are received and processed each year. With such potential, research indicates little about your brain computer's capacities. Its capacity could easily learn four different languages, take all the required courses for a dozen University Degrees, and memorize a complete encyclopedia. Brain Research Institutes have come to the conclusion that humans possesses enormous unused mental capacities, which actually could be infinite.

The capacity of the brain computer is so amazing, that if you were to flip through pages of a thirty-volume encyclopedia, glancing at each page, your brain "registers" everything your eyes "see" instantly. This is commonly called a "Photographic Memory."

The physical construction of the human brain consists of two main lobes or hemispheres, separated in the middle by a thick tissue called "the corpus collosum." It is commonly believed that each hemisphere of the brain is responsible for different mental functions. Though the subject of some debate, the left hemisphere is regarded as primarily logical, and is used for analytical mental tasks, such as mathematics. Persons of a scientific nature are usually considered left-hemisphere dominated, while those who perform well in subjects of art, music, creative writing, etc., are considered right-hemisphere dominated.

These facts are accurate in relation to how an individual uses their brain, but from an anatomy standpoint there exists a crisscross of nerve ganglion directly from right to left hemisphere. The design affords an operational connection between the two sides of the brain. In other words, the brain-computer is anatomically designed to function as a whole unit, just like the computer on your desk is designed to function as a whole. This fact must be considered in developing Right Brain/Left Brain Hypnotherapy Techniques.

Hypnosis seems to teach us to direct and control the tremendous capacities of that brain-computer inside our head. Some research has been done. Dr. Norton Price (of Harvard Medical School) was one of the first to probe the subconscious memory banks of hypnotized persons. He describes an experiment: A full page of The Wall Street Journal was displayed before a hypnotized person student at the university to peruse. The hypnotized subject was told to open his eyes, gaze at it for a minute and memorize the entire page. The Wall Street Journal was removed, and it was suggested the subject would bring to conscious recall, what he has subconsciously recorded. The subject recalled and recited the entire page from memory. He had created "eidetic imagery" or a memory of a visual image from one minute of observation. Your fabulous brain-computer works with incredible speed to recall in great detail any knowledge, any information, or any experience that has been recorded in its memory banks.

Your brain-computer can probe your genetic history, and withdraw the accumulated survival information that has been stored there for time immemorial. Your incredible brain can extract, analyze, organize, correlate, and otherwise process any part, or all, of the data that has ever been stored therein, in order to come forth with the best possible instant solutions to any problems with which you may be faced.

If your mental powers are not infinite, they indeed stretch a long way towards infinity. What is really amazing is that this remarkable brain-computer is only an instrument you use. There is nothing immortal about it. No computer is ever self-operating; something outside of its operation has to program it into required operation. That outside something is called the programmer. Your mind is that programmer, and your mind is immortal.

Just as the computer on your desk operates, if you want to make a decision, solve a problem, invent something new, or otherwise make use of your brain-computer, all you need to do is press the right buttons to program it into operation. The directive use of hypnosis directs your mind to press the right buttons.

Right Brain/Left Brain Hypnotherapy always upgrades mental powers and belongs to the realm of talent development. It will start your client on the way to using their talents.

Right Brain/Left Brain Hypnotherapy serves a dual purpose:
1. Amplifies
   It amplifies the special abilities invested in the right and left hemispheres.
2. Unifies
   It unifies left and right brain abilities in working as a holistic unit, thus increasing
   the abilities of each.

Right Brain/Left Brain Hypnotherapy is easy. You don't need to know how it works. You just need to know how to make it work. Hypnosis provides the way to press the right buttons.

MODUS OPERANDI: RIGHT BRAIN/LEFT BRAIN HYPNOTHERAPY:
You Will Need:
The *Serenity Resonance Sound* as background to the operation

Hypnotize the client producing a somnambulistic state.

Face the hypnotized client and place the palm of your right hand on their left temple. Place the palm of your left hand on their right temple. Press in firmly. Maintain this pressure while presenting the following directed operation instructions to computer-brain of the client:

"Your computer-brain will be programmed to holistically operate in perfect cooperation between your right and left brain hemispheres. Your right brain and left brain hemispheres will operate with greater and greater perfection. Submerge yourself in Serenity Resonance Sound now as this programming by your mind goes into effect. Sink deeper and deeper into hypnosis, and absorb."

Go silent, and allow the hypnotized client to submerge into the sound for some minutes. (Release pressure on temples.)

"When this programming of the brain-computer has become the case, subconscious mind arouse the person with remarkable control of their mental powers."
Your client arouses from the hypnosis.

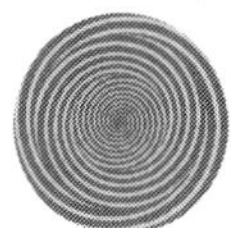

~ *Chapter 95* ~
COUNT YOUR BLESSINGS
HYPNOSIS

As a Hypnotherapist, a client may come to your office woe-begone! Their life is going to pot! They have nothing to be happy about. They come for help. What can hypnotherapy do? Goodness gracious what a lot of imagined nonsense they conjure. To help such a client, never say they are wrong. Just listen with a sympathetic ear. Then start their session.

MODUS OPERANDI: COUNT YOUR BLESSINGS HYPNOTHERAPY

Hypnotize client. Then directly tell the subconscious…

"Thank you for your confidence in me to turn your life around from being unhappy to recognizing how fortunate you are. Together let us count your blessings instead of non-blessings. Absorb this deeply:

You can see. If that is true nod your head.
(Wait for response.)

What a wonderful blessing you have just affirmed that you have.

You can hear. If that is true nod your head.
(Wait for response of affirmation and acceptance of this fact.)

What a wonderful blessing you have just affirmed.

You can smell the odor of beautiful flowers. If this is true nod your head.
(Wait for response.)

What a wonderful blessing you have just affirmed that you have.

You can taste. Hmm, how good things can taste. If this is true nod your head.
(Wait for response.)

You can feel. How countless wonderful things you can handle. You can feel so much to enjoy beneath your touch. If this is true, nod your head.
(Wait for response.)

You can think. How fortunate you are that you can think. You have told me of many depressing things you think about. That is perfectly okay. The important thing is that you can think whatever the thoughts may be. If this is true, nod your head.

(Wait for response.)

Most importantly of all you exist. And you will exist eternally. How fortunate you are. Understand? If you know this is true, nod your head.

(Wait for affirmation.)

Now, fill your mind with your blessings, and count your blessings. Then give thanks to your existence that you are.

When you leave my office you will be filled with so many blessings there will be no longer room in your mind for any thoughts other than the many things that you are blessing. Blessings. Blessings. Blessings. You stand in the midst of a flower garden of your blessings. Let this truth sinks deep inside yourself. Take your time. When it has become your reality then arouse from the hypnosis. You will leave my office with a bounce to your step and a smile on your lips."

Allow time for the client to come out of trance. A remarkable transformation has occurred. The client who leaves you office has reversed their polarity.

Good hypnotherapy? Too simple? In the simple is the most complex.

Does it work? The proof of the pudding is in the eating.

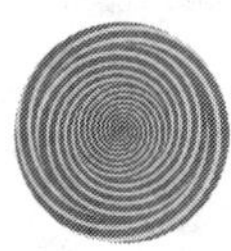

~ *Chapter 96* ~
YOUR LITTLE THEATER
OF THE MIND

Hand your client an eyeshade and take them to the theater.

You help them by pulling the eyeshade down and as you do, telling them that they are closing a curtain that will take them into their special theater. If you hold their hand during this process you will notice a slight tremble in their hand when the theater show begins. Then you can give them the direct suggestion of the results you want to happen.

MODUS OPERANDI: YOUR LITTLE THEATER OF THE MIND
You Will Need:
Eye Shades

As you place the eyeshades down over their eyes:
"This is the front curtain to the little theater of your inner mind. As it gently descends and closes over your eyes, you enter an inner space and watch the show begin. A curtain is closing down now. Give it no direction at all. Let it happen and just observe the boats of a swirl. Sometimes you may see almost nothing until you find a light. When you do, go to it and discover an opening. This is hypnosis that works spontaneously on its own, without any effort at all.

Things are getting dark now and the inner show is about to begin. All the fantastic things, like a golden tree dissolves as gradually you discover that you gain control of them. When this happens you drift deeply into the inner sanctum of your mind.

Enter a blue light in the blackened space. When it comes and is seen, you will go even deeper. When this has happened, when you see or sense the blue light in space, go deeper, and grip my hand."

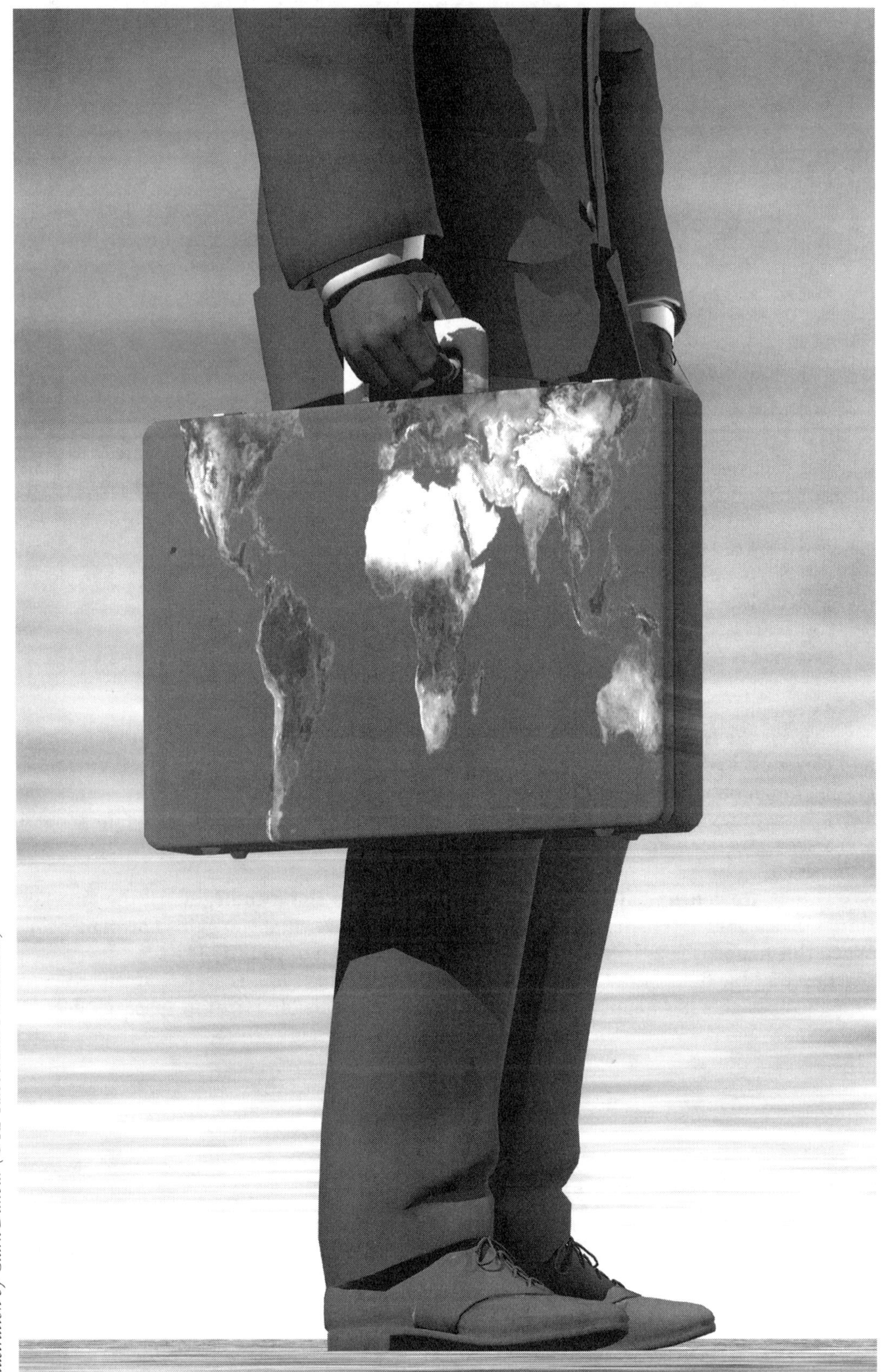

Illustration by Clark Dunbar (© RF RubberBall Productions)

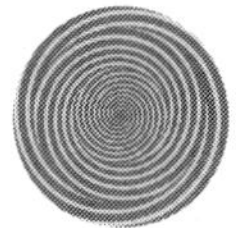

~ *Chapter 97* ~
NLP HYPNOTHERAPY

Includes
William Horton On Strategies

NLP was a name given to an objective way of performing hypnotherapy. The "N" for "Neuro" refers to mental activity, as a functional activity of cellular structure of nervous tissue. The "L" for "Linguistic" refers to communication, including the units, nature, structure and modification of language. And the "P" for "Programming" refers to learning what to do by being instructed. It is like programming a computer for specific responses. In some places the "P" in NLP stands for "Psychology."

NLP lets you determine what is going on inside the client by their outer action. The body speaks a language that tells how the inside dweller prefers to communicate. For example, if the client tends to look upward when talking, it indicates that they are visual minded. Such a client would be best presented hypnotherapeutic suggestions in graphic form.

If a client tends to look from side to side (ear to ear) when communicating it indicates that they are auditory and can be most readily reached through skillful use of language.

If the client tends to look downward (toward the body when communicating, it indicates that they are kinesthetic and are best reached through feelings.

For some hypnotherapists such objective aids are helpful in their work.

With NLP, the hypnotherapist subtly imitates the client's actions to automatically produce rapport. Such must be very subtle, as clients tend to pick up that they are deliberately being imitated and that brings in critical mind and is anything but subjective.

NLP is a methodical way of handling hypnotherapy. It offers "dealing strategies" for tackling problems by relating how to handle them in everyday situations. NLP strategies in designing suggestion formulas is a down-to-earth academic approach to hypnotherapy.

WILLIAM HORTON ON STRATEGIES

Hypnotherapist, and NLP expert, William Horton, PhD wrote an interesting article, "Introduction to NLP Strategies: How You Decide What To Do" that says;

"Every person has their own strategy for everything they do. They will use these strategies when they communicate and you can then use this feedback for more successful suggestions. Persons visual, auditory or kinesthetic strategies when buying a car is easily observed when you listen and map visual cues. Do they: 'SEE' a car they like?' 'HEAR' good things about the car? 'FEEL' how good the car feels when they drive it?

When they ACCEPT the right input they buy the car."

For clients with weight issues Horton asks, "How do you know it's time to eat? And then evaluates their response.

Do they "SEE" food, "SEE" others eating or "SEE" the time on the clock?

Do they "FEEL" that they must eat to "FEEL" good or eat when the "FEEL" bad.

Most overweight people rarely use physical "hunger" as their cue; naturally thin people always do. A naturally thin person will not eat if they are not hungry."

If you like a practical approach with precise patterns to help the client, NLP works fine…if you have the time. It has some rather round-about methods. Who can say what approach is best? That depends on you the hypnotherapist. Do what works best for you.

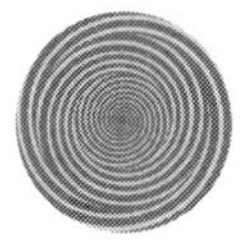

Chapter 98

STOCKWELL-NICHOLAS NLP
(Neuro Linguistic Programming)HYPNOTHERAPY

By Shelley Stockwell-Nicholas, PhD

Includes
MIRRORING & MATCHING
>**Dominant Senses**
>**Eyes Watching**
>**Breath Pacing**
>**Word Pacing**
>**Body Pacing**
>**Body Language**
>**Voice Matching**

MANIPULATING or LEADING
CHUNKING: THE HIERARCHY OF IDEAS
>**Chunking Up**
>**Chunking Down**

ANCHORING: STIMULUS/RESPONSE
SQUISH A CONFLICT
SWISH-SWAP A HABIT OR FEAR
SWISH-SWAP WITH SOUND
SNAP SHOT SWISH-SWAP
INSTALLATION
CIRCLE OF EXCELLENCE

NLP

If you met-a-four, count its legs
Then divide that by blades of grass
Chunk your images, feel your toes
Hear your hair grow in your nose.
Use your words to sway each thought.
It costs $6000 to be taught that…
change takes place in the altered state
as you control, confuse and manipulate.
>—Shelley Stockwell

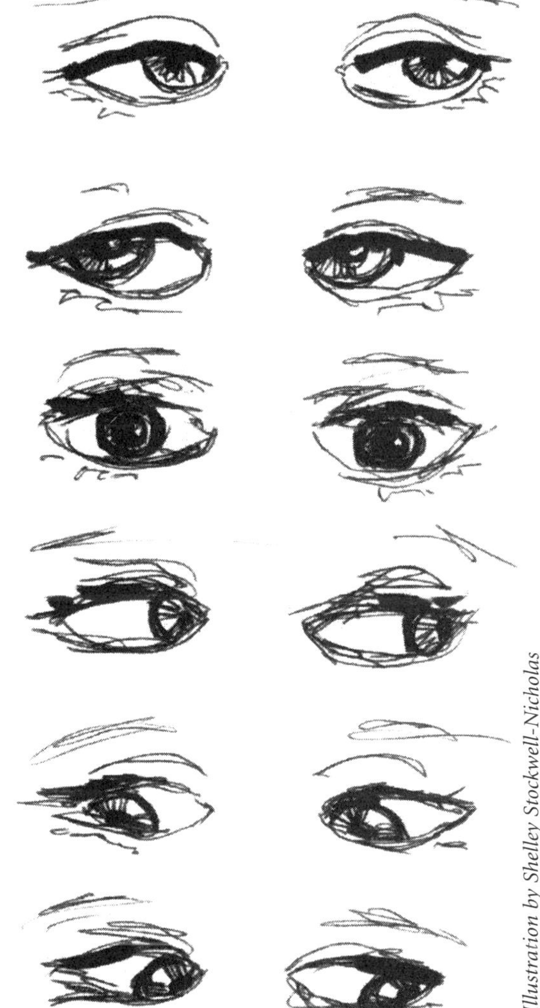

Illustration by Shelley Stockwell-Nicholas

The name NLP was coined by A. Korzybski in 1931. The books of John Grinder and Bandler and Motivational Speaker, Tony Robbins more recently popularized NLP.

NLP is a patterned hypnosis system designed to aid communication, rapport and then mold behavior via mirroring, manipulating, re-framing, "chunking," "squishing" and "anchoring." New ideas are "installed" and the future is reviewed as "future pacing."

Similar to Eriksonian Hypnosis, NLP thrives on vague metaphoric language. The procedure can be a long drawn out one or streamlined to a few minutes. Tidbits of NLP in your Hypnotherapy salad are delicious. NLP re-trains neuro-response to stimuli. Logic and reason usually do not override a compulsive problem behavior as well as reprogramming physical responses does.

MIRRORING of MATCHING

We all naturally imitate those around us. Children model their caregivers, students mirror their teachers, athletes copy the coach and the Beatles meditated as the Maharishi Mahesh Yogi showed them.

We all learn as the big people instruct us: "do what I do." In all hypnosis, the subconscious enjoys following along with a skilled hypnotist.

NLP imitates, matches, mirrors and synchronizes as you mimic eye movements, body language, breathing and speech style (voice tone, pacing, volume and phrases).

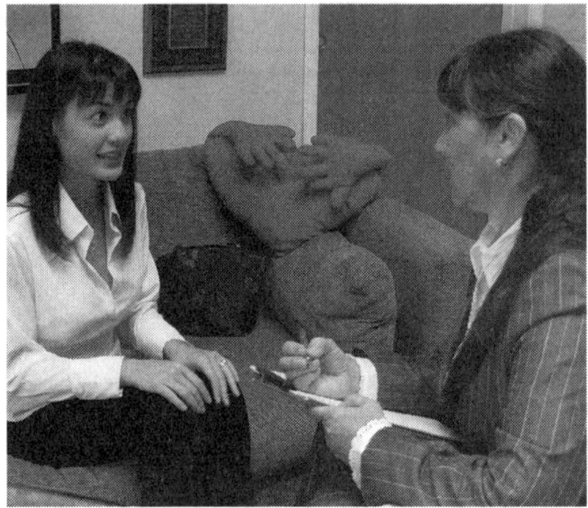

Let's reflect on mirroring.

Photo by Jon Nicholas

Dominant Senses

NLP originally assumed that each of us are dominantly visual, auditory (sound), kinesthetic (touch). Visual, auditory and kinesthetic in NLP language is "V-A-K". Recently "olfactory/gustatory" and "self talk" were added to the NLP list. I add "beyond the senses."

Check in with your client and note their dominant senses. Their words or phrases will tell you…if you "see" what I mean. When you play to your client's dominant senses, you speak to them where they live.

Eyes Watching

Eye movements indicate a person's sensory processes. The direction someone looks and the clarity of their eyes tell you if they are:

1. Organizing incoming sensations and information
2. Recalling the past
3. Imagining or construction something not previously experienced
4. If they are dominantly visual, auditory or kinesthetic

An eye movement might be a flicker or held for several minutes. The way a person moves their eyes is called "accessing cues." NLP practitioners study eye movements and say that you change your mind by changing your eye movement patterns.

If someone is "making something up" or untruthful, their eyes will generally go up and to their right (your left if you are facing them). But you'll need to know if the person is left handed to really be sure because left handed people look up and left when fibbing.

HER RIGHT

HER LEFT

VISUAL (UP)

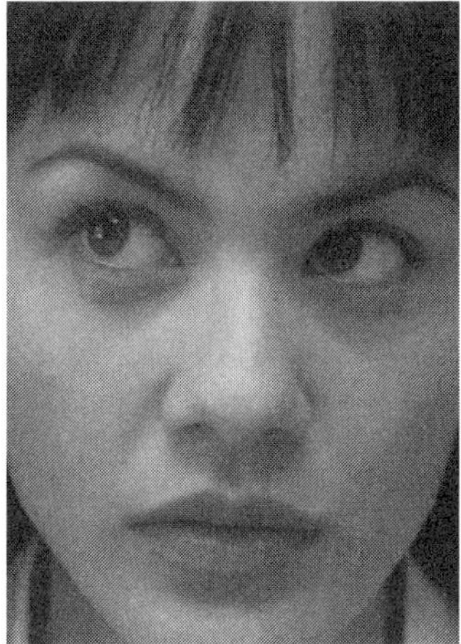

VISUAL CONSTRUCT
Visualizing Something New, Lying

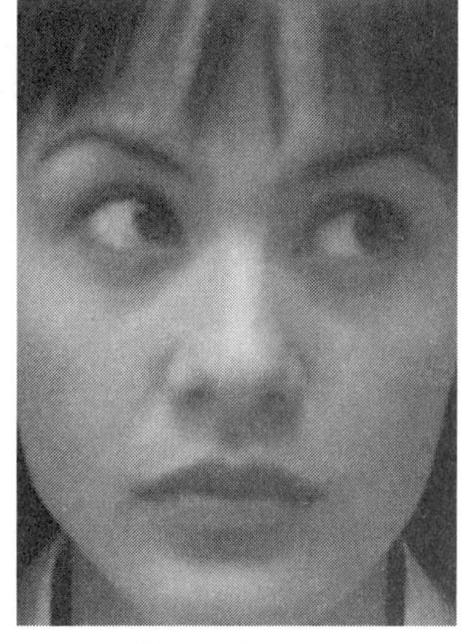

VISUAL MEMORY
Recalling Something Seen

AUDITORY (STRAIGHT)

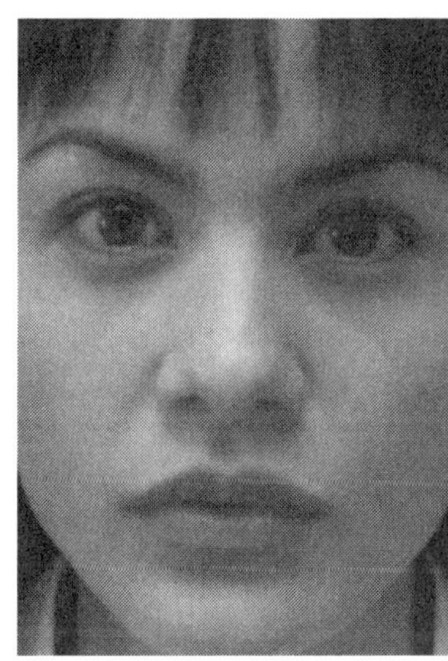

AUDITORY CONSTRUCT
Imagining Sounds

STARING DILATED
Trance

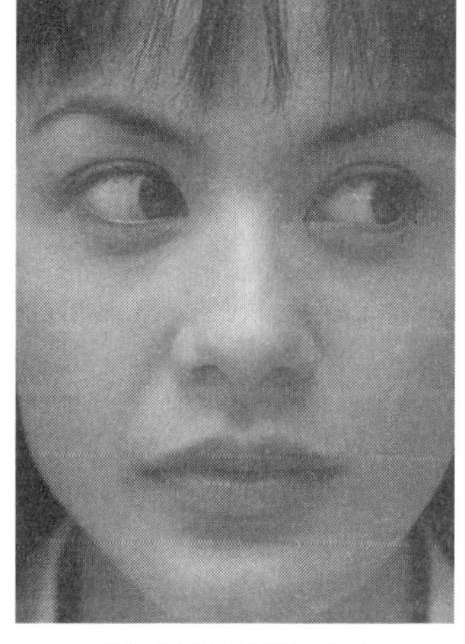

AUDITORY MEMORY
Recalling Sounds

KINESTHETIC (DOWN)

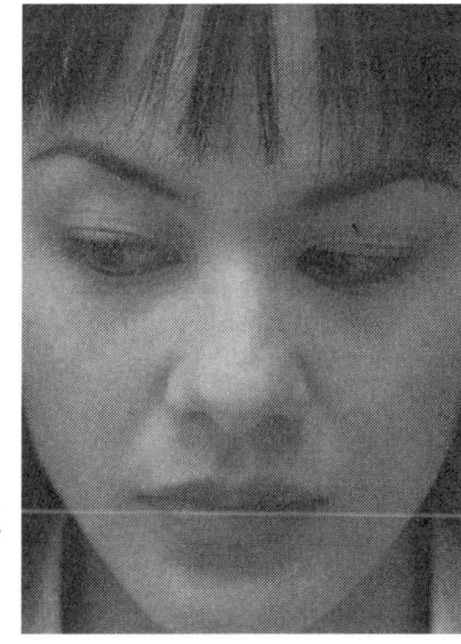

KINESTHETIC CONSTRUCT
Talking and Listening to Yourself

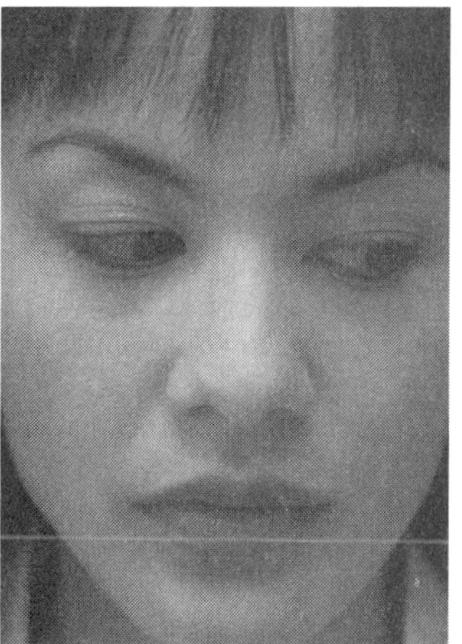

KINESTHETIC
Sensing How the Body Feels

Photos by Jon Nicholas

Breath Pacing

Feel the rhythm! Your breath is an unconscious indicator of your mental state. NLP teaches you to breathe in sync with the client to establish rapport. Babies learn to breathe with mom. Lovers often breathe at the exact pace. Mediators may feel that they are literally breathing the same breath with others.

NLP teaches you to breathe in and out when your client does. You can practice this skill with your family or in the grocery line and you'll be more popular!

Word Pacing

Use your client's words and phrases and report what they know as facts. This puts you in harmony with them. Then, when you add a new idea, it is more readily accepted as a logical progression of truth.

Here is an example of word pacing, **"You are sitting in a chair with your hands at your side and as you said, 'you are learning to relax.'"** Now, lead them into new thoughts.

"As you sit in this chair with your hands at your side and say to me, 'I am learning to relax'" (Word pacing.)

…you notice how your eyes grow heavy and you want to close them down.'" (Leading.)

Body Language

Subtly imitate your client's posture and gestures. Tilt your head the way they do, match their body position. When you repeat back a phrase use their same accompanying gesture. You'll be amazed how this comforts your client.

Voice Matching

In the conversation imitate or match the client's voice tone, rhythm, rate (fast or slow), volume (loud or soft) and pitch (high or low). Use their exact language and phrases.

MANIPULATING or LEADING

NLP now moves to "influence" the client into a more relaxed state. This is done by subtly shifting the rhythms and patterns you've been imitating. Model a more relaxed posture and the client will follow suit. Slow down your breathing and your client will too. If you close your eyes so will they. (You can open your eyes to see if it is so.)

If you speak in a higher or lower voice tone or increase the speed of your speech and they follow, you have succeeded!

The simplest leading is with a physical gesture. Once you are in sync, sit back and they will, too. Reach for a glass of water and so will they. The subject is now ready to take on your non-verbal and verbal suggestions and come around to your helpful way of thinking.

CHUNKING: THE HIERARCHY OF IDEAS
A problem is a common noun
Chunk 'em up and chunk 'em down
Neuter gender solves the case
to laugh in problem's funny face
                    —Shelley Stockwell

NLP chunking moves the mind to grasp the biggest and smallest picture. Big pictures are like using a wide-angle lens and is called "chunking up."

Zooming in spotlights the little pictures and is called "chunking down." You can also chunk sideways which mean that you recall related categories that are on the same level.

MODUS OPERANDI: CHUNKING UP (Divergent Thinking)
Abstracting an idea or moving into the BIG picture is used to override inner conflict.

You can ask your client sweeping questions like "what do you really want in your life?" "Of all people living and dead, who do you hold as your ideal person?" and "What message or lesson can you take from them and apply to you?"

This chunking up exercise can be done either in or out of trance:
"Think of a problem that bothers you. Good.
Now answer these questions with the first thing that comes to your mind:
1. What purpose does this problem have?
2. What is your positive intention here?
3. What's the greater purpose?
4. What is the higher function here?
If you have that _______ (higher function), what does that give you that is greater?"

MODUS OPERANDI: CHUNKING DOWN (Convergent Thinking)
Abstracting an idea or moving into minute detail is also used to override inner conflict. This can be done either in or out of trance.
"Think of a problem that bothers you. Good.
Now answer these questions with the first thing that comes to your mind:
1. What specifically do you mean?"
2. According to whom?
3. Why do you say that?
4. What do you mean by that?"

ANCHORING: STIMULUS/RESPONSE
Do you salivate when you smell cinnamon rolls?

Remember how Pavlov's dog was conditioned to salivate when he heard a bell? He anchored the stimuli of the bell and the response of the saliva together.

You can anchor positive feeling in your hypnosis session using this principle.

Let's say that your client expresses a positive emotional "state" like laughing. Touch their wrist and laugh with them and then quickly release the touch. You have "set" an anchor. Joy and a touch on the wrist, are now linked. Later in the session you can "fire off" the anchor by touching their wrist and saying, **"You now happily accomplish your goal."**

You can also anchor in negative feelings in a form of aversion therapy. **"Every time you see a candy bar you think this vile, gross, disgusting thing. This vile, gross, disgusting thing and the candy bar are all mixed up in your head."**

In trance you can suggest a waking trigger like, **"It is safe in your world. There is always a bubble of protection that surrounds you. To remind yourself, all you need to do is to touch your thumb to your forefinger and that invisible protective energy will encapsulate you completely."**

Other anchors:
When you see a color, see a T.V., turn on a light, brush your teeth, flush the toilet, walk into a classroom, enter a market, open the refrigerator, ride your bike, or take a bath.

MODUS OPERANDI: SQUISH A CONFLICT

The Squish Technique helps an unresolved conflict or something the client wants to change. Have your client put both of their hands out in front of them. Each hand represents one side of the conflict (or the behavior they want to change). For example: "I don't want to go to school" vs. "I want to go to school." "I always want dessert" vs. "I don't want any dessert." Here's how it's done:

1. HANDS IN FRONT "Put your hands out in front of you, palms facing upward. Choose one hand to represent the part of you that holds the attitude of _____________ (state the behavior or attitude on one side of the coin or the positive change you want to make). Which hand is it? Very good."

2. SIDE ONE SPEAKS "Now, in your mind's eye, imagine this point of view there on your hand looking the way it looks, sounding the way it speaks, feeling the way it feels, smelling, tasting and being this attitude and viewpoint. What is its point of view? What would it like to say to you? Just report what comes to mind and don't concern yourself if it makes sense or not.
(Pause) **Good.**
What gift does this viewpoint bring you?
What is its positive value? (Active listen their responses and dialogue until you feel they have said what needs to be said).
Good. Now if there are any emotions or ideas that you need to let go of now, do it. Good."

3. SIDE TWO SPEAKS "Turn your attention to your other hand and place your other point of view (or the part that doesn't want to change) **there. Let it look the way it looks, sound the way it speaks, feel the way it feels, smell, taste, intuit and be this attitude and viewpoint. What would it like to communicate to you? Report what comes to mind and don't concern yourself if it makes sense or not.**
(Pause.)
Good. What gift does this viewpoint bring you? How does it benefit you? (Active listen their responses.)
If there are any thoughts or ideas that you need to let go of now, do it. Good."

4. UNDERSTANDING EACH OTHER "Look straight ahead so that you can easily see both hands stretched there before you. Good. And let your two palms face each other. I am speaking to each hand, do you understand what the other hand had to say. (Pause for a response.)
Each is starting to understand each other better. Now, one at a time, let each tell us what they notice and appreciate about the other. Or, what gift their job brings that could offer a positive solution." (Pause.)

5. SQUISH INTO-GREAT-NESS "You've listened well to both parts of yourself and now it is time for them to integrate what is most useful to you. Watch, listen, feel, smell, taste, and intuit them as they now come together and blend what is useful and important to both parts, so they learn from each other. Let them come together. Good. They now work as a team. Take a moment and enjoy this new more productive attitude."

6. MENTAL REHEARSAL (NLPers call this future pacing.) "Imagine yourself sometime in the future in a situation where these new positive qualities will assist you to feel great. Excellent."

MODUS OPERANDI: SWISH-SWAP WAKING SUGGESTION

This simple rapid behavior modification technique changes limiting habits, and eliminate upset and fear. It allows your client to disassociate from negative feelings and responses and re-associate them into good feelings and responses. You don't even need a formal trance state to do a simple Swish-Swap; a simple waking suggestion works perfectly.

1. "Think of the most beautiful being that you can imagine. It can be a beautiful human or animal friend, a religious figure, a place in nature or a peace of art. Whatever you find most beautiful. Good.

2. Now in a moment you will think about the thing that has been disturbing you and when it comes to mind you will instantly hear your mind say 'SWISH' and the image will change to that beautiful thought, that beautiful being. And that is how it will be always from this point forward. Let's try it…"

MODUS OPERANDI: SWISH-SWAP WITH SOUND

Sound dominant people like this simple process that eliminates fear or upset. Hypnotize your client and suggest:

"Think of sounds that are very pleasant to you. Enjoy them thoroughly. How good you feel as you enjoy these sounds with your inner ear. You can turn them on or turn up or down the volume as you choose. Notice the 'you' that hears such fine and rewarding sounds and imagine that you can create these sounds any time you like.

Now think of sounds you associate with your upsetting experience (or fear). Turn the sound down as you hear now.

Far away the good sounds are coming to you. You hear them as they come closer and closer. Soon you can only hear the good sounds. The other sounds are gone.

In the future (Future pacing.) if you ever hear those old unpleasant sounds you immediately turn them off and you hear the pleasant sounds fill your whole body and mind.

MODUS OPERANDI: SNAPSHOT SWISH-SWAP

Visually dominant folks like this one!

"Close your eyes and in your mind's eye, visualize a photo the represents to you the moment in time where you act the way you no longer want to act (smoking, over-eating etc). Put that picture on one of your hands. Good.

Now, visualize and imagine a second photo of yourself reacting the way you'd rather react instead. (Breathing fresh air, drinking a glass of water, etc.) Put that picture on the other hand. Good.

Look at the first picture in your _____ hand. (The one with the negative behavior.) **and imagine it melting away until it disappears. Let me know when it is gone. Good.**

Look at the other picture in your _____ hand (The one the results you want.) **and imagine the photo getting so big and the colors so radiant, that you step right into the picture. Feeling just marvelous. Let me know when it is so. Good."**

Repeat step 3 and 4 several times, each time faster and faster five to eight times. Finally, **"take a deep breath and relax, feeling terrific."**

MODUS OPERANDI: INSTALLATION

If you want to exchange a limiting belief for a positive belief it is easy to do:

For example" "I can't say no to chocolate" is exchanged for "I could care less about chocolate."

1. Yes Identity

"Let's start with something you know to be true like 'I am a human,' 'I am on the earth,' '1 plus 1 equals 2'. Good. Now decide where this true belief is 'located' in space and through which senses you perceive it."

2. Dubious/Uncertain Identity

"Mention something you aren't sure is true like 'the president is eating right now,' 'I live on Mars,' '1 plus 1 equals 3' and then decide where this dubious belief is "located" in space and through which senses you perceive it."

3. Limiting Belief

Next, have them state their limiting belief and then decide where this dubious belief is "located" in space and through which senses they perceive it. They might say, "I can't resist chocolate is up to the left."

4. Empowering Preferred Belief

Have them state their empowering belief that they would like to embrace as the new truth. And then decide where this preferred belief is "located" in space and through which senses they perceive it. They might say, "I don't like chocolate in the middle and up."

5. Release the Limiting Belief

"Imagine the limiting belief now moving toward the horizon and getting smaller and smaller and then snap it into the place where dubious ideas are located for them. Now, permanently glue it into place so it can never be removed. Snap goodbye."

6. Install Empowering Preferred Belief

"Imagine the empowering idea (that you want to install) **and move it toward the horizon. At the count of three, snap it into the certainty space. One, Two, Three, Snap Hello! Welcome you are now where you belong. Secure in the truth that it is now your reality."**

7. Future Pace

"Anytime from this moment forward when you think about this subject, you are certain that this belief is true and positively right for you."

MODUS OPERANDI: CIRCLE OF EXCELLENCE
Thanks to William Horton, PhD, for this idea

This simple powerful way takes you beyond limits into success. Try it, you'll like it! Allow time for your client to embrace each suggestion. Begin by having your client stand with their eyes closed and instruct them to:

"Imagine a circle on the floor in front of you about a foot from where you stand. In the circle are all the feelings and thoughts that you associate with excellence. You might think of a time when you were pleased with your own excellence…a big or small moment when you were filled with confidence and self-satisfaction…a time of great pride inside yourself. When you think of special a moment of personal excellence let me know with a nod of your head…very good.

Be there 100% and notice what it is like for you to be in your excellence. Notice how you breathe, what you say to yourself. Notice how you feel in your arms, your chest, your heart and your stomach. Give your excellence a color, a sound. Notice the energy of excellence and put that into the circle.

In a moment, but not just yet, you will want to step forward into this circle of excellence and when you do you will notice wonderful changes inside yourself as you become one with excellence.

All right now at the count of three; one, two, three…take a step forward. Excellent.

You are completely infused with excellence you can feel, see, hear, taste, smell and intuit it. Imagine now a perfect song for this powerful feeling; your own personal theme of excellence, strength and energy…good. And now a gesture that symbolizes for you your power.

In the future, whenever you use that gesture, you'll immediately enter into this circle and know that you are completely excellent from head to toe; mentally, physically, spiritually and emotionally.

All right, take a deep breath and return to the room, eyes open and feeling great."

Reinforce the suggestion this way:

"Close your eyes again, imagine the circle on the floor, step into it and automatically you will think of your theme and do your gesture and all those wonderful feelings will fill you from top to bottom…very good. In the future you will use this wonderful technique and every time you do it, you will feel even more elated in excellence. Ok open your eyes again.

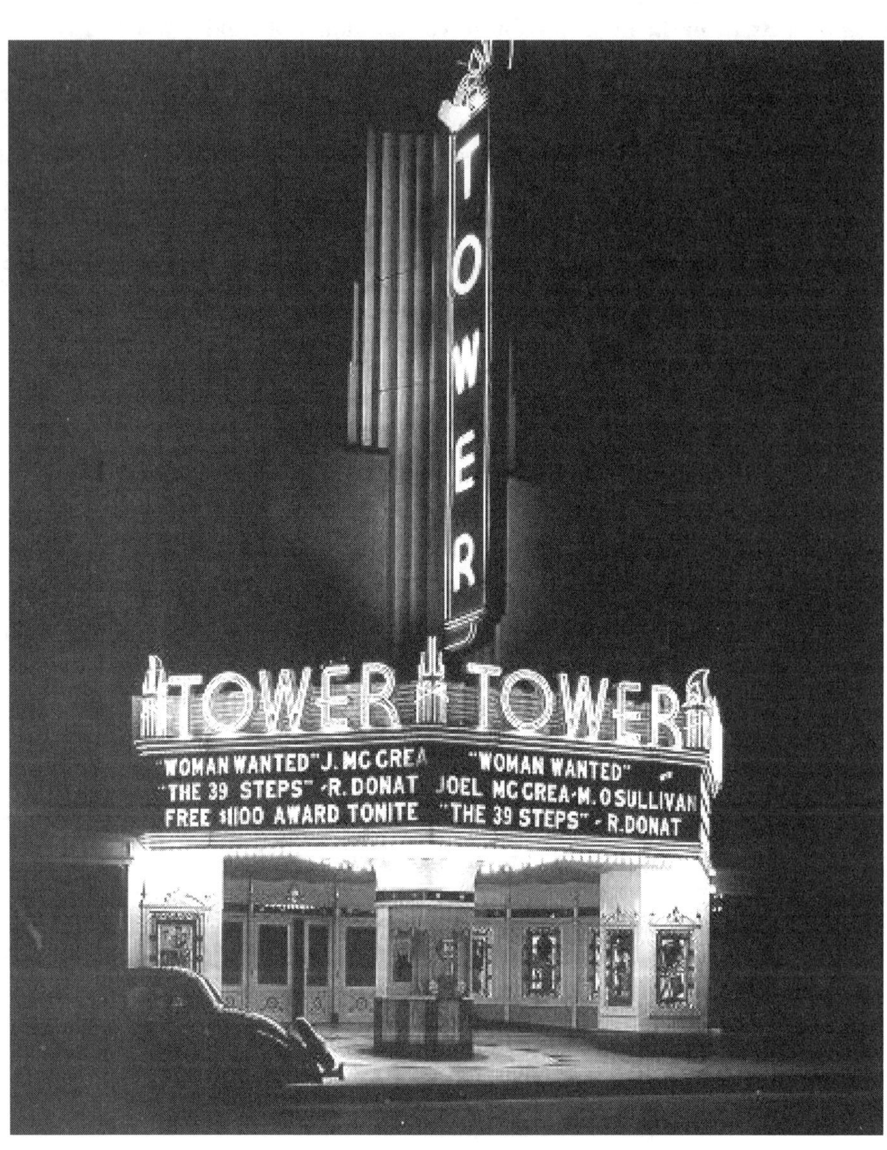

TOWER
TOWER
TOWER
TOWER
"WOMAN WANTED" J. MC CREA
"THE 39 STEPS" ·R. DONAT
FREE $1100 AWARD TONITE
"WOMAN WANTED"
JOEL MC CREA·M. O'SULLIVAN
"THE 39 STEPS" - R. DONAT

Photo by Jon Nicholas

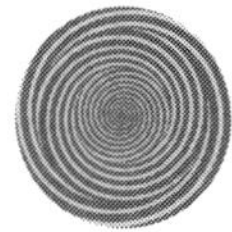

~ *Chapter 99* ~
NLP MOVIE THEATER TECHNIQUES

Includes
Dr. Stockwell-Nicholas Instant-Change Movie
Dr. Neves' Phobia Release Theater
Cartoon Movie That Mends

NLP MOVIE THEATER TECHNIQUES

NLPers use a lot of movie theater imagery. This disassociates or detaches the client from the stories they tell themselves and works well for dominantly visual people. The movie analogy can be swapped for reading about yourself in a book or listening to a song that tells the positive story.

MODUS OPERANDI: DR. STOCKWELL-NICHOLAS INSTANT CHANGE MOVIE

"Diminishing your fear and finding your courage is an adventure in self esteem. The only thing you have to lose is the heavy yoke that fear imposes."
> —Captain T.W. Cummings,
> Author of Help for the Fearful Flyer

How rapidly your brain learns!

Most phobias and compulsions are imprinted in a single, dangerous (or seemingly dangerous) experience. They can be unlearned as rapidly. An imprinted pattern is often eliminated in one re-learning experience.

Phobias usually begin with a traumatic event that brings up vivid internal images, sounds or statements within us. These are sometimes exaggerated or distorted by imagination. At this time a trigger is created. Usually a trigger is a fragment of the original trauma or thought to be part of the original stimulus. We often don't consciously remember the trauma or the trigger.

Use this exercise to instantly change limiting behavior. Here's how:

1. Pretend:
"Assume that you are sitting in a seat in a movie theater with your eyes open or closed. Look at a black-and-white picture of YOU projected on the screen."

2. Projection Room:
"Take a deep breath. Imagine yourself in the projection booth. At the same time continue to sit in your seat in the theater observing the picture on the screen. You are safe. You are in charge of the projection."

3. Re-View:
"Run a short clip of yourself just before the trauma or phobic or compulsive reaction. Watch the whole event, from beginning to end…then, a little bit farther, until things are OK again. If you have any emotional response that takes you from your chair or the projection booth, simply un-focus the picture a bit or stop and start the film again."

4. Happy To Be Me:
"Project a photo of yourself feeling great on the screen."

5. Repeat Until Complete:
Repeat numbers 3 and 4 until they really do feel great.

MODUS OPERANDI: DR. NEVES' PHOBIA THEATER

Richard Neves, PhD, teaches this very effective phobia intervention to clear any instantaneous or spontaneous fear that results from a specific stimulus: insects, heights, birds, snakes, water, needles, elevators… You can also use it for many problems that are not generally thought of as phobias, like traumatic responses to past/post traumatic stress like accidents, abuse, illness and drug flashbacks.

Start by finding out what fear or issue they want to release. You may ask, "What do you want?" and "How will you know when you get it?" You could even let them begin with what Dr. Neves calls *end result imagining* by suggesting "Imagine yourself the way you want to be in the future."

Each step of the process is orchestrated to almost rewire and defuse emotional upset. The device of eyes opening is a separator state. The eyes are left open. As you run the movie forward your eyes are closed. Only run it forward once. Eyes open. Show them a picture. You can actually draw a picture of the process.

1. **Focus on Fear** (Eyes closed.)
    Select an unpleasant memory, fear or trauma to neutralize. During the process, pay close attention to the watch for "Biological Manifestation of an Internal Response" or what NLP calls "BMIRs." When you see a BMIR, shift the pattern to snap them out of it. Have them open their eyes or stand up and look up. It will instantly bring them back to a peaceful state. Then say:

    "Tell me a little about your issue." Get specifics during the interview about the issue. You could say: **"If you were imagining this happening now what is the problem?"**

    "In this simple process you will follow my instructions. This is going to be easy and quick. You don't have to do too much. You will just do certain things in your head. OK, lets begin."

2. **Comfort Zones** (Eyes closed.)
    You now move them to two "comfort zones" one before the incident and then to one after the incident:

    Prior to the response
    "Close your eyes and imagine that you are sitting in a movie theater and see yourself in a black and white still picture…not a moving picture…on the left side of the screen. The picture is of you any time *before* you ever had this fearful response (fear or issue). **As you look up and to the left, you are comfortable and relaxed. Good."**

After the response

"Now look up and to the right and see on the right side of the screen, another black-and-white still picture of you taken just *after* this fearful response (the fear or issue). **Good. Now open your eyes. So now that you are comfortable and relaxed looking up to the right and comfortable on the left."**

3. Detachment
    "Alright, close your eyes again and imagine yourself sitting in theater, looking up and to the left, seeing that black and white picture. Now, let's just pretend that you could leave your body and rise up above and float out and stand at the back of the theater. So, there you are standing in the back of the theater seeing yourself looking at the black and white picture up to the left. From behind your body, you watch yourself, watching yourself on the movie screen with the picture up and to the left before the incident or to the right, after the incident."

    Or

    "Imagine now that you are the projectionist who can control the picture's speed and clarity upon the screen. See yourself, seeing yourself watching the photo up on the screen."

4. Quick Trauma Review
    "In a moment, I'm going to ask you to throw a switch and the black-and-white picture on the left is going to change to a black-and-white movie until you see the picture on the right. You understand. Good. It will happen very quickly; boom, boom, boom, boom…very quickly, all the way through. It's going to run through real fast. Good. When you have gotten all the way to the picture on the right."

5. Quick-Time Trauma Run
    "Ok, still looking at yourself looking at yourself looking at the still picture on the left, let it become a black-and-white movie that shows you in _____ (the experience that you have selected to neutralize). **Run this part very quickly. Excellent. Ok, throw the switch… go! Run the movie very quickly."**

    Or

    You could count from 1-5 so that they run it quickly. Say, **"As I count from one to five you run it very quickly through to the picture on the right and will stop the movie. Ok Very quickly run the movie 1, 2, 3, 4, 5 stop the movie. Stop. Are you all the way to the picture on the right? Excellent. Stop the movie."**

6. Reverse It Out
    "Now run down and jump into your body and go up to the screen and stand in front of the picture on the right. Looking up at the screen. Imagine that you can jump into the screen and it will run the movie backwards with all the colors and sounds and feelings.

    Good, now jump into the picture and turn it into full color and run the picture backwards, in full color, with all the sounds and feelings. Do this very rapidly. It will be like seeing a movie backwards, with you inside it, as if time has reversed direction."
    You could reverse your count and count from 5 to 1.

7. **Test**
   "Think of _________ (the event or memory) **and notice if you think about it more comfortably. If so! You are done. Very good!"**
   (If not, have them do it two or three more times.)

8. **Future Pace**
   Take them into an hypnotic state and instruct, **"See yourself now doing _______** (What they want to do) **now and in the future."** Be sure to watch for physical confirmation of their positive change.

MODUS OPERANDI: CARTOON MOVIE THAT MENDS

1. **Baseline**
   "Imagine me and you in the front row seeing a film of what you did yesterday on the screen. Good.

2. **View The Problem**
   "Now pretend that we are watching a black and white movie taken when you felt safe before your problem happened to you…the problem you came here to release."

3. **Detach and Rewind**
   "Now float out of your body up to the projection booth high up at the back of the theater and see me and you watching this black and white movie. Put on the movie of just before the upset and then the upset and when the film gets to the end, freeze frame it and press the rewind control and very quickly see the film going backwards until it gets back to the pleasant beginning.

4. **Cartoon**
   "Now edit the film making changes along the way, and turning any figures you like into cartoons. You can shrink them to the size of little ants and dress them any way you please. Then run this movie back from the end to the beginning. Do this several times."

5. **Movie Star**
   "Now move back into your body and step on to a film set as the lead actor in a fabulous color version of this cartoon running backwards. You do everything backwards, and the movie is a bit like Charlie Chaplin jumping around. Do this a few times."

6. **Direct Success**
   "Now be the film director as well as the lead actor and remake the scene as though everything happened exactly as you would want it to be done ....everything is perfect...and run a film forward in real time as you notice how calm and confidence you feel as you reorient yourself and watch this terrific movie."

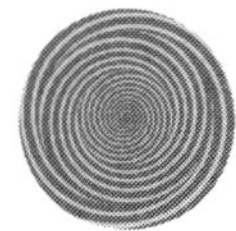

~ *Chapter 100* ~
HYPNOTIC DREAM WORK

"We often get a more accurate picture of the significant changes in the client's life from the subconscious symbols he molds and recreates in dreams than from what he consciously elects to express."
　　　　　—Rollo May, Psychologist

Includes
Stockwell's Hypnotic Gestalt Dreamwork
Stockwell's Shamanic Hypno-Dreaming

Dream work has been used since the beginning of recorded history and most likely way before that. Shamanic teachers and healers are the earliest known dream workers and obtained knowledge from the guiding spirits who appeared in dreams. They strongly believed in the power and knowledge of the dreamtime. In our more sophisticated modern Hypnotic Dream work, the client is lead into an inner communication with his or her psyche where their inner guidance uproots limiting personal depreciation of misconceptions.

Hypnotic Dream work is an artful blend of dreams and hypnotherapy. Dreams provide expression for the subconscious. Trust the inner guidance of the dreamer. They offer important "in-formation" and suggestions.

MODUS OPERANDI: STOCKWELL'S HYPNOTIC GESTALT DREAMWORK

In Hypnotic Gestalt Dream work, every person or an object, is considered a projected part of the dreamer. Skillful Gestalt dialogues between dream characters consistently reveal themselves to be parts, viewpoints or sub-personalities regarding significant issues. The process leads to insights from each energy or strength of each character that can be positively integrated to empower the dreamer. Weaving of hypnotic deepening, suggestion and other hypnotic techniques into the dream further grounds and integrates insights derived from Gestalt methods.

Shelley Stockwell, in her book *Denial is Not A River In Egypt*, says **"Imagine yourself as each character in your dream and retell the dream from each viewpoint. Then have each character converse with each other. This re-frames or puts a new frame around uncomfortable images and underscores and celebrates positive ones."**

Let's say you dreamt, *'Two people are riding on horses. One looks good from the outside but is really in bad shape. My horse is sick and tired and can't go any further. He is dying. I realize I am dying.'*

1. **MAGNIFY YOUR DREAM**
    Instruct the client to, "Look more closely at the dream. What is it trying to tell you?" In the case of the above horse dream ask, "Is this dream about two horses or is it talking to you about something else?"

2. **BECOME THE ELEMENTS OR CHARACTERS IN THE DREAM**
    "Speak from the voice of each part of the dream." In the example "Speak from the voice of the horse, and then the voice of each of the two people. Tell the dream from each of their viewpoints."
    "Have each element talk to the other characters."

3. **ASK**
    "Ask yourself; "What do these images tell me about my feelings. In this horse dream, do you feel sick and tired on the inside, as if you want to quit?"

4. **PLAY IT AGAIN, FRITZ**
    "Make a new script that creates the story the way that you want it to be." In this case, "Bring your horse to a gorgeous brook, let him rest, brush his coat and feed him a fresh apple. If you do, both you and your horse will be revitalized."

STOCKWELL'S SHAMANIC HYPNO-DREAMING

Here's what Stockwell says about The Shamanic approach:

"Some societies believe that your waking state is the dream and your sleeping state is reality. Aborigines travel the dreamtime and heal. Patricia Garfield studied the Senois society in her book *Creative Dreaming*.

The Senois are happy, peaceful, well adjusted and thought to be "too magic to fight" by their aggressive neighbors. The key to Senois "magic" is their deep respect for the dream state. A Senois is taught from birth to manipulate their dreams into a positive outcome. The positive goal of Senois dreaming is to fly, receive gifts, or have sex to orgasm. In pursuit of these goals, there are no taboos.

Dreaming in western civilization is often a nightmare, repeated. Let's say you are being pursued by a big, nasty, ugly brown bear to the edge of a cliff. You fall off the precipice, and awaken in a cold sweat. Fear never gets a resolve. Learn to reconnect with your dream world and reframe old pain.

A Senois child with the same big nasty brown bear chasing him to the edge of a cliff tells his family the story. His aunt says, "That was a wonderful dream, but you should not have awakened. The next time you have such a dream, make sure you hit the ground. And if you die, be sure to ask the bear for a present. Or you could turn around and fight the bear. And if you kill the bear, be sure to ask for a present. The next time you have the dream, everyone wants to hear about it." That day is spent celebrating your *gift*. Songs are sung, dances are danced, and paintings are painted; all to celebrate your dream.

Embrace these same goals. Each night, fly anywhere and any way you want. Have sex with any recipient you want, any place, and any time. There are no taboos when you're deep in sleep. If dreams frighten you, the trick is to not wake up but to take the dream to its completion and then, ask for a present. Before you go to sleep, request beautiful, restful slumber, flying, sex to orgasm, and to remember your dream. Ah. Zzzzzz."

Hypno-Helper

"Hypnosis Dream Interpretation Series" by Liz Fortini
"Become The Dream" by Randal Churchill
"Creative Dreaming" by Patricia Garfield
"Denial Is Not A River In Egypt" by Shelley Stockwell

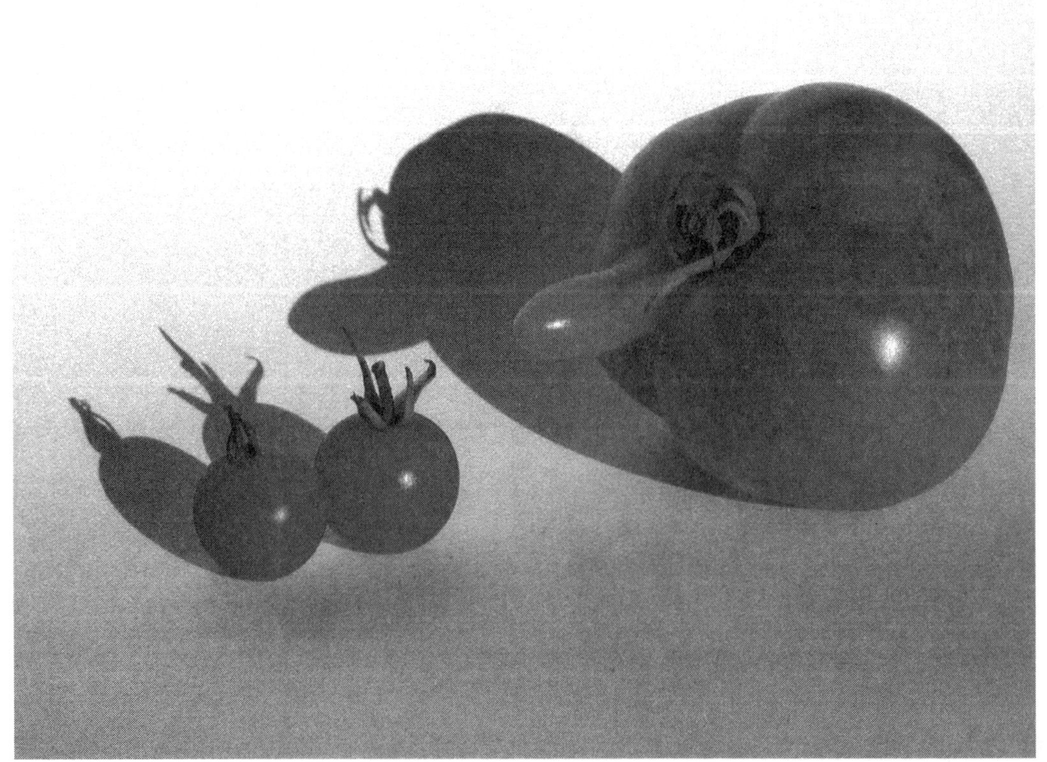

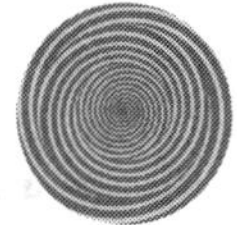

~ *Chapter 101* ~
HYPNOTHERAPY OF IMAGINATION

Our future may well depend upon the constructive use of imagination

Imagination is the KEY to unlocking the advancement of hypnotherapy and all progress humans create in the 21st century. Give your clients the gift of imagination. You bring in the Serenity Resonance Sound as a gentle background as you tell of imagination and present these suggestions to your client in profound hypnosis

MODUS OPERANDI: HYPNOTHERAPY OF IMAGINATION
You Will Need:
The Serenity Resonance Sound

Induce somnambulism in your client and present these suggestions directly into the subconscious to become reality for knowing and behavior.

"As you are told of the power of imagination, you will drop deeper and deeper into hypnosis. As you learn of power of imagination every difficulty you have ever imagined will vanish like water on a hot tin roof.

Come to know the power of imagination for it is like magic. In countless ways you can use it to benefit your life.

Using the power of imagination is the way to learn and do it to make it so…Listen, listen, listen."
Bring in the Serenity Resonance Sound as a gentle background.

"Imagination is the creative function of your mind. Everything you KNOW within yourself and outside your self originates in imagination. Everything GOOD comes via imagination. But equally everything UN-GOOD comes via imagination too. Imagination is a two edged sword that must be wielded with discrimination. Come to know this that you will always use your imagination to create what is good."
Bring in the Serenity Resonance Sound up a bit then let it fade again into the background.

"Recognize that what you are in this space and time begins with imagination. Feel the power…"
Pause

"Imagine you are walking alone in a desert with the blazing sun beating down on you. It is HOT, HOT, HOT. Imagine this scene in your mind so powerfully that you feel the heat! That is the way imagination operates. It becomes so real that it is transformed into your reality. That is what imagination hypnotherapy is all about. It is the great power within

yourself to make yourself what you wish to be. Now take a gentle breath and let your temperature be perfectly comfortable.

Whatever you wish to improve your life, imagination can produce that improvement. Through your learning of this truth in your subconscious phase of mind, while you are in hypnosis now, increases the power of your imagination by leaps and bounds."

Pause

"Imagine the improvement. Then you experience the improvement. And finally the improvement becomes your reality."

Pause

"This is the gift of hypnotherapy to you. The hypnotherapy of imagination is yours to use henceforth for the benefit of yourself in every way. The power will increase continuously with every breath you take. You will come to know and feel this truth deep inside yourself."

Pause

"Accept this gift. When you know that this gift has been accepted, nod your head (ideomotor response). Take your time. There is no hurry. Let this truth set in deeply."

Pause and wait until the client nods, then proceed with arousal from the hypnosis and turn off the Serenity Resonance Sound.

"One, two, three, four, five. You are fully aroused. You are fully alert. You feel wonderful and fine awakening with an inner realization of the amazing transformation that has occurred within yourself."

Pause

"You have become master of your imagination and you will always use it to create that which is good!"

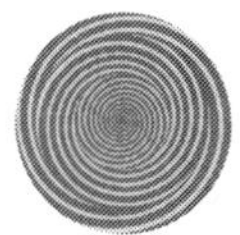

~ *Chapter 102* ~
ALADDIN'S ARABIAN
HYPNOTHERAPY

"Shaharazad's stories, still told today, are the center of miracles; the sole, unparalleled."
—W.E. Henley

Includes
Make a Wish Hypnotherapy

An Encyclopedia of Hypnotherapy would not be complete without mentioning the oldest, and possibly the most important, hypnotherapy textbook in the world THE ARABIAN NIGHTS. It first presented itself during the reign of Sultan Haroun-al-Raschid in Baghdad somewhere around 786-808 A.D.

The stories are actually case histories told in symbolic form. The Sultan is the hypnotherapist who may cut off the head of unwanted ideas. Cutting off the head symbolizes removing (going beyond) critical mind, releasing the GENIE. The lamp is the process of hypnosis and the magic power of the GENIE is, of course, the powers of the subconscious mind.

Illustration by ?????

Sultan = hypnotherapist
Head = critical mind
Genie = subconscious mind

This most overlooked form of hypnotherapy seemingly disappeared much like Poe's "Purloined Letter." All searched in every nook and cranny for that missing letter, only to discover it in plain sight upon the table all the time. It had been overlooked. It was temporarily invisible to perception.

The "Arabian Nights" contains the story of *Aladdin & The Magic Lamp*, in which the young hero finds a Magic Lamp that, when rubbed, produces a GENIE. The wonderful GENIE grants him his fondest wish. "But be careful, for once the wish is used up, there would be no more." What should Aladdin wish for?

It dawned on me, like a flash of lightening, what hidden truth hypnotherapy this story held? What is your fervent wish that you would like granted? Is it love, money, health, success? What is your heart's greatest desire? The Magic Lamp is your means to achieve your greatest desire. What you wish for may be difficult or simple.

The power of belief makes it so. No humans are more responsive to belief than children. Adults sometimes learn to be skeptical and have miracle healings at Holy Shrines for example when they move into the realm of childhood and expect a miracle.

I thought and thought, and suddenly it dawned on me: why not go back to the source of the inspiration, the wonderful story of Aladdin and the GENIE! When you rub the Magic Lamp, which can be named "hypnotherapy," out pops the GENIE to grant your fervent wish. This GENIE is your subconscious mind, which the hypnotherapy brings forth. This GENIE grants your wish. Remember, only one wish. You'd better choose carefully. What a wonderful form of hypnotherapy. Think it over carefully. What is that wish to be? That wish will be granted. *Wishing makes it so.* This is a splendid hypnotic technique when working with children. And always remember, there is a great big child in every adult just screaming to get out.

MODUS OPERANDI: MAKE A WISH HYPNOTHERAPY
You will need:
A Pencil & Paper
A Candle
Tibetan Bowl Music (Peter Blum's music is recommended) **or soft meditative music**

I call my office, "The Chamber of Realized Dreams." If your session room is fitted in Oriental style, so much the better: an altered atmosphere takes a person from the ordinary and enhances the method.

As this is an Eastern approach to hypnotherapy, I have found the sounding of a Tibetan singing bowl as an effective background to this induction. The singing bowl seems to increase the response to therapeutic suggestions. A tapestry, a flowing fountain, incense or a statue in the room can promote the oriental atmosphere.

1. Purpose
"Decide what you wish most to be granted. What wish would you like to become your reality? Make it a careful decision."
Decided!

2. Repeat Your Wish: 3 Times The Charm
"Write your wish three times on a sheet of paper."
Physically affirmed!

3. Sit Back and Relax
Go into your private session room or relax where you are. Darken the session room and light a candle on a table before you both, as you sit side-by-side. The light of the candle is the only light in the room. While meditative music softly plays in the background, both you and your client concentrate your gaze upon the candle flame.
"Sit back comfortably where you are."

Remain quiet and establish silent communication with the relaxing client as they quiet their mind and enjoy the atmosphere and the music. When ready, instruct the client **"Relax and enjoy this moment as you close your eyes and enjoy this moment. Relaxation comes to your body and mind. How enchanting it feels in this pleasant state of being.**

Now, drift, drift, drift down into the realm of sleep and dreams. Drift into hypnotic reverie and open wide the memories of your childhood when you pretended and believed in

the story of Aladdin and the magic lamp. Enter the happiness of these early times in your life when you believed and so enjoyed pretending."

Be quiet for a few moments for these suggestions to sink in

"Go back in your memory and believe in the power of magic, just like Aladdin did…and you have a magic lamp of your very own which you can rub to bring forth your very own GENIE to grant your wish…the wish we chatted about together in my office.

With your eyes still closed, visualize and imagine your GENIE touching your eyelids. Believe that they are stuck together so firmly they cannot be opened."

As long as the client believes their eyes will not open, they will find it quite impossible to open their eyes. Allow some moments to thoroughly test this physical response to this mental belief. Their eyes will not open; try as hard as they will. Critical mind has been bypassed and subconscious mind takes over. Hypnosis awaits without resistance, as critical mind is not threatened by fantasy, while subconscious mind loves to accept fantasy as reality. Childish? Of course…returning to childhood is one of the more important times of lifetime. In this state of mind, miracles occur.

"The GENIE will now cause you to become completely relaxed, and you will quickly drop into hypnotic sleep. When your inner Self knows this state has been reached, give me an audible sigh."

When you hear the "sigh," you will know the client is in the proper depth of hypnosis to allow the GENIE to perform the magic. Give the GENIE the credit. After all, they are the GENIE. In hypnosis, the client wide-openly accepts beneficial suggestions.

"Believe, believe, believe in the magic power of your genies to grant this wish this very minute. Now, we'll test the power of the GENIE who grants your wishes. As you go back in your mind to when you were very young, and loved to pretend. You pretended so strongly what you pretended actually seemed real and recall the story of ALADDIN AND HIS MAGIC LAMP, when he rubbed the Magic Lamp and out came a GENIE to grant his wish." Most everyone can recall this story, as Disney Studios recently did a great job of producing it in their ALADDIN animation.

"Drop into a state of reverie as you recall, and pretend that you have the Magic Lamp. Pretend to rub the Magic Lamp and out comes the GENIE, who will grant you your most desired wish. Pretend. Pretend. Pretend. And as you do, drop off into the realm of sleep and dreaming. In this reverie, the GENIE comes forth, your subconscious mind to grant your heartfelt wish.

Now, place your hands over your ears, and speak your wish out loud three times just as you wrote it on the paper.

"Your wish rrrrrrrrrrruns through your head, and commands the GENIE to make it so."

Wishing makes it so, you know.

"Go deeper and deeper into hypnosis, and let the GENIE do his job, as you drift and dream of your wish's fulfillment."

End the session with the suggestion:

"When you arouse from hypnosis, you'll feel wonderful and fine. The magic has been accomplished. Thank you GENIE for granting the beneficial wishes. When it has been fully granted, arouse __________ (client's name) from hypnosis when they wish to arouse, they will consciously know that their wish has been granted, and feel wonderful and fine."

How will you know it has worked? Trust the GENIE to grant the wish; however, do not expect to observe an instant transformation. This kind of hypnotherapy is invisible, but lasts a lifetime and possibly many lifetimes.

The magic is complete.

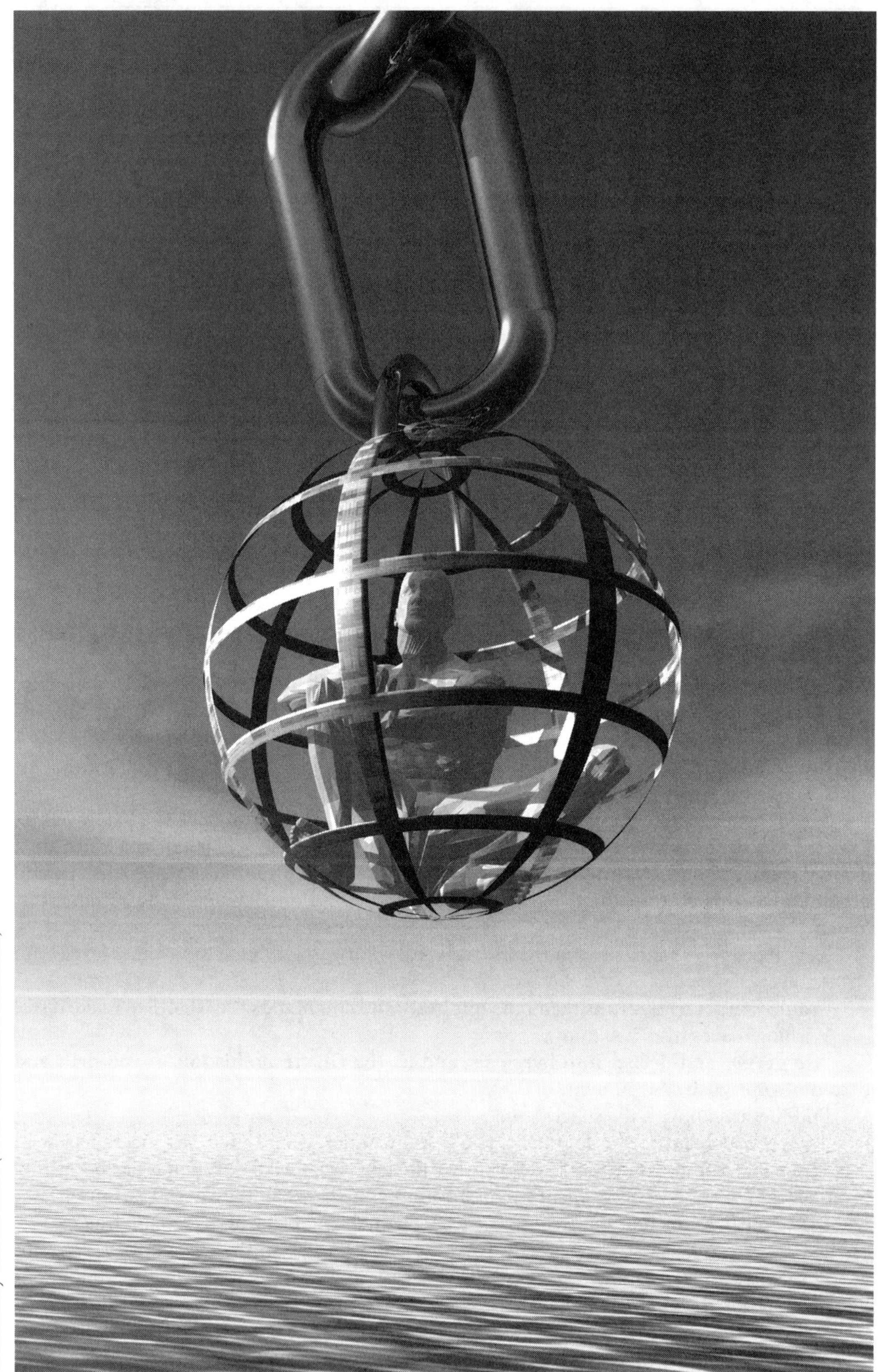

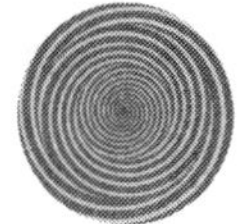

~ *Chapter 103* ~
# THE HYPNOTIC SEAL

Includes
How To Break The Hypnotic Seal

The hypnotic seal is a funny thing that is not so funny. For many years it has been a subject of controversy. It is a matter of ethics really and an ego problem of the hypnotist.

When a client, submerged in hypnosis, is told by a hypnotist, "no one but myself will be able to hypnotize you," the client is said to "seal off." Hypnotists using "the seal" are un-American and undemocratic. It opposes the real purpose of hypnosis, which is to increase the client's mastery of himself or herself, not to decrease their mastery.

The dictatorship of trying to force the choice on a subject to work exclusively with this hypnotist has no place in hypnosis. The only time a hypnotic seal may have usefulness is if the subject seems to become overly susceptible to inadvertent hypnosis and then only if they make a request should the seal be made. Giving a subject freedom of choice to do what they wish is okay but forcing choice upon them assuredly is not.

Fortunately, the power of the seal is more fanciful than factual.

When the hypnotist suggests in hypnosis "Only I will be able to hypnotize you- no one else can"…the hypnotist is in fact asking a "favor" of the subject. The inner mind of the subject picks up the suggestion and the subconscious agrees, "Okay, he is my friend, if he wants it that way…it's okay with me." In this response is the recognized rule of hypnotic behavior: **The hypnotized person endeavors to accommodate and please the hypnotist.** The responsibility of being trustworthy when you hypnotize someone is obvious.

The seal works because of an innate social situation exists between the hypnotists and the subject and the subject has the power to break the seal at anytime if the hypnotist gives cause to reject the friendship.

A hypnotic seal is only difficult to break if the subject believes in its power and is willing to allow it to be and then, after repeated use, it sets in as a behavior habit repeatedly acted out.

HOW TO BREAK THE HYPNOTIC SEAL

Breaking the Hypnotic seal is really quite easy when gone about in a sensible manner.

For a suggestion to be accepted by the mind, it has to more or less reasonable. Under the seal, a conflict develops in the mind of the subject. "To allow being hypnotized, even in profound hypnosis, the subject still has choice to accept or not accept a suggestion. If the seal is obeyed, it may appear that there is no choice when in truth choice is still present. "Accepted" means that the subject "wants" to accept it and that is an element of choice.

If you have choice to accept or not accept a suggestion why would the seal work? It works because of a social situation. In the hypnotizing process there develops a close rapport or a form of friendship between the client and the hypnotist. The hypnotist has asked the person for a favor, the favor of allowing only him to be the only one who hypnotizes. Can you imagine one close friend asking another close friend for a favor and the favor not being granted?

Do not push. Do not demand the seal be broken. Do not attempt to hypnotize the person on the moment. Tell the person, **"Relax and reflect on your own feelings."** As relaxation sets in, the subconscious becomes amenable. This type of suggestion does not conflict with the seal. When you sense the time is right ask; **"How do you handle life? Do you do most things in life because someone else told you what to do or do you make your own choices?"**

Allow this wisdom to sink home for some moments. The person is at choice. The seal is broken.

Hypnosis is a state that occurs through their conscious or subconscious willingness to be hypnotized. If the inner mind says "yeah" the seal is broken and hypnosis can proceed.

Interesting, this approach demonstrates the often overlooked, but important logical reasoning of the subconscious. Using this logic to beat the hypnotic seal is trivia. Using this same logic for the countless ways it may benefit your clients is very valuable. It reminds us to address the brilliant unlimited subconscious mind as a child still open to the wonder of it all and not as an adult who is set in one pattern and has grown skeptical.

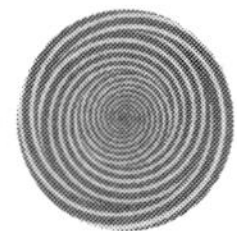

~ *Chapter 104* ~
ABREACTION MANAGEMENT

Thanks to Hypnotherapists, Gerald F. Kein and Shelley Stockwell-Nicholas
for their ideas on this subject:

Includes
What is an Abreaction?
Gateway Release
What Stimulates an Abreaction?
Four Abreactions
Guidelines for Facilitating An Abreaction

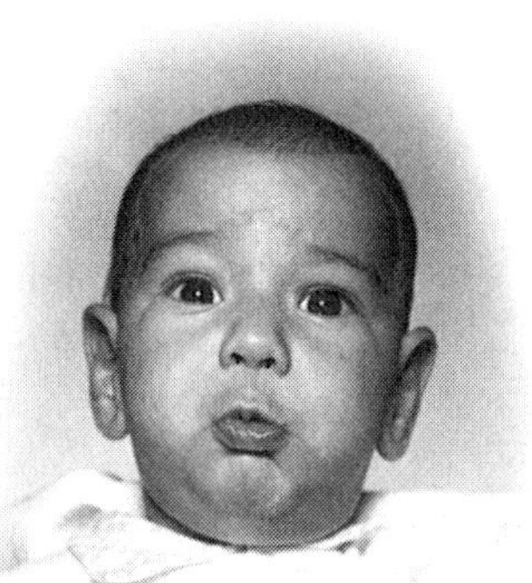

Old Emotions Revisited

Simple suggestions may not be enough to deal with deep core issues. No hypnotist wants a client to leave saying, "I tried hypnosis but it didn't work for me." An abreaction helps people to correct unfathomable underlying problems so that they leave saying, "Hypnosis really worked for me."

The subconscious buries a memory from conscious awareness if it perceives that you won't cope well with it. Upsetting and pitiful physical, mental, sexual and verbal events may be blocked from conscious memory. Loss may be glossed over. An abreaction allows a person to "re-call" and release trauma that underlies frustrating thoughts, actions and reactions. It is quite a relief to express such deep emotions. It is cathartic.

A good Hypnotherapist needs to know how to instigate, use, and defuse an abreaction.

WHAT IS AN ABREACTION?

The outward signs of an abreaction run the gamut of a tear trickling down the cheek to dramatic deafening screams. Your client may sob and flail about. During an abreaction a person doesn't just recall a traumatic event, they "re-live" it in full living color. They see, smell, taste, hear and feel it. A key event is perceived all over again, just as it was the first time.

Sometimes, powerful energy will have no conscious connection to specific events. This can happen during a spiritual emergency when enlightenment energy (the kundalini) opens the body chakras. It can also happen during a "rebirthing" when you energetically release primal memory.

GATEWAY RELEASE

"What did the grape do when it was squished"
"It lets out a little wine."

Don't let a gateway release confuse you. Sometimes when you start an induction, or relaxation comes, a person will laugh, or yawn, or cry. This is usually not an abreaction. It may be more like taking the lid off of a pressure cooker…they are just letting go of trapped energy.

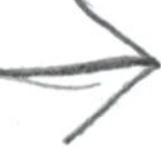

The best thing that you can do for this person is to let them express and comfort them by saying, **"That's fine. Go ahead and let this out and go deeper"** and they will go deeper into the trance. This may be all you have to do to have them leave your office feeling like a million dollars. An abreaction expresses an even stronger emotional release.

WHAT STIMULATES AN ABREACTION?

An abreaction can happen spontaneously when you least expect it or can be stimulated by simple hypnotic procedures. You could go your whole career and never have one happen, or it could happen five or more times in one week. Even someone who appears to be "always up" can on the other end, be very down and need to express the repressed emotions they've covered with a smile.

FOUR ABREACTIONS

Here are four ways an abreaction takes place:

1. Directed or Therapeutic Abreaction

A hypnotist regresses a client back to a known emotional situation and this past event causes the abreaction. The hypnotist looks to this event to discover what happened and who the players are. In other words, who of significance is involved in the event. Once this information is discovered, the abreaction is terminated and the transformational therapy started.

2. Non-Directional Abreaction

This is a modified directed regression. The hypnotist directs the client to go back in time, as far as need be, to the first situation or event that caused the issue that the client needs to resolve. Since the hypnotist doesn't know where the client is going, it is called non-directional.

3. The Spontaneous Abreaction

Hypnotized clients who look for balance and harmony may spontaneously snap themselves into an abreaction. A simple hypnotic relaxation induction could be enough to release the repression and have that memory come up to the conscious level.

4. The Recreational Abreaction

Many clients are interested in exploring past lives. They enjoy being regressed to a previous life as an exploration of their consciousness. Whenever you use a regression technique, there is the possibility that the client may regress to a highly charged emotional situation in that lifetime or in the current one that causes a strong abreaction.

GUIDELINES FOR FACILITATING AN ABREACTION
Stay Calm

Keep calmness in your voice even if you have to raise it over the noise so the client can hear you. Radiate that you are in control. Do not radiate apprehension or your client will know it. Hypnotized people are super sensitive. Stay in center. You might give yourself the suggestion, **"I am calm and attentive. I hold the mirror steady so this precious one can express and cleanse the past."**

Get Permission

An abreaction may startle a client especially if they came to you to solve a seemingly simple issue like smoking or nail biting. Yet it may be at the heart of the issue. Ask permission to proceed by saying, **"Take a deep breath. That's right. Good. Now I am speaking to your higher self. You came here to quit smoking and now we are dealing with a very deep issue. Higher self is it acceptable to you to heal this deeper issue at this time?"** If you get the green light you may proceed. **"Good. You're going to feel a lot better once this comes out."** Make sure however that you resolve the session with suggestions that address the presenting issue as well as the abreacted issues.

Avoid Touching the Abreacting Client

Touching an abreacting client may anchor them to the memory. Meaning that after you get past the abreaction, some time later, they could be at the local pub having a good time, when someone comes by and taps him on the shoulder the way you did and triggers them right back to the abreaction and they may not know what is going on.

Stopping An Abreaction

You would want to stop an abreaction if:

1. The client or the higher self says that they don't want to "do this." Or "There is no need to deal with the issue at this time."

2. They have sufficiently released the trapped energy.

3. They have gleaned the information they came to find.

4. If emoting becomes a "game" of repetitive high drama with no resolution. The client's subconscious mind knows best.

It is easy to stop an abreaction. Just say these nine words and they will stop every time, **"The scene fades and you tend to your breathing."**

or

You may say, **"When you have received the gift of this memory, take a deep, slow full breath and rise above it. Taking all of the good and none of the bad."**

Or address the Higher Self:

"Higher Self, _______________ (their name) is expressing and releasing some strong feelings. Guide them to receive the beneficial lessons from this experience so that they never have to do this again and can put this memory to rest. Let me know when it is so."

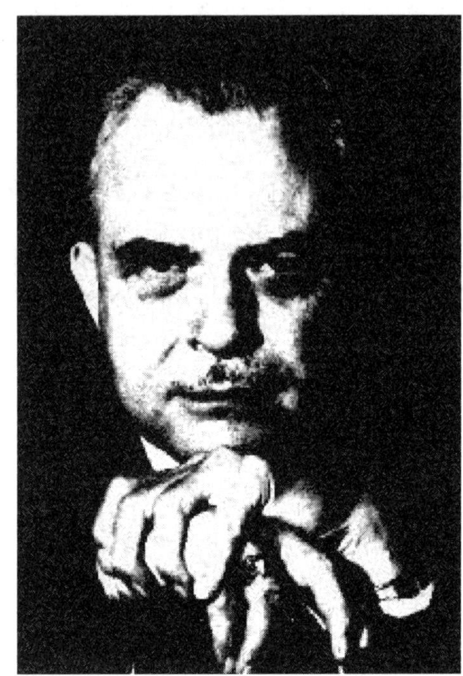

Milton Erickson

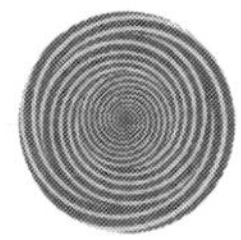

~ *Chapter 105* ~
STOCKWELL'S ERICKSONIAN HYPNOTHERAPY

By Shelley Stockwell-Nicholas, PhD

Includes
Indirect Suggestion
Indirect Induction
Erickson's Environmental Induction
Metaphor And Allegory
    Indirect Suggestions to Stop Alcohol
    Milton's Paradox
The Teaching Tale
    Trust Your Timing
Use Everything To Your Advantage
The Gift Of What You Resist
Stockwell's King Of The World Game
Imbedded Commands

"You are here to learn."
        —Milton Erickson

Dr. Milton Erickson, Ph.D. and M.D. wove true and fantastic stories to serve as metaphor and indirect trance induction. His hypnosis style which he named "unconscious learning" was a Zen-like art form based on symbolic language, imbedded commands and suggestions that allowed the subject to attach their own meaning and conclusions. He also enjoyed manipulating for positive results. A famous story tells of Erickson assisting a schizophrenic who claimed to be Jesus;

"I understand you're a carpenter." Erickson said.

"Yes" replied the fellow.

"Good I need you to build me a bookcase"

The young man was put to the task of actually building a bookcase, in the here and now, which was said to help him greatly and gave Erickson a bookcase.

INDIRECT SUGGESTION
Ericksonian hypnosis uses roundabout suggestions to overcome resistance.

INDIRECT INDUCTION

An indirect trance induction suggestion might be,

"Now you might be able to remember back to a time when you were more relaxed…or more comfortable…I really don't know. But somewhere in your background you have experienced relaxation and you have experiences of comfort. I know that if you consciously believe that you will go into trance that you can go into trance. I really don't know if you are certain how deeply you could go into a trance. And if you really know how quickly you could go into trance."

ERICKSON'S ENVIRONMENT INDUCTION

Milton was famous for using every day observations to bring about altered states. Here is a simple way to do it;

"Notice three things you see right now. Good.

Now pay careful attention to three things you hear. Good.

Now focus upon three things you feel. Excellent.

Now two things you see…two things you hear…two things you feel.

Deeper and deeper as you now put 100% of your attention on one thing you see… one thing you hear…one thing you feel.

And I wonder if you are starting to wonder how deeply you will relax with this heightened awareness and if your eyes will close now or with the next breaths you take."

METAPHOR AND ALLEGORY

Erickson enjoyed veiled suggestion. If well done, the client listens and creates mental images and external responses. An example, **"I know a man your age who was able to remember back to a time when his back felt perfect in every way. Somewhere in your background you have experiences of relaxation and comfort."**

A clever process is to instruct your client to, **"Create a story with the first thing that comes into your mind."** After they are complete ask, **"If this story was actually about you and your situation what could you learn from it?"**

If they say that they don't know what it means ask them to guess at what it might mean. **"Just make up a story about what the story means in your life."**

Indirect Suggestions to Stop Alcohol

"A cactus is special plant that doesn't need to drink for very long periods of time as life goes on. The cactus easily controls its thirst and remains quite beautiful. How blessed it is when pure water comes from the heavens to truly nourish it to the core of its being. As you think about the cactus…"

Milton's Paradox

Milton Erikson, the famous hypnotherapist, discovered this principle when he was a small boy. His father was trying to pull a stubborn calf into the barn by tugging on his ears. The cow wouldn't budge until Milton tugged even harder in the other direction on the calf's tail. The poor mooing soul bolted into the barn.

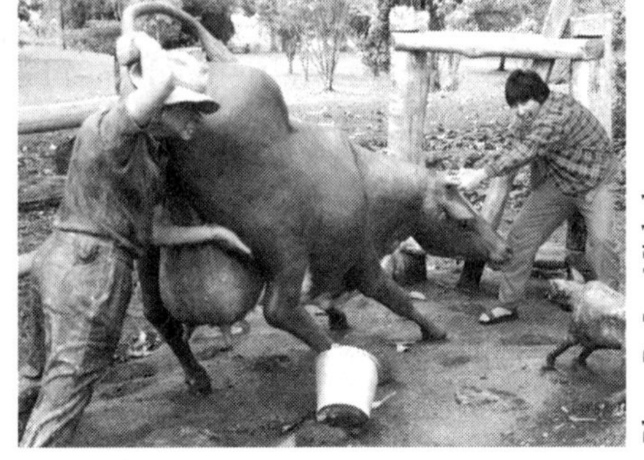

Erickson would sometimes do the unexpected and break limiting patterns forcing someone to detach, muse and exaggerate a contrary action. A famous story is told about a hopelessly obese woman who told him, "I have to lose 150 pounds."

"I will help you only if you promise to do exactly as I tell you. Do I have your word?"

"Yes Doctor, whatever you say."

"Very good…come back when you have gained another 35 pounds."

She forced herself to follow his directions and became so disgusted with eating that she easily lost all 185 pounds and then some.

Erickson was actually employing the "Law of Reverse Effect" he had learned as a boy when his father was trying to get a stubborn calf into the barn by tugging its ears. The cow wouldn't budge until Milton tugged even harder on the tail in the opposite direction. The poor mooing soul bolted into the barn.

THE TEACHING TALE

The teaching tale is an allegory told by tribal storytellers worldwide. Teaching tales have been written on ancient temple walls, told in nursery rhymes and fables (like Aesop's), bibles and books like "Alice In Wonderland," "The Little Prince," "The Wizard of Oz" "Siddhartha" and, my newest favorite, "The Knight In Rusty Armor." Movies like the "Truman Show" also weave a thread that can help mend your life. When you tell your client one of these open-ended stories, they use their gift of intuition and observation to imbue the tale with their own wisdom.

I sometimes use teaching tales to underscore a situation. They are delivered during waking hypnosis or while the client rests with eyes closed. Here a few tales I created to solve specific issues.

Trust your Timing Tale

"Imagine an apple tree that is about 40 years old and lush with apples. What color are the apples? Good. Notice how the apple ripen in their own and perfect time. Some may be ripe now and others still in the process of becoming ripe."

Use Everything to Your Advantage Tale

"My friend Carl spent hours commuting to work every day. It was a long drive on crowded freeways. Carl was a follower of a wise guru of some faith or other, you can imagine. Anyway his guru told him that his personal sacred meditation was to talk with god while driving. God had given him lots of time to enjoy commuting and communing. Soon Carl looked forward to going to work and discovering the gifts his sacred devotional to work brings."

The Gift Of What You Resist Tale

"Imagine your office building as a big Christmas tree and every person and every experience a gift just for you."

Get Over It Tale

"One day I was complaining to my friend Dennis, 'I am having such a tough time…everything is going wrong and so on and so on…' you can imagine. And Dennis said, 'What do you want?' 'I want to be happy' I replied. 'Then be happy' he said."

STOCKWELL'S KING OF THE WORLD GAME

I use my "King of The World Game" to empower and evoke self-discovery. Try it you'll like it!

"We are going to play a game. Just make it up as you go along. Tell me the story you just told me but this time, pretend that you are king (or queen) of the universe. As king (or queen) you have created everyone and everything in the story for your own advantage."

IMBEDDED COMMANDS

Imbedded commands are sentence fragments intended to impact a person without their being consciously aware that the suggestion was made. To be most effective, you "mark" the command by doing something different while you say the word. You might lower or raise your voice pitch or volume, tilt your head, look directly into their eyes, point to them, smile or touch the person you are talking to when you speak these ideas.

Imbedded Commands to be Slimmer

At a seminar Erickson was asked, just before lunch, "What do you tell an obese person?"

His response, **"I hope every one of you enjoys lunch today. I'd like you to enjoy it thoroughly and well. You know it's as easy to enjoy a small portion as a large portion. In fact, those of you who eat a small portion will enjoy a small portion much more than you would a large portion. And you really will, because you won't even have to feel guilty about that small portion. You'll be perfectly delighted with it. And so, good appetite!"**

Let's break this down:

"I hope every one of you enjoys lunch today." ("Enjoyment" overrides guilt and rewards)
"I'd like you to enjoy it thoroughly and well." (Implies that the food is properly chewed and digested for more enjoyment.)

"You know it's as easy to enjoy a small portion as a large portion. In fact, those of you who eat a small portion will enjoy a small portion much more than you would a large portion." (Sells the benefits of less, overrides resistance and implies that because there is so little of it, it is easier to enjoy.)

"And you really will, because you won't even have to feel guilty about that small portion. You'll be perfectly delighted with it. And so, good appetite!" (A 'future pacing' seals the outcome and makes you feel good about your selection.)

More Imbedded Commands

You may give a string of facts that they say, "yes" to and then put in the fact you'd like to imbed (i.e. "you are sitting in this chair and enjoy and the lovely day as your mind drifts off into pleasant far away places").

"Maybe you will _____________." ("…find new ways to have fun.")
"Maybe you haven't _________ yet." ("…decided to enjoy eating fresh vegetables yet.")
"How would feel if you _________ ("…stopped eating chocolate cake?")"
"I wouldn't tell you to __________ ("…stop eating chocolate cake") **because …"**
"When you __________, then you _____________." ("When you forgive yourself then you feel happy.")
"I was wondering _____________." ("…what it would be like for you to not eat the cake tonight.")
"You probably already know ____________." ("…many ways to let the weight go.")
"Don't ________ too quickly." (…go into trance too quickly.")
"Can you imagine _________?" ("…yourself 40 pounds slimmer?")

"You might notice how _______." ("…much more you relax with this next breath.")

"One could (a person or people might) _______." ("…permanently change their eating patterns because they are having so much fun.")

"I don't know if _________" ("…you will raise your left or your right hand first.")

"You might notice how good_______ feels, when you _________."

"You may not know if ______________. ("…you are going to enjoy weighing 130 pounds and then you'll find you are delighted and giggling all the time.")

"It's easy to _________, isn't it?" ("…relax")

"You are able to _________. ("…relax completely with the next thought you have.")

"_________told me, __________. ("Henry Ford said/told me 'If you think you can or you can't, you're correct.'")

"A person may _______, when _________." (… remember all the good reasons donuts make them sick when they have an urge to eat one.")

"Eventually __________. (…it will be second nature to only eat fresh vegetables.)

I could tell you that ______ but _______. ("…you are self-assured in your new slim body but I wouldn't do that")

IMBEDDED QUOTES

Fragments of quotes also impact a person without their conscious awareness. Here are some you may want to use:

"The best way to get even is to forget."

"Some marriages are made in heaven but they ALL have to be maintained on earth."

"Standing in the middle of the road is dangerous. You get knocked down by traffic from both ways."

"You can make a mountain out of a molehill by adding a little dirt."

"The mighty oak was once a little nut that held its ground."

"Words are the windows to the heart."

"It's all right to sit on the pity pot now and then; just be sure to flush when you are done."

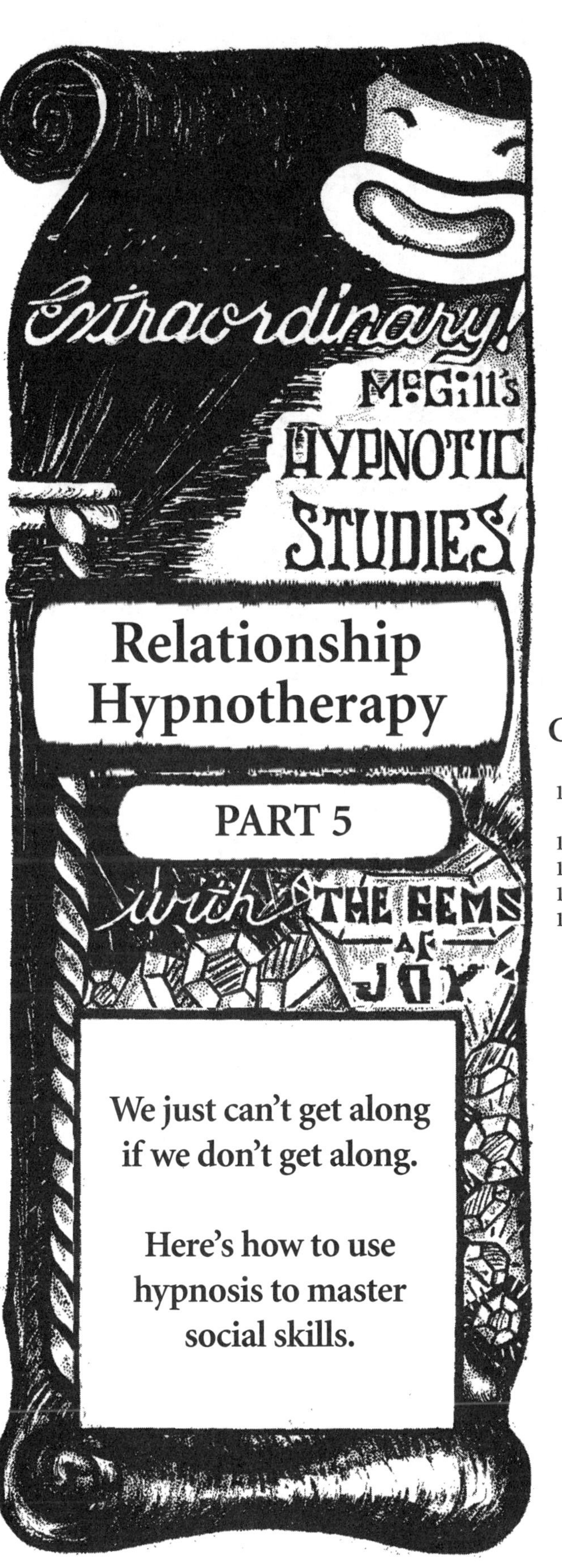

CHAPTERS IN PART FIVE

106. Developing Personal
     Magnetism ....page 375
107. Matrimony Hypnotherapy 381
108. Heart-Mending Hypnosis 383
109. Mind Trap Hypnotherapy 387
110. Stockwell-Nicholas Cognitive
     Hypnotherapy...391

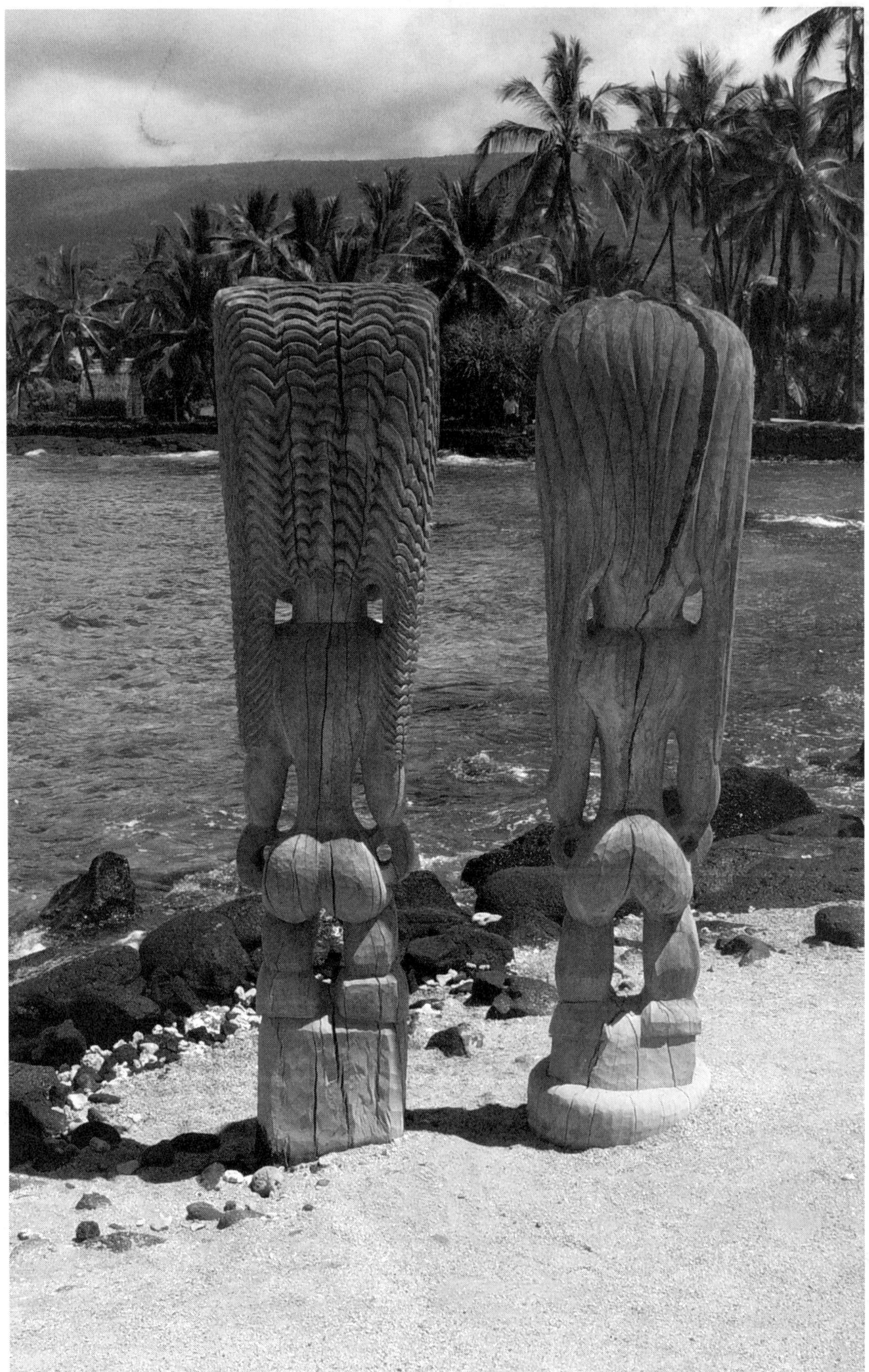

Photo by Jon Nicholas

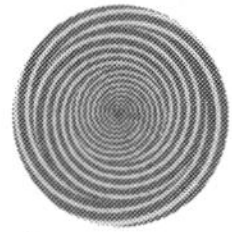

~ *Chapter 106* ~
DEVELOPING PERSONAL MAGNETISM

Includes
Personal Magnetism for Professionals
    For The Lawyer
    For The Physician
    For The Minister
    For The Salesperson
    For The Politician
Cultivate Self-Control
Techniques Of Personal Magnetism
Cultivating Determination
Cultivating Self-Control
Reinforcing Self-Hypnotic Suggestions For Home

Personal Magnetism is essential to your outstanding success in life and as a hypnotist. The instructions in this chapter and your own WILL make it so. Persevere; practice and you will cultivate personal magnetism.

Shall we say your personal magnetism is imaginary or shall we call you charming?

Charisma is a synonym for personal magnetism. It is charm. It is exerting your personality to influence. In that sense it is a form of hypnotism. Charisma might be interpreted to mean "exerting a hypnotic influence over others without arousing the least bit of apprehension."

For the hypnotist, charisma makes you a really GREAT hypnotist. People obey your commands through this mental influence. The more you develop your personal magnetism the better hypnotist you will be…also, the more charming hypnotist you will be.

Franklin D. Roosevelt is an excellent example of personal magnetism in action. His personality influenced the entirety of America. A great entertainer like Maurice Chevalier is another example. Chevalier was never much of a singer, but his personality was so powerful that the entire world loved to hear him sing. Charisma boils down to the PERSONALITY OF YOURSELF. As a matter of fact most top ranking people have personal magnetism.

Some people are naturally endowed with it; others acquire it by persistent practice. One may win some degree success without personal magnetism but they never attain great heights of the truly successful without it.

This mighty power brings many friends, for everybody thrills to a magnetic personality. There is something irresistibly fascinating about a magnetic personality. It is felt…invisible-like and compels admiration. A person may carry magnetism in their voice. It may be carried in the eyes. Others manifest it in their gestures, smiles and self-confidence of bearing. Some develop it in one direction and others in another, but everyone can become magnetic to some extent by following the instructions in this chapter.

PERSONAL MAGNETISM FOR PROFESSIONALS

Belief in the value of having a magnetic personality has even invaded the business world. Opportunity!

Personal Magnetism and hypnotism are invaluable to the various professions. No great professional success can be attained without the practical employment of this wonderful power. Its use benefits you in every way, PLUS be of great value to your clients whether a business person, physician, politician, actor, lawyer or salesperson. Personal magnetism, or charisma, is a gift to acquire.

For The Lawyer

Every successful lawyer, especially criminal lawyers, pleading their case before a jury, uses hypnotic suggestion. The judge and jury's attention is skillfully drawn to them as every ounce of will power and magnetism is directed towards the attorney's view of the case. A lawyer can attain full use of The *Power of Suggestion* when combining it with personal magnetism.

For The Physician

No profession can use the power of personal magnetism more than the physician. In connection with their medical knowledge, hypnotism and magnetism make them paramount in their profession. In addition to being a doctor they become a *healer*. Personal magnetism can effect cures that would otherwise be impossible. The physician who uses it gains the full confidence of patients who embrace their ability to evoke wellness. Herein lies a great secret for the healing the sick.

For The Minister

The minister has a wonderful opportunity to use the power of suggestion and personal magnetism. The minister who has Personal Magnetism fills their church and knows how to keep and attract the attention of the congregation. They are magnetic and emanate forceful and powerful thought waves each time they deliver a sermon. Such personal magnetism attracts people to their pews like bits of iron attracted to a magnet.

For The Salesperson

The most far sweeping field for the use of Personal Magnetism and hypnotic influence is in the profession of salesmanship. The "knight of the grip," the insurance solicitor, the canvasser, the clerk behind the counter, the merchandise salesman, the real estate broker, everyone connected with salesmanship…the list goes on and on…could easily double their sales using hypnotic suggestion combined with cultivated personal magnetism. All persons engaged in the business of selling would do well to study this text thoroughly, and master what it tells.

For The Politician

With the media and the political climate of what we expect from a leader, charisma and magnetism will win or lose an election.

Self-Hypnosis For the Use of All Professions

You can use self-hypnosis, and design your own charismatic suggestion-formulas, that apply especially to your work as a hypnotherapist. You can teach your clients self-hypnosis and let them design their own personal suggestions for personal magnetism as well. A bit of thought, a little effort and the results achieved are excellent.

GREAT STUFF! Try it for yourself. Then, teach the process to all your clients. Ever think about holding a "Magnetic Personality Development Clinic"?

MODUS OPERANDI: CULTIVATE SELF-CONTROL & AFFIRMATIONS

1. Personal Self Control

You cannot expect to control others unless you can control yourself. Remember this. Learn to know yourself…find your faults and correct them. Find your good qualities and amplify them. This helps you become magnetic. In other words, self-control increases charisma. It increases your charm. And, so the first essential for developing a magnetic personality is your personal self-control.

"You have excellent self-control. I become a master of any anger in self. If you feel anger, immediately…STOP and TAKE THREE DEEP BREATHS. Anger becomes rational and you deal with it and do not allow it to undermine your personality. Anger takes away your vitality and weakens well-being. Conversely, cheerful thoughts are infective and their radiance produces corresponding actions in the minds of others. Your Magnetic Personality radiates sunshine and good will and thought waves are contagious. You greet others with a smile.

2. Be Confident

The second essential for charisma is confidence in yourself and in your ability to develop a magnetic personality. This is a matter of will power. You must have the necessary will power to carry out your desire. Your must be strong and firm in the mastery of yourself. To be strong and firm does not mean you should be egotistic. An egotist is usually stubborn. Stubbornness is a sign of a weak will. A person who will not be amenable to others from pure stubbornness, denies everything, is anything but strong-willed. The person with a magnetic personality can always master one who is stubborn.

"You are confident. If you want to influence a stubborn person never argue with them. For 'Where ignorance is bliss, it is folly to be wise.' Lead them with something that interests them. Play on their ego and you will accomplish your purpose. A vacillating unsteady disposition is anti-personality. You cultivate the faculty to get the facts, make a quick decision and then stick to it. Do not change a decision until you are convinced you are wrong."

3. Be Tactful

Most people are magnetic to some extend, but their use of language destroys their influence. Some people talk just to hear themselves talk, without really saying anything. They are boring and boredom is anti-personality. Use tact and study the characteristics of the person you wish to influence. You then gain their confidence and confidence begets confidence.

If you are in company and there is discussion of things of which you are well informed, you do not force your views; you remain a good listener. You avoid debate unless you are absolutely sure of your ground.

Magnetism's power can be enhanced and developed. The basic principle of Personal Magnetism is strong will power. Personal Magnetism is a nerve force, which is produced and directed by the will of the producer. Will can be strengthened by exercising it. You cannot expect will to be strong without training. Hypnosis provides a remarkable way to exercise the will and develop WILL POWER.

MODUS OPERANDI: TECHNIQUES OF PERSONAL MAGNETISM

This technique employs the ideomotor response idea; that every thought produces an accompanying subjective response in the body. That is to say, if we consciously think an idea we subconsciously tend to move in that direction. Using this process effectively increases personal magnetism. You can use it as a self-hypnosis process or with your clients

SESSION ONE: SELF EMPOWERMENT

Here are suggestions for session number one:

Place your client in a trance and suggest:

Yawn Induction

"Take a seat and think about yawning and actually yawn. As you do, you will find yourself really yawning, and yawning is very relaxing to the body, and moves you in the direction of sleep. Deliberately thinking of going to sleep moves you into hypnotic sleep, wherein mind becomes activated to accept suggestions. Now, close your eyes and think of how relaxed all over you are becoming. Think of how receptive your subconscious mind is becoming to accept and act upon the suggestions you are going to implant in it that will increase your personal magnetism.

Continue on, relaxing, and think 'sleep.' Think 'going to sleep.' Think 'Sleep.' You will find yourself becoming very sleepy, but just let your mind drift and don't allow yourself to actually go to sleep. You are close to sleep yet still not asleep. You have placed yourself into Self-Hypnosis.

In this receptive and passive condition of mind, place the palms of your hands over your ears and press in a little. Now, speaking out loud to yourself, present these suggestions three times, and each time they will seem to ring inside your head: 'I am a man (or woman). I have strong will power. My will is powerful. I believe in myself and my ability to succeed. My personality is becoming magnetic and nothing can prevent me from succeeding. My will is strong. My confidence in myself is unlimited. I rely absolutely on myself. My confidence cannot be shaken.'

'I am a man (or woman). I have strong will power. My will is powerful. I believe in myself and my ability to succeed. My personality is becoming magnetic and nothing can prevent me from succeeding. My will is strong. My confidence in myself is unlimited. I rely absolutely on myself. My confidence cannot be shaken.'

'I am a man (or woman). I have strong will power. My will is powerful. I believe in myself and my ability to succeed. My personality is becoming magnetic and nothing can prevent me from succeeding. My will is strong. My confidence in myself is unlimited. I rely absolutely on myself. My confidence cannot be shaken.'

Having repeated these suggestions in this special mental state, three times, drop your hands from pressing on your ears to relax them in your lap and go to sleep if you wish. Awaken when you will."

MODUS OPERANDI: CULTIVATING DETERMINATION

Next day or the next session apply the same Yawn Induction method to induce Hypnosis and present these suggestions for cultivating Determination:

"Think about yawning and actually yawn. As you do, you will find yourself really yawning, and yawning is very relaxing to the body, and moves you in the direction of sleep. Deliberately thinking of going to sleep moves you into hypnotic sleep, wherein mind becomes activated to accept suggestions. Now, close your eyes and think of how relaxed all over you are becoming. Think how receptive your subconscious mind is becoming to accept and act upon the suggestions you implant into it as you increase your Personal Magnetism. Continue, relaxing and think of going to sleep. Think going to sleep. Think Sleep. You will find yourself becoming very sleepy, but just let your mind drift and don't allow yourself to actually go to sleep. You are close to sleep yet still not asleep. You have placed yourself into Self-Hypnosis.

Now say these ideas inside your head so that they become your very own: 'I am developing a magnetic personality. I am determined to succeed. I am a complete success in everything I start out to do. I have the ability to influence people. People respond to the influence of my personal magnetism. People respond to the power of my will. I am determined to radiate cheerfulness at all times. I have powerful determination to do whatever I set out to do. Nothing can deter me. The power of self-confidence is mine. The power of determination is mine as well.'

'I am a man (or woman). I have strong will power. My will is powerful. I believe in myself and my ability to succeed. My personality is becoming magnetic and nothing can prevent me from succeeding. My will is strong. My confidence in myself is unlimited. I rely absolutely on myself. My confidence cannot be shaken.'

'I am a man (or woman). I have strong will power. My will is powerful. I believe in myself and my ability to succeed. My personality is becoming magnetic and nothing can prevent me from succeeding. My will is strong. My confidence in myself is unlimited. I rely absolutely on myself. My confidence cannot be shaken.'

Having repeated these suggestions to yourself three times while in the state of hypnosis, go to sleep. Awaken when you will."

This ends the session of this day.

MODUS OPERANDI: CULTIVATING SELF-CONTROL SESSION THREE

"Think about yawning and actually yawn. As you do, you will find yourself really yawning, and yawning is very relaxing to the body, and moves you in the direction of sleep. Deliberately thinking of going to sleep moves you into hypnotic sleep, wherein mind becomes activated to accept suggestions. Now, close your eyes and think of how relaxed all over you are becoming. Think how receptive your subconscious mind is becoming to accept and act upon the suggestions you implant into it as you increase your Personal Magnetism. Continue, relaxing and think of going to sleep. Think going to sleep. Think Sleep. You will find yourself becoming very sleepy, but just let your mind drift and don't allow yourself to actually go to sleep. You are close to sleep yet still not asleep. You have placed yourself into Self-Hypnosis.

Now say these ideas inside your head so that they become your very own: 'I have full control of myself at all times. I never lose my temper. No one can ruffle me. I always have a smile when needed. I never discourage or be nervous. I am the controller and master of myself. I am cheerful and happy. My WILL POWER is vast and supreme and I have a magnetic personality that influences others, as it is my will to cause. My eyes exert this power. My voice exerts this power. My body exerts this power. My entire BEING exerts this power. I have developed a magnetic personality.'

'I am a man (or woman). I have strong will power. My will is powerful. I believe in myself and my ability to succeed. My personality is becoming magnetic and nothing can prevent me from succeeding. My will is strong. My confidence in myself is unlimited. I rely absolutely on myself. My confidence cannot be shaken.'

'I am a man (or woman). I have strong will power. My will is powerful. I believe in myself and my ability to succeed. My personality is becoming magnetic and nothing can prevent me from succeeding. My will is strong. My confidence in myself is unlimited. I rely absolutely on myself. My confidence cannot be shaken.'

Having repeated this three times we conclude this session. Awaken when you will. Use this process daily for a few weeks. The results will amaze you in the qualities of Personal Magnetism it will cultivate in yourself."

MODUS OPERANDI: REINFORCING SELF-HYPNOTIC SUGGESTIONS FOR HOME

After each of the above exercises give your client this assignment while in trance.

"On a piece of paper, write suggestions for today's will-power and self-control session that you want to give yourself. (Or you can give them a written copy of the affirmation used in that session) **Later, in your private room tonight, just before going to bed, darken the room and place a lighted candle on the table before a comfortable chair in which you seat yourself. Position the candle up high enough so you have to open your eyes wide in looking at the flame. Now study the suggestions. As you read the message, speak it out loud to yourself. Read it and speak it several times committing it more or less to memory. Then relax back in the chair, stare directly at the candle flame and as you do, repeat verbally what you have memorized. When your eyes get tired, close them and relax yourself even more. Now mentally review what you have been speaking. Continue this until you can absorb no more and just want to go to sleep. Blow out the candle. Go to bed and have a good night's sleep. Sometimes, after looking at the candle flame for awhile, it will seem to become very large and you will see the suggestions written in the flame. If this illusion happens, it means your self-suggestions have very much become your own."**

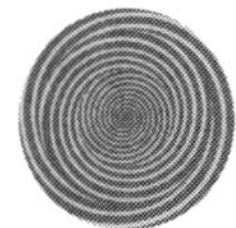

~ *Chapter 107* ~
MATRIMONY HYPNOTHERAPY

Includes
Saving A Marriage That Is Right

Matrimony Hypnotherapy= Hypnotherapist As A Marriage Couch

Often a hypnotherapist is called upon to harmonize matrimonial issues. The hypnotherapist is well qualified to do this. Marriage counseling is a profession in itself. The majority of marriage counselors handle matrimonial difficulties in an objective manner. The hypnotherapist handles them in a subjective manner and love squabbles are mainly subjective.

Consider the Wedding Ceremony as a hypnotic induction session: The minister is the hypnotist. The bride and groom are the clients. Marriage is highly charged with feelings, and feelings are the domain of the subconscious. A responsive subconscious is hypnosis– a state of mind that is hyper-suggestible. The wedding ceremony is loaded with suggestions:

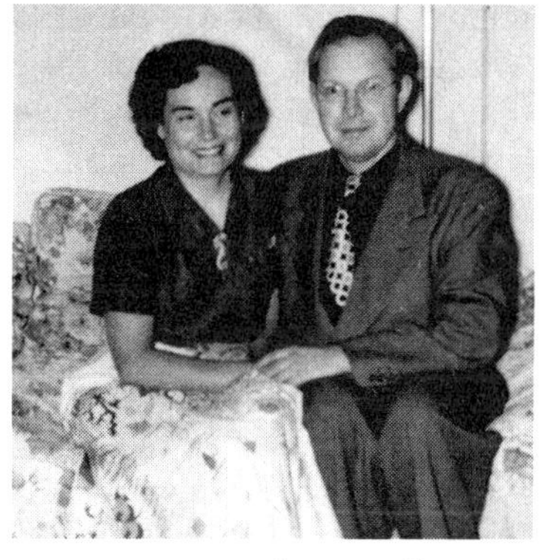

Ormond McGill
with his beloved wife,
Delight

"We are gathered here in the sight of God, to join together this man and this woman in holy matrimony.

This man (give name) **and this woman** (give name) **are to be united in marriage. All others forever hold their peace that their love may reign."**

Marriage vows include:
"To have and to hold from this day forth."
"For better or worse."
"For richer or poorer."
"In sickness and in health."
"To love and cherish each other until death do you part."

Wow! Suggestions. Suggestions. Suggestions. At the time of the marriage some couples are so deeply entranced they scarcely recall the ceremony. It was performed subconsciously.

Yet, humans are humans, and in the course of time, domestic difficulties can arise; some so serious that divorce is intimated. Often it is then that the couple comes for counsel.

If a marriage is right it should be saved. If a marriage is wrong, divorce is just as well. When you look upon marriage as a hypnotic induction, you are the perfect expert to save the marriage. Saving a so-called marriage made in heaven is wonderful hypnotherapy.

When basic love and harmony (call it "chemistry," if you like) is there, such togetherness is one of life's greatest treasures. When the basic "chemistry" is not right, divorce is just as well. Then both can be free to seek out better happiness. One mate may want to retain the marriage while the other wishes it terminated. The suggestion-formula of Matrimony Hypnotherapy helps a couple decide from the most aware state, that of hypnosis, what is truest for them.

Divorce is not easy, as the marriage vows remain imprinted in the subconscious. If it is decided that divorce is right then hypnosis can help the couple with a peaceful divorce. But let's find out the inner truth and save the marriage that is right:

MODUS OPERANDI: HYPNOTICALLY SAVING A MARRIAGE THAT IS RIGHT

Have the couple sit side-by-side, and hypnotize both together and induce a somnambulistic trance. Then suggest they join hands as you direct:

"Let your energies flow between you through your hands. If your chemistry is right for each other, you will grip hands tighter and tighter. If not, you will release hands immediately, and drop even more deeply into hypnosis. Let your subconscious mind decide what is right for you. If you find it best to release hands, it causes no distress; it simply means that as a married couple it would be best for each to go their way and this is appreciated without remorse of any kind."

If the couple is right for each other, their hands grips will tell the story. Hands carry a powerful "bond of love." You can then solve current difficulties for the couple by suggesting:

If they do release hands, suggest that they work things out amicably with no remorse.

"The difficulties you have been experiencing are all passing events that will automatically correct themselves. The love you share together is what is of real importance. Go back in your mind now and experience the love bond between you on your wedding day— to the space and time when you were married. and These vows of eternal love were implanted in your subconscious, and became your reality of togetherness.

Go back. Go back. Go back to your Wedding Day. Kiss now with passion while still in deep trance, just as you were in a trance when you were married.

Kiss, kiss, kiss with passion and let your love energies flow between you. All surface thoughts of disharmony and divorce are gone…and the harmony you feel flowing between you glows through your being.

Feel your love, and when you both are ready, come back out of hypnosis – returning to the here and now– with the glow of love shining brightly between you. You are so glad, for you now know you are right for each other.

Arouse now when you are ready… join hands and go on your way together following a path of love which spreads before you."

When they are ready, the couple returns to the here and now. They smile, grip hands, and go on their way.

You watch them take their leave, and you know you are a master of Matrimony Hypnotherapy.

382

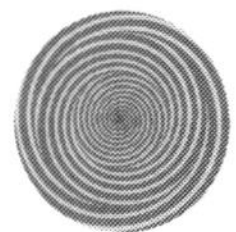

~ *Chapter 108* ~
HEART-MENDING HYPNOSIS
By Shelley Stockwell-Nicholas, PhD

"You done stomped on my heart and mashed it flat.
How the heck can I get over that?"
—Shelley Stockwell

Includes
Pre-Hypnosis Pointers For The Broken Hearted
Kate Ellis' Broken Heart Hypnosis
McGill's Trust Method

Have you been jilted, dumped and devastated? Or, even worse, been the one who dumped another? What happens when your bed of roses turns to thorns? How do you help a client mend a broken heart?

PRE-HYPNOSIS POINTERS FOR THE BROKEN HEARTED

Loss of love creates an ache in the heart, obsession of the mind and a hollow feeling in the pit of the stomach. As the expert, here are some pointers that point your clients to sooth, comfort and put themself back in the driver's seat. You can give them these as a pre-hypnosis pep-talk or after they have entered trance:

1. **Love Is Forever**
   "Just because you are not going to be together doesn't mean you have to stop loving. One of the glorious things about love is that it lasts forever. Each relationship allows you to reflect on your loving emotional self. Love belongs to you not to someone else. No one can take your loving heart away. Put your love for that person in a special heart compartment. They were a gift that has prepared you to love even more the next time."

2. **Love Is A Mirror**
   "All love starts with self-love. If you were not beautiful you would never have noticed the beauty in another."

3. **Forgive And Live**
   "Stored resentment hurts you more than it could possible hurt anyone else. If someone has harmed you with insensitivity, they will have to heal and live with that. If you have hurt some one with insensitivity, make amends and then forgive yourself. You let it go because, above all else, you choose to feel terrific."

4. Love is Therapy
    "Relationships are always an opportunity to look at your 'stuff.' Your childhood patterns, and what Mommy and Daddy showed you about love, is not always what you want for your relationships when you grow up. Some relationships are training wheels to show what works and doesn't work in love so you can let go of the wheels (the past) with a new and more compatible bicycle built for two.

    Now is your golden chance to observe what did work so you can do it even better in the future and what didn't work so you can give that pattern up. If you're not sure what healthy love is, now is the perfect time to become a love scholar. We go to school to learn all sorts of things."

5. Lopsided Love Loses
    "Love is both giving and receiving. If you've just been only giving, it's like breathing out and never breathing in. No wonder this relationship keeled over. Practice giving and receiving on yourself right now breath in and bathe yourself with loving thoughts: inspiration. Breath out cleansing: exhalation. Ask yourself for what you want and then generously give it to yourself and say 'thank you' or if you've only been receiving, it's like breathing in and never breathing out."

The most profound words ever written on this subject comes from a country and western song:
"You got to know when to hold 'em.
Know when to fold 'em.
Know when to walk away.
Know when to run.
You never count your money while your sittin' at the table.
There'll be time enough for counting when the dealin's done."

Hypnotist Kate Ellis uses a gorgeous NLP (neurolinguistic programming) technique. It works well with someone with a keen imagination and who is visually dominant. Try it, you'll like it:

MODUS OPERANDI: KATE ELLIS'S NLP HEART MENDING THEATER
Here is my version of Hypnotherapist Kate's approach.

"Imagine yourself sitting in a posh chair in a movie theater. On the screen is a super big color photo of YOU. What is around you? What are you wearing?

Next, imagine yourself in the projection room, about to show you a movie about your 'relationship.' When both the you in the theater and you in the booth are ready, run a movie about the great things that happened in your romance- the fun, the passion, the gentle moments, all the sweet memories. If you get misty watching the movie, that's fine.

Now rewind that movie all the way back to before you ever met. Take it off the projector and put on the next feature: A movie about all the bad parts of your relationship: your pet peeves, injustices, hurts, and disappointments. It's OK to growl watching this movie.

When it's done, rewind that movie too and just relax in your comfy seat. How happy you are as you look up at the screen and see a happy picture of yourself smiling at you saying: 'I'm glad that's over.'

Finally, project a movie of yourself five years from today; happy in a new life surrounded by love. That old relationship is the past. You are now in a new moment of joy. And you say 'thank you' to that person and that relationship that didn't work out five years ago. 'You taught me so much about loving myself and making healthy choices in love. All the past is forgiven and I have matured and grown into a happy, successful and loving one.'"

Leave the theater and enjoy a beautiful night sky and, if you happen to see that old flame again, you feel comfortable and complete."

MODUS OPERANDI: McGILL'S TRUST METHOD

Sometimes a person in pain would love to give their pain away. They come to you to help them and this Trust Method relieves their suffering.

Here is how Ormond describes it:

Trust is a very powerful suggestion. "I trust you" makes it personal. Ambroise Liebeault is regarded as one of the greatest Hypnotherapists that ever was because trust was his talent. He instilled in his patients the knowing that he could be trusted to solve their problem. You can do the same.

Following your consultation directly ask your client: **"Do you trust me enough to help you let go of this problem?"** (Place your hand on their shoulders) **"Look deep, deep inside my eyes and see if you completely trust me to take away your hurt** (disappointment, or whatever problem they presented). **If you find you completely trust me tell me, 'I completely trust you.'"**

Maintain continuous eye contact. If they say "Yes" (usually the case) proceed on, otherwise end this approach on the spot.

"Good, since you trust me deeply, I will take your concern from you and place it in myself. You will be cleared as it will become my obligation to myself and not yours. All you have to do now is relax, close your eyes and go to sleep. Your are all cleared. How free you feel…now that I have taken your trouble…you are clear of it forever. Now I must clear myself. It is going, going, going …It is gone. We are both cleared. We are both a well and fine…a happy team. Awaken when you wish and you will go your way happy and peaceful. Thank you for your trust."

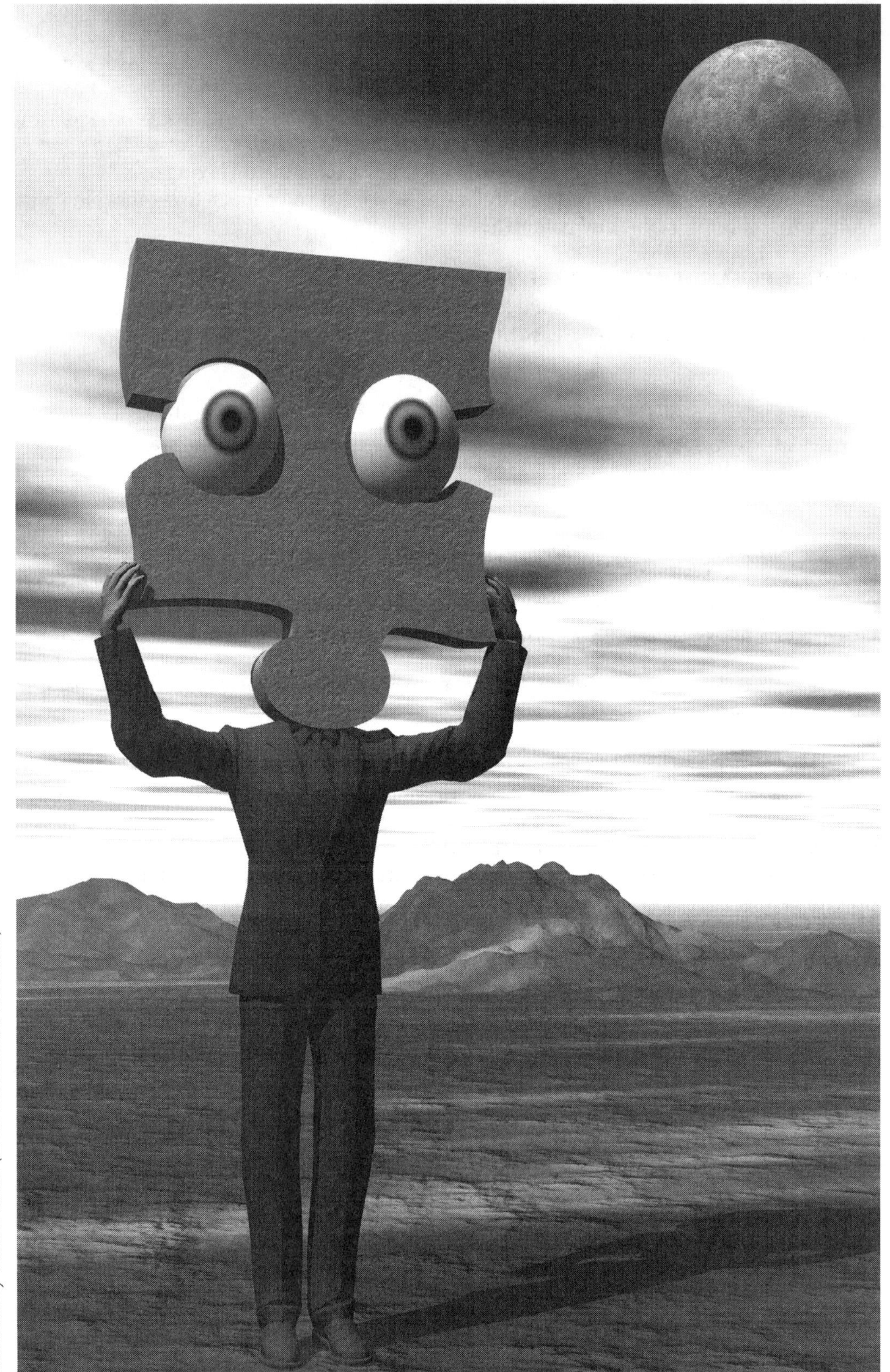

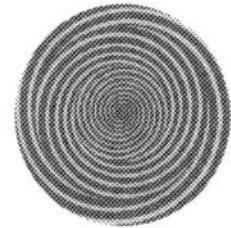

Chapter 109
~ MIND TRAP HYPNOTHERAPY ~

Includes
Sexual Dysfunction
Stuttering
Fear of Heights
Releasing Mind Traps
The Bulldog Approach
Mind Trap Hypnotherapy

Have you ever heard of a mind trap?"
Hypnotherapists recognize them as the mental blocks to mental-healing. To get around a mind trap become familiar with their nature. They are a hypnotic, or subconscious phenomena. Any unwelcome behavior, over which people lose their own control, is an example of a mind trap. Mind traps are illogical.

Releasing clients from mind traps can become a specialty for the professional hypnotherapist. It can become a hypnotherapeutic business in itself.

Here are some good examples of mind traps…

SEXUAL DYSFUNCTION
Let's say that a client reports being sexually molested as a child, which has produced a blockage of normal sexual response ever since. The molestation took place some thirty years back in time. Other than the trauma, no physical injury was been done; no social condemnation. They are physically healthy. There was no impairment of their normal sexual activity; yet the early trauma continues.

After thirty years there is no rational reason to hang on to the childhood trauma. Yet caught in the "Mind Trap" the trauma/drama persists, and no amount of intelligent reasoning will remove it.

STUTTERING
A client stutters. She started stuttering years back, for one reason or another, and it became an annoying, distressful habit of defective speech. It has remained year after year, when there is actually no physical cause for it. Is it a product of "mental cause?" It is a "Mind Trap".

You can reason with a stutterer and they know that there is no need for them to stutter. They can even understand the reasons why they developed the distressful habit, and that there is no reason why they have to continue, yet they still stutter. Why? They are caught in a "Mind Trap."

FEAR OF HEIGHTS

A client has a great, unreasonable fear of being in high places. Every time they get in a situation where they might fall, vertigo grips them, and they feel an impulse that they are going to plunge into the abyss below. You reason with such a person, that their current situation holds no danger of falling, yet they still feel like they are going to fall. It is a dreadful fear. They may even recall a past time when a fall would have cost then their life and understand the origin of the fear. He can know that he is now in this time in no danger of falling, yet the fear of falling persists. He is caught in a "Mind Trap."

RELEASING MIND TRAPS

Clients caught in "Mind Traps" present difficult cases. The entrapped pattern of mind may be so ingrained that neither conscious reason nor subconscious suggestions "springs" the trap. Traditional regression back to the source of the trauma may only increase the disturbance.

What can you the hypnotherapist do to help your client release a disturbing persistent past pattern of behavior? You need to deal with mind traps differently than conventional problems.

First, understand that "Mind Traps" are the personal creation of the person. They are very personal.

Second, understand that "Mind Traps" exist entirely within the mind of the person. They seem tangible, but actually they are intangible phantoms. In other words, while they seem to exist, they do not actually exist in the client's current time and space.

THE BULLDOG APPROACH

A "Mind Trap is like a bulldog's grip." It hangs on tenaciously.

How do you get a ferocious bulldog to release his grasp? You hit him sharply on the nose, which makes him open his jaws and release his grip, and the person is free. The release has to be aggressive.

You release the client from "mind traps" in precisely the same way. Hit them "right on the nose," as it were, by bringing the REALIZATION that actuality belongs to the <u>here and now</u> – it does not belong to the past. "Mind traps" are not reality in the here and now. Thus, they really are nonexistent. Establish that recognition in the subconscious of the client, and you free the client on the instant.

Hypnotize the client and relate to their subconscious the past is over and done. In your suggestions (instructions) to the subconscious) hit it right on the head. In assimilating this basic truth, mind transforms it into thought within the biocomputer brain of the client, which commences a new track of behavior for the client. In recognizing that it no longer exists in current space and time, the "mind trap" is opened, and the client is released.

In the process, you bring in a realization that a "mind trap" is but a traumatic past memory that persists. <u>The past is but memories that will never happen again. Only the here and now is real.</u> Get that point across to the client's subconscious and the trap loses its power. You've helped them spring a mind trap! This can be a specialty or a hypnotherapeutic business in itself.

MODUS OPERANDI: MIND TRAP HYPNOTHERAPY

Appreciate that an entirely different mental realm is used in releasing a client from a "mind trap" than in any other hypnotherapy.

"Trauma is just an unwelcome memory, which has been allowed to continue. The past is but memory that will never happen again, only the here and now is real. There is no need to go back to release a disturbance from the past, your life is in the here and now– it does not belong to the past. The past is gone and in truth, no such disturbance even exists. You now REALIZE that any __________ (sexual limits, stuttering, fear) are not your reality. Your reality is in the here and now. The past has no reality in the present and its existence in the present is entirely a delusion. The past is really nonexistent.

Because your subconscious mind now recognizes this fully, you are free in this instant. This is a truth in fact. You now instantly and automatically have a new happy, healthy track of behavior. You function perfectly, as God intended you to in the here and now."

One thing more about "mind traps." As they open and the person is being released from its jaws energy is needed to open the trap fully. They have been in the same position for so long that they are probably rusty. For that purpose, the client and the hypnotherapist perform the OM MANTRA together. The sound of OM starts a Cosmic Energy Flow, which is mentally directed for the purpose of opening fully the "Mind Trap" to release the client.

"So now, to open the flow of energy entirely so that you are feeling perfect in every way, let's tone this sound "OM." Let it resonate and vibrate you from bottom to top and you will feel the great freedom of the cosmic flow of energy which is your reality in the here and now. Let's begin: OM." (Begin and they will follow your sound. It makes you feel great. too.)

Too simple to work? Try it and see what results you get. It's not difficult at all, as actually a "Mind Trap" is cause for continual mental tension (stress), and mind is most happy to let it go within the energy realm of AUMMMMM.

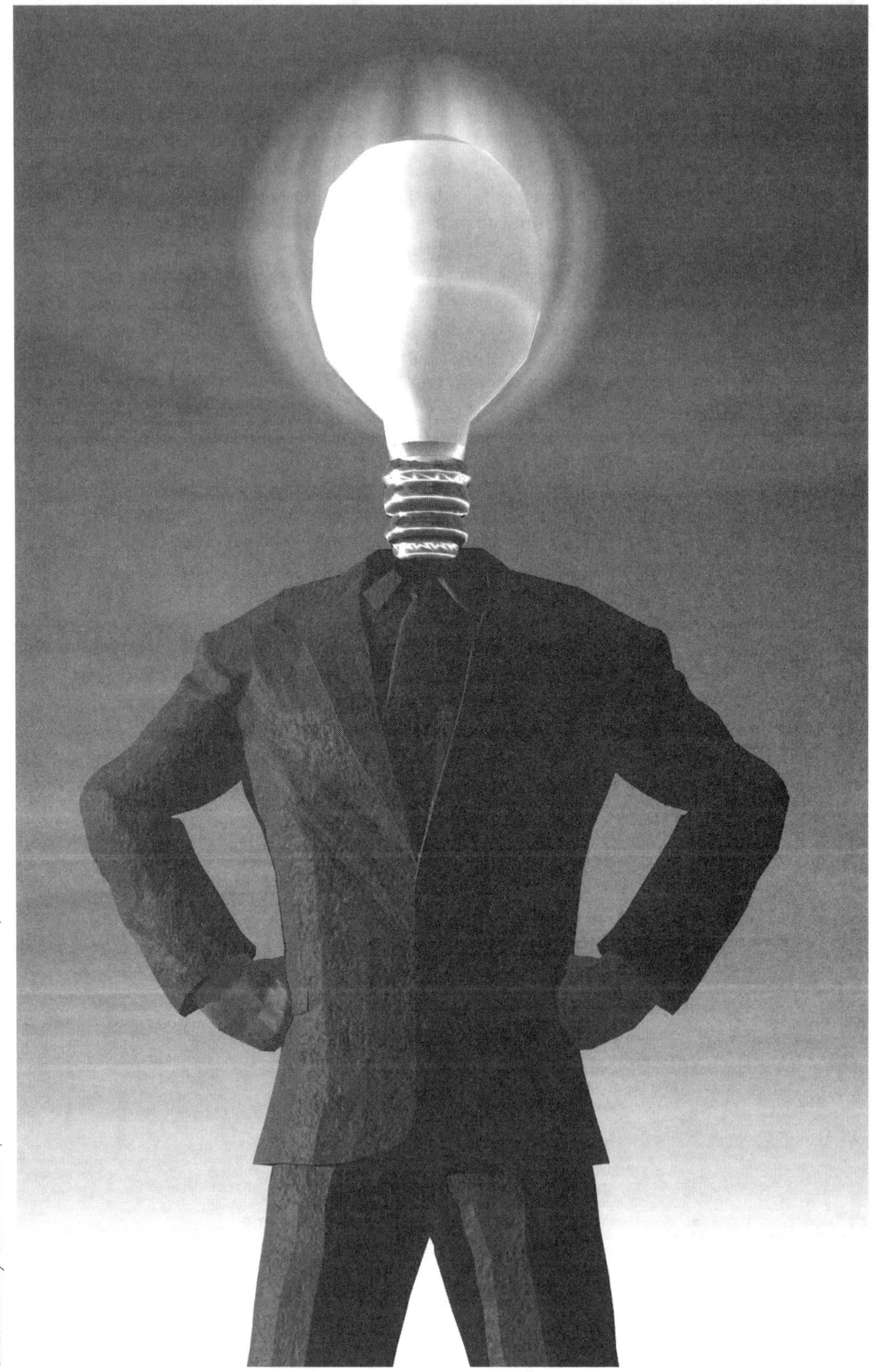

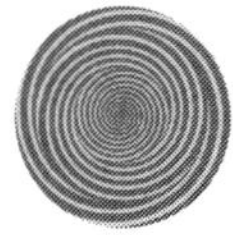

~ *Chapter 110* ~
STOCKWELL-NICHOLAS
COGNITIVE-BEHAVIOR HYPNOTHERAPY

By Shelley Stockwell-Nicholas, PhD

Conscious + Subconscious Awareness = Cognitive-Behavior Hypnotherapy

---

Includes
Cognitive-Behavior Hypnotherapy
Mind-Trap Games
> **Labeling and Name-Calling**
> **Locked-In, Black and White Thinking**
> **Sweeping Generalities**
> **Nit-Picking Negativity**
> **Positives Don't Count**
> **Perfectionism or Nothing**
> **The Great Mind Reader Concludes…**
> **Big Mistakes, Little Successes**
> **Power & Control Game**
> **Coulda/Woulda/Shoulda**
> **Broken Record**
> **Worry Game**
> **Complain Game**
> **Blame Game**
> **A Hypnotic Game To End All Mind Trap Games**

"Real-eyes" your thoughts and actions and you get a grip on joy!

I created Cognitive-Behavior Hypnotherapy (CBH) (also called Conscious Awareness Hypnotherapy (CAH) or "Conscious/Subconscious Behavior Modification") for clients who like a logical/rational spin for positive change. This profound learning experience helps your client consciously understand and remember to change dysfunctional thinking. It offers automatic coping skills through self-observation, mental rehearsal and post hypnotic suggestion.

The precursor to Cognitive-Behavior Hypnotherapy was Cognitive Therapy (Developed by Ellis-1962, Bandura-1969, Mahoney and Arknoff-1974, Aaron Beck-1976 and Meichenbaum-1977) that contended that emotion results from how you *interpret* what you feel. You shift underlying emotion by consciously analyzing self-talk and behavior goes the theory. But how do you get an undisciplined person or a person lacking self-control and will or won't-power to systematically analyze conscious thoughts and actions?

That's where hypnosis comes in.

Hypnotherapists know that thought, behavior and emotion *originate* in the subconscious mind. If you ask your aware mind to change a pattern that has its origin in the inner mind, it's a little like calling in a plumber to fix your electricity. Cognitive Awareness Hypnotherapy conditions the veiled mind to report limiting thoughts and behavior to the aware mind so they work together to create right thinking and right action. Additionally, bumps on point-of-view lane come from past imprints. Hypnosis is the direct route to the subconscious and the source of limiting imprints, behavior and self-talk. It makes for a smooth ride.

Sessions focus on fourteen "mind trap games" (distorted or limiting thought patterns). You may pinpoint a mind trap game by actively listening to your client as they speak. For example, if they say, "nobody ever cares about me" suspect a "sweeping generality" mind trap. You could also employ an old Gestalt technique and focus on a habitual gesture to underscore a mind trap game. Let's say that during your pre interview, you notice your client regularly bite their lip, you could say, "as an experiment, notice your teeth biting your lip. What are your teeth saying to your lip? What is your lip saying to your teeth?"

You can discuss and reveal mind traps both in and out of trance. Perhaps the easiest way to discover and dispel a mind trap is to hypnotize your client and ask their mindful self if they have that specific pattern. If one is revealed, offer overriding suggestions for it. I like to pinpoint one or two mind traps per session.

In general this approach, like all hypnotic behavior modification, teaches the client to accentuate the positive and eliminate the negative.

MODUS OPERANDI: STOCKWELL'S COGNITIVE-BEHAVIOR HYPNOTHERAPY

Interview the person and listen for and write down exactly any negative or limiting comments they speak. You will use their words as examples.

PRETALK

To begin a Cognitive-Behavior Hypnotherapy session, explain to your client:

"Cognitive-Behavior Hypnotherapy, trains your thoughts for right thinking and your behavior for right action, so that you achieve your goals and are happy. It helps you rethink assumptions and knee jerk responses."

For golfers, I like to say, **"Thoughts are like playing golf. Limiting thoughts are sand traps that keep you from your dreams. Positive thoughts make dreams come real and when you learn to automatically shift the way you speak to yourself, you easily stay on the fairway and may even get a hole in one! What you are about to learn keeps you on course and out of the hazards."**

At this point, you may teach what contributes to our point of view by using the memory peg **PRETAB**:

Perception
Rules (that you use to explain your perception to yourself)
Expectation
Thought
Assumption
Belief

"How you use your perceptions, rules, expectations, thoughts, assumptions and beliefs (PRETAB) determines how happy you are. When they are aligned for your highest good, life works perfectly. If they are negatively distorted, life becomes difficult. The hypnosis we are about to do helps you be positive and proactive in your viewpoint and your life."

THE SESSION

Induce trance using your favorite induction and when they are deeply relaxed, talk to them about "Mind Traps." If they are resistant to trance tell them to just breath fully and close their eyes as they answer questions: **"As you embark on a new way of thinking, a new attitude, you learn to consciously monitor what you hear yourself say both inside your head and to others. As you hear your words, check in with yourself and notice how your thoughts settle with you; how they feel. If a thought sits well, that's fine. If it makes you upset or uncomfortable you will instantly replace it with a more realistic and logical sentence. Hypnotists call this reprogramming.**

To resolve ______________ (your issue) **you'll identify any limiting thoughts you say. We call these mind traps. For example, one mind trap is 'All or Nothing Thinking.' Things are all or nothing, right or wrong, never or always, either/or. An example would be if you say to yourself 'I can *only* be successful or I'm a failure.'** (or use an actual all or nothing statement they made to you). **With no middle ground and no shades of gray, this game certainly could limit possibilities.**

Not every mind trap is unacceptable. You will be the judge. Imagine that you hear yourself say an all or nothing statement like *"I will never, ever, ever as long as I live use heroin."* **That will perfectly acceptable, whereas, the remark "I'll never trust a man** *(woman)* *again"* **may not sit too well. As you listen to your self-talk and what you say to others and yourself you check in and notice how that phrase or thought sits with you. Does it work to bring you harmony and joy? Ask yourself 'how do I feel** (or if they are a man, 'how do I think') **when I say a particular thing?' Then instantly change any limiting thought to a positive, practical one. Hypnosis uses the power of suggestion to help you do this. Here is a perfect affirmation for you. Go deep into yourself and let these ideas become your reality:**

You are a positively developing personality…learning new and better ways to think, act and react. Positive change is exciting. You positively change your words, thoughts and actions. You claim joy and vitality. You find positive ways to release frustration. You stay aware and express easily your truth and yourself. You do good things for yourself. You are awake to your thoughts and actions. You seek out and enjoy others. You choose healthy people who are safe to talk with. You are natural, outgoing and spontaneous. You release any thought or behavior that harm you. You are kind to yourself and others. You release energy in healthy ways. You feel good. Every day in every way you feel better and better. You are your own perfect mommy, daddy, best friend, lover and cheering section. You are 100% responsible for everything you create in your world. You choose joy. Joy is your compass. You are free to live life joyously in the here and now. You are responsible for your joy. You choose to feel great. You free yourself to be happy."

THE MIND TRAPS

Then define each mind trap and underscore any heard in the interview.

If you discover a phrase that fits a specific trap, ask the subconscious mind to change it right now to a more accurate truism, read the appropriate suggestions that follows each trap. And/or reverse any mind traps you heard in the interview. Take your time. Give the subconscious time to analyze and replace a hurtful word pattern with one that brings accomplishment. I use the "I" form in the suggestion formula because it helps my client identify more closely. You could write a suggestion formula as an "affirmation" and tell your client to recite it daily. Or, you could let their own subconscious mind issue the correct affirmation for themselves as a "homework" assignment.

Now continue:

"If you always do what you've always done, you'll always get what you've always gotten. You determine if what you say to yourself brings happiness or not. If you are unhappy, upset, stuck in the past, or bored most likely your self-talk is not working. You'll be the judge of that.

Here are the Mind Trap Games one by one. If you think you might play one let me know by saying, 'familiar' (or if using finger signals: 'lifting your finger'). We'll explore each in detail.
1. **Labeling & Name Calling**
2. **Locked-In, Black and White Thinking**
3. **Sweeping Generalities**
4. **Nit-Picking Negativity**
5. **Positives Don't Count**
6. **Perfectionism Or Nothing**
7. **The Great Mind Reader Concludes…**
8. **Big Mistakes, Little Successes**
9. **Power And Control Game**
10. **Coulda/Woulda/Shoulda**
11. **Broken Record**
12. **Worry Game**
13. **Blame Game**
14. **Complain Game"**

1. LABELING AND NAME CALLING
"You are an idiot."
"I am so stupid"
"I'm a loser."
"Liar, liar pants on fire."

"Labels are like writing fiction. Childhood labels call out names like good girl, trouble maker, slow learner, genius, crippled and have consequences on your behavior. As we get older we often characterize others and ourselves by the work we do, our shape and the way we dress. The problem in living up to a label is that it may hold you back from being and feeling genuine. The problem with labeling another is that you may miss their magnificence."

"Do you label or name-call? (Pause and wait for response.)

Give an example. (Let them give you an example or you lovingly cite one you heard them saying in the interview.)

What does that negative name or label mean to you? (You can wait for them to speak)

Where did you get that idea? (You can allow them to answer.)

How does it benefit you? (Wait for response.)

Is it in your best interest to keep that label? (Pause for response.)

If it doesn't benefit you, are you willing to let it go?" (Get their agreement.)

RE-MARK-ABLE AFFIRMATION
"Here is your affirmation. Repeat it now and if ever you hear yourself using negative name-calling, 'Immediately I positively re-label things with a better name…one that makes you feel better, and affirm I take each person and situation on an individual basis. I think and speak from the heart. I speak kindly to myself. I think kindly toward others. I notice if I made a mistake and I correct it. I am authentic with myself and others.'"

2. LOCKED-IN, BLACK AND WHITE THINKING
"I am absolutely not stubborn and I won't budge on that one an inch."
"Because I'm I'll never _________ (get married…again/lose weight/find a job…)"
"Nobody like me, everybody hates me, guess I'll eat some worms…"
"I'll either go to school or I'll be a failure."

"With locked-in thinking, things are right or wrong, black or white, never or always, either/or and you are either a success or failure. We all vow 'never again' so that we don't make the same mistakes twice, and that is good, but when locked-in thoughts become an excuse and stands between you and happiness, you know it. Never/always thinking can disempower freedom of choice and narrow your scope. It has a faulty assumption that there is only one potential outcome."

"**Do you use locked-in thinking?** (Pause and wait for response.)
If so, give me an example. (Let them give you an example or you lovingly cite one you heard them saying in the interview.)
Go inside yourself and honestly decide if that thought benefits you. (Wait for response. If they say yes you could move on to another mind trap. You decide. If they say no, continue.)
What does that locked-in thought mean to you? (You can wait for them to speak.)
Where did you get that idea? (Allow them to answer.)
Is it in your best interest to keep that either/or thinking? (Pause for response.)
If it doesn't benefit you, are you willing to let it go? (Get their agreement.)
Okay, repeat this affirmation now and if and if you ever hear any such thoughts or words inside yourself:

SHADES OF GRAY SUGGESTIONS:
"I discover an unlimited range of possibilities, choices and outcomes. I enjoy the subtleties of life and open my mind to new possibilities. I open to the now with all its surprises and unlimited possibilities. Life is dynamic. Each day is a new day. Each experience is a new experience. I lighten up. I am flexible. I have fun. I am an artist of life. I widen my scope."

3. SWEEPING GENERALITIES
"All _________ are jerks."
"I have bad Karma."
"Nobody cares about me.
"I can't take tests."
"I don't know."

"With over-generalizing one single glitch becomes a never-ending proof of failure or defeat. Over-generalizing is oversimplification.

Do you use sweeping generalities? (Pause and wait for response.)

If so, give me an example. (Let them give you an example or you lovingly cite one you heard them saying in the interview.)

Go inside yourself and honestly decide if that thought benefits you. (Wait for response. If they say yes you could move on to another mind trap. You decide. If they say no, continue.)

What does that over-generalizing thought mean to you? (Wait for them to speak.)

Where did you get that idea? (Allow them to answer.)

Is it in your best interest to keep that sweeping thought? (Pause for response.)

If it doesn't benefit you are you willing to let it go? (Get their agreement.)

Okay, repeat this affirmation now and if you hear any such thoughts or words inside yourself."

DETAILING SUGGESTIONS:

"I am keenly aware of my thoughts and words. I take things on an individual basis; one at a time. My viewpoint is well balanced. I enjoy positive tenacity. If my mind goes to sweeping generalities, I say to myself 'enough! I choose joy. Joy is my compass' and think of new ways to move forward in my thoughts and my life."

4. NIT-PICKING NEGATIVITY

"The story I wrote was no good. I didn't dot the 'i'."
"Throw the loaf away there is one sesame seed on it."
"I look hideous, I have a pimple on my arm."

Finicky nit-pickers dwell on the negatives and discard the positives.

"Do you nit pick? (Pause and wait for response.)

If so, give me an example. (Let them give you an example or you lovingly cite one you heard them saying in the interview)

Go inside yourself and honestly decide if that thought benefits you. *(Wait for response. If they say yes you could move on to another mind trap. You decide. If they say no, continue.)*

What does that nitpicking thought mean to you? (Wait for them to speak.)

Where did you get that idea? (Allow them to answer.)

Is it in your best interest to keep that nitpicking thought? (Pause for response.)

If it doesn't benefit you are you willing to let it go? (Get their agreement.)

Okay, repeat this affirmation now and if you hear any such thoughts or words inside yourself."

NOT TO NIT PICK SUGGESTIONS:

"I am keenly aware of my self talk and the words I speak. I quickly and easily change any negative to positive. I lighten up. Any negativity becomes fertilizer for flowers growing in my beautiful garden of mind. I approve of myself. I choose joy. Joy is my compass.' I think of new positive ways to move forward in my thoughts and my life. I move my body, make new positive statements and get a life."

5. POSITIVES DON'T COUNT
"He is only nice to me because he thought I was someone else."
"I got the job 'cause I faked them out."
"My accomplishments don't mean a thing."
"My positive qualities aren't that big a deal."

Negative becomes an excuse not to try and positives are discarded.

"Do you discount positives? (Pause and wait for response)
If so, give me an example. (Let them give you an example or you lovingly cite one you heard them saying in the interview)
Go inside yourself and honestly decide if that thought benefits you. (Wait for response. If they say yes you could move on to another mind trap. You decide. If they say no, continue.)
What does discounting positive thought mean to you? (Wait for them to speak.)
Where did you get that idea? (Allow them to answer.)
Is it in your best interest to keep that discounting thought? (Pause for response.)
If it doesn't benefit you are you willing to let it go? (Get their agreement.)
Okay, repeat this affirmation now and if you hear any such thoughts or words inside yourself."

YES! I'M POSITIVE SUGGESTIONS:
"I celebrate all the good inside of me. I am proud of my mini and maxi successes. The world is in a conspiracy to do me good. I deserve good. I am worthy. If my mind discounts the positive, I say to myself 'enough! I choose joy. Joy is my compass.'" I think of new ways to positively move forward in my thoughts and my life. I accentuate the positive, eliminate the negative and don't mess with Mr. In-Between."

6. PERFECTIONISM
"What if I made a mistake?"
"If you can't do it right; don't do it at all."
"I'm so overwhelmed I don't know where to start; so I don't."
"I'm waiting until _______ (get married when the relationship is perfect) the time is right."
"I can't start 'til all the ducks are in a row."

"Doing things right is important. But pushed to excess, perfectionism destroys spontaneity, wastes time and is perfectly boring. The three P's in the PPP game stand for perfectionism, procrastination and paralysis. The PPP dance begins, 'I must do it perfectly.' 'I won't tolerate mistakes.' Rather than fail, 'If I can't do it perfectly, I'll put it off until I can.' Then finally, "If I can't do it perfectly, might as well not do it at all.'
Perfectionists judge their worth, potential or ability as superior and will not settle for less. This is similar to negative thinking. Perfectionists focus on what has not been done. Instead of praise, they generally offer criticism to themselves and others."

"Do you stall out because of your demand to be perfect? (Pause and wait for response.)
If so, give me an example. (Let them give you an example or you lovingly cite one you heard them say.)
Go inside yourself and honestly decide if that thought benefits you. (Wait for response. If they say yes you could move on to another mind trap. You decide. If they say no, continue.)

What does that perfectionism mean to you? (Wait for them to speak.)
Where did you get that idea? (Allow them to answer.)
Is it in your best interest to keep that perfectionistic thought? (Pause for response.)
If it doesn't benefit you are you willing to let it go? (Get their agreement.)
Okay, repeat this affirmation now and if you hear any such thoughts or words inside yourself."

BEST IS BETTER AFFIRMATION

"I am my journey. The destination is the journey. I am beautiful because I 'am.' I realistically accept myself as a human, coming to balance. 'Mistakes' are opportunities to learn. I am realistic. I am in action. 'Persistence, patience and perseverance' is new motto. I move my body and thoughts in positive ways. I move my face to a smile. When I'm in action I feel terrific. I break tasks into small action steps. I start with part I want to do least and get it out of the way. I do something every day for at least ten minutes. After I do my ten minutes I can decide if I want to keep at it. As I progress I reward myself with a walk, a sip of tea or a glass of water. I enjoy beginnings, middles and endings. Life is an adventure. I love to move my body and my mind.

I reach my own goals. I enjoy the journey to my goals. I do what I want to do. I do what you request only if I want to. If not, I do something else. I am in action. Other's goals are their business. I support others when they request my help, otherwise I back off. I make sure that my children have guidance and REALISTIC expectations from me. If something must be done perfectly for realistic reasons, I make sure that I am diligent and accurate. I honor each person's right to live their own life, learn their own lessons and choose or not choose their own goals. I focus my attention on learning, growing and I lighten up. I have all the resources to meet all of life's challenges. I value myself. I believe in my self. I can. I will. I am.

If I don't try, I fail before I begin. Either I win the race or I don't. Either I make the deadline or I don't. Either I get the job or I don't. Either I lick this thing or I don't. Either way, I can handle it. I'm just experiencing life. I like completing tasks. I do them step by step until they are complete. I'm terrific at doing things well. I allow myself to grow and learn with each new task. I open myself to each new challenge. I do my best. I develop and learn as I do."

7. THE GREAT MIND-READER CONCLUDES…

"I know you don't think about me and will never ask me to marry you."
"I know that things will turn out badly."
"A catastrophe can strike at any time.
"When I see someone whispering I know that they are gossiping about me."

"Negative fortunetellers predict negative outcome as fact. This works fine if you want to be sure that you are going to have a miserable vacation. Negative predictions distort and exaggerate the worst possible conclusion."

"Do you mind read? (Pause and wait for response.)
If so, give me an example. (Let them give you an example or you lovingly cite one you heard them saying in the interview.)
Go inside yourself and honestly decide if that thought benefits you. (Wait for response. If they say yes you could move on to another mind trap. You decide. If they say no, continue.)
What does that mind-reading conclusion mean to you? (Wait for them to speak.)

Where did you get that idea? (Allow them to answer.)

Is it in your best interest to keep that mind-reading conclusion? (Pause for response.)

If it doesn't benefit you are you willing to let it go? (Get their agreement.)

Okay, repeat this affirmation now and if and when you hear any such thoughts or words inside yourself."

BE HERE NOW SUGGESTIONS:

"My life is now and in this moment I choose to be happy. I get the details and facts. I plan for the most positive conclusion and am not attached to the outcome. I enjoy sweet spontaneous fate to unfold unlimited possibilities for me. What are the odds of a bad thing happening? Really? This moment is the only truth. I live in this moment and make positive choices about what and how I think. I hold other people capable of having their own thoughts. I only know for sure what I think. The future is made up of possibilities that change instantly with my positive thoughts."

8. BIG MISTAKES, LITTLE SUCCESSES

"She can speak perfectly. I always make mistakes."

"This mind trap looks at mistakes through a microscope and successes through the back end of binoculars. A little glitch is blown out of proportion to a gigantic scale or a lovely success is shrunk to the size of an ant."

"Do you see mistakes as big and success as little?" (Pause and wait for response.)

If so, give me an example. (Let them give you an example or you lovingly cite one you heard them saying in the interview.)

Go inside yourself and honestly decide **if that thought benefits you.** (Wait for response. If they say yes you could move on to another mind trap. You decide. If they say no, continue.)

What does that big mistake, little success mean to you? (Wait for them to speak.)

Where did you get that idea? (Allow them to answer.)

Is it in your best interest to keep that big mistake attitude? (Pause for response.)

If it doesn't benefit you are you willing to let it go? (Get their agreement.)

Okay, repeat this affirmation now and if you hear any such thoughts or words inside yourself."

CELEBRATE SUCCESS:

"I now discover the gifts God has hidden inside of me. I celebrate every success in this moment by putting my hands on my heart and saying 'I am proud of you for __________.' And I congratulate myself for five baby steps of goodness I have done for others or myself. One goodness is saying this affirmation. If my mind goes to this limiting pattern, I say to myself 'enough! I am a winner.'"

9. POWER & CONTROL GAME

"I am toxic waste"

"Everything I touch turns to junk."

"I make my mommy very unhappy."

"It's my way or the highway"

"The power and control mind trap makes you personally responsible for all the evil in the world. Sorry to say, you are not all that powerful. You cannot control the Mother Earth, God and what others do or don't do. The trick is to know when and what you can control."

"Do you think that you control the world? (Pause and wait for response)

If so, give me an example. (Let them give you an example or you lovingly cite one you heard them saying in the interview.)

Go inside yourself and honestly decide if that thought benefits you. (Wait for response. If they say yes you could move on to another mind trap. You decide. If they say no, continue.)

What does a power and control thought mean to you? (Wait for them to speak.)

Where did you get that idea? (Allow them to answer.)

Is it in your best interest to keep that power and control attitude? (Pause for response.)

If it doesn't benefit you are you willing to let it go? (Get their agreement.)

Okay, repeat this affirmation now and if and when you hear any such thoughts or words inside yourself."

LIVE AND LET LIVE SUGGESTIONS

"I nourish myself and others. I take responsibility for only that which I truly influence. I learn what I can and can't control. I control how I drive my car but I can't control a spaced out driver in front of me. I control how I react to the spaced out driver.

I don't control my actual age, the calendar or the number of hours in the day. I control how old I act. I control how my day is spent and how much time I spend on a particular project or activity. I control what I do. I control my goals. The outcome is influenced by my action but I cannot control what will happen. I choose what action I will take or not take. I take right action.

I control my thoughts and what I say to myself. I decide how I react to my emotions. My self-talk determines my belief and behavior. So ultimately, I control my behavior."

I choose my friends and who I spend time with. I control how I treat others and what I say to them. The words I use impact my relationships with others. I control communicating my needs to others. I control how I raise my children.

I choose how much money I make and spend. I am in charge of the job I choose to do. I decide whether I stay or go in that job. (I don't usually choose if I get laid off or not).

I control my health by my diet, habits, sleep and attitudes. I choose whether or not to smoke, drink or take drugs. I control my exercise habits. I control how I react to illness and pain. (I cannot control another's health or death.)

I control how I live my life and fill my time. I choose the activities I do or don't do.

I book my own dance card.

I hold everyone (except little children) fully capable to run their own life. I empower myself. I am response•able for running my own life. I allow spontaneous fate to co-create exciting change and adventure. Others do themselves perfectly. I give up the myth that I can change others. If they change they choose it. No matter how many times I replay the scene, if I play my old part, 'they' will always play the flip side of my part. I stop playing the game."

10. COULDA/WOULDA/SHOULDA

"You should have ___________."

"I would if I could. I could if I would."

"If grandma had wheels she'd be a bicycle."

"You ought to…must…have-to…

"Criticizing yourself and others with should/shouldn't statements make you feel terrible."

"Do you 'should' on yourself? (Pause and wait for response)

If so, give me an example. (Let them give you an example or you lovingly cite one you heard them saying in the interview.)

Go inside yourself and honestly decide if that thought benefits you. (Wait for response. If they say yes you could move on to another mind trap. You decide. If they say no, continue.)

What does a coulda/woulda/shoulda thought mean to you? (You can wait for them to speak.)

Where did you get that idea? (Allow them to answer.)

Is it in your best interest to keep a coulda/woulda/shoulda attitude? (Pause for response.)

If it doesn't benefit you are you willing to let it go? (Get their agreement.)

Okay, repeat this affirmation if you hear any such thoughts or words inside yourself."

CUT YOURSELF SOME SLACK SUGGESTIONS:

"I stop 'shoulding' on myself. I change 'I'll try' to 'I will' or 'I won't.' 'I choose' to 'I choose not to.' I change 'Woulda, coulda, shoulda' to 'I did,' 'It was,' and 'Oh well.' The change is a relief."

11. BROKEN RECORD

"You remind me of___________."

"…and now ladies and gentleman, once again for the very first time may I present the same story."

"A broken record always comes back to the same drama with the same actors no matter the situation.

Do you play a broken record? (Pause and wait for response.)

If so, give me an example. (Let them give you an example or you lovingly cite one you heard them saying in the interview.)

Go inside yourself and honestly decide if that thought benefits you. (Wait for response. If they say yes you could move on to another mind trap. You decide. If they say no, continue.)

What does a broken record thought mean to you? (Wait for them to speak.)

Where did you get that idea? (Allow them to answer.)

Is it in your best interest to keep a broken record attitude? (Pause for response.)

If it doesn't benefit you are you willing to let it go? (Get their agreement.)

Ok. Repeat this affirmation now and if and when you hear any such thoughts or words inside yourself."

UNSTUCK AFFIRMATION:

"I am present. I enjoy the now. I stay conscious, awake and alert. I easily listen to others without adding my story. It is safe in my world. You experience each moment as a new delicious one.

12. WORRY GAME

"Worrywarts are highly creative and dream up any situation to ruminate about; being too fat, too slim, too poor, what others are doing or not doing. Worrying can become a very hazardous mind trap."

"Do you worry a lot? (Pause and wait for response.)

If so, give me an example. (Let them give you an example or you lovingly cite one you heard them saying in the interview.)

Go inside yourself and honestly decide if that thought benefits you. (Wait for response. If they say yes you could move on to another mind trap. You decide. If they say no, continue.)
What does worry mean to you? (Wait for them to speak.)
Where did you get that idea? (Allow them to answer.)
Is it in your best interest to keep a worrying attitude? (Pause for response.)
If it doesn't benefit you are you willing to let it go? (Get their agreement.)
Okay, repeat this affirmation now and if and when you hear any such thoughts or words inside yourself.

WHAT, ME WORRY?

"Worry shows that I have a creative mind. I now turn my creative mind toward interesting pursuits. Drawing, painting, building, designing, writing, sculpting or making positive plans that put me in the driver's seat. I thoroughly engage myself in things I enjoy. If I learned to worry from someone else, I give this pattern back to him or her. It's theirs. I don't want it and I don't need it. The instant I fret, I deliberately direct my mind to pleasant activity. I get out of my chair and walk around, pet the cat, hug someone, wash the dishes, talk with a friend or think of something else to do. Sing 'pack up your troubles in your old kit bag and smile, smile, smile.' Or sing 'Don't worry, be happy.' I choose to enjoy my life. Nix on the News. I choose to listen to, read and watch pleasant things."

13. THE COMPLAIN GAME

"Every silver lining has a cloud."
"I'm so tired/sleepy/overworked/underpaid."
"My hair is coming out by the handfuls, what should I do?"
"He/she/I never come home on time."
"Life/school/work sucks."
"I've got troubles, I've got worries, I've got my gal who could ask for anything more."
"Oh, my aching bones."
"Poor me."
"Sufferin' succotash! If you've heard these kinds of messages from yourself you've tuned into a painful victim game. Complaining may engage people in conversation…for a while. Then it becomes boring. We usually learn to complain from caretakers. If you get stuck in this trap your whole life can be a never-ending saga of doctor visits, "woe is me" and "ain't it awful."

"Do you complain? (Pause and wait for response.)
If so, give me an example. (Let them give you an example or lovingly cite one you heard them saying in the interview.)
Go inside yourself and honestly decide if that thought benefits you. (Wait for response. If they say yes you could move on to another mind trap. You decide. If they say no, continue.)
What does complaining mean to you? (Wait for them to speak.)
Where did you get that idea? (Allow them to answer.)
Is it in your best interest to keep a complaining attitude? (Pause for response.)
If it doesn't benefit you are you willing to let it go? (Get their agreement.)
Okay, repeat this affirmation now and if and when you hear any such thoughts or words inside yourself."

AN ATTITUDE OF GRATITUDE SUGGESTIONS:
"I'm thankful that I have been able to complain. It proves I'm alive. Indeed everything in my life is miraculous. The fact that I think, see, hear and speak are all part of the miracle of me. As I reflect on these precious gifts, I am filled with pleasure. I submerge every muscle, nerve and ligament in pleasure. How fortunate I am to be alive. I experience pleasure. I enjoy pleasing myself. I enjoy celebrating my life. It's a lot of fun to have positive exchanges. I now enjoy getting attention in positive ways. If something bothers me, I enjoy discovering why and enjoy creating positive solutions. I find creative solutions. I enjoy telling others what's on my mind so we can brainstorm solutions together. I listen to the ideas of others. If their advice is good for me, I take it. My problems belong to me. My solutions belong to me. I don't wear others out with my problems. I enjoy overcoming challenges. I get attention from others and myself in positive ways."

IF ANOTHER PLAYS THE GAME OF COMPLAIN
Don't get engaged in the game. Give them a hug. Say only once: "It sounds like you're having a rough time," or offer a helping hand solution. Then notice their response. If they discount your ideas and continue playing say: "You're wise. I'm sure you'll figure out what you need to do to be happy." If they appear eager to negotiate a solution, jump right in, the game is over. If not, disengage from the downer; they are boring and depressing.

14. THE BLAME GAME
"It's always my/your fault."
"The computer (car, bus, computer, traffic, internet...) is at fault"
"My secretary (boss, husband, wife, kids, democrats, republicans, evil spirits, God...) screwed up"
"I drink (eat, smoke, cry, yell) because of my wife (boss, mother, father, my illness...)"
"If it wasn't for __________ I would have what I want. It's not my fault…it's theirs"
"I'm depraved because I was deprived."
"My darn shoe slipped on the step."
"It's not the kids fault, they 'act out' because of the divorce."
"If it wasn't for you, I would have (not have) divorced your father/mother long ago."
"We'd divorce but no one wants you kids."
"I have bad Karma."
"I beat my kids because I was beaten."

"Blame shifting is a cultural pastime. Drunks aren't drunks they have a "disease." Criminals aren't bad they have dysfunctional families. With yourself, the blame game is played two ways:

1. **You are responsible for something that you weren't entirely responsible for. You build a case against yourself. This can be a great way to make excuses for not doing something you are avoiding or a way to get negative attention from yourself.**

2. **Mostly blame gamers live life by default: "de fault ain't mine." Blaming others for your attitudes and behavior, make them wrong so you feel right, takes the heat off of you or lets you overlook how you contribute to a problem. Usually, when you point a finger at someone else, three fingers point at you. You may blame that "SOB" but secretly you blame yourself.**

Either way you let the fickle finger of fate focus fallaciously. In fact, it's easier to learn from mistakes and take responsibility than to put out the energy to blame. Some things are beyond our control. But how we react is within our power. Let the buck stop here and buck the blame game.

"Do you regularly blame yourself? (Pause and wait for response.)

If so, give me an example. (Let them give you an example or lovingly cite one you heard them saying in the interview.)

Do you regularly blame others or circumstances?

If so, give me an example. (Let them give you an example or lovingly sight one you heard them saying in the interview.)

Go inside yourself and honestly decide if that thought benefits you. (Wait for response. If they say yes you could move on to another mind trap. You decide. If they say no, continue.)

What does blaming mean to you? (Wait for them to speak.)

Where did you get that idea? (Allow them to answer.)

Is it in your best interest to keep a blaming attitude? (Pause for response.)

If it doesn't benefit you are you willing to let it go?" (Get their agreement.)

THE GAME OF GIFT

Okay, repeat this affirmation now and if or when you hear any such thoughts or words inside yourself.

I play 'The Game of Gift' and learn from every situation in my life. I take full responsibility for my behavior and actions. If I make a mistake, I honestly admit it. I notice what I learn and congratulate myself for taking charge of my life. If necessary, I apologize. I right wrongs. I honestly own up to the situation as my responsibility. I forgive myself. I am sensitive to others. I am sensitive to myself. I congratulate myself for growing in wisdom and responsibility. I hold others to be responsible for running their own lives. I forgive others, they were doing the best they could given who they are. They do themself perfectly. I enjoy sweet spontaneous fate. I enjoy others and their own way of doing things."

A HYPNOTIC GAME TO END ALL MIND TRAP GAMES

1. **"Replay a scene where you Name Call,** (or play any of the other traps) **but this time pretend that you are in power of your thoughts."**

2. **"Ask yourself, 'What was my payoff in creating those thoughts?'"**

3. **"If you hadn't played this mind trap game, how would you tell yourself the same story? Then tell the story again without the game."**

4. **"What did you learn from this scene?"**

5. **"Situations from the past gave you a gift. What is the gift? An insight…strength…an awareness?"**

6. **"If the same circumstances happen again, what would you do differently?"**

7. **"Promise yourself right now that if it ever happens again you will automatically do it the way you'd rather do it."**

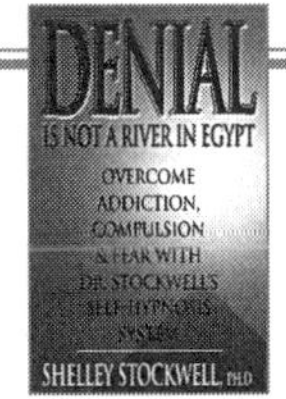

Hypno-Helper
"Denial Is Not A RIver In Egypt: Overcome Addiction, Compulsion and Fear with Dr. Stockwell's Self Hypnosis System" available on the order form at the back of this book.
"Been There, Done That, Do This" by Sam Obitz

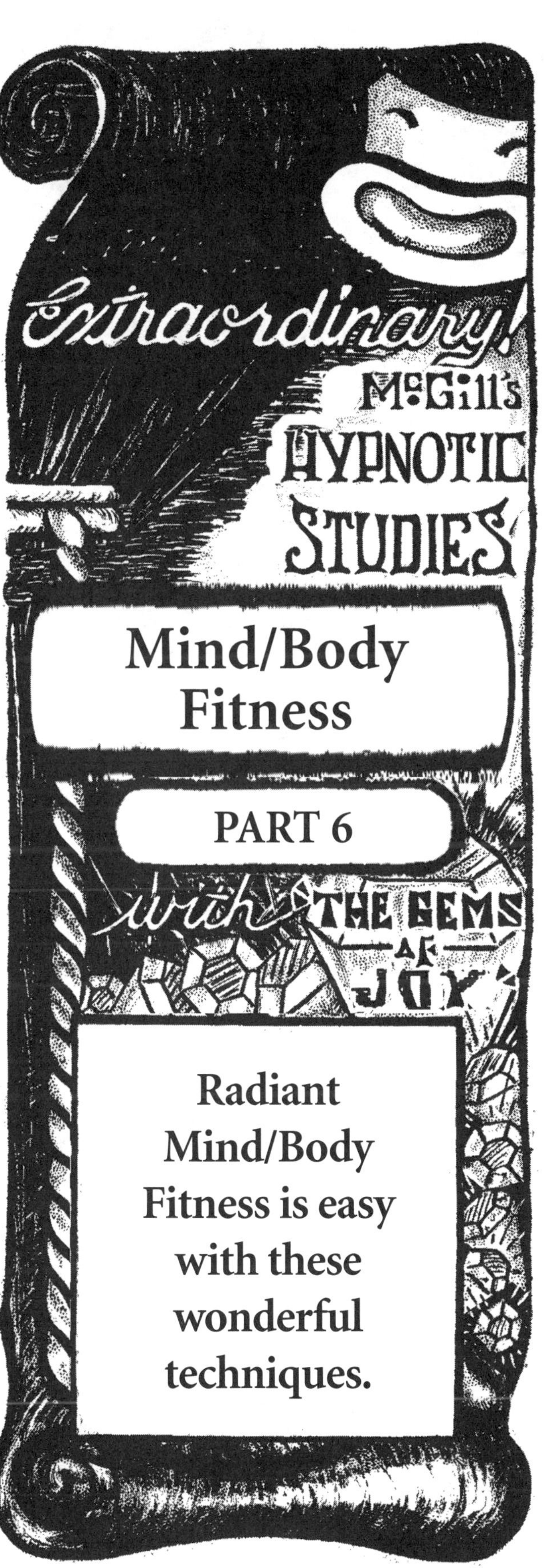

CHAPTERS IN PART SIX

111. Mental Set Hypnosis ....page 409
112. Mental Set Your Weight 411
113. Stockwell-Nicholas Joy Therapy..........413
114. Coue's Autosuggestion For Wellness ..417
115. Good Health Hypnotherapy 421
116. Anti-Aging Hunza Breath 423
117. Hypnotherapy Of Death 427
118. Common Sense Hypnotherapy 431
119. Stockwell's Hypno-Wellness 433
120. Astral Hypno-Healing 441
121. Ellner's Neuro Linguistic Healing 445
122. Reflexology Hypnotherapy 447
123. Stockwell-Nicholas Sleep Program 451
124. Vitali's Hypnoaesthetics
     For Beautiful Skin................................457
125. 3-D Hypnotherapy 461

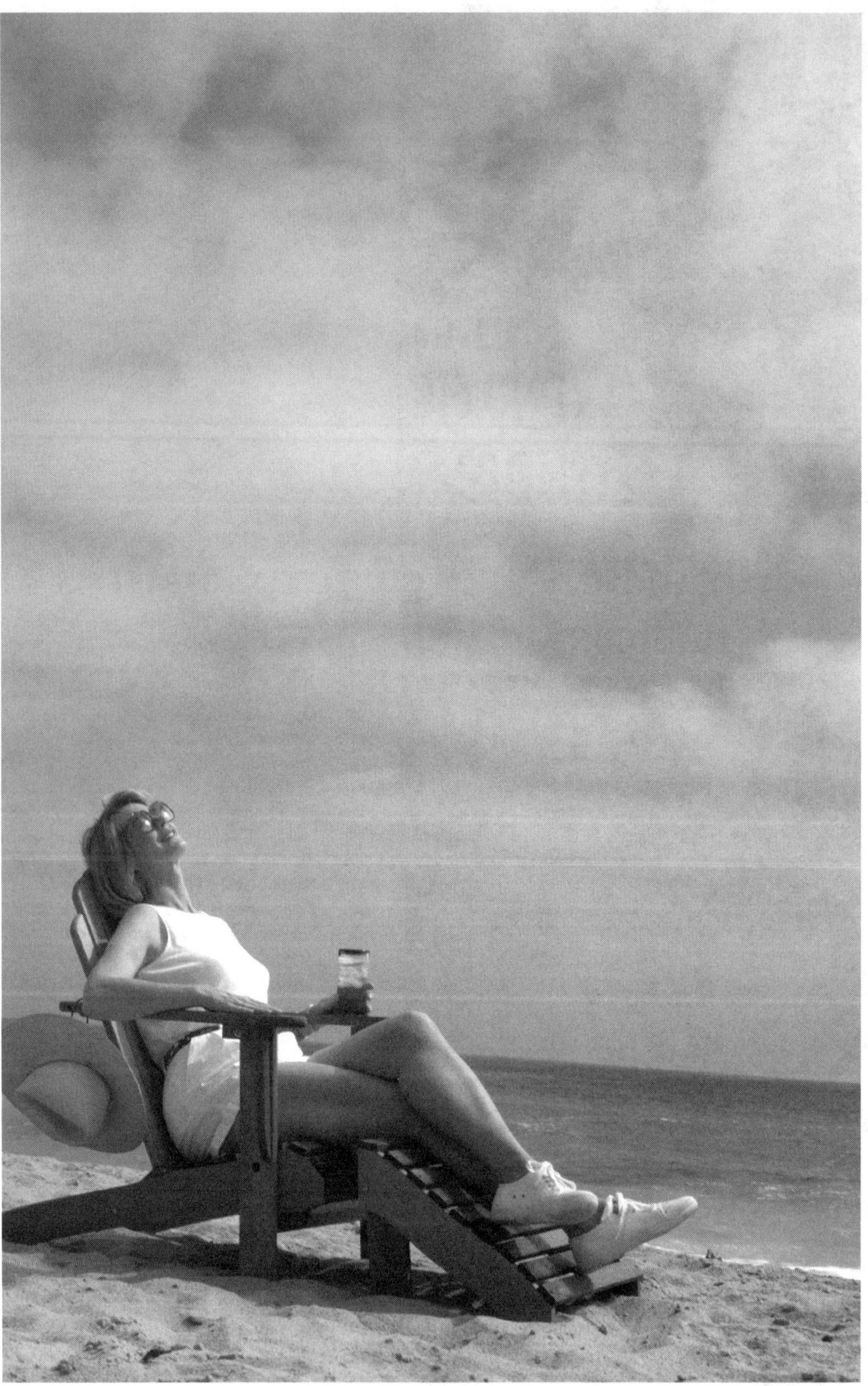

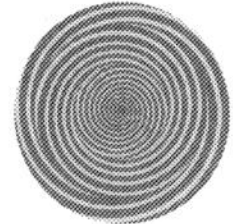

~ *Chapter 111* ~
MENTAL SET HYPNOSIS

The easiest way is to relax your mind is to let your body muscles relax. Your state of mind will mirror your muscles. Your relaxed mind in turn causes your body to relax more. Physical action causes a mental response and thoughts express themselves in physical response. It is a nice circle.

Simply the idea of calm can also bring about relaxation. Think of the word "calm" as your key word to bring relaxation into yourself. Hold a firm underlying conviction that recalling the word 'calm' will re-induce relaxation every time and anytime. Sincerely expect to relax when you think calm! Expectancy speeds up the learning and makes results certain.

Like waking hypnosis there is no formal hypnotic induction used in the 'mental-set' method. Applying its power of suggestion not only works for weight control but also in the dentist chair, to replace the need for a local anesthetic. With practice, some become so efficient in it; they use it to master pain when surgery is performed.

Use mental-set hypnosis for yourself and teach it to your clients. Let's practice this remarkably effective skill:

MODUS OPERANDI: MENTAL SET HYPNOSIS

Have your client close their eyes to shut out distractions. If your chair reclines do so. If not, then just sit easily in a fairly upright position.

"Relax your body while thinking over and over: calm...calm...calm. Visualize it; see it upon your screen of mind and feel it bringing relaxation into the muscles of your body. Make this key word stand for relaxation and establish it as a direct connection between your mind and your body. Do this association deliberately at first, and shortly you will find that every time you think 'calm' you will automatically commence to relax. Experience how pleasantly the word calm affects you.

Think of the word calm and you are calm all over in mind and body. Relax all your muscles deliberately. Let them go soft and limp. Remember that relaxing is letting go! Do not try to do anything...just let go! Complete relaxation is complete doing nothing.

Sigh and feel as if you breathe out all tension; a sigh of relief. Sighing relaxes the diaphragm. Now, take a deep breath with a great feeling of calm entering...a great feeling of calm, of utter peace. Sigh again...and again...and again.

Make all the muscles of your chest loose and limp. Relax all through the abdomen. Relax the muscles of your back. Let go all the body muscles. Relax more and more. You are becoming so calm and relaxed that you sink down into the chair more and more...

Feel as if a wave of relaxation goes down each arm right to your fingertips. All those arm and hand muscles become soft. Do it more. Now a wave of relaxation goes down your legs out to the toes. It is as if you had no bones. You make yourself soft as jelly.

Now your head…relax all the muscles around your mouth…let all the muscles of your cheeks relax…and relax those muscles around your eyes and forehead…all the muscles of your head become more and more relaxed.

Calm has taken hold of your whole body, spread all over you. It is like resting on a cloud. You are calm through and through– calm everywhere. Your body is relaxed and your mind is calm. You are quiet, calm, and peaceful. You help this feeling of calmness grow even more by thinking of something very soothing, very calming, and very tranquil. Think of a beautiful outdoor country scene…perhaps a place where you like to fish by a beautiful lake. See yourself there, quietly happy, absolutely relaxed. See again the beauty of the spot– the water, the trees, and the sky. Think how quietly beautiful it is. Imagine yourself there: calm, contended, at peace with everything.

Give yourself up wholly to the idea of calm, and know and expect that at any future time when you but think the word calm, it will bring back peace of mind and relaxation of body; just the right amount of relaxation. Set your mind so this will occur whenever you think calm, wherever you are, whatever you are doing, under any conditions. Remember that a set of expectancy brings results. Expect wholeheartedly that thinking calm will make you as calm as you need be. Think to yourself, 'Anytime, anywhere, under any circumstances, when I want to be calm all I have to do is think calm and I'll be that way.'

When you are complete, take a nice deep breath and stretch. Very good."

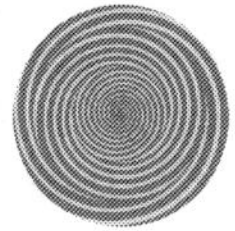

~ *Chapter 112* ~
MENTAL SET YOUR WEIGHT

Pavlov's conditioning reflex method caused a dog to salivate when a bell was rung. Humans undergo a similar conditioning process. When someone speaks of delicious things to eat, a conditioned reflex occurs; your mouth waters and an urge to eat comes in. In fact, just thinking about juicy steaks or your favorite pie makes your mouth water. This especially happens with someone who obviously enjoys eating. The spoken word does for them what the bell-ring did to the dog. The thoughts and/or spoken words have become associated with eating actual food.

People most commonly put on weight because they overeat or eat the wrong things. They do that to combat tension. Unfortunately hypertension gets worse with excess pounds.

How then is the best way to combat tension?

Relaxation!

If you want and need to release weight, cultivate a habit of being relaxed all the time. As you release hypertension you release fat. Dispose of stress and dispose of excess bulk. Learn to ring the relaxation bell instead of the dinner bell.

This induction is the same as the chapter before with added suggestions that curb the habit of overeating. **"When you sit down to a meal, think 'calm' and tension will disappear and the tendency to overeat will diminish in direct ratio."**

MODUS OPERANDI: MENTAL SET YOUR WEIGHT

Have your client close their eyes to shut out distractions. If your chair reclines do so. If not, then just have them sit easily in an upright position.

"Relax your body while thinking over and over: calm…calm…calm. Visualize it; see it upon your screen of mind and feel it bringing relaxation into the muscles of your body. Make this 'key word' stand for relaxation and establish it as a direct connection between your mind and your body. Do this association deliberately at first, and shortly you will find that every time you think calm you will automatically commence to relax. Experience how pleasantly it affects you.

Think of the word calm and you are calm all over in mind and body. Relax all your muscles deliberately. Let them go soft and limp. Remember that relaxing is letting go! Do not try to do anything…just let go! Complete relaxation is complete doing nothing.

'Sigh' and feel as if you breathe out all tension, a sigh of relief. Sighing relaxes the diaphragm. Now, take a deep breath with a great feeling of calm entering…a great feeling of calm, of utter peace. Sigh again…and again…and again.

Make all the muscles of your chest loose and limp. Relax all through the abdomen. Relax the muscles of your back. Let go all the body muscles. Relax more and more. You are becoming so calm and relaxed that you sink down into the chair more and more…

Feel as if a wave of relaxation goes down each arm right to your fingertips. All those arm and hand muscles become soft. Do it more. Now a wave of relaxation goes down your legs out to the toes. It is as if you had no bones. You make yourself soft as jelly.

Now your head. Relax all the muscles around your mouth…let all the muscles of your cheeks relax…and relax those muscles around your eyes and forehead…all the muscles of your head become more and more relaxed.

Calm has taken hold of your whole body, spread all over you. It is like resting on a cloud. You are calm through and through– calm everywhere. Your body is relaxed and your mind is calm. You are quiet, calm, and peaceful. You help this feeling of calmness grow even more by thinking of something very soothing, very calming, and very tranquil. Think of a beautiful outdoor country scene…perhaps a place where you like to fish by a beautiful lake. See yourself there, quietly happy, absolutely relaxed. See again the beauty of the spot– the water, the trees, and the sky. Think how quietly beautiful it is. Imagine yourself there: calm, content, at peace with everything.

Give yourself up wholly to the idea of calm, and know and expect that at any future time when you but think this word, it will bring back peace of mind and relaxation of body; just the right amount of relaxation. Set your mind so this will occur whenever you think calm, wherever you are, whatever you are doing, under any conditions. Remember that a set of expectancy brings results. Expect wholeheartedly that thinking calm will make you as calm as you need be. Think to yourself, 'Anytime, anywhere, under any circumstances, when I want to be calm all I have to do is think calm and I'll be that way.'

WHEN YOU SIT DOWN TO A MEAL, YOU THINK CALM, AND ALL TENSION DISAPPEARS, AND THE TENDENCY TO OVEREAT WILL DIMINISH IN DIRECT RATIO.

When you are complete, take a nice deep breath and stretch. Very good."

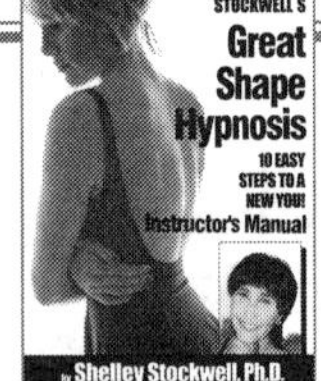

Hypno-Helper

"Stockwell's Great Shape Hypnosis: Ten Easy Steps To A New You" Instructor's Manual by Shelley Stockwell-Nicholas. This book has over 50 scripts, techniques, quizzes, exercises, helpful facts and detailed instruction on how to make money as a weight control specialist.

"Lose Weight," "No More Sugar Junkie," "Peace and Calm," "I Love Exercise" audio tapes and "Stockwell's Lose Weight Hypnosis" video tape.

All are available at the back of this book or by calling (800) 366-7908

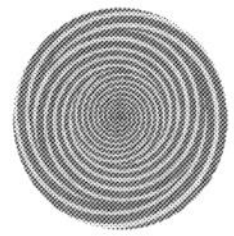

~ *Chapter 113* ~
STOCKWELL-NICHOLAS JOY THERAPY

By Shelley Stockwell-Nicholas, PhD
©2001 from "Denial Is Not A River In Egypt:
Stockwell's Hypnosis System to Overcome Depression, Addiction, Compulsion & Fear."

Includes
Love to Laugh, Laugh to Love
Laughing: The Aphrodisiac of the Mind
Stockwell's Happiness Hypnosis
Smile Homework For Clients

"Everybody's got a laughing place, a laughing place to go."
—Uncle Remus

"A human is the only animal who truly laughs…or needs to."
—Richard Lederer

Joy Therapy is a hoot. Everyone leaves laughing and loving themself. After all, love and laughter, go together.

Your client's biggest problem is acute seriosity and the ONLY reason they come for help is to FEEL GOOD. Laughter makes that happen. Laughter lets you play, helps you cope and brings joy. Humor lightens any emotional load and makes you more positive. People who laugh are less likely to be upset by negative situations.

A real or imagined smile or laugh tickles the release of positive chemicals into your brain. The "endogenous" opiates you release, (endorphins, dopamine and seratonin) are the same ones that you experience during orgasm, peak experience, an "ah ha" or runner's high. Laughing chemicals peek under the skirt of depression by suppressing stress-related hormones. That is why, after the guffaw, stress is reduced, muscles go limp and blood pressure drops.

John D. Petegrew, a neuro-biologist at the University of Queensland in Brisbane, Australia, found that the vibration of laughter reverberates your brain to re-balances and more easily use your right and left hemispheres. Every few seconds we usually see though one eye, then the other. A good belly laugh obliterates or reduces this binocular rivalry so you see simultaneously through both eyes, for up to an hour and a half. In other words, when you laugh you make a balanced spectacle of yourself.

SMILE…NOW.

A smile is a God hook that lifts you up. Smiling feels good, relaxes you and puts others at ease. If you "wiped that smile off your face" paint it back on. Have your client smile while in a trance. Have them smile as they report their biggest tragedy. They will rewire their bio-chemical response and reframe the pain. Do it yourself. All you have to lose is misery.

A LAUGHING MATTER

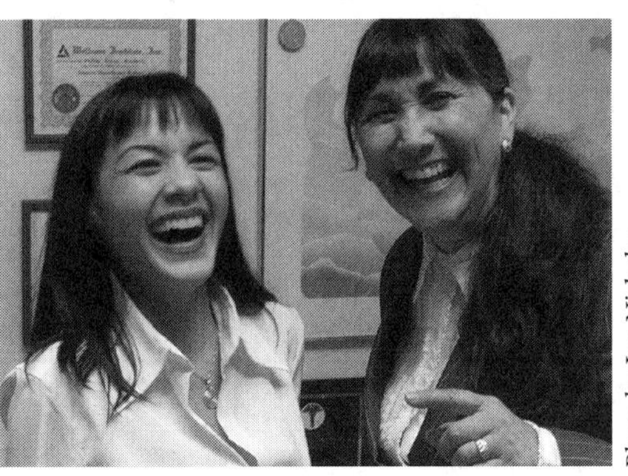

Babies start laughing at ten weeks. Navajo Indians say that a baby's first laugh is sacred and the person who evokes that laugh will be forever connected to them. An Apache Indian myth says that the Great Spirit who created us wasn't satisfied until we laughed. The Navajo Indians have a "First Laugh Ceremony" when baby laughs their first laugh.

Laughter is contagious and brings people closer together in chuckle-belly bonding. It gives us a time-out from problems. In business and in life, a good laugh cuts the tension of serious issues and tough decision-making. When you come back to a problem after laughing, you see it more clearly. 98% of CEO's say that they would hire someone with a sense of humor over a serious person any day.

LAUGHING: THE APHRODISIAC OF THE MIND

Paraplegics, paralyzed from the waist down, can achieve orgasm by stimulating their mind with glee. Some say that having sex while laughing is the highest high (seriously)!

LAUGHTER: JEST, THE BEST MEDICINE

Laughter is contagious but not infectious. In fact, laughter literally fights infection. Blood tests show that laughing releases and increases antibodies, white blood cells and molecules like immunoglobulins, which find and destroy tumor cells and viruses.

Laughter helps your body fight bacteria and infection.

Studies at the Loma Vista University School of Immunology show that laughter increases your body's natural toxic-attack killer cells (T-lymphocytes) and helper receptive cells. Laughter lowers cortisol levels, which keeps you healthier.

Patch Adams (played by Robin Williams) was right; laugh just for the health of it. A University of Maryland study says that laughter relieves the pain of arthritis and hypertension.

Norman Cousins (*Anatomy of an Illness*) cured himself of an "incurable connective tissue disease" by checking himself out of a hospital and into a hotel (the hotel's lower cost would make anyone feel better). Norman only invited uplifting people who told him funny stories and read funny passages. He watched amusing movies (Candid Camera and the Marx Brothers), took vitamin C and discovered that for every 20 minutes of laughter, he had several minutes pain-free. Within a short time, his "incurable" illness vanished. He died of old age, many years later, and a happy man.

SEVEN DAYS WITHOUT LAUGHTER MAKES ONE WEAK

Studies show that most adults laugh less than fifteen times a day, while the average five year old laughs 250 times a day! The delight of a child makes YOU your best.

OUR TICKLE ATE

Laughter aids digestion by stimulating enzyme secretions. It even acts as a mild laxative, cleansing you more. Laughter neutralizes acid/alkali imbalance in the body.

414

HILARIOUS WORKOUT

Called "internal jogging," laughter works like aerobic exercise. A hearty chortle a hundred times a day equals ten minutes on a rowing machine.

A belly laugh improves muscle tone and breathing. Research by William Fry and Lee Berk of Loma Linda Medical School, reports that a good laugh improves circulation, increases heart rate and afterwards, lowers blood pressure. More oxygen is delivered to your blood and brain, refreshing your mind and relaxing stress-cramped muscles.

Long bouts of laughter can temporarily make you less coordinated and weaken bladder control. A small price to pay for a great time!

LAUGHTER, THE HEALTHY ESCAPE

"When you have a dilemma, make de lemonade"

Enjoying yourself is a delight-full escape from problems. Humor is anything that you think is funny. What tickles you and makes you laugh reflects your inner attitude. My friend Steve Bhearman (aka Swami Beyondananda) says it perfectly: *"If you don't laugh you may be suffering from humorhoids or hardened attitudes, which may actually lower your laugh expectancy. I suggest taking a laughative daily and restore your regul-hilarity."*

MODUS OPERANDI: STOCKWELL'S HAPPINESS HYPNOSIS

Hypnotize your subject and then take them through the following steps to feeling great:

1. **"Think of a time when you laughed real hard; a funny incident, scene in a movie or television or a joke you heard. Even if you can't remember what was so darn funny it doesn't really matter, does it? As you think about it, relax your jaw and tip up the corners of your mouth. COME ON; SMILE."**

2. **"Now let yourself YUK IT UP. Go ahead let out a little chortle. It doesn't really matter. Ha, Ha, Ha. That's right. You are doing fine."**

3. **"Now, if you can, think of a problem…and then laugh. Really let out a good hearty laugh… What happened to your problem?"**

4. **"Repeat these words with me. 'I lighten up and lighten up. I give up suffering…and have fun. Fun as a lifestyle suits me. Fun may be a tough job, but someone's got to do it. I love to laugh. I live to laugh. I am the laughter.'"**

SMILE HOMEWORK FOR CLIENTS

Assign these smile exercises to yourself or your clients and enlighten up

1. Keep a humor journal.
2. Write down a pet peeve and think of five delightful ways to deal with it.
3. Collect cartoons that make you laugh. Write your own captions for them.
4. Make a collection of absurd newspaper captions.
5. Write down funny things that you hear.

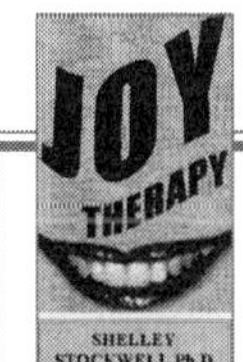

Hypno-Helper
"Joy Therapy" video tape by Shelley Stockwell-Nicholas

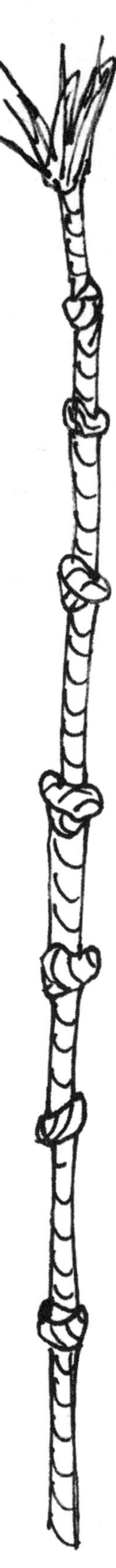

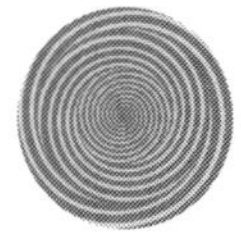

~ *Chapter 114* ~
COUE`'S AUTOSUGGESTION
FOR WELLNESS

Includes
Coue`'s Twilight "Good Knot" Autosuggestion
Coue`'s Well-Being Suggestion Formula

French clinician, Emile Coue` was the most famous mental healers in the world during the first quarter of the 20th Century. Following his highly successful tour across the United States, his suggestion-formula "Everyday, in every way, I am getting better and better," became a household slogan.

Coue` developed a method of using suggestions with no formal induction. He simple applied "the power of suggestion" which he called "autosuggestion." Coue` made it easy for the average person to use hypnosis to benefit their every day life. His process is easy because it operates automatically without having to think about how it works.

Critical mind is thinking. Subconscious mind is emotion. Coue`'s method required no thinking, just doing…and in the doing the critical mind is bypassed and selective thinking established. Precisely like Dave Elman.

The sovereign rule to successfully using Coue`'s autosuggestion is to make the effort without effort. If this is observed, one will intuitively fall into the right attitude. It becomes an art. Such generalized suggestions, handled this way, are sufficient for the performance of "autosuggestion" that can do a great deal of good especially when used night after night and day after day.

As pianist Arthur Schnabel puts it *"The notes I handle no better than many pianists. But the pauses between the notes ah, that is were the art resides."* Ah, yes, the pauses in between is where the subconscious is to be found.

There occurs two pauses in every day for every person that Coue' called: "The Outcropping of the Subconscious." One pause is in the morning just upon awakening. The other is in the night just before falling asleep. Those are special times to readily implant new beneficial suggestions into the subconscious or remove old unwanted ones.

MODUS OPERANDI: COUE`'S TWILIGHT "GOOD KNOT" AUTOSUGGESTION
You Will Need:
A String Tied with Twenty Knots

Coue`'s autosuggestion works by counting and repetition. He uses a simple device, a string tied in twenty knots. The number twenty has no intrinsic virtue; it is merely adopted as a suitable number. Upon retiring and arising, the person counts the knots and repeats the affirmation. The counting itself is hypnotic. Prayer beads and rosary beads have been used throughout time in this same manner. Each knot becomes a trigger to repeat the suggestion.

Coue` says do this:
"Take a piece of string and tie it in twenty knots. By this means you can count with a minimum of attention. Once in bed, close your eyes, relax your muscles, and take up a comfortable posture in preparation for going to sleep. Now repeat twenty times counting by means of the knots: 'Day by day, in every way, I am getting better and better.'

Uttered these words aloud; that is, loud enough to be audible to your own ears. In this way, the idea is reinforced by the movements of lips and tongue, and by the auditory impressions conveyed through the ears. Say it simply, without effort, like a child absently murmuring a nursery rhyme. When you become used to this exercise and can say it quite unselfconsciously.

Begin to let your voice rise of fall, it does not matter which, on the phrase, 'in every way.' But at first do not attempt this accentuation; it will only needlessly complicate the procedure.

Do not try to think of what you are saying. On the contrary, let the mind wander whither it will. If it rests on the formula, all the better. If it strays, do not recall it.

As long as your repetition does not come to a full stop, your mind wandering will be less disturbing than would be the effort to recall your thoughts."

Repeat this process in the morning, before you arise, exactly the same manner. Repetition is the foundation of this autosuggestion method. You may also design your own generalized "suggestion formulas" and use them via autosuggestions.

MODUS OPERANDI: COUE`'S WELL-BEING SUGGESTION FORMULA

Emile Coue` detailed a wonderful suggestion formula for perfect well-being. Read it out loud to yourself during periods of "The Outcropping of the Subconscious," (going to sleep or upon awakening). Use it with your clients. But don't concentrate on what you are reading, just read it with little thinking in a monotonous singsong fashion, just like a mantra – all given to yourself or your client in first-person narration.

Or, even more powerful, record it to play to yourself over earphones. Relax in a chair, close your eyes, start the tape and listen. Use the process often and the effects are compounded.

"All the suggestions given here to benefit yourself will be fixed, imprinted, engraved deep within your being.

Every day, at my regular mealtimes, I am pleasantly ready to eat. I will eat healthfully with excellent appetite and enjoy my food while eating exactly the proper amount my needs for perfect nourishment. I keep myself at exactly at my ideal weight and in radiant good health. My metabolism and assimilation is perfectly performed for my healthy and happy living of my life.

As new cells are created within my body, they will be healthy normal cells. My created cells grow normally and heal all damaged or worn-out tissue...providing normal growth and development in the entire organism that is me.

My excretory functions will be normally performed; each morning, throughout the day, and in the night, as my good health requires.

Every night I will fall asleep at the hour of my choosing...and I will sleep healthfully through the night. I awaken with my vitality renewed. My sleep will be calm, peaceful and profound...and on awakening in the morning I will eagerly face each day.

My mind will be peaceful and serene. I feel friendship towards the successful and compassion towards the miserable. I feel joy towards the virtuous. This provides me a peaceful mind. I am alive and I live fully to the hilt.

I have confidence in myself. I radiate it to others. I bring abundance into my life in every form and in every way. Success in every way is becoming my reality.

Now I sink down into the pleasant lassitude of relaxation, and allow these beneficial suggestions to go deep into my subconscious and become my way of life. Truly, day-by-day, in every way, I am getting better and better.

Each morning, just when I awake, I repeat this formula of well-being and start each day upon it. Each night, just before I fall asleep, I repeat this formula of well-being, and it goes deep into my subconscious while I sleep."

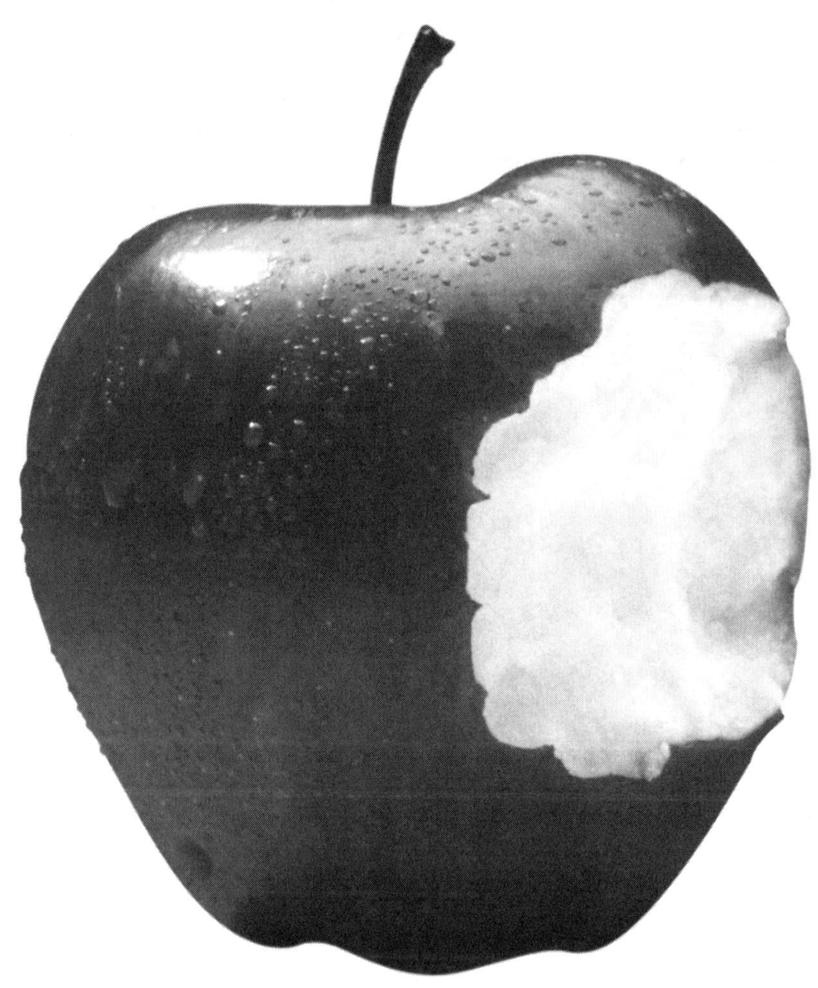

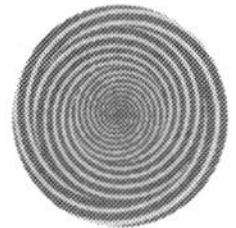

~ *Chapter 115* ~
GOOD HEALTH HYPNOTHERAPY

Includes
Good Health Hypnosis For Clients
Good Health For Yourself

Never mind specifics as to what your health should be. The subconscious knows instinctively how your health is and what should happen to be your best.

A peaceful mind leads to health in the body. Yoga teaches that there is a "Center of Being" within the body of each person that is located behind the navel within the solar plexus. Some call it the "abdominal brain" or "the mid brain." This place is the seat of your feelings. Reflect upon it.

If you feel fear, you feel it in your torso. Happiness also. Indeed, all feelings seem centered there. When the mind is peaceful this "center" is a realm of serenity. Hypnotherapy for good health is designed to take the mind into this private space. Use this process for yourself via Self-Hypnosis or for clients via Hetero-Hypnosis. It is of great value.

MODUS OPERANDI: GOOD HEALTH HYPNOSIS FOR CLIENTS
a) Have your client recline and close their eyes.
b) Request them tosition the body comfortably and relax
c) Play the *Serenity Resonance Sound*® for five minutes, at high level and have the enter the sound. It produces a subjective state of mind.
d) Reduce the sound level to soft background.
e) Hypnotize your client.
f) Present this Suggestion-Formula:

"In hypnosis now, let these suggestions become reality. Conscious mind move to one side. Subconscious mind come to the front.

This person seeks good health. Let them now go deep inside themselves and enter their center of being. Within their private space let all peace reign. Any and all stress is gone, and the body basks in an aura of good health. The mind is totally at peace, and the body commences to glow with radiant good health. The glow increases more and more with every breath that is taken, as the vitality of prana enters the body.

Your mind is quiet. Your body is relaxed. All that is old and limiting dissolves and is gone, and is replaced by that which is new and in radiant good health. Good health manifests through you with every breath you take. Every cell in your body is functioning to perfection. You are generating good health and well being in every way.

When this matter of ever-increasing good health produced by your peaceful mind has been accomplished, return with me to the here and now feeling wonderful and fine, in radiant good health."

MODUS OPERANDI: GOOD HEALTH FOR YOURSELF

a) Recline and close your eyes.

b) Position your body in comfort and relax all over.

c) Listen to serenity resonance sound for five minutes. Enter the sound allowing it to generate a subjective state of mind within yourself. You could record the following message and then play it for yourself if you like.

d) Lower sound level to a soft background.

e) Hypnotize yourself using whatever self-hypnosis you prefer.

f) Place hands over your ears and press in gently. As you read this suggestion-formula out loud to yourself (or play the recording of it that you previously recorded).

"I am in hypnosis now, and these suggestions which I give myself become my reality. My conscious phase of mind moves to one side and my subconscious phase of mind comes to the front.

I am going to obtain good health for myself by obtaining a peaceful mind. I go deep inside myself to dwell within my center of being, where all is peaceful and serene. I dwell within my personal private space and my body basks in an aura of good health. My mind is totally at peace, and my body is becoming aglow with radiant good health. All that is old and limiting within me is replaced with the new. Every cell in my body functions to perfection. The glow within me increases more and more with every breath I take, which brings in the vitality of prana into myself.

My mind is quiet. My body is relaxed. All tension, in every way is gone from me. I am free. I am free. I am free.

My body manifests good health and well being ever growing with every breath I take. I am generating good health and well being for myself from my inner peace of mind.

Subconscious mind when you know this objective has been accomplished, return me to the here and now feeling wonderful and fine. I am in radiant good health.

Arouse. Arise. Turn off the sound. The session for you is complete. You can use it as often as you please. Obtaining a peaceful mind for good health in the body can never be overdone. Always it is a benefit."

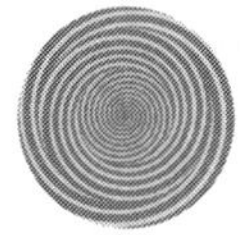

Chapter 116

ANTI-AGING HUNZA BREATH

Includes
The Hunza Prahna Method

"People think that 100 years is something of an achievement [but] if you stick around long enough, it will happen to anybody."
        —Margaret Rawson
        Who turned 100 years old in July, 1999
        Her study on dyslexia was published at age 96.

Everyone matures, ripens and comes to bloom. Many clients seek ways to counter aging and wish to promote longevity. As baby boomers move into twilight years, Rejuvenation Hypnotherapy allows them to activate their bio-computer for vitality and personal growth. If you advertise "anti-aging hypnosis" don't be surprised if you get swamped!

The use of prahna is one of the Hunza peoples great secrets of the fountain of youth. Prahna is an Eastern term meaning "vitality of life," and this has to be, as breathing IS life.

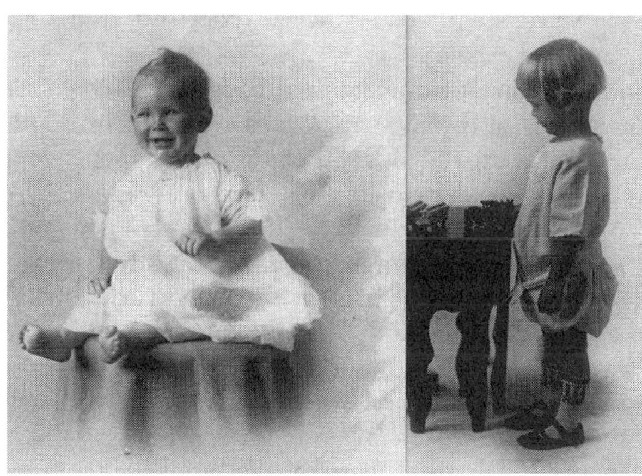

Ormond McGill

In prahna, mind and breath become closely associated. Prahna is bioenergy that enters the body with each breath. It is not air. It comes into the body with air. The human organism does not produce Prahna. It is cosmic and universally present.

As you teach your client each breathing method, have them visualize the in-taking of prahna. Prahna is stored in the solar plexus, which acts as a reservoir. It is then directed by mind for whatever purpose is required. To understand prahna is to imbibe the fountain of youth.

The better the breath, the more the intake of prahna. Prahna is life force. Scientists who seek the source of life will find it in the study of prahna.

The Hunza way of breathing is holistic. You commence by practicing it until you know it well and it is established in your subconscious. It becomes instinctive. IT IS THE WAY TO A LONG LIFE.

MODUS OPERANDI: THE HUNZA METHOD
You Will Need:
Soothing Music

Place the client in a state of light hypnosis and tell them this story with soft music playing in the background. You begin by explaining the Hunza Method of complete breath established it in the subconscious…the home of habits:

"Finding the fountain of youth was the dream of Ponce de Leon, the Spanish explorer. In his quest he found Florida. He didn't find the Fountain of Youth in Florida but had he searched a beautiful valley in the Himalayas he would have met the Hunza people and they knew the secret. These youthful people retain their vigor and live long and healthful lives. By following the ways of these peaceful people you can give this treasure to yourself.

The Hunza Method is based on learning the art of breathing. As you bring in air you bring in Prahna or life force energy and then direct it with mental energies into various parts of your body. You do this by visualizing its perfect function for retaining youthfulness.

This process of complete breathing is performed as a continual inhalation in which the entire chest cavity, from the lowest part of the diaphragm to the highest part of the chest, is expanded in a continuous steady action. The Hunza complete breath method; becomes your habitual way of breathing."

HUNZA COMPLETE VITALIZING BREATH
"Sit or stand erect as we practice full vitalizing breath. It is easy to learn to properly inhale and exhale.

The Hunza complete breath, combines low, middle and high breathing, in which the upper part of the chest and lungs are used, the diaphragm is pushed forward, drawn in and the chest is expanded and then the diaphragm is depressed downward completely filling the total cavity of the lungs.

Let's begin by visualizing this action in your mind."
(You do the breath with them so they learn by your breathing)
"In this moment, breathe through your nostrils inhaling steadily. Draw in the air to fill the lower part of your lungs, which pushes out your hips, breastbone and chest. This action continues now in filling mid and higher portions of your lungs and the seven pairs of ribs. As it does, the lower abdomen is slightly drawn in which gives your lungs support and helps fill the highest parts of your lungs…low, middle, high, as the abdomen is drawn in for support. Retain this breath in your lungs for a moment and then exhale slowly while holding the chest in a firm position and drawing the abdomen in a little lifting slowly upward as air leaves. When the air is entirely exhaled, relax your chest."

Now bring your client back to room awareness and practice this method of breathing together. With practice it becomes a regular and natural way of breathing. It becomes instinctive. Mastering it shows your client the way to the Fountain of Youth.

THE CLEANSING BREATH
Next you will teach your client to master the cleansing breath. You teach this in the same procedure as the complete vitalizing breath. Place your client in light hypnosis while giving the initial instruction and then practicing the process with full awareness.

Breathing is instinctive and is habitual. Once established, it is subconscious in its performance. By combining subconscious and conscious mastery you teach your client to easily master this training.

"The cleansing breath is used to ventilate and cleanse the lungs. It is refreshing to the

entire body. Here is how you do it. Inhale a complete breath and retain the air in the lungs for a few seconds and then compress your lips close to your teeth with your teeth close together, while leaving a narrow slit between them. Now exhale a little of the air with force between the teeth. Then pause a moment, retaining the air and repeat this forceful expulsion of air from your lungs, a little at a time until all the air is exhaled from your lungs.

As you do this visualize the air as being purified as it is forced from the lungs. Hunza breathing always combines the mental and physical."

Having instructed subjectively in hypnosis, bring your client back to the objective state and practice this together.

THE NERVE REVITALIZING BREATH

Next, teach your client the subjective/objective nerve revitalizing breath. This provides a powerful stimulant to the nervous system. It develops a "nerve force" that revitalizes. It requires plenty of vigor in the action. Begin by putting your client in a light trance so that the action becomes conditioned in the subconscious and begin:

"Make your hands into fists and hold them against your chest. While you inhale and keeping your muscles tense, forcefully push your clenched hands out full length from your body and then draw them back to your chest. And again force your fists outward. This drawing in and out action as you inhale is performed with vigor. Then allow your hands to drop to your sides and relax while exhaling through your mouth."

Perform this process several times each time allowing the fists to spring out from the chest and then end with the cleansing breath.

RHYTHMIC BREATHING

Rhythmic breathing brings in large quantities of prahna into the system. The secret of rhythmic breathing is its vibration. Rhythm is vibration. Everything in the universe is in a constant state of vibration. This method is used to harmonize your client's vibration or body rhythm with cosmic vibration.

Do this:

"This special rhythmic breathing makes a connection between you body and universal energy. As you establish its rhythm in hypnosis your subconscious relates to it and you will sense it as a tide of psyche-energy within yourself.

This very moment, while still in hypnosis, tune into the rhythm of your heart. Check your pulse and count the beats in units, one, two, three, four, five, six… one, two, three, four, five, six. Get this rhythm firmly in your mind so that you know it instinctively. (Which is the same as saying you know it subconsciously.) This way you will be able to reproduce the count easily as you breath.

Now, assume a straight-line posture. Sit erect, head and chest up, shoulders back, hands resting on your lap as you inhale a Hunza Complete Revitalizing Breath (Low, middle high, as the abdomen is drawn in for support.) taken to the count of six heartbeats. Retain the breath in your lungs for three heartbeats and then exhale the breath while counting six heartbeats. Inhale and exhale through your nostrils.

Do this over and over again as you establish this natural rhythm in your breathing. As you master this, you will sense the flow of vibratory effects that it produces throughout your body. This is definitely something you are experiencing.

Now inhale a complete breath counting six heartbeats, hold it for three heartbeats and then exhale for six heartbeats.

Now, while still in hypnosis, lie prone upon your back and rest your hands on your solar plexus just beneath your rib cage and as you breath rhythmically you build up the energy within yourself. With each inhalation, visualize prahna coming into you and being stored in your solar plexus reservoir. When you sense it is full, each time you take a breath WILL this energy to be taken up by your central nervous system and distributed throughout your body to every organ and cell, every muscle and artery, from the top of your head to the soles of your feet. WILL that prahna that you are imbibing to invigorate and strengthen your body in every way. You are imbibing the fountain of youth. Perform the process using effort without effort. Your subconscious knows exactly how to do this. Just use your WILL and mentally direct the prahna to flow as you direct it.

Distribute it throughout your body and then you are ready to perform the Hunza Grand Psychic Breath.

THE HUNZA GRAND PSYCHIC BREATH

"This Hunza method of breathing is an advanced process of breath control. It is often referred to as "breathing through the bones" as it saturates your entire system with prahna and you emerge with every bone, nerve, organ and part energized. Still in hypnosis, rest quietly upon your back. Relax completely and totally let go. Commence with rhythmic breathing until you sense the vibration in your body.

Now while you are inhaling to the rhythm of your heartbeat, visualize your breath being drawn in through the bones of your legs. As you exhale force the breath out of the bones of your legs. Continue this until you develop the full sense of breathing through your bones of your legs.

Next visualize your breath being drawn in through the bones of your arms. As you exhale force the breath out of the bones of your arms. Continue this until you develop the full sense of breathing through your bones of your arms.

Next visualize your breath being drawn in through the top of your skull. As you exhale force the breath out of the top of your skull. Continue this until you develop the full sense of breathing out the top of your skull.

Next visualize your breath being drawn in through your stomach. As you exhale force the breath out of the top of your stomach. Continue this until you develop the full sense of breathing through your stomach.

Next visualize your breath being drawn in through your reproductive organs. As you exhale force the breath out of the top of your reproductive organs. Continue this until you develop the full sense of breathing through your reproductive organs.

Next visualize your breath being drawn in through your skin. As you exhale force the breath out of your skin. Continue this until you develop the full sense of breathing through your skin.

Finally, visualize your breath being drawn up and down your spinal column. Continue this until you develop the full sense of breathing through your spinal column. Practice this well.

As you lie quietly, you will commence to experience vitality of life surge up within you. Visualize the prahna current going through your entire body. Feel it especially in your forehead and at the base of your brain. Then start moving this feeling to your internal organs, your heart, stomach, kidneys, liver, to every organ of your body. You are learning to use your mind to move prahnic energy of life through your entire body. You are partaking of the fountain of youth.

Finally, you are ready to complete the process. Lie quietly for some moments while you visualize the prahna sweeping through you from head to toe. Then perform the cleansing breath. (Inhale a complete breath, retain the air for a few seconds and then exhaling the air with force between the teeth a little at a time until all the air is exhaled from your lungs. As you do this visualize the air as being purified as it is forced from the lungs.)

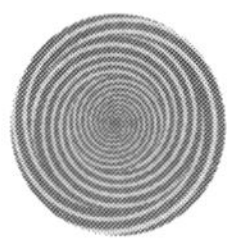

~ *Chapter 117* ~
HYPNOTHERAPY OF DEATH

"As the embodied self continually passes in this body from childhood to youth to old age, the self similarly passes into another body at death. A person who has realized spiritual identity is not bewildered by such change."
—Bhagava Gita

This chapter is presented to help those close to dying appreciate how wonderful death really is. It is an important form of hypnotherapy. Look upon death as a Christmas present long awaited, not something to be shivered over.

Death and dying is not a great-unknown mystery. Actually each person has been through the experience many times. Most simply do not remember yet, all are there stored in their subconscious memory banks ready to be recalled. The

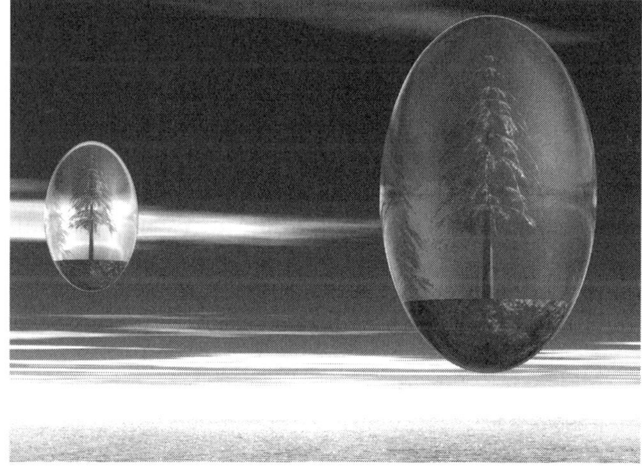

Hypnotherapy of Death helps a dying person recall what a truly wonderful adventure the transition of going from form to formless really is.

Lord Krishna said, "Life in the body is as nothing compared to the freedom death offers." Think of existing in a multidimensional body; no more pain, no more limitation of three-dimensional space. And always you will know yourself, as the individual that you are. Indeed, you are the only one of your SELF in the entirety of the Universe.

To be of value to dying client, simply present that the experience of death in no more than going from one room of a house to another.

The Hypnotherapy of Death removes all fear from dying and represents an understanding of what death is all about to help your client recall previous transitional experiences and appreciate a personal eternal continuum.

Present it while in hypnosis with a sense of no importance. The process is refreshing and reminds the subconscious of what is important.

MODUS OPERANDI: HYPNOTHERAPY OF DEATH

You Will Need:

"The Serenity Resonance Sound" or

"Entrancing Music" (See order form at the back of this book)

Turn on the Serenity Resonance Sound or Entrancing Music at soft volume as you present these reminders to your client about what death is all about.

"As you rest in profound hypnosis now, relax completely and let this understanding of your true nature of death refresh your inner memory of the immortal nature of your SELF. As you enter your subconscious mind, you continue going deeper and deeper into hypnosis. (Pause)

Remember that which you already know; the concept of death as an end to yourself is the greatest lie that humanity has ever created. In believing this lie great fear has evolved; a fear that forms the root of all fears. The truth is that YOU are eternal and it is impossible for YOU to die. The body in which you dwell for a brief span in time can die, but never your SELF. Death is a lie. The remembering of your subconscious in recalling life after life knows this is true.

Come to look upon the true nature of death and know it well. Look upon death is the culmination of life. Life is just a process and death is the crescendo of the process. Life is just the moving while death is the reaching. Both are one. Your subconscious knows this well.

Death is the flowering of life…death is the flower, life is the tree and the tree is there for the flower. The flower is not there for the tree. The tree will dance when the flower comes. Feel this, then death will be accepted and welcomed as a divine guest. When death knocks at the door, it means that the universe is ready to receive you back.

Absorb this; 'only when you drink from the river of silence shall you indeed sing. When you have reached the mountaintop then will you climb. When the earth shall claim your limbs then shall you truly dance.'

Death is a door. It is not a stopping. Your awareness of your SELF moves but your body remains at the door. The body is left outside the temple, but your awareness of yourself enters the temple. It is a most subtle phenomenon. The life you thought so important is nothing before this greatness. Appreciate that basically life is a preparation for dying. If at the thought of death you feel fear it only means that you have not yet known LIFE because life never dies.

Life cannot die. Trembling at the thought of death means that somewhere you have become identified with the body only. You have identified with the mechanism. The mechanism depends on many things as it is a conditioned phenomenon. Your consciousness is unconditional; it does not depend on anything. Your subconscious, your awareness of SELF is YOU.

You have been told that you must learn the art of living.Now, more importantly you learn the art of dying. To learn death fully you must give up control of your physical body when it is no longer suited for YOU to dwell within.

Death is ever coming and it can happen at any time. The very essence of the art of dying is being ready, at any moment in your earthly life, in the midst of the fullness of living, to make the transition from this life to the next phase of life and to do this willingly, joyfully and with confident serenity. To attain this inner attitude, understand that the body is but a temporary housing which is occupied by your SELF, your individual consciousness, which is immortal and exists eternally.

Let this be repeated to refresh your memory of this transition. All physical life is transitory and temporary and a continuum that can pass at anytime. LIFE as YOU is never ending. Let this true nature of death go deep into your subconscious and refresh your memory. You are calm and joyous. You take this in like the refreshing drink it is."

(Pause)

Rest deeply now in hypnosis and allow what has been given to you to become your reality. All fear of dying is gone. You look forward to wonderful adventures ahead. When you are ready to go you remember that you have simply passed onwards. Most make the transition while asleep. If you manage to make it consciously, it is deliciously emancipating.

Arouse yourself from hypnosis anytime you wish. Come back with joy filling your heart at the great blessings that you are."

The session is complete. You have given someone a most valuable service that is seldom offered.

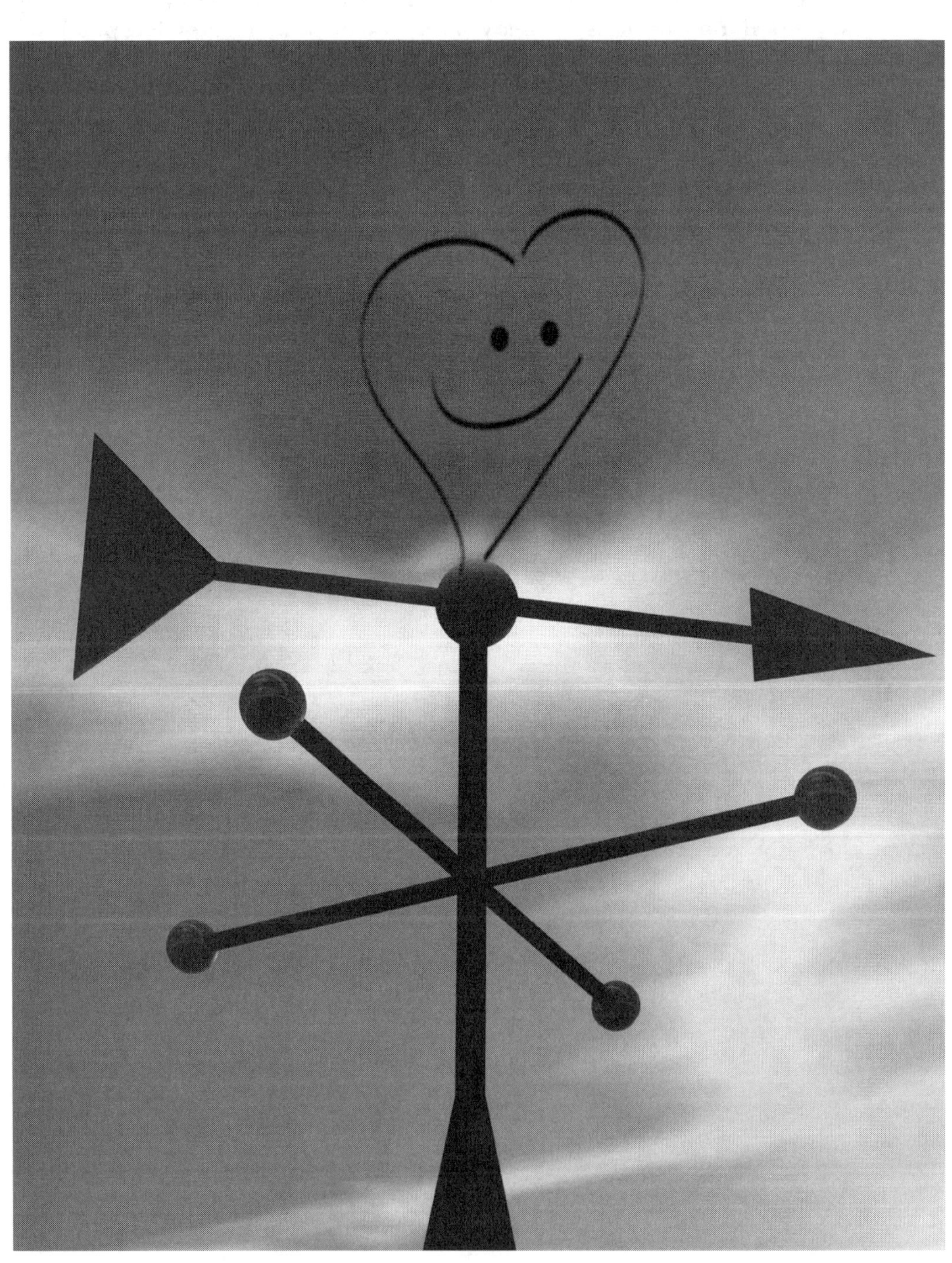

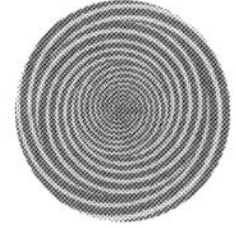

~ *Chapter 118* ~
COMMON SENSE HYPNOTHERAPY
Common Sense= Timeless Wisdom

Includes
Common Sense and the Abdominal Brain
Abdominal Brain Hypnotherapy

Common sense is a valued commodity.

Proficient hypnotherapists appreciate the value of common sense. Sometimes a client comes to your office full of complaints and stuff and stuff that scarcely makes any sense. The best hypnotherapy for such a client may be to give them their common sense. Instilling common sense into their subconscious with hypnosis is perfectly.

Common sense is actually far from common; it distills wisdom passed down through ages to become instinctively employed and appreciated.

Good health of the mind aids the body and good health of the body aids the mind. Even with mental abnormalities, good health is important to move someone from insanity to sanity. It is common sense.

Physician and hypnotherapist come closer together as healing becomes more holistic. The physician aims to heal the body, the hypnotherapist the mind. Cooperation of physician and hypnotherapist promotes subconscious motivation which directly influences the body's organic functioning. The value of working together is obvious. It is common sense.

COMMON SENSE AND THE ABDOMINAL BRAIN

Hypnosis directed toward the solar plexus stimulates the action of any organ, which has fallen into a habit of poor function. It is the action of mind upon body and body upon mind. The solar plexus is the seat of the subconscious mind within the body. It is sometimes referred to as the abdominal brain.

Make any sense? Common Sense.

Think about it.

The subconscious deals with feelings. Where do you experience your feelings most? You feel them in your gut.

Give the instinctive mind of the solar plexus proper direction and you do not need to rely on medical knowledge. This seat of your feelings knows what is needed to promote healing. It possesses common sense. After all, its very nature seeks good health. Nature itself does much healing when allowed freedom. The hypnotherapist does not have to direct nature to the place in need of wellness. Any malady in need of correction strongly impresses the solar plexus to improve its condition. Yet, when you draw attention to a malady and impress the solar plexus to make it right; it has an obligation to improve a condition. After the request, give it a free hand to do this job willingly. If your requests make sense- common sense- this approach complements medical efforts. To best use this approach you will want a physician's diagnosis of a problem and what correction is needed.

MODUS OPERANDI: COMMON SENSE (ABDOMINAL BRAIN) HYPNOTHERAPY

Induce trance and then inform the subconscious what correction is required.

Suggest:

"With your permission, I will place my hand on your solar plexus and, of course, I will be most respectful."

Then with your hand resting on their belly (or above it if they would not like you to touch them) recount the physician's requirements for improvement. Use the client's first name as it increases rapport.

"________ (Name) you know what the trouble is. Let's get busy and improve it. Your doctor and I will cooperate with you in every way to bring excellent health to you. Get busy now and direct the healing energies of your body to heal your body and restore it to perfect wellness."

Press firmly on the solar plexus as you continue:

"We will see to it that your body is given proper nourishment, water and required aids to assist in you internal healing. If this is agreeable, give me a signal that it is by automatically lifting your right forefinger."

This language of the subconscious can be any signal agreed upon, like the nodding of the head or even a smile. When the signal is given, proceed by giving suggestions as to the corrections needed and when you are complete end the session by suggesting

"When you return to the here and now, good health of both your body and mind is on its way."

Release pressure on the solar plexus and arouse the client knowing that improved health is just around the corner. IT IS THE CASE!

When you accept the idea that the subconscious mind is centered in the body rather than the head, this process is priceless. If not, bypass this approach and do another process.

Make any sense?

Common sense.

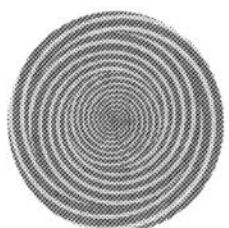

~ *Chapter 119* ~
STOCKWELL'S HYPNO-WELLNESS
By Shelley Stockwell-Nicholas, PhD

Includes
The Goals Of Hypno-Wellness
Stockwell's Hypno-Wellness Script
How Illness Can Benefit You
Stansberry's Healing Script
Mozart's Musical Meditation

"There is no illness of the body apart from the mind."
—Socrates, 6 Century BC

"Hypnosis doesn't cure you, it stimulates your body's natural healing power. Your wonderful mind-body constantly maintains, repairs and renews itself without conscious effort."
—Shelley Stockwell

Can hypnosis really help you be well?
Yes!
Hypnosis assists you to tap your optimal state of mental, physical, spiritual and social well-being. If you are not at optimum, Hypno-Wellness…also called Therapeutic Visualization or the Placebo Effect…taps your innate ability to "well" yourself and perks you up!

You enter into a relaxed and receptive mind state of trance to support your body with its own flow of balanced energy and receive your body wisdom and wellness suggestion. Hypnotherapists dialog with symptoms, discovers the source of the malady and what steps you need to take to solve it, motivates you to take those steps, and then gives affirmations for radiant health.

You were born without conscious effort and with a natural, innate immune response. This amazing non-specific defense mechanism fights imbalances, or illness, and regularly returns you to homeostasis or wellness. If you cut your skin, your blood quickly clots so that you don't bleed to death and the wound reseals itself. If toxins enter your body, your blood calls out special cells and organisms to destroy hostile invaders. If you are exposed to a toxic virus or bacteria, your system develops antibodies that protect you if they show up again. That's why most of us only have the mumps once.

If you feed yourself junk food, smoke, don't sleep or take drugs, over-stressed adrenals and your liver say "enough already" and you experience pain, stress, depression or illness causing your body works overtime to "well" you. That's where hypnosis comes in. Hypnosis taps your innate body wisdom via your sub and super conscious mind for cells, mind and spirit to work in harmony. On this level, you know exactly what you need to do to revitalize your body. Often a simple attitude, life style or dietary change restores radiant health.

The behavior modification of hypnosis eases dis-ease, extinguishes fear and grief and alleviates chronic discomfort. For a person suffering from degenerative illness, hypnosis can help detoxify, cleanse and fortify their immune response.

In other words, your same innate intelligence that made and organizes your body, lets you adapt, grow and develop, also has the power to heal it.

Illness and emotions are similar. When suppressed, they travel deeper into our being and increase discomfort. As we get healthy, such putrefied tensions unravel much like a ball of yarn. Hypnosis offers the honesty and positive thinking that cleanses the mind of denial, illusion and destructive patterns and releases symptoms and sickness.

When ill, your brain secretes chemicals that affect your mood and personality making it challenging to get a clear perspective on how to proceed. Hypnosis helps you focus on a positive action plan.

Inadvertent Hypnosis

Doctors and nurses as authority figures are amazing hypnotists that we unconsciously empower. They are top dog; we are bottom dog. They are parents; we become a yielding child. What they suggest is often realized and literally helps us live or die.

Hypnotherapists are trained to use verbal and non-verbal suggestions to actively enlist the body-mind to solve problems.

Medical arts practitioners are trained in problem diagnosis and are often unaware of their powerful verbal and non-verbal communications. What they say becomes accepted suggestions that profoundly impact a patient with closed or open eyes and can become a self-fulfilling prophecy. What is said under anesthesia makes a deep and lasting impression on wellness too. The famous Hypnotherapist of the 50's Dave Ellman put it well, "Doctor if you present positive suggestions of healing, it is guaranteed you will compound the healing…"

GOALS OF HYPNO-WELLNESS

Hypnotists assume the following regarding illness:

1. Hypnosis Evokes Balance

Pain, stress, negativity, hurtful habits, resistance to change, and/or the need to be nurtured, cause imbalance. With hypnosis, you examine the problem, its cause & effect, and enlist new strength and your individual healing resource. That strength manifests in thoughts, brain chemistry and your body as homeostasis.

2. Hypnosis Moves You

Hypnosis releases you from the trance of past painful souvenirs that block positive energy flow. You learn to be to live your life now being true to your natural rhythm; your genuine self. Illness then becomes just a fleeting blip on the radar screen of your happy life.

3. Hypnosis Accentuates the Positive and Eliminates The Negative

Hypnosis and the power of suggestion easily change (or reframe) negative habits, thoughts and behavior, into positive habits, thoughts and behavior. Hypnotic suggestions motivate you to say and do good, kind and nourishing things to and for yourself and seek positive action and positive healthy emotional payoffs. Hypnosis affects better results for medical and dental treatments. It reduces bleeding and minimizes drugs.

4. Hypnosis Puts You In Charge Of Yourself

Do you act as if you're a brain with a body dangling from it? If your body gets sick, do you get angry? Being alive requires you to accept and own your body. You are your body. You are every cell, muscle, nerve and organ. Hypnosis puts you in the driver's seat of your body and in charge of your thoughts.

5. Hypnosis Calls In The Big Guys

In hypnosis, your profound inner knowing, silent witness, or a higher self, tells you exactly what you need to do to renew and restore mental/physical/emotional harmony. It motivates you to embrace a healthy diet, life style and exercise.

6. Hypnosis Relaxes and Heals

The side effects of hypnotic trance is profound healing relaxation that, similar to sleep, regenerates and renews. Fear and stress often the culprit of illness step aside when we relax. Hypnosis accelerates healing & recovery time. The placebo effect of hypnosis can make physical changes in your body.

7. Hypnosis Helps Us Let Go

We gain terrific freedom when we let go. Finally we enter a place of quiet acceptance and celebrating what each moment brings. Grief when processed becomes an emotional gateway to the garden of the soul.

8. Hypnosis Eliminates Pain

You attitude has a lot to do with whether you experience pain and suffering. Hypnosis teaches how to rise above, reinterpret, divert or eliminate pain. That is why drugless anesthesia for childbirth and surgery are so successful.

9. Hypnosis Is The High Road

There are many options to feel well and overcome illness. Drugs and surgery are the most dangerous options. A healthy diet, exercise and life style are the best approach. Hypnosis motivates you to take the high road with no adverse side effects. That's why hypnosis is astounding popular as a legal alternative health care modality.

STOCKWELL'S HYPNO-WELLNESS SCRIPT
Pre Talk

"You and your body are miraculous. You are in a constant state of renewal and regeneration. Every 4 days your stomach lining regenerates and your gastric juices renew every 5 minutes. Your skin replenishes itself every 4 weeks, your liver every 6 weeks, and your bones every 9 months! Hypnosis and your intention can help your body renew and restore itself to its optimum state of well being."

Induce trance using your favorite induction and then suggest:

"Everything you've ever done began as a thought. The work you do, the place you live and the clothes you wear, are results of a thought that you manifested into action and reality. Because you choose wellness, joy and peace, you now choose to think wellness, joy and peace with all of your senses and all our being. Let's begin.

What would you do if you took excellent care of yourself? Take a minute and tell yourself exactly what you'd do and listen well to your answer.

(Pause)

Good. What wouldn't you do if you took excellent care of yourself? Take a minute and tell yourself exactly what you wouldn't do and listen well to what you answer.
(Pause.)

What does a nourishing life style mean to you? Take a minute and tell yourself exactly what you'd do and listen well to what you answer.
(Pause.)

What is full wellness like for you? How does it taste? How does it smell? How does it sound? How does your body feel? What does it look like?
(Pause.)

As you listen to the small voice within you, hear the cause, results and solutions for your current health challenges. From this point of wisdom you are now prepared to hear other theories, and solutions and see if they truly fit into your reality.

What proactive steps are you willing to take right now today to take excellent care of yourself and feel great?"
(Pause and let them tell you their suggestions. Then affirm their ideas. Continue with these suggestions.)

"You choose to live. You are healthy. Repeat these words out loud or to yourself:
'I choose to live. I am healthy'
I choose to live. I am healthy
I choose to live. I am healthy
I do what creates good health for myself. When I am awake, I create wellness. When I am asleep, I create wellness. I am perfectly healthy.

I am true to my natural rhythm, my real self.

I release any habit or emotions that cause issue to my tissue. I'm healthy and unlimited.

If I spring a leak I examine it and recognize its cause. I discover new personal strength and this heals. I completely and absolutely release any and all limits I am unlimited. I return to balance in my body, brain chemistry and mind.'"

"Here is a terrific way to solve a problem.

First identify what is wrong. Subconscious, come forward and reply with the first thing that comes to mind.

1. Does this condition serve a useful purpose? If so, what?
2. Did it serve a useful purpose at another time? If so, what?
3. Pinpoint the part of you that will now heal. Thank you. Go deep to that very place.
4. What do you notice? Describe it. What shape? What color? What texture?
5. Become keenly aware of that place that needs renewal. What do you need to do to help and let it restore itself? Do you need to cool it down, warm it up and bring more blood there? Less blood? Do you need to just let it go?
6. Do what needs to be done. Notice when this is complete. Great!
7. Is there anything else that needs to happen? If so, I do it now.
8. All levels of your body, mind and energy now make a promise to do whatever is necessary right now to be at your peak performance.

Focus all levels of yourself upon a molecule in the part of your body that needs renewal. I speak directly to that molecule, that cellular structure;
(In a firm voice:)

I know that you will hear me and accept this clear communication:

It is God's will that you and all other cells to go back to your innate healthy coding. Return at once to the blueprint that allows you to do your job most effectively. Return in full balance, fullness and harmony. Restore your original and most perfect imprints, coding and function as it was meant to be. Restore your natural ability to function efficiently. Your protein receptors, your cells, your DNA your muscles organs and ligaments are now restored to full and perfect functioning. Molecule do you understand?

(Pause and wait for an affirmation.) **You are now restored renewed and regenerated.**

I speak now to your endocrine system:

Glands and immune chemical responses, you now return to your perfect state, the way God intended you to be. **Heal ______** (give specific instructions).

Your body is now fully activated and produces all you need to be entirely renewed, restored and invigorated. You have accomplished a lot and are very proud of yourself. Congratulations."

HOW ILLNESS CAN BENEFIT YOU
Is illness as a statistical mistake or an unfair finger of fickle fate.
That illness pains and irritates is not a subject of debate.
But, illness too is a wake up call;
A chance to love yourself warts and all.
An invitation for transformation,
shedding the old: regeneration,
counting blessings, honoring life,
slowing down and avoiding strife
—Shelley Stockwell

Some unconsciously create physical and emotional problems for attention, caring, or to go home again. Some create illness to resolve inner conflict. Constant stress is like putting your foot on the brake, while stepping on the accelerator full throttle and can cause unhealthy "stress fractures." A German study of 2,000 people over a thirteen-year period found that those who kept emotions bottled up, experienced anger, depression, hostility and despair and were more likely to get cancer and heart disease.

Illness can result from the environment we create for our body. Habits and stuff we stuff in our mouth for pleasure can make us sick. So can hypnotic suggestions we give ourselves when traumatized. Sometimes illness is just bad luck followed by secondary gains like attention that we begin to enjoy. Sometimes none of these payoffs are true.

There is only one person who knows the truth of an illness and that is YOU.

Hypnosis literally stops us from being sick with worry. Hypnosis reveals to your conscious mind repressed causes, excuses or ignored self-destruction and the best proactive solutions to heal. It sets the record straight on illness and what we conjure up subconsciously.

In all cases, I see illness as a transformative opportunity for self-love and spiritual openness. The shock is a wake-up call for change so we face inner demons and discover inner resources. Some transform and give up a lifetime of bad habits. Some change stifling jobs, relationships and locations. Illness forces you to slow down, take responsibility for joy, change behaviors that aren't working and refocus on a bigger picture. For those who have made pain their gain; giving up pain, means giving up the suffering lifestyle as well. It reminds you that even if you have pain you don't have to be one.

Illness may be just what your inner doctor ordered for you to dump toxic attitudes and habits, and connect with your higher self. Welcome it as a wake up call that alerts you to what you need to do to free yourself from limits. Honor it as your teacher who allows you to discover your inner and outer resources.

Shamanistic societies say that the holiest person is the wounded healer. For in their wounding, the gods were summoned for the healing to take place, gifting them with a God power to heal others. Shamans respect physical, emotional and spiritual energy as inseparable.

If you are feeling ill or upset, the safest and easiest is option is hypnosis.

STANSBERRY'S MULTIPLE SCLEROSIS HEALING SCRIPT

Hypntherapist Barbara Stansberry of Milwaukee, Wisconsin shares this wonderful script for wellness for those suffering from multiple sclerosis. It is terrific for whatever else ails:

"Let the searchlight of your mind move and shine on your brain, spinal column and nervous system and to the glistening myelin sheaths covering each neuron. Sense if there is any damaged area. Trust yourself; your mind knows where to go. Your mind is your body. As you shine your light, look upon any place that needs repair, use all of your senses. Notice the textures, smell, sound called forth in your imagination. Notice the color. We begin by cleaning that area so that it will no longer cause any symptoms. Do it any way that makes sense to you: you can sweep, scrape, sponge or wash as you clean your nervous system. When all is new, strong and healthy, wrap new hearty myelin around and around each neuron; new, strong, healthy myelin wrapping round and round each neuron. This clean and repair process is natural and happens if ever you have a symptom. Symptoms just fade- gone completely and you are strong, and healthy in every way.

We now move to your immune responses and your white blood cells. They are now working perfectly to defend and protect your body. Any confused white blood cells that hurt any good healthy cells are now instructed to stop altogether and shrink in numbers. Bless you confused cells. You are confused you may not reproduce any more. Confused cells will die as all cells do. Only clear and understanding white blood cells prevail. Healthy white blood cells now recognize what is friend. Blood recognizes now that myelin sheaths are friends and are loving and kind to your neurons.

If you are using any treatment or medication decide if the treatment is helping. Is it quieting symptoms so that you have a chance to cleanse and renew? If so, imagine the treatment effectively. Review any substances that you take into your body are they helping you if so that is good. If anything hurts you say good-bye to it now. You don't need it any more. You now avoid what you know hurts you. You don't want or need it.

Now become aware of your deep state of relaxation and calmness, your auto immune system works perfectly and you are free you are healthy and strong and whole and this wonderful feeling saturates your entire body. You congratulate yourself for this terrific wellness and relaxation."

MOZART'S MUSICAL MEDITATION

Thanks to Sharon E. Toole, MTC and the great composer Mozart for this idea. Mozart was said to use this thinking process when composing. It is especially useful for those who are sound dominant.

"Be aware of the feeling in your body...notice the symmetry of your hands...your body...your feet...your left side...your right side...Good.

Now, take a deep breath inside your self and focus your awareness upon the part of you that is most healthy and vital. It may be a part that you haven't paid much attention to lately. Maybe it's your heart...eyes...lips...legs...or ears. As you scan your body you can easily identify it. Good.

(Pause)

As you notice that part feel its vitality and healthy. Imagine this part of you as a musical instrument...with its own unique sound and melody. Listen, listen, listen to that sound. Listen to the sound of that part of your body as it incorporates its vitality into all your energy. As you hear it, you feel strong, healthy, vital and alive. This feeling spreads through every molecule of your entire body. Nod your head when this is so.

(Wait for them to nod their head and continue)

Continue to hear the melody and feel the vitality as you turn your attention to the unique smell of that sound. Smell that sense of aliveness, and vitality...let it fill up your senses. Excellent.

(Pause)

Now as you continue to hear the melody, feel the vitality and smell the delicious smell of energy, notice its distinct flavor and taste. Smell and taste that vitality as it spreads any place on your body you'd like it to go.

It is as if you are a symphony and every part of you is a piece of music as you allow the sound, feeling, smell and taste of vitality and health to dance within you. It spreads inside you like a beautiful light. Notice the color that brightness brings as it dances in rhythm in the music of your body...spreading and massaging every part of your radiant body.

This profound symphony the dance continues from now on in the back of your mind all the time. Even tonight, in your sleep and dreams, that music spreads its light, color, warmth, smell and flavor all through you. This vitality and wellness is always there for you- 24 hours a day, seven days a week.

This symphony is always there directing your unconscious mind to the most appropriate things to eat, see, hear and do. The light of this fine symphony shines out through your pores and through your eyes. Its tones spill out through the tones of your voice and easily and naturally spreads to others.

This process continues in all ways that are best for you...as you now accept these ideas and make them your very own. Each morning you rise with energy and vitality, feeling relaxed and alert. Good. When you are ready, allow your eyes to open and you will notice that you are filled with the beauty of this wonderful music of yourself.

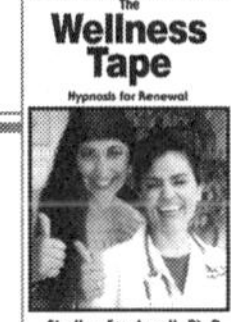

Hypno-Helper
"The Wellness Tape" by Shelley Stockwell, PhD and Lily Prado, D.O.
is available on the order form at the back of this book.

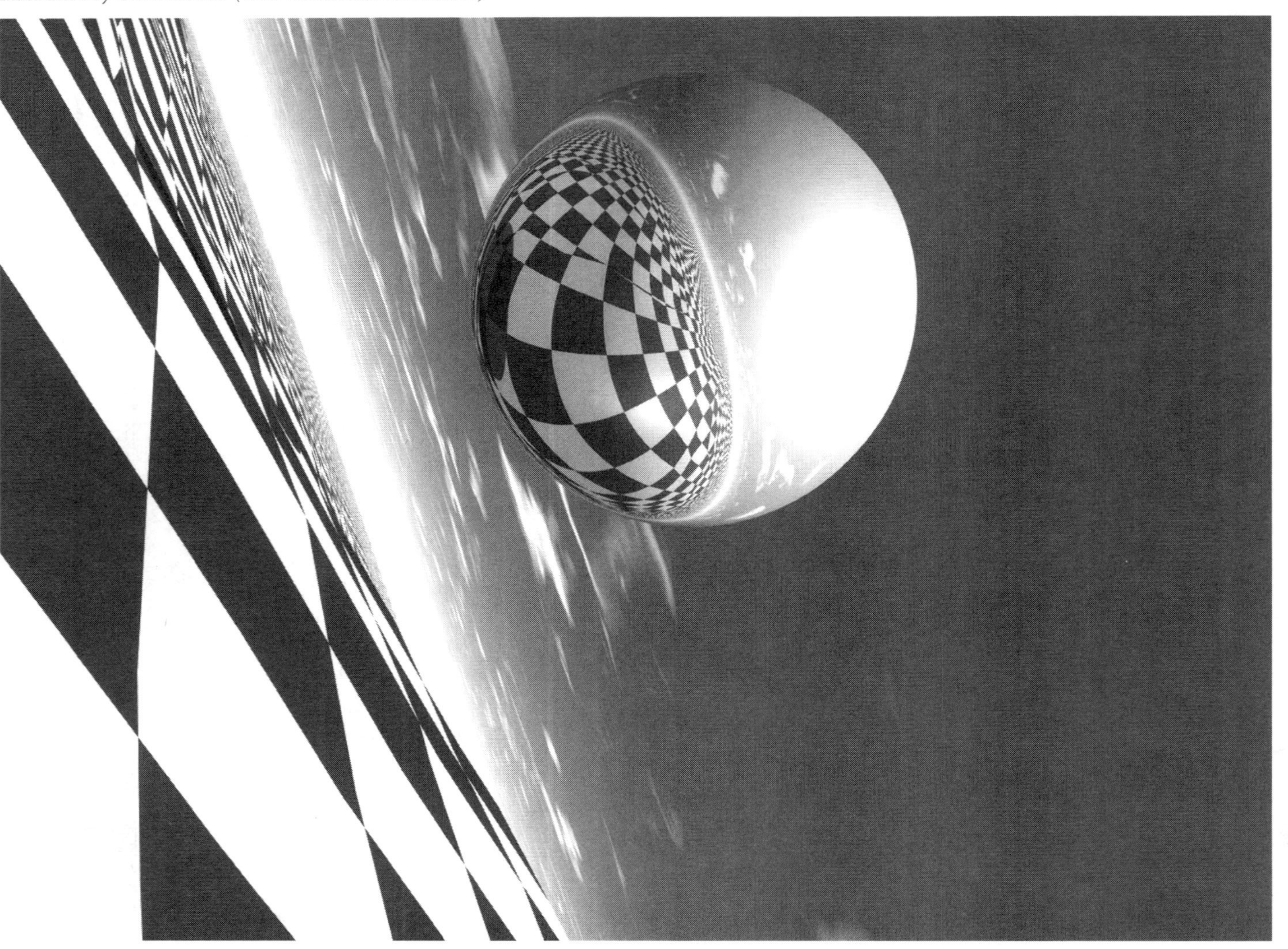

Illustration by Clark Dunbar (© RF RubberBall Productions)

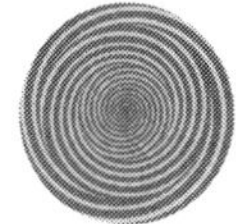

~ *Chapter 120* ~
ASTRAL HYPNO-HEALING

Includes
Curing Illness
Distant Healing
Suggestions For Astral Healing

CURING ILLNESS

Usually we identify so closely with our body that if the body is mentally or physically sick we feel that we are sick. In reality we are not sick– only our body is. Your body in due time can and will die but YOU will not die. You will simply leave the body that dies. If the SELF (soul) can leave the body at the time of death (as numerous persons who were declared clinically dead and returned to their bodies to live testify), there is no reason why it cannot leave the body during the period of the body's life span. After all, the same astral body that leaves at the time of death sometimes leaves during periods of deep sleep.

It is more difficult to cure yourself from a disease when you are close to the disease. You feel like you are part of it. When you distance yourself from disease you can treat it in an objective manner. This breakthrough point is the remarkable result of out-of-body hypnotherapy.

The SELF comes to recognize that it is actually *not the body* but controls the body. An out-of-body experiencing brings to awareness automatically. The SELF comes to recognize the body for what it actually is: a wonderful machine that lives and is operated for a time. The SELF may further come to realize that as the operator, it can readily repair the machine (or make desired changes) as it elects.

Correcting a problem from an out-of-body position causes a more objective viewpoint A new self-image and diffuse negative emotion. In other words, the problem is taken less seriously. This psychosomatic effect lessens serious problems and more readily achieves a cure. In knowing that IT is the real controller behind what the body does, the SELF comes to know itself as the master of what disturbs the body as well. SELF has "housed" itself during this lifetime and can control its environment.

The positioning of SELF outside the body to view the body as points of view rather that being confined to a point of view is an advancement in consciousness and provides a most effective form of hypnotherapy.

MODUS OPERANDI: DISTANT HEALING
Various religious practices make use of distant healing. This belongs to the realm of the hypnotherapist.

A time for the treatment is arranged and the client reclines and become passive and receptive to receive the healing influence that the practitioner sends from afar. The healer also becomes passive and visualizes the client as being close, and then sends positive curative thoughts mentally to the person. These suggestions in the form of thoughts are thus received by the client's subjective mind and, since they have absolute control of all the functions of their body and are amendable to the suggestions, (whether oral or mental) a cure if often obtained. The essential part of cure is the earnestness of purpose on the part of the healer and a passive condition of willingness of the client. Call it rapport.

SUGGESTIONS FOR ASTRAL HEALING
Hypnotize the client and give these suggestions:

"Conscious Mind of MYSELF stand to one side. As you now invite the Subconscious MIND OF SELF to come to front. Say to this part of the subconscious mind of myself stand at attention. I have some information to give you, which very possibly you already know. However, I want to repeat this information to you here and now. I want you to use, to act upon, and put this information into immediate operation.

Look upon yourself as being dual in nature. Your SELF exists as both body and mind. You exist in the body but you are not the body. You know this as truth. Mind goes where the SELF goes. As you know you, SELF and the body are separate, it is easy to leave the body when you wish to, and is equally easy for you to return to the body when you wish to. It is easy for you to do this, as you have done it many times.

Search your 'memory banks' and review this process so you can instantly project your astral body from you physical body on the post-hypnotic cue, which I now give you. Every time I say to you, while you are in hypnosis, 'Astral body project outside' you will automatically detach your astral FORM– containing yourself and mind– from your physical form, and you will project outside of your physical body. It is easy for you to know when this has occurred, as the experience to you will be that you are hovering above and looking down upon your physical body, which is sleeping below yourself. It is a real experience."

Is this experience real, or is it imagination or hypnotic hallucination? The astral body is so tenuous in structure that no one on the physical plane (except the very psychically sensitive) can see it. How, therefore, do you know it is real? You don't, but the experiencing is real, and that is all that is required for this form of hypnotherapy. If you want to look deeper into the matter, how do you really know that anything in life is any more than experiencing? You can say that you experience it as real; therefore you know it is real. If that is the way you reason, then you will very much feel that your out-of-body experiencing is real.

Continue now with the suggestions applied to this form of hypnotherapy:

"When you are out of your body you will be in your astral form above looking down upon your physical body enwrapped in hypnosis. Now you can give the body any suggestions you wish in order to make of it whatever you wish. You vacate that body for the moment. It lies before you like clay and you are the artist who can mold it in any form you wish. From your position outside of you body, you can remove any and all imperfections and make it perfectly as you wish it to be.

See a new image of your body, which is made perfect in every respect. See your body as a new body, which you are proud to exist in, in the here and now. You are in complete command of that body, and now that you are out of it, it will do exactly what you tell it to do and to become. As the operator of the body machine, you will now make the body exactly as you wish it to be so it performs perfectly and operates perfectly, and will be perfect for your use in every way when you reenter it and take up occupancy again.

Form the body, which belongs to you, as you want it to be. From your astral position in time and space you do this easily and to perfection. Start the processes of making the body perfect now.

When this is complete, reenter the body and awaken from the hypnosis knowing that the processes that you have put into operation, while out of the body, are now in effect. Your new body, as you desire it, is shaping up and becoming precisely the way you imaged it while you are in-body. It is your perfect body. Make this reality."

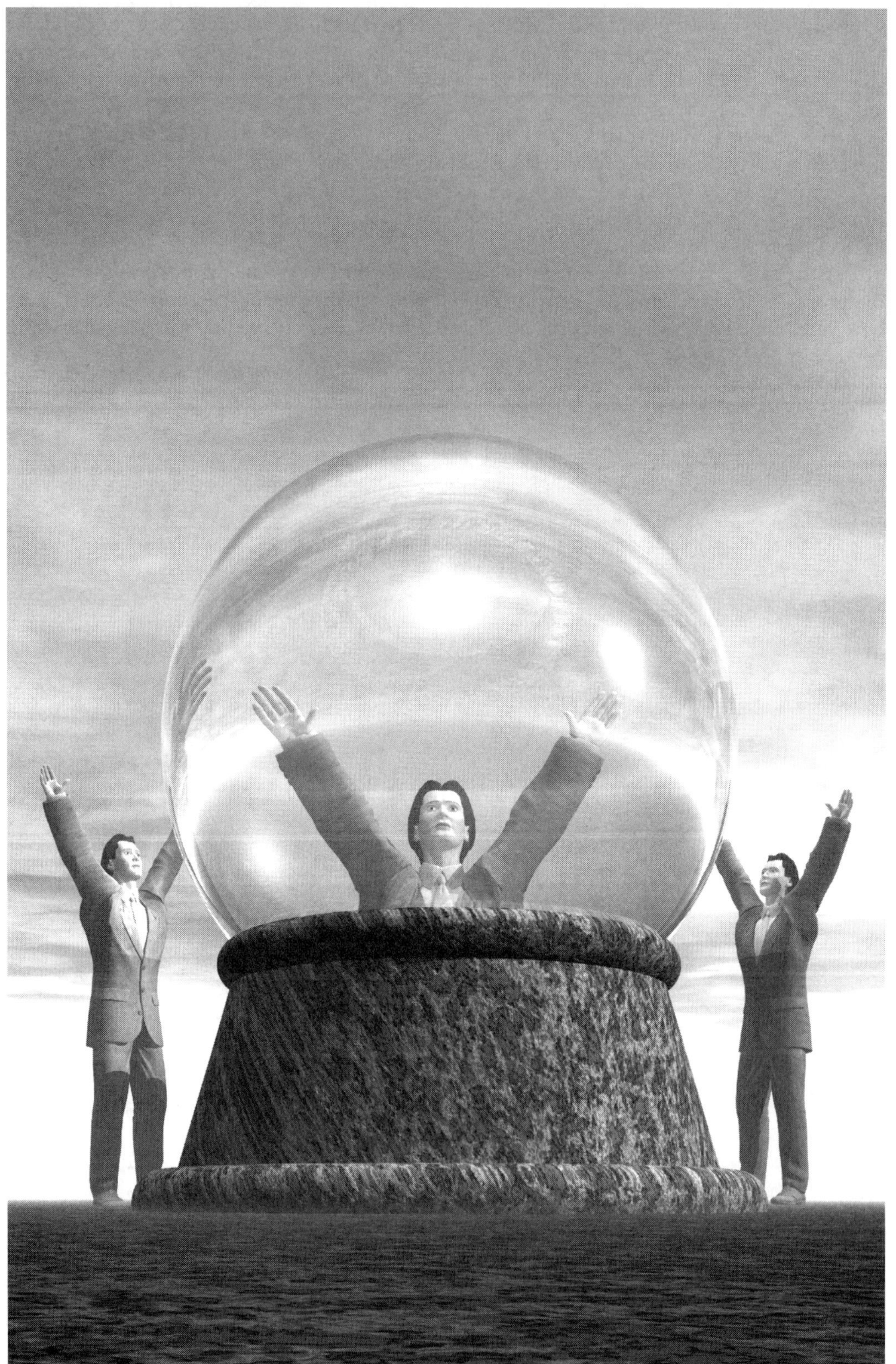

Illustration by Clark Dunbar (© RF RubberBall Productions)

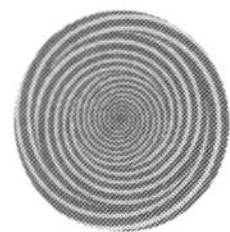

~ *Chapter 121* ~
ELLNER'S
NEURO LINGUISTIC HEALING (NLH)

By Michael Ellner, PhD

NueroLinguisticHealing™ or NLH is an emotionally detoxifying technique created by Michael Ellner, PhD of New York. It liberates someone who is stuck and unfeeling and helps them take charge of their life and wellness. Ellner crafted this approach from the teachings and techniques of Milton Erickson.

MODUS OPERANDI: EMOTIONAL DETOX

1. Pretalk

"Before we start, I want to assure you that you can be hypnotized. In fact, you have a veritable black belt in self-hypnosis. When you think about it; most of the time you are completely unaware of actually being asleep when you are dreaming. And, in the same way, most people don't even notice that they have moved into hypnotic states, when they are day-dreaming, fantasizing or are just plain pre-occupied.

During the session, feel free to space out any time you feel like it. That's right. During our session you can enjoy a favorite fantasy, take a mental nap or listen to everything that I have to say. Your subconscious mind will be doing all the work anyway.

Soon you will be able to hear the sound of my voice, while you time out everything else, without even thinking about it. As you begin to withdraw from this environment, every sound, thought, beat of your heart and breath you take will all work synergistically to help you feel more and more peaceful and calm. Its really automatic and you can slip into a profound trance state without even trying to do so.

Before we start, I want to remind you that no one can go back in time and start again, but any one can seize the moment and change their future: right NOW. All right get comfortable and feel free to shift your position any time that you feel you want to. Good.

Inhale and exhale deeply and let's release all of the unnecessary tension in your body. Starting with the left side of your body; mentally scan the toes on your left foot…now scan your foot, your ankle, calf and shin. That's it.

Now scan your knee, thigh, hip, the left side of your solar plexus and your left lung. Scan the left side of your neck and face. Now scan your right side of the body. Soon there will be no unnecessary tensions in your body at all. They are gone and that feels so right.

Good we are almost ready to start."

2. Unload Toxic Emotion

"Now for the purpose of off loading toxic emotions and feelings, close your eyes and let yourself feel any and all of your fears, doubts, anger and confusion so that we can detoxify them. Make a fist with your right hand. Release the fist and inhale and exhale deeply. Now vigorously shake those feelings right out of your system. That's it! Shake 'em out. Now gently open and close your eyes. Good.

Now picture yourself in your mind having a great hair day; you are at your ideal weight; your skin is glowing with health; your eyes sparkle with confidence and there is a big smile on your face because you feel centered and balanced. Excellent.

Now enjoy these feelings as you make a fist with your left hand and release it. Now inhale and exhale deeply and gently open your eyes. Okay, now count to ten and at the count of ten make a fist with both hands at the same time.

(Wait until they have done so.)

"You can actually feel yourself feeling better as you drift into the an image of yourself three months from today. You can see yourself clearly having a great hair day; you are at your ideal weight; your skin is glowing with health; your eyes sparkle with confidence and there is a big smile on your face because you have learned that when you have a happy heart, peaceful mind and playful spirit, life is on your side!

Enjoy these feelings and at the count of three, in the privacy of your mind, quietly shout 'life is on my side!' Let it vibrate in every cell in your brain. Wonderful!

Now, before you bring yourself back to everyday time and space, take another few moments to process today's session. Notice that a shift has occurred deep inside you. No matter how hard you try, you can't get in touch with any of the stuff that was disturbing you when you came to see me today. The reason is that you have successfully put those feelings and emotions behind you and you are feeling too good to be bothered by stuff that you have put behind you. You will continue to feel better and better during the next 48 hours as your subconscious mind continues to push those toxic emotions further and further away. In 48 hours, tomorrow will be yesterday and you will be feeling ready willing and able to take charge or your life and wellness.

When you leave the office today and the air touches your face, you will notice that everything is lighter and brighter. You'll be amazed by how much better you feel. Okay, finish up and bring yourself back to every day time and space."

Give them a moment or two and when they open their eyes, ask them to **"Try as hard as you can to reconnect with your toxic feelings and you'll notice that they won't go there; there is no desire to be there and this is proof that today's session was a great success."**

This is an ideal time to recommend a follow up session.

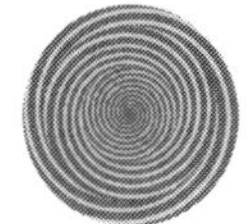

~ *Chapter 122* ~
REFLEXOLOGY HYPNOTHERAPY

Includes
Quick Reflexology Relaxation
Quick Reflexology Induction Formula
Reflexology Hypnotic Deepening
Reflexology Suggestion Formula

Reflexology is a timeless art and science of healing. Feet map our entire body and mental processes. The thousands of nerves are reflex triggers that correspond to every organ, function, and system within the body. Simply pressing on a reflex point can remarkably revitalize, balance body's energies, and create overall well being. Stress, pain and fatigue, headaches, insomnia, and depression are quickly relieved by reflexology.

Applying pressure to these points stimulates the functions of mental and physical performance, in relation to the pressure point areas show in the chart.

Hypnosis is a psychological/physiological process. Reflexology is a combination of both. The mental process of hypnosis is centered in the brain, which functions like a bio-computer within the head, which through its many wires (nerves) manipulates the body and motivates the behavior.

Reflexology and hypnosis are a good match, each greatly amplifies the other. Manipulating the feet can induce hypnosis and hypnosis advances the effectiveness of reflexology. Both hypnosis and reflexology induce trance and control the state it induces.

As in hypnosis, reflexology helps the person bypass critical (conscious mind) and establish selective thinking and receptivity to suggestion in the subconscious phase of mind. In other words, old unwanted ideas are easily replaced by the new wanted ideas with reflexology-hypnotherapy.

The hypnotherapist applies pressure upon the specific spots that relate to the person's issues and simultaneously give verbal hypnotic suggestions.

Illustration by Ormond McGill

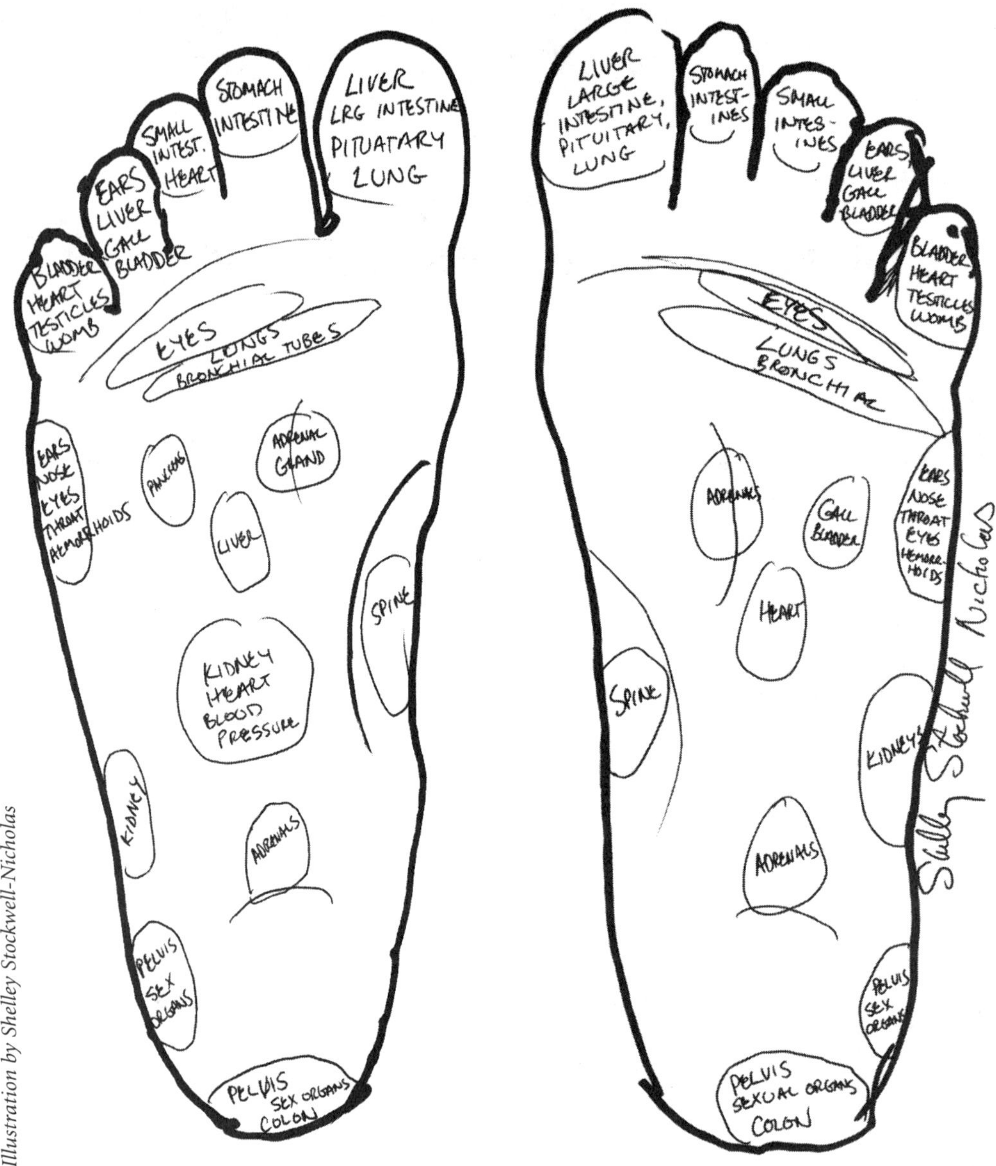

Look at the reflexology chart above as it relates to organic functioning of the body.

MODUS OPERANDI: QUICK REFLEXOLOGY RELAXATION

You Will Need:

Something to Wash and Dry the Client's Feet
Dusting Powder
New Age Music

Wash your hands. Have your client thoroughly wash and dry their feet or you can do it for them if you are so inclined.

Dust the feet generously with talcum powder. Feet so prepared are a pleasure to work with and "feel so good." Feeling good is very important to successful hypnotherapy. A relaxed client produces a reverie state of mind. Have the client lie outstretched on their back on a couch or reclining chair, with their bare feet projecting out towards you.

Music like "Golden Voyage," "Ancient Echoes," or better yet, use the specially produced "Hypnotrance Music" or "Entrancing Music."

The induction is ready to begin:

QUICK REFLEXOLOGY INDUCTION FORMULA

Tell the reclining, barefooted client:

"You will rest quietly without moving once hypnosis commences. So, get comfortable now, and remain still. Breathe deeply and think how comfortable you feel. Relax your body all over, as you rest with your feet comfortably relaxed. How nice it feels to be bare footed. For a few moments, concentrate on how good bare feet feel. As you listen to the pleasant meditative music.

THINK of how relaxed you are becoming. THINK of how sleepy the music makes you feel; how nice it is to have bare feet. Now, just drift away with the music.

Now, pick up the client's right foot and hold it between your hands, with a palm of hand flat against each side of the foot, as it is cradled between your hands. Now, vigorously and gently massage your hands up and down on each side of the foot. As do, suggest:

"How sleepy this massaging of your right foot makes you feel. It makes you feel relaxed all over, and you are dropping off to sleep… going deep into hypnotic sleep. As I release your right foot now, and massage your left foot… you will continue going to sleep.

Go to sleep. You feel relaxed and serene all over.

I now gently release your left foot and place it comfortably beside your right foot.

Now, I will pick up one foot at a time, and gently bend your toes between my hands, back and forth. As your toes bend back and forth in this pleasant way, you drop deep, deep into hypnotic sleep. Go into hypnosis now."

REFLEXOLOGY HYPNOTIC DEEPENING

Release the client's bare feet. To rest side-by-side upon the couch. Direct your attention now towards the background music. Suggest:

"You are dropping down into hypnosis now. Just listen to the music and go to sleep. Experience the sleepiness. You are so sleepy. Sleep. Let yourself go to sleep. It feels so good to go to sleep. Breathe deeply now and go to sleep… and every breath you take sends you down deeper and deeper to sleep. All you hear is the beautiful music claiming your attention and lulling you to sleep. It is so soothing to go into the music and go to sleep, to sleep in pleasant hypnosis. You are breathing deep and full… deep and full in the rhythm of sleep."

Watch the client's breathing now, and observe how they enter hypnotic sleep. You are now ready to present Reflexology suggestions for benefit.

REFLEXOLOGY SUGGESTION FORMULA

Study the Reflexology chart of the areas of the feet related to organic functioning of the body. Depending upon the purpose of the session, apply pressure upon these specific spots simultaneously combined with hypnotic suggestions.

"Drop down into deep hypnosis now, as the music slowly fades away, and you relax. (bring the music volume down). **Relax as I apply beneficial pressure upon your feet and give you beneficial suggestions."**

First I am going to stimulate your biocomputer brain by pressing on the tips of your BIG TOE, SECOND TOE, and THIRD TOE of each foot. This intensifies the operation of your brain center. Is this agreeable, subconscious mind? If it is agreeable, nod your head."

Get a subconscious acceptance nod. Then press in firmly on the tips of those toes on both feet.

"You are in hypnosis now, in which every suggestion given you becomes amplified in effect. I am going to press in on every area of the soles of both your right and left foot. As I do this, your entire body will benefit with good health and well-being. Every organ in your body functions perfectly. Reflexology Hypnotherapy benefits you in every way. Relax and go deeper and deeper into hypnosis as the music plays."

Allow some moments of silence, as the music volume level rises. As the music plays, proceed to press in firmly in every area of the client's feet. Take your time in doing this; there is no hurry. Press in on each spot firmly, hold for a couple of seconds... then release and proceed on to the next spot on the foot to be pressed upon.

The hypnotic suggestions you have given the client will increase the effects of Reflexology. Covering all pressure spots provides tremendous benefits to the client.

When both feet have been completely activated, fade the music to play softer, and give these suggestions to the client's subconscious:

"Subconscious mind, has the activation of the organs of this person been properly stimulated for maximum operation and benefit? If so, nod your head."

If all has been done correctly, you will get a nod of affirmation.

"Now, I am going to carefully go over every area on each of your feet – pressing in upon every point activating every organ in your body to perfection. Your body and mind function in perfect harmony with each other. You are alive and vital in every way. In your entirety, you function to perfection.

You are ready to come out of hypnosis now, and return to the here and now. I will count slowly from one to five... and by the time I reach the count of FIVE, you will be wide-awake, alert, feeling wonderful and fine. You will be in perfection of well-being.

When you leave my office, you go on your way...amazingly benefited from your enjoyable session in REFLEXOLOGY HYPNOTHERAPY."

Music fades out. Client arouses. The session is complete.

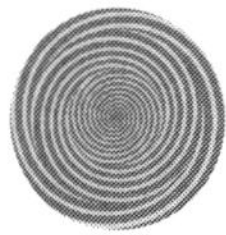

~ *Chapter 123* ~
STOCKWELL-NICHOLAS SLEEP PROGRAM

By Shelley Stockwell-Nicholas, PhD

Includes
Why Do You Sleep?
Call Me A Somnambulance
How Much Sleep Do We Need To Feel Refreshed?
For The Sleepless Client
Sleep Apnea
Narcolepsy
Eating To Exhaustion
Sleeping Pill Problems
Get The Picture: Get Sleep!
Honor Circadian Rhythms
Peaceful Slumber Script

Hypnosis is a miracle for those who have trouble sleeping!

The dictionary defines sleep as *"A periodic suspension of conscious awareness during which the body rests and restores itself."* This could be a great hypnosis definition as well.

WHY DO YOU SLEEP?

Sleep takes up a third to half of your life and nobody is really sure why. We do know that it seemingly paralyzes the body, activates the brain and renews. Your muscles relax, you digest, your pituitary gland manufactures more seratonin and you more readily synthesize protein and growth hormones. Cortisol, the hormone your adrenals release as your fight, flight, fright or excite response, is lowered. This may be why sleep helps you cleanse stress. If you do not sleep, cortisol levels remain high. This stress damages and shrinks the part of your brain (hippocampus) that remembers and learns. That is why you don't think as well when sleep deprived

Sleep cycles four or five times a night into quiet, dreamless sleep (non-rapid eye movement; NREM) and dreaming sleep, (with its rapid eye movements or REM's). Hypnotists know REM and eye fluttering as outward signs of a trance. Trance also seemingly paralyzes the body and activates the brain.

Millions of years ago humans ate every two hours and slept afterwards, the same way primates do today. Night was a dangerous time to forage for food, so people learned to sleep at night and stay awake during the day. This conserved energy and kept them safe during darkness. The ancestors' two-hour sleep cycles is probably why we daydream in a waking trance (alpha state) every two hours and enter dreamful sleep (theta state) every two hours while asleep.

CALL ME A SOMNAMBULANCE

Sleep-deprived folks talk about sleep the way starving folks talk about food. These folks come to a hypnotherapist for help and hypnosis is terrific help.

The word *insomnia* used to mean the "total inability to sleep." Now it describes difficulty in falling asleep, waking during the night, or getting up too early in the morning. Those who have disrupted sleep for over three weeks are said to have insomnia.

Extreme temperatures, odd schedules, jet lag, poor breathing, lack of exercise, late strenuous exercise, a lumpy bed, noise (like the TV), pain, stress, loss, poor eating habits, an uncleansed bowel, alcohol, caffeine, sugar, artificial sweeteners, processed food, salt, soy, dairy, meat, and drugs, (like sleep medications and nicotine) unwind your body clock and disrupt sleep. So does obsession about work, family, money or anything! Recent studies say that sticking to a regular bedtime and waking schedule, not watching television in bed, healthy eating, and the right mental attitude gets the best results. Hypnosis helps reestablish new healthy patterns.

HOW MUCH SLEEP DO YOU NEED TO FEEL REFRESHED?

How long you sleep doesn't depend on how tired you are; it depends on your body's natural rhythm, your environment and what you have in your system.

The more sleepless nights you have, the more catnaps you take. If sleep-deprived for two to three days, we micro-sleep and doze for a few seconds with eyes opened or closed. When your body clock returns to a normal cycle you crave a good night's rest.

Newborn babies sleep sixteen to eighteen hours a day. By age two or three sleep drops to twelve hours and by age five naps usually stop. Adults sleep anywhere from four to ten hours, with the majority sleeping seven to eight hours per night. As people age, they often get less sleep but they still need seven to eight hours. The elderly tend to be more "early birds" than "night owls." Only a small percentage of people function well with only four to five hours of sleep.

MODUS OPERANDI: FOR THE SLEEPLESS CLIENT

During your interview have your client conduct an informal self-study to determine how many hours of sleep they actually need per night. Then hypnotically set a sleep goal. Do a thorough interview and discover what outside factors come into play, so you help them become consciously aware of anything they do that interferes with sleep. Heavy meals, caffeine, sugar, alcohol, allergies, excessive exercise, tobacco and other drugs, especially after 4 p.m., mess up sleep rhythms. As you discover their sleep disrupters give simple suggestion formulas to reverse them.

EATING TO EXHAUSTION

Check out what goes in their mouth. Sleep difficulties are often a reaction to binging and boozing. A tasty dinner and dessert, innocently eaten hours ago, may stoke a metabolic furnace to increase body temperature instead of lowering it for sleep. Gas and indigestion interrupt sleep. A University of Chicago study had healthy subjects sleep four hours for six nights straight. The result was an inability for their body to break down sugar, which produced a rise in serum glucose and serum insulin levels. This risks adult onset diabetes and weight gain. Suggest: **"I eat lightly in the evening, and avoid caffeine, nicotine, alcohol or exercise** (whatever vexes them) **four to six hours before bedtime. I enjoy a good night's sleep. My body is bio-chemically balanced and renewed."**

MODUS OPERANDI: SLEEP APNEA

Poor breathing disrupts sleep and deprives the brain of oxygen. Stoppage of breath and collapsed airways is called sleep apnea. If that's a problem, ask your entranced client,

"Subconscious Mind, what is causing _________ (Their name) **sleep challenges? Is it the result of a physical issue or obstruction? If so, please shrink any enlargements so that** _____ **can sleep soundly through out the night."**

Some folks have great results using little nose shields that football players wear. Others attend sleep clinics, or wear a mask that shoots air up their nose. Surgically removing enlarged tonsils or adenoids or righting a deviated septum may be a good strategy for some so you might suggest that they see their doctor.

MODUS OPERANDI: NARCOLEPSY

Narcolepsy, or nodding off to sleep at the wrong times, is a sleep disorder helped greatly by diet, hypnosis and biofeedback.

SLEEPING PILL PROBLEMS

It is estimated that 4.3% of Americans take prescription sleeping pills and even more buy sleeping aids over the counter. If your client is one of them, they know the price they pay in stress.

Sleeping pills, sedatives (barbiturates) and hypnotics (benzodiazepines), actually make sleep problems worse, because they backfire and disrupt sleep. Meds like alcohol and sugar knock you out only to wake you up mid-sleep. Over time, the body develops tolerance and requires more and more drug to get the same effect...a true nightmare. Because of their addictive nature, stopping usage can cause insomnia,.

Even if sleeping pills increase the number of hours of sleep, they decrease deep REM sleep essential for wakeful clear thinking and coordination. That's why folks on downers (that's what sleeping pills really are) feel confused after a drugged night's rest. Older folks on downers have a higher incidence of falling down and hurting themselves.

Such addictions eventually contribute to illness and injury. When this happens, folks tend to move on to different medications. A sleeping pill junkie who has tried to stop, knows how addictive these drugs are. Withdrawal often causes a kind of healing crisis, where sleep problems worsen for a short time, excessive REM sleep occurs, and nightmares may ensue. Hypnosis and its placebo like effect helps to kick away the pill mill.

MODUS OPERANDI: SLEEPING PILL ADDICTS

Recommend that your client talk to their doctor about "weaning off of their drugs." Quitting some sleep medications cold turkey can be deadly.

Ask your client while in entranced:

"Is your issue with sleep the result of anything that your are eating, drinking or taking into your body?"

Wait for their reply.

"Thank you. What action step can ______(their name) **take right now to let that behavior change for the good?"**

GET THE PICTURE: GET SLEEP!

Daily exercise deepens sleep. A Stanford University study said that people who exercised 30 to 40 minutes, four times a week showed "significant improvement" in the duration and quality of sleep. Some say that gentle stretching before bedtime is helpful. There is a hot debate on whether exercise just before bedtime helps or hinders sleep. Let your client's subconscious mind tell what is best for them.

A glass of warm milk, with its natural l-tryptophan, the same amino acid found in mother's milk, beans and turkey helps drowsiness. If sex comforts your client, it's a great nightcap. Some say a warm bath is a terrific bedtime ritual.

Insomniacs frequently lack thiamin, riboflavin, B6, B12, folate, pantothenate, potassium, magnesium and iron. Some swear that the right vitamins are the ticket to a great night's sleep. I prefer hypnosis. Hypnosis helps you develop healthier habits.

HONOR CIRCADIAN RHYTHMS

Sleep, at regular times, and in a darkened room, allows normal body rhythm.

Morning sunlight has one hundred times the intensity of indoor light. It interacts with melatonin, a neurotransmitter that your body releases when you sleep. If you expose yourself to light at six a.m. melatonin releases earlier the next evening to make you sleepier sooner. My friend swears that melatonin tablets, taken just before bed, counteract jet lag and sleep pattern disruptions.

Night owls are more suited to shift work than morning folks are. Rotating work shifts that move from day to evening to night (clockwise) are easier on sleep patterns than counter-clockwise shifts. It's easier to keep regular sleeping patterns by maintaining the same schedule on days on and off work.

MODUS OPERANDI: Peaceful Slumber Script
1. Recognize a sincere desire to positively change patterns for the good.
2. Discover what their sleep patterns are, what is their sleep environment; is the room too cold, noisy or is their bed lumpy?
3. Reverse them out with their own subconscious solutions or use your own reversals
4. The following are presenting problems and helpful suggestion formulas for each:

PRESENTING SLEEP PROBLEM	**SUGGESTION FORMULA**
"I worry at bedtime."	**"Leave a list of concerns and to-do's in another room."**
"I eat a heavy dinner."	**"Eat lightly at night and eat earlier in the evening. You lower your body temperature and metabolism when you close your eyes to sleep."**
"Caffeine, nicotine, alcohol."	**"None after 4pm or none at all."**
"I exercise at night."	**"Exercise, morning, noon or at least 4 hours before sleep. You enjoy light stretches before sleep."**
"I watch the clock all night."	**"Turn the clock away from the bed"**
"I have a crazy schedule."	**"You create a regular bedtime and rising schedule. You go to bed and get up at the same time each day, even on weekends. You factor in extra sleep time to regulate your body clock and adjust to shift changes, jet lag and time zones. If you choose, schedule an extra 30-60 minutes sleep treat weekends or vacation."**
"I have trouble falling asleep."	**"As soon as your head touches the pillow you relax all over. When you move your pillow you hypnotize yourself to fall asleep and sleep even more deeply, Listen to McGill's *Sleeping Pill Tape* or Stockwell's *Sleep Beautiful Sleep* tape."**
"There is too much noise."	**"The sound of the room goes on & you don't notice it at all"** or **"You block out the sound with the white noise of a fan or a hypnosis tape. Move noisy clocks away."**
"I sleep with the TV/radio on."	**"Put the television (radio) in another room or turn it off or enjoy soothing music instead."**
"My bed is uncomfortable."	**"You manifest the perfect bed for yourself. You have the right amount of covers."**
"My medication keeps me awake."	**"Talk to your doctor immediately and let them wean you off the medicine or find a more beneficial one. The best sleeping aid is pleasure seeking and doing good kind and relaxing things for yourself all day long. Self hypnosis and meditation are terrific relaxers. You find new ways to take it easy."**
"I have nightmares."	**"Your dreams are pleasant and fun. They have comfortable beginnings and middles and interesting and rewarding endings. While you dream you will meet a special helper guide who gives you a gift. Your actions and words in your dream are positive and you feel great."**

"You enjoy restful slumber. It is easy for you. You always enjoy a good night's sleep. Your bedroom is a cozy sanctuary. You tell your body when it's time for bed and your body easily relaxes and complies. You take an honest inventory of any action or behavior that disrupts perfect slumber and let them go. You don't need those anymore. You embrace thoughts and actions that encourage sleep. You love sleep and you love yourself. You easily drift into sleep and sleep soundly. The sounds of the night go on as you enjoy renewing and restoring your body and mind. If for any reason you must arise to attend to something, you do so quickly and efficiently and then easily return to slumber within 2 minutes. You picture pleasant scenes in your imagination. You take pleasant thoughts to bed with you and leave negative things outside. Your time in bed is a reverent time.

Say this loving prayer 'bless me to sleep full and soundly so that I do the work and play I came here to do. Thank you for this sacred time of deep renewal and love. Amen. Awoman. Ah Life.'

Now imagine yourself in your bedroom. The clock says that it is your bedtime; the time you choose to get a delicious night's rest. You have just completed a lovely bedtime ritual and you how good your room looks, feels, smells, tastes, sounds. Notice the ceiling as you experience yourself snugly nestled in your bed. You enter into deep hypnosis as your head touches your pillow.

That's right. As I count now from five to one, say to yourself, I go deeper and deeper into this beautiful room of relaxation. Five…four…three…two…

When you reach the number one you will be there entirely and fully relaxed in your bed…one…very good. You experience yourself completely rested and relaxed, as you lie comfortable in your bed. You are at peace. Notice how you so easily drifted into drowsy slumber. As you sleep you go deeper and deeper inside yourself. You so enjoy this special time with yourself. It is fun for you to sleep soundly. The clock is now three hours from the time you drifted away into such a profound sleep. It is so restful as you sleep hour after hour after hour and you remain asleep until it is your time to get up. You awaken in a terrific mood, full of energy and happy to be you."

Hypno-Helper
"The Sleeping Pill Tape", Ormond McGill
"Sleep, Beautiful Sleep", Shelley Stockwell
Two audio tapes that help you sleep.

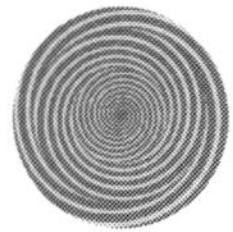

~ *Chapter 124* ~
VITALE'S HYPNOAESTHETICS™
FOR BEAUTIFUL SKIN

By Anna Vitale, A.C.H.

When I was first certified as a hypnotherapist in 1987, I willingly immersed myself into all the literature my thirsty mind could soak up. I read voraciously about the studies that demonstrated that hypnosis could accelerate healing in burn victims, create healing of serious skin conditions and increase breast size!

Experimentation on my favorite subject (myself) took me into wonderful altered states of mind travel, glimpsing other realities and experiencing hypnotic phenomena through self-hypnosis.

One day, in an exceptionally deep state, I noticed a very powerful sensation that felt like electricity. In my deep state, I questioned what I was experiencing. I heard a voice reply "You are experiencing electrical thought energy." It was a strange feeling yet I wondered if I could make it work for me.

I directed the energy to my face, then my scalp, then my bloodstream, then my internal organs. Low and behold, the energy would slowly but steadily flow to the part of my body I directed it to. I remembered the small facial wart on my left cheek. I directed the energy to the wart. I asked it to dissolve the wart. I sensed the energy following my directions, pinpointing itself on the tiny unwanted growth. Then I visualized my face without wart.

Every day I took the time to do this and would glance in the mirror. Day by day, I saw the wart becoming smaller. After about a month, not only did the wart disappear but the brown spots on my cheek did too!

After that success, I decided to send the energy to my entire face and scalp. My thinning hair came to life and my facial skin looked healthier than ever. My enthusiasm with the results gave birth to the technique I call Hypnoaesthetics. (Hypnosis for Aesthetic Enhancement.)

New applications came flowing. First for face and hair, then facial skin alone, then concentration on hair, then the entire body, then cellular health, then vision, breast enhancement and longevity. My Hypnoaesthetics audio tape series was born.

MODUS OPERANDI: VITALE'S HYPNOAESTHETICS ™

1. Ask the client, **"Do remember waking from a particularly vivid dream or nightmare with your rapid heart beat or drenched in perspiration?"**

2. **"Close your eyes and visualize your favorite meal. Imagine the aroma as you do."** Then have them open their eyes and ask them, **"Did you sense your salivary glands creating more saliva?"**

3. **"Now sit quietly and think about your left thumb."** After about a minute **"Notice the sense of throbbing or tingling."**

4. Talk about how blood flow is affected by thought.

5. Talk about how the world programs us to believe that aging means physical deterioration.

6. Bring your client into the deepest state of hypnosis with an induction of your choice. Here is a generic example of the kind of suggestions that can be applied to any physiological goal. Make sure you take a long pause between suggestions to allow your client to experience the sensations:

    "Become aware of your right toe. Sense a feeling of energy or awareness in that right toe."
    (Long Pause.)

    "Now sense that the energy is expressing itself with a tingling feeling in all of your toes."
    (Long Pause.)

    Now sense that energy and tingling feeling in your fingers. Sense the energy becoming stronger and stronger."
    (Long pause.)

    "This is your own electrical thought energy creating change. Now sense that energy tingling as it travels up your arms."
    (Long pause)

    "Now sense that energy or tingling feeling traveling up your legs."
    (Long pause)

    "Sense that it is becoming stronger and more powerful. You are taping into the powerful energy of change. Now send that energy to the area of your body you wish to enhance or heal. Feel that energy traveling to where you are directing it to go. Feel the power of your own mind to create change. Sense the energy as it makes its journey to the area of your body you wish to improve. Feel it, experience it."
    (Long pause.)

    "As you experience this electrical thought energy-generating change in your body, know that this energy is created through the power of your own mind. Welcome that energy and allow your mind to create an image of yourself achieving your goal. Visualize that change in you."
    (Long pause.)

    "Sense it, feel it, imagine yourself achieving that goal now.
    You realize that your body is a precious gift that needs attention, nurturing and care. This is your wonderful home in this lifetime. You allow your body to consume as much water as possible. You choose to live a healthier lifestyle with your choices of food, activities and attitudes. You are helping your body to enhance itself in every way. You are creating changes within your body that will enhance your well-being and result in the healthiest lifestyle

possible. You are allowing your mind to create the changes you desire…now. I will wait a few moments to allow your energy to make the changes you desire."

(Give the client at least sixty seconds of silence.)

"Now whenever you think of the word (choose one based on the goal) you will sense your energy going to work for you."

After your session, ask the client what they felt during the session.

Have them come back for more sessions or record the session so that they may continue doing the method at home.

Hypno-Helper
"Hypnoaesthetics" Audio Tape by Anna Vitale

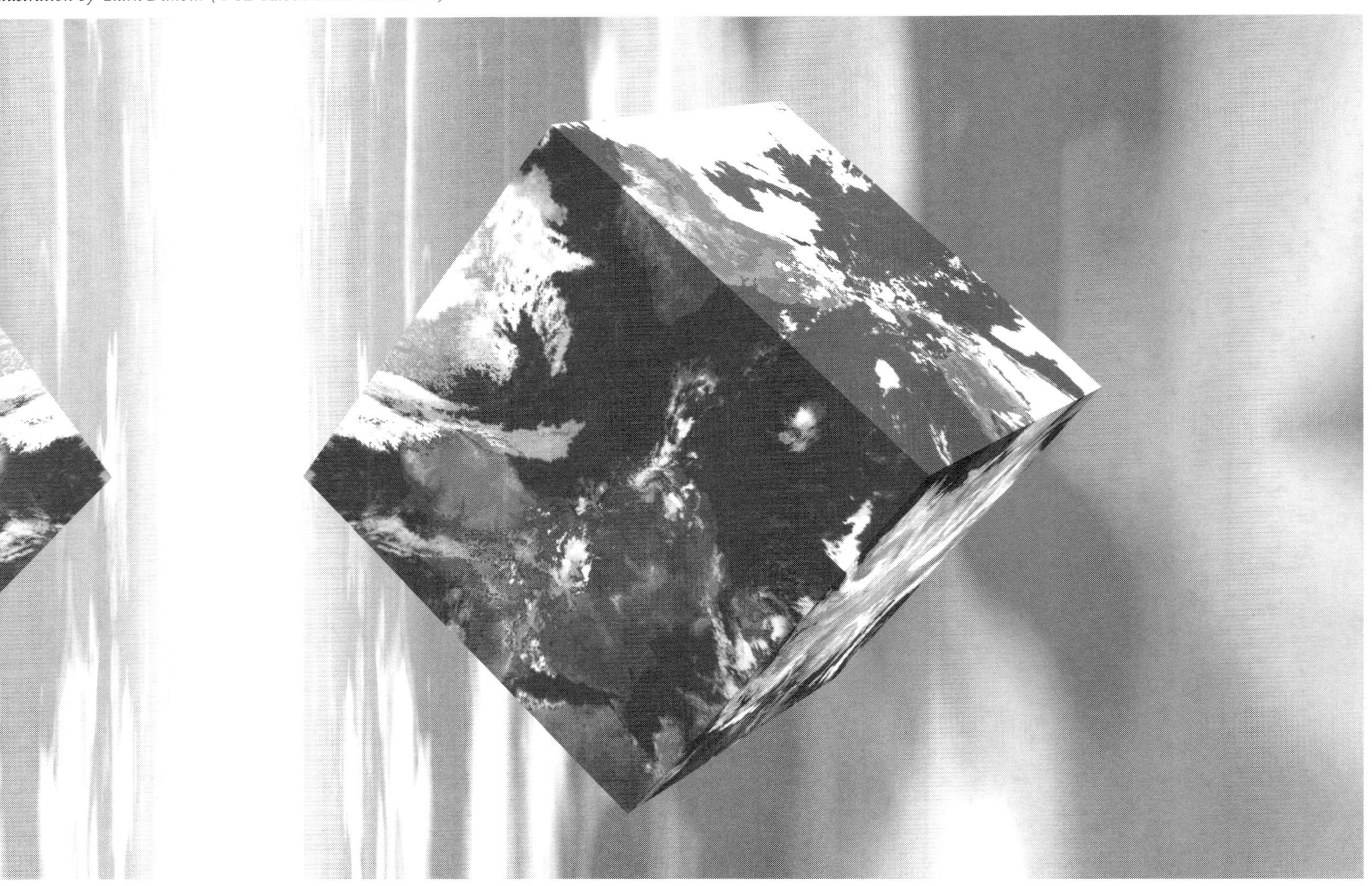

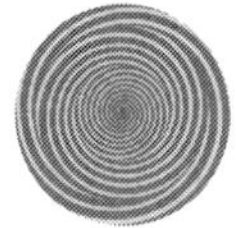

~ *Chapter 125* ~
3-D HYPNOTHERAPY

Includes
Playing The Game Of Life

3-D adds a new dimension to what you perceive. You become a witness to life. Here is great Hypnotherapy. The 3-D way for playing the game of life is to recognize that the life you are currently living is just a game, and a game is to be played while enjoying the playing. When you appreciate that this is the case and observe your life from a 3-D perspective, you have taken a quantum leap in consciousness.

For a start, appreciate this story:
Buddha was dying. His followers gathered around and asked,
"Master, now that you will be leaving us soon, please tell us how we can have the peace and serenity you possess."
Buddha looked up and smiled, "Just change your attitude."
Buddha told the entire process in that one sentence. When you are in control of your attitudes, you have become a master of your mind. You have taken control. A PEACEFUL MIND IS A MIND UNDER CONTROL.

The Hindu Sage, Patanjali gives four directives for having a peaceful mind:
1. Be friendly towards the successful.
2. Show compassion towards the miserable.
3. Enjoy the virtuous.
4. Be indifferent in your opinion as to what is evil and what is not evil.

Establishing these four tenants into the subconscious, as the way to handle life, is wonderful hypnotherapy. Give them to your clients. It is establishing 3-D Perception, which is to relax into Existence, and view life from a vertical position rather than a horizontal.
For centuries many have conjectured what the Master meant in telling you to PLAY THE GAME OF LIFE with a peaceful mind. In this, 3-D Hypnotherapy is being spoken of. It is the mental therapy for obtaining serenity.
Absorb the Buddha story.

The subconscious loves to get absorbed in stories. Absorption is to get totally with something…to completely feel it, to get at ONE with it. The subconscious is "the feeling mind." The famous hypnotherapist, the late Milton Erickson told metaphors to his clients/patients as a major part of his work. The use of metaphors as a hypnotherapy healing method is what this chapter is all about. In 3-D Hypnotherapy, a story is given as an instruction in narrative form to the subconscious. The professional practice of 3-D Hypnotherapy opens a whole vista of mental healing.

Most who find their way to the hypnotherapist office are seeking relief from some inner conflict of one kind or another. That is to say a battle of life rages within the individual. They would give their eyeteeth to move from a battlefield to a playfield…a playground in which life is enjoyed just for the playing. What happens in a playground? Games are played in a playground, and games are meant to be enjoyed. When the pattern of life is turned into a GAME, one's entire philosophy of living is transformed. The hypnotherapist can do this for his or her clients. You can call it 3-D Hypnotherapy of Hypno-philosophy, as you choose. Whatever you call it, use your skills to cause clients to come to know how to joyfully PLAY THE GAME OF LIFE.

What truly great Hypnotherapists Buddha and Patanjali are saying is to relax into existence and view life from a vertical position to successfully PLAY THE GAME OF LIFE.

The vertical means one rises above the horizontal happenings of ordinary perception and becomes a witness to it all, as an interesting panorama of miracles unfolding below in <u>knowing</u> that all life is a miracle, and YOU…to yourself…are the greatest miracle of all. No ego involved; simply as Patanjali puts it, "It is the case." To RELAX INTO EXISTENCE what a wonderful symbolism of hypnotherapy that is. And to use it for training the mind for PLAYING THE GAME OF LIFE…that is 3-D HYPNOTHERAPY.

MODUS OPERANDI: PLAYING THE GAME OF LIFE

Hypnotize your client by any method you prefer. When the person is in that receptive subjective state, implant this suggestion-formula: **"As you drift along in this pleasant reverie open wide the vistas of your subconscious and allow these suggestions to become your way of responding to life. They become your very own as you instinctively come to know how to PLAY THE GAME OF LIFE. You KNOW that life is a game we play that goes on and on with never an ending. You recognize this truth about eternity, and through this knowing the better you play the game.**

Now ask yourself a question or two or three…

How do you play a game?

What is the root purpose of a game?

How do you become master of a game?

Just let the answers come from the KNOWING that is deep inside yourself…

You play a game by first learning its rules and then by following the rules. KNOW THIS! A game at its roots is just a game and basically is something to be enjoyed. KNOW THIS!

Combine this KNOWING and you commence to live life fully to the hilt and with a merry twinkle in your eyes.

Now as you drift along in this pleasant reverie of hypnosis, within your mind's eye see before you a vast game-board upon which the game of life is played. It is like a huge chessboard that unfolds out into space with its furthest rim lost in distant infinity.

Lifetime after lifetime you have played upon that game-board, so you really know it well. And upon that game-board of THE GAME OF LIFE many pieces have come and gone in the persons that form the game-pieces of the game you play.

One can get so caught up in the game that you, yourself, at times seem to become one of the game-pieces that move upon the board.

But that is not the truth you know…for you KNOW that no game is ever played upon the board by the player, as the real player sits beside the game and watches and makes the

game-pieces move. The more expertly this is done, the more is your mastery of THE GAME OF LIFE.

And yet in your mounting wisdom, you know how intensely we do become sometimes enmeshed in the game we play, as so much is to be found within THE GAME OF LIFE. Just think:

There is happiness there…there is sadness there.

There is love there…there is unlove there.

There is health there…there is illness there.

There is success there…there is failure there.

On and ever on, the possibilities of experience go. Just come to know they are but adventures you have along the way, as you play GAME OF LIFE. Yin and Yang…positive and negative…ever the pendulum swings:

On and on and ever onward THE GAME OF LIFE IS PLAYED. How deeply it captures attention that we oft forget that it is but a game we play, and how seriously we take it all.

BUT NOW YOU KNOW THE TRUTH!

And you will ever know that life is but a game we play with existence as our partner. And remember, always that a game to be most enjoyed must be played for the sheer fun of playing.

AND YOU WILL KNOW…

All persons that enter your life and come and go upon your game-board are but players as game-pieces in the game, you watch. You are a witness to the game. Some game-pieces become so seemingly important they stay upon the board, while others are more flitting. But remember, one of wisdom, the truth is that they are but game-pieces…they are not the player. YOU ARE THE PLAYER.

And so it is with everyone. Each is the player of their own game of life. And even the player can at times seem to become a game-piece in the life of others. In and out, up and down, and as the game advances, the 3-dimensional it becomes.

AND SO JUST KNOW…

It is when you recognize the multidimensional possibilities of THE GAME OF LIFE, which you can play in the eternity of Existence divine BEING that you are. When you really come to MASTERSHIP, let this become your KNOWING.

Then you will come to know, as the game-player seated on one side of the vast game-board that spreads into infinity before you, that EXISTENCE is your friend and nothing can really harm you at all. So play the game with love in your heart for all that is and smile at your fellow layers. YOU PLAY THE GAME IN HAPPINESS AND THOROUGHLY ENJOY THE GAME OF LIFE. It is lots of FUN!

AND NOW YOU KNOW!

Now rest…resting in the deepest of relaxation…in hypnosis…so very close to sleep…and experience yourself as one who knows HOW TO SUCCESSFULLY PLAY THE GAME OF LIFE.

When your subconscious has completely absorbed these truths and formed them into your way of life, gradually, very gradually arouse from hypnosis and return to me in the here and now feeling wonderful and fine in every way. You have become a master of 3-D PERCEPTION."

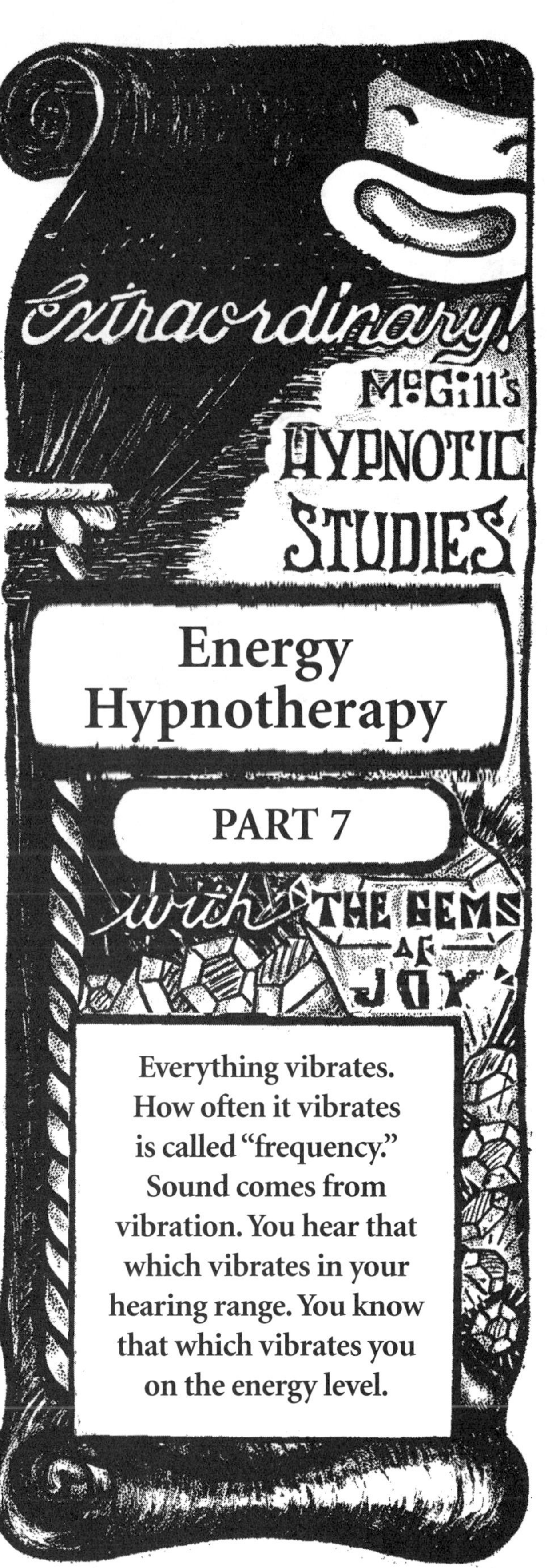

CHAPTERS IN PART SEVEN

126. Hypnosis History And Energy
Overview ....page 467
127. Acupressure Hypnotherapy 473
128. Mesmerism/Hypnosis 477
129. Mesmer On Mesmerism 481
130. Mesmer's Fantasy & Facts 485
131. Bio Magnetic Hypnotherapy:
Baron von Reichenbach 489
132. Magnetic Healing 491
133. Hypno-Reiki 499
134. Tapping Techniques 503
135. Vogel's Energized
Hypnotherapy Couch 507
136. Light & Sound Hypnotherapy 509
137. Psycho Acoustic Hypnotherapy 511
138. Vitality Hypnosis 513
139. Stockwell's Biochemistry
of What You Feel 517

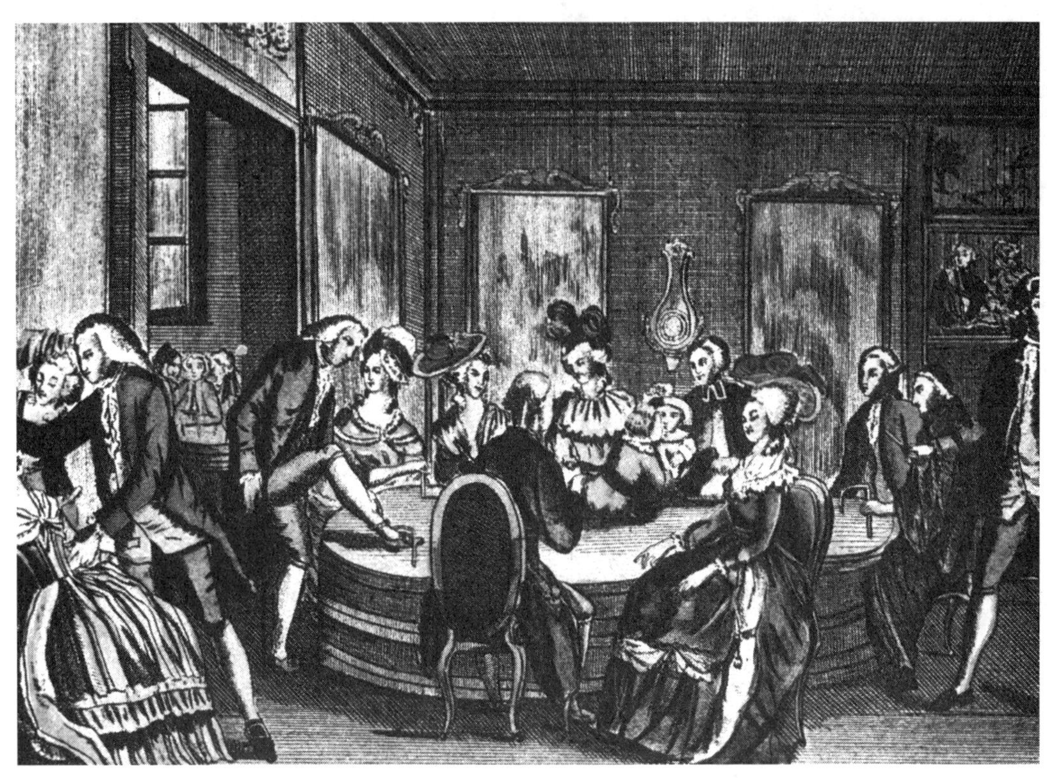

1887 Painting of Mesmer's Baquet
by Richard Bergh

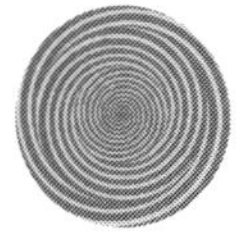

~ *Chapter 126* ~
HYPNOSIS HISTORY AND
HUMAN ENERGY OVERVIEW

By Ormond McGill and Shelley Stockwell-Nicholas

Mesmerism=Animal Magnetism=Zoomagnetism=Somnambulism=Electromagnetism=
Lucid Sleep=Induced Sleep=Artificial Sleep=Braidism=Neuropnology = Hypnosis!

Dr. Franz Anton Mesmer
Dr. James Esdaile
Baron von Reichenbach: Od Theory
Prana Theory
Reiki Theory
Energy Divining Rods

"Take a boy and sit him upon another brick, his face turned to the lamp. Close his eyes and recite into his head seven times what is written. Make him open his eyes and say 'Do you see the light?' When he tells you he sees the light in the flame of the lamp, cry at this moment 'Heoue' nine times and you may ask him concerning anything you wish."
> —3rd Century Egyptian Papyrus
> Found in Thebes

"I became a genius because I learned how my brain worked and then I used my brain."
> —Leonardo Da Vinci
> 1452–1549

Dr. Franz Anton Mesmer (1734 to 1815)

Mesmerism is an energy form of hypnosis in which the subject is hypnotized by your raw human energy, the energy of thoughts, your hands, magnets and the energy of the oceans and planets. Mesmer's animal magnetism theory speculated that if the "tides within the body" become unbalanced, fluid energy could cause illness. Conversely, balanced energy creates wellness.

We can thank Mesmer for originating self-hypnosis, healing support groups and pain free childbirth. You'll learn how to use his approach chapters 128, 159, and 130.

Mesmer came to Paris in 1778 from Vienna and opened an elegant salon to treat and cure. The rich paid handsomely and he treated the poor for free. He recorded seeing over eight thousand patients in 1784! To accommodate such large numbers, he used a "baquet," a large covered tub filled with water, organic material and magnets. Music was played, as some thirty people held a protruding rod coming from holes in the contraption. The group was tied together by a silver cord and Mesmer, robed in lilac, walked about touching the troubled part of each person's anatomy.

Dr. James Braid (1795 Manchester, England-March 25th 1860)

Braid graduated as a physician and surgeon in Edinburgh in 1795.

On November 13, 1841, Braid saw a "séance" demonstration of mesmerism, by a "magnetizer" named La Fontaine. He found that he could produce the same effects without using passes and without the belief in "magnetic fluid." He had his subjects gaze at a bright object and, in his early work, used no verbal instructions to amplify trance. Later he added suggestions. He used his procedures (that he called "nervous sleep" and some referred to as "Braidism") in his practice from the 1840's through the 1850's and reported that it cured or improved deafness, rheumatic disorders and paralysis. In 1842 he renamed his process "hypnotism" after the Greek word "hypnos" for the "god of sleep" and called the reawakened state "dehypnotizing." Later in life he realized that "hypnosis was not true sleep, but concentration of the mind" but it was too late, the name hypnosis and hypnotism were known all over Europe.

Braid believed hypnosis to be a "powerful tool with no great danger, pain or discomfort" that was capable of curing many diseases for which there had been no remedy. He wanted to study and research the phenomenon thoroughly.

James Esdaile, MD (February 6th 1808 Scotland, to January 10th 1859)

Dr. James Esdaile, who received his MD from Edinburgh in 1830, used Dr. Mesmer's animal magnetism while performing surgery on a Hindu convict on April 4th, 1845 in Hooghly, India. This was the first of over 3000 major surgical operations he performed in India using hypnosis. When he began there was no chemical anesthesia. (Later chloroform and ether came along.) Under Mesmeric influence, he reported that his patients were "insensitive to pain" with "magnetic fluid flowing between physician and patient." He said that under certain conditions of their respective systems, irregularity in the distribution of nervous energy causes all mesmeric phenomena. The mesmeric influence was a physical power which one animal exerts over another:

"There is good reason to believe that the vital fluid of one person can be poured into the system of another. There is a communicable life-giving curative power in the human body. When two persons are found together, the one in health may often be able to relieve his sick companion, by imparting to him a portion of his vitality.

In the first stage there is stimulation; in the second, confusion of the mind with exhalation of some organs and depression of others, while in the third stage, coma, with complete extinction of sensibility occurred."

Esdaile claimed that no remedy rivaled Mesmerism's influence on the nervous system was as safe for successful treatment that abolished and prolonged sleep. He successfully treated many different forms of local inflammation pain by this "prolonged sleep."

Esdaile observed that inflammation and sympathetic fever disappeared during mesmeric trance, and that the pulse and temperature became normal. Esdaile did 19 amputations and removed dozens of scrotal tumors, common among Indian men because of the prevalence of elephantiasis. In one astonishing case he excised a one-hundred-and-three pound tumor. It was so large that to operate he had to "cut with a two-edged knife while the tumor was wrapped in a sheet attached by a rope and pulley to the rafters." He wrote that his "patient did not even quiver."

He wrote about many other uses for hypnosis in his books "Mesmerism in India" and "Hypnosis in Medicine and Surgery."

"I had today the honor of being introduced to one of the most famous magicians in Bengal, who enjoys a high reputation for his successful treatment of hysteria and had been sent for to prescribe to my patient, but he came too late: the success of my charm MESMERISM, having him nothing to do."

Ambroise-August Liebeault, MD (1823, France to 1904)
Dr. Hippolyte Bernheim (same time frame)

Liebeault began using Braid's verbal hypnotism methods in 1848 while still in medical school (He graduated in 1850). He took two years to write a book on his hypnosis work and sold only one copy to Hippolyte Bernheim who was eager to prove Liebeault a "quack." When Bernheim paid the author a visit, he was so impressed that he became his devoted student and together they wrote and published the famous book "Suggestive Therapeutics" and founded the Nancy School of Medical Hypnotherapy in Nancy, France.

Liebeault reportedly greeted patients wearing "old slippers, a threadbare bathrobe, tie twiddled around his crumpled collar, tousled hair and looking more like a cobbler than a doctor." He induced trance with a rapid induction like a simple hand pass and a quick "Sleep" or "Sleep, my little kitten."

Bernheim preferred to say, "Look at me and think of nothing but sleep. Your eyelids begin to feel heavy…your eyes are tired and they begin to blink…they are getting moist…your eyes cannot see distinctly and they are closed." He repeated his suggestions until he got results. If not he said, "Sleep is not essential…hypnotic influence is easily exerted without it."

They used of hypnosis with verbal suggestions for everything and recognized that a deep trance was not necessary to effect results.

Liebault and Bernheim said, "Somnambulism (hypnotism) is universal to all humanity" "Most people can be hypnotized," and "Healthy people made the best subjects."

Many famous names in the field became their pupils including Freud, Wettesstrand, Van Eeden, Von Schrenk, De Jong, Moll, Noltzing, and Babinsky.

Dr. Jean Martin Charcot (1825 to 1893)

At the same time as Liebault and Bernheim, the famous Dr. Charcot started the Salpetriere Hospital of Hypnotism, the largest hospital in Paris. It was an asylum for hysterical women who were declared "crazy." In his lectures he asserted that the "morbid condition" of hypnotism was one that only "neurotics and hysterics could enter." His remark that "Hypnotism is a pathological state that weakens the mind" was disproved by the work at Liebeault and Bernheim's School of Nancy. After Charcot's death, Babinsky retaliated by denouncing Charcot's "cures" as "faked" or as "figments of Charcot's imagination."

Dr. Jean Martin Charcot

Sigmund Freud
(May 6th, 1856 Freiberg, Austro-Hungary to September, 1939)

Freud studied with Charcot and Bernheim and used hypnosis in his work. He named his eldest son "Jean Martin" after Charcot. Josef Breuer's writings changed Freud's emphasis from using hypnosis to remove symptoms of "hysteria" to the using hypnosis to discover the cause of the symptoms. In 1895 Freud and Breuer co-authored the book "Studien uber Hysterie" which said that hysterical symptoms develop from suppressed damaging experiences and when

Sigmund Freud

released from the subconscious mind, via "mental catharsis," can be eliminated." Breuer used hypnosis to accomplish the catharsis. Freud, said to be a poor hypnotist, preferred what he coined "psychoanalysis" and "free association and dreams." Nonetheless, Freud used many hypnotic techniques in his work. He constantly "touched the patient's forehead; called for the "concentration of the patient's mind" and bid them "to relax on the couch" and "use their imagination."

Publicly Freud discredited hypnotism as "only employing direct suggestions." Of course, all excellent hypnotists do so much more than just directly suggest; they evaluate, synthesize and offer rapid resolution via direct and indirect transmissions, Freud's Psychoanalysis and free association approach eventually evolved into years of sessions and offered no direct suggestions.

In essence, Freud's Id, Ego and Super-Ego Theory described you as born with a leering libido "Id" trying to get its way, a slowly developing "Ego" (subconscious) to modulate it and, somewhere around six, Freud added, a judgmental sensoring "Superego" that morally puppets your upbringing and represses or disguises subconscious desire.

He wrote, "The Interpretation of Dreams," that maintained that dreams result from "repressed sexual instincts and desires" and that our sexual instincts are chauvinistically male dominated with all females pathetically harboring "penis envy" making us all schmucks.

Baron Von Reichenbach: "Od Theory" (mid 1800's)

Baron von Reichenbach used the Universal "Odic" Force Theory, which he nicknamed "Od." The great healing power of the ODs therapeutic magnetism was said to originate from the Aurora Borealis and practitioner's mind. Directed or channeled to the client, it evoked universal healing. His book, "The Dynamics Of Magnetism, Electricity, Heat, Light, Crystallization And Chemistry In Their Relation To Vital Force" was written in 1846 and translated from German into English in 1855. You'll learn more about Von Reichenbach in chapter 131.

Prana Theory

Yogis say that prana (or prahna) is the vital cosmic source energy (life force) that enters the human body with breath. It can be brought into the body and stored to promote good health via a special breathing practice called "pranayama." Prana's combined "animal magnetism" and "odic force" produces remarkable healing when used in hypnotherapy. Prana oversaturates the brain with oxygen, producing a swoon-like state. A suggestion of sleep given at that time rapidly induces hypnosis. One explanation of pranic power is that as we breathe we absorb the electrical vibrations of the earth's frequency.

Reiki Theory

The application of Reiki is similar to Mesmerism and the Od. Reiki is said to not be generated by the practitioner but from a cosmic source channeled through their "healing hands."

Energy Divining Rods

A simple device to objectively show the presence of human energies. The device could be as simple as holding the long side of wire hangers (or bend a couple of foot long stiff wires at right angles). Hold these loosely in your hands, side by side, straight out pointing towards your subject. Now approach the subject. As you move within the range of the aura, the extended wires will move apart, in opposite directions in response to the energy.

The Aurameter

In 1926, a famous dowser, the late Verne L. Cameron, created a spring-balanced rod called a "water compass." His mother taught him to use a forked switch, or wand made of green wood, to find well water. He took the best features of this and other directional devices like L-rods, weighing devices (that bobbed up and down on numbers or letters), gravity pendulums, upright pendulums and inverted wand pendulums and in 1952 created the "Aurameter," to detect the invisible outlines of the human body, the etheric body and even thought forms of people! Many great hypnotists became enthralled with his device and used it in their practice to read and harmonize the energy around their clients.

MODUS OPERANDI: USING THE AURAMETER FOR HYPNOSIS

Your Will Need:

A Cameron Aurameter (or Simple Dowsing Device)

1. **Decide What You Want To Do**

   The aurameter begins with the logical mind setting up what you want to do. You develop a code for "yes or no" or letters and numbers to give you the answers.

2. **Tune In**

   Get into center and hypnotize yourself to suspend your critical mind, so you create a feeling, intuitive experience and a free flow of information between your left and right hemisphere. Read your client's vibration, energy or wave front (called the "vatic" body/mind projector), their aura and energies (Sanskrit called this the "nadis").

3. **Scan The Client With The Aurameter**

   When a location emits more or less energy the aurameter will bob accordingly. When it does, ask, **"What is going on here** (name the region)?" "Wings" or a large discharge of energy from their back may be an antenna for danger or say that their survival "back is up." You can then give suggestion that they, **"Go to a safe place."** If a bubble of energy is perceived over the heart and extend several feet, reinforce that with, **"Your heart is wide open. That's very good."**

Hypno-Helper

"Ambroise-August Liebeault: The Hypnological Legacy of a Secular Saint"
by Laurent Carrer, PhD

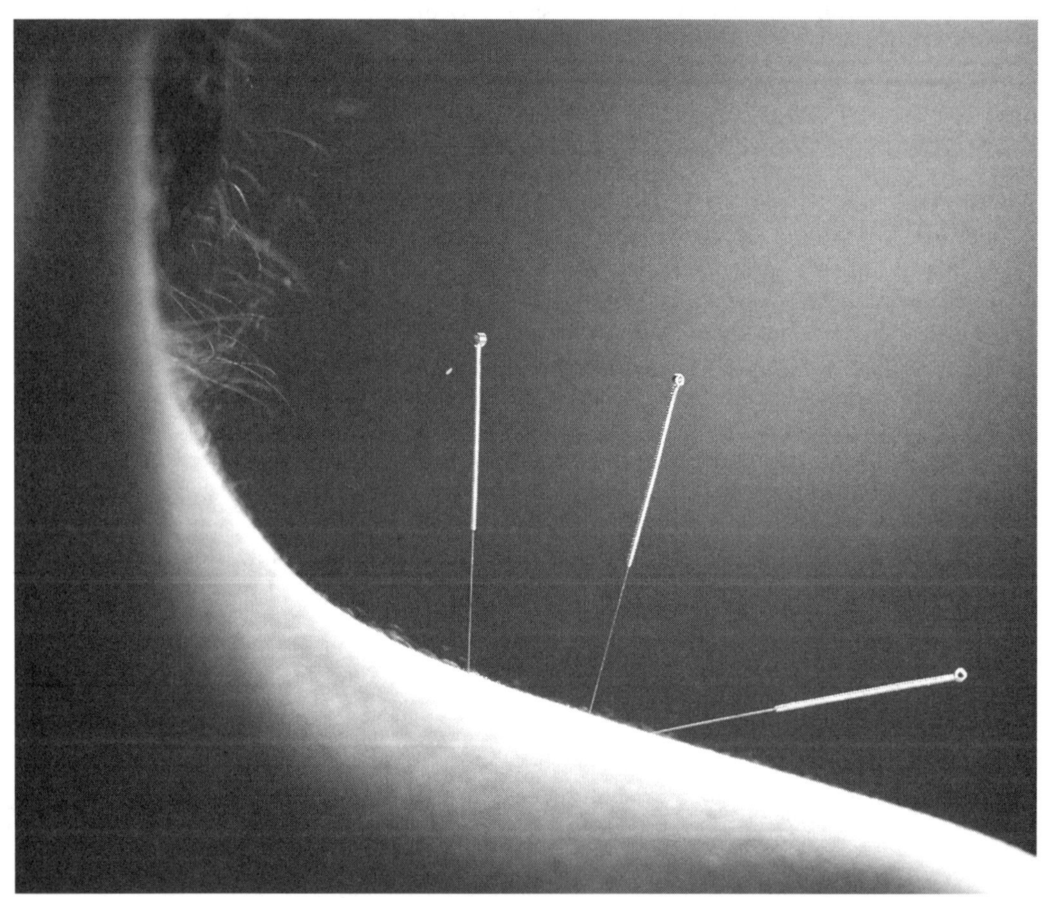

Acupuncture

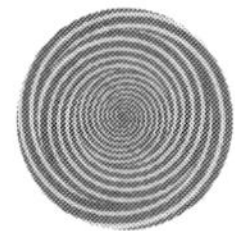

~ *Chapter 127* ~
ACUPRESSURE HYPNOTHERAPY

Includes
The Twenty Steps To Acupressure Hypnotherapy

Acupuncture is a form of Chinese healing that dates back thousands of years. The Chinese physician maps over three hundred acupuncture points, masters the twelve "pulses" and balances life energy within the body via the meridians to produce wellness. It works!

Acupressure is a terrific hypnosis specialty that uses finger pressing on meridians and not needles. Deep hypnosis is achieved when 20 major meridians are depressed or tapped. This automatically amplifies the healing suggestions you give. A simplified form of hypnotic acupuncture popular today is called "tapping" or EFT (these "Emotional Freedom Techniques" are found in another chapter).

There is a close connection balancing meridians, what the Chinese call chi and what Mesmer called animal magnetism. Acupuncture produces an effective anesthesia, similar to the mesmerism used by Dr. James Esdaile for painless surgery before the advent of chemical anesthesia.

Most meridians can be felt as little depressions in the body. Some are quite sensitive and a slight pain sensation may be felt when pressed or tapped.

The consultation for ACUPRESSURE HYPNOTHERAPY, is simply an explanation that you will be appropriately touching them for the purpose of balancing their meridians and their self. Of course, if you think that your client would greatly benefit by a telling their "troubles," lend a sympathetic ear.

These are litigious times. Because this is hands-on help, it is practical to have a massage license or be certified as a minister of a hands-on discipline. Of course, you have a moral obligation to always remain appropriate and respectful.

MODUS OPERANDI: THE 20 STEPS OF ACUPRESSURE HYPNOTHERAPY

Wash your hands thoroughly. Have the client remove their shoes, loosen any tight apparel, and relax in a comfortable position sitting or lying down with hands resting at their sides and feet slightly apart.

Some hypnotherapists use this process without verbal suggestions. I like to use it with the verbal approach.

STEP ONE: EXPLANATION

"In using acupuncture hypnosis, I will apply pressure or tap various meridian centers using scientific points. Of course, I will be very respectful of you at all times. This process will cause you to relax automatically and, very likely, you will doze off to sleep. Just let yourself relax and GO!"

STEP TWO: CROWNING BREATHS

"Close your eyes and as I touch the center of the top of your head, roll your eyes upwards under your closed eyelids as though looking at the point I am touching on your head. Then take three deep breaths. Internally, keep looking at this spot.

In this position, you will find it physically impossible to open your eyes, and when you notice this, just relax your eyes downward and drift off into sleep. Each touch and sensation sends you down deeper and deeper into profound hypnosis."

Begin by energizing your hands. Shake them vigorously or rub them together. Feel them tingle. Then place your hands palm-to-palm, and slowly separate them. There is "energy" that flows between your "charged" hands when they are ready to be applied to the meridian centers of the client.

STEP THREE: THE BALL OF THE FOOT

Locate the point of the left foot just behind the ball of the foot in line with the middle toe. Press firmly (or tap vigorously) on this point for five seconds, while softly suggesting, **"You will notice how relaxed this causes your foot to become. It may possibly feel numb. Good."** (Do the same with their right foot.)

STEP FOUR: THE ANKLE

Locate the point on the left foot just below the bulge of the inner ankle and press firmly (or tap) on this point for five seconds. **"Notice how relaxed this makes your foot become."** (Do the same with their right foot.)

STEP FIVE: INNER SHIN

Move your fingers up the leg about three inches above the ankle and press or tap on the inner edge of the shinbone. This may cause numbness. Continue doing this for five seconds. **"Any numbness you feel here moves gently up the leg, relaxation moves up, up, up."** (Do the same with their right leg.)

STEP SIX: OUTER ANKLE

Locate the point on the left foot just before the outer bulge of the left ankle. Press in or tap vigorously for five seconds. **"You grow numb and relaxed."** (Do the same with the right leg.)

STEP SEVEN: BELOW THE KNEE

Locate the point on your left leg just below the level of the kneecap. Press or tap firmly at the top of the calf muscle. This is tender, so be firm but gentle. **"Your legs become relaxed and numb."** (Do the same with the right calf muscle.)

STEP EIGHT: BELLY

Locate the point on front of the body midway between the pubic bone and the navel. Press firmly. Do not tap here. Suggest, **"You will drift away to pleasant sleep. This is a powerful meridian center and your breathing depends and takes you deeper. Good."**

STEP NINE: BREASTBONE

Locate the point on the front of the body just below the end of the breastbone. Touch or tap here in a slow, gentle rhythm while suggesting, **"You can go to sleep now. Just drop off to sleep. Breathe deeply and freely, and drop off to sleep. Sleep. Sleep. Sleepy sleep. Go to sleep now."**

You can tell by the deepening and rhythmic breathing of the client that hypnosis is being induced. You can continue this beneath breastbone tapping until this breathing is achieved.

STEP TEN: HEART

Locate the point on the front of the body, three inches over towards the left side. You will find a soft, depressed spot here over the heart. Press or tap this meridian center. Suggest, **"You are dropping into sleep now. Go soundly to sleep, as I press (or tap) on your heart meridian."**

STEP ELEVEN: SHOULDER BONE

Using both thumbs simultaneously at the points located in depression at the end of the shoulder bones where the arms and shoulders meet, continue suggesting, **"Sleep, deep sleep. Drift away into sleep, as you feel the pressure. The pressure will melt away, as you drift away into sleep. Breathe deeply and sleep."**

STEP TWELVE: INNER ELBOW

Tap or press what is called the "Joy of Living" point at the inner crease of the right elbow. Bend the elbow and place the tip of your thumb in the crease. Then, unbend the arm and press in firmly. Press on relaxed tissue, always. Suggest, **"Sleep. Deep sleep. Go into deep sleep."** (Perform the same on left elbow.)

STEP THIRTEEN: OUTSIDE ARM

Move your hand down the arm from the inner elbow to the point located two inches down the arm on the outside of the right arm. Press in firmly. Suggest, **"You can feel your arms becoming numb, and you go to sleep. Sleep. Deep sleep."** (Perform the same on the left arm.)

ALLOW SOME MOMENTS HERE FOR THE CLIENT TO RELAX BETWEEN THE NEXT ACUPRESSURE.

STEP FOURTEEN: LOWER ARM

Move on down the right arm further on the outside to a point two inches from the wrist, in line with the little finger. Press in firmly. Suggest, **"Sleep. Sleep. Go to sleep. Deep sleep."** (Perform the same on the left arm.)

STEP FIFTEEN: HAND

Locate the point on the back of the right hand between the bones of thumb and the index finger. Press in deeply. Suggest, **"Sleep. Deep sleep. Go deeply into a hypnotic sleep."** RELAX THE PRESSURE. Press in deeply again on this point, and suggest, **"Sleep. Deep sleep. You are sleeping deeply in hypnotic sleep, as the meridians of your body become perfectly in balance."** Repeat this press in – relax the pressure – five consecutive times. (Perform the same on the left hand.)

STEP SIXTEEN: INSIDE WRIST

Locate the point on the crease inside of the right wrist in line with the little finger. Press in firmly and maintain pressure. Suggest, **"Go on deeply into hypnosis now. Sleep. Sleep deeply in hypnotic sleep."**

Release all pressure and allow the client to drift alone quietly into profound hypnosis.

STEP SEVENTEEN: TOP OF SHOULDER

Locate the point at the top of each shoulder, midway, between the neck and the top of the shoulder. Press in deeply, with both hands, at these points. Hold pressure for thirty seconds, then release, and start tapping on these points for a full minute. Suggest, **"Every tap and touch aligns you. You are in balance. The meridians of your body have aligned. You are healed."**

STEP EIGHTEEN: UPPER LIP

Locate the point on the face between the upper lip and the tip of the nose. Gently tap (in rhythmic tapping) on this point. Suggest, **"Each tap sends you deeper and deeper into hypnosis, and balances the meridians of your body in perfect sequence."**

STEP NINETEEN: THIRD EYE

Locate the point between the eyebrows (Third Eye Center) and gently tap for thirty seconds. Suggest, **"With each tap upon your Third Eye Center, go deeper and deeper into profound hypnosis, as the meridians of your body are in perfect balance."**

STEP TWENTY: CROWN OF HEAD

Locate the small depression in the crown of the head. Tap on that point for a full minute as you suggest, **"Cosmic energy comes into you. Both your mind and body are in perfect harmony. The meridians of your body are in perfect balance now. You are well and healthy in every way. You have achieved what was your purpose to achieve.**

When your inner mind knows that your wish is achieved, you will arouse from the hypnosis, fully awake and alert...feeling wonderful and fine. Take your time; there is no hurry. Arouse when your inner mind tells you it is time to arouse."

The session is complete.

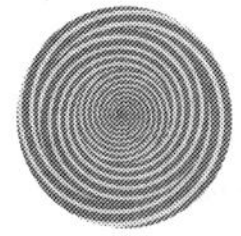

~ *Chapter 128* ~
MESMERISM/HYPNOSIS

Includes
Animal Magnetism and Human Energy Hypnotherapy
Mesmerism/Hypnosis For Wellness

Human Energy Hypnotherapy is a dynamic energy between you, the hypnotherapist, and your client. In a vigorous exchange, you give your energy to the client and remarkably receive even more energy for yourself. That's how the flow of universal energy operates.

Every communication between people involves the exchange of human energy. In hypnosis this is particularly notable, especially when you and the subject are in close proximity and your auras and energies intermingle. All hypnotherapy (often unconsciously) includes such human energy. The more skillful you become in manipulating these energies, the better a hypnotherapist you become.

In the 20th Century, Dr. Franz Anton Mesmer (1734–1815) may have been omitted from a book about hypnotherapy because many discredited him as a charlatan. In 1784 King Louis XVI sent out a commission to investigate Mesmer. Benjamin Franklin, a United States diplomat in Paris at the time, along with others concluded that, "animal magnetism is nonexistent" and "any reported cures were the product of a stimulated imagination."

Today it's an entirely different matter. Not only is Mesmerism respectable, its study is fashionable. Scientists are investigating his approach and Mesmer is considered the venerable father of hypnotherapy.

Dr. Franz Anton Mesmer

In Mesmer's time, mind and body were considered separate. Physical influences were "mesmeric" and psychological or mental influences "hypnotic." The two of course intertwine since mind affects the body and body affect the mind.

Today we understand that all human behavior, both mental and physical, is an energy phenomenon. In fact, each simultaneously evokes and augments each other. Psychological and physiological processes both produce discharges within the brain that transmit energy. Scientists and researchers are starting to explore these subtle spectrums of energy.

The Mesmerism/Hypnosis Approach
"The difference between hypnotism and mesmerism will be found to consist only in the different ways of giving suggestion. Hypnotists usually employ oral suggestions. Telepathy is actively employed by mesmerists."
> —Albert Olston,
> "Mind Power and Privileges"1902

Mesmerism/hypnosis artfully combines the physiological and psychological. This energy form of hypnosis hypnotizes the client with your raw human energy and the energy of your thoughts. Use it with a new client on their first session (following the interview), or anytime and it revitalizes and amps energy without verbal suggestion or other hypnotherapy techniques. It may be all that is necessary to help someone and could well be the specialty of your practice.

Two energies come into play in the hypnotism/mesmerism:
1. Raw human magnetic energy is called "animal magnetism."
2. Your specifically directed thoughts as telepathic energy is called "human magnetism."

Mesmer's method for treating the sick deserves careful study. He believed that a person was sick because their vital energy was low and in need of revitalization or balancing. He generated a "power" within himself, which he named "animal magnetism," that he then transmitted to his patients for curative effects. As a source of magnetic energy, he could build up the reserves of the sick and they in turn, could use this energy to overcome disease. Calling this "animal magnetism," shows rare insight. You are surrounded by an electro-static (electromagnetic) aura. Though subtle, it can be measured and photographed using the right equipment.

Mesmeric entrancement is conveyed subconsciously and strongly recharges your vital force, which you directly transfer to stimulate your client's energy. Hypnosis is the wordy process using the verbal "the power of suggestion." Mesmerism is a thinking process mind-to-mind between the hypnotherapist and client that creates "the power of energetic expression."

In mesmerizing, you think about the verbal suggestions you would give if you were performing standard hypnosis. These same suggestions are given mentally rather than verbally. In other words, you think, **"body relaxing, eyes getting heavy and closing, breaths deepen and you are dropping off into the realm of sleep."** Mesmeric trance is induced nonverbally.

MODUS OPERANDI: MESMERISM/HYPNOSIS FOR WELLNESS

First, conceive of yourself as an energy source.

Stretch out the fingers of your hand. Now, think of your energy as flowing down your arms and passing out of your fingertips. Use your imagination in doing this. At first it will be imagination, but soon it will become reality, and you will actually note a physical sensation of an energy flow out of your hands. It will feel like your hands have become alive with energy and there is an electrical-like tingling in your fingers. The more you concentrate upon directing that energy in your hands, the more you will sense the energy you are projecting. Once you become aware of the energy flow within yourself, then you can project it to others via hand contact, contact and non-contact passes, and from your eyes.

To test the influence, request a subject to, **"Close your eyes."** Then direct the energy out of your fingertips as you pass your hand, without contact, over their forehead and down the sides of the cheeks. A sensitive subject will distinctly feel the electrical-like tingling sensation from your fingers. You can now use this method to hypnotize (mesmerize) the client. Here is how:

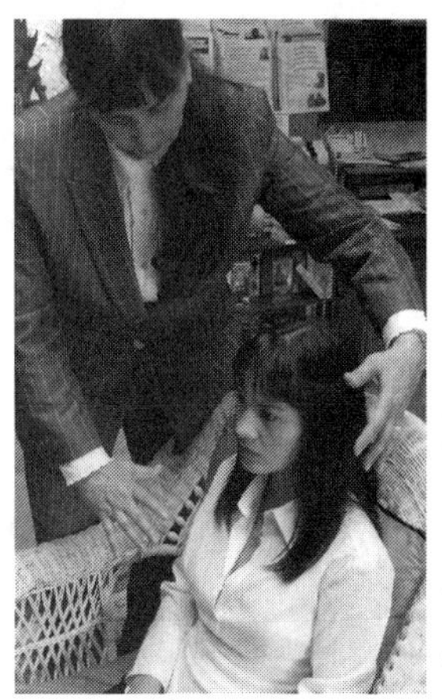

Photo by Jon Nicholas

Sit in front of your client so that your knees touch.

Explain: **"I will actively send my energy to you, as you take a passive role and receive the energy I transmit. I will use very few words, as I send you healing thoughts. As you ride upon the energy flow you will pass down into a subjective (hypnotic) state. You will experience a tingling in your hands as I hold them and you will notice that you are filled with energy. You can freely use this energy in anyway that is helpful to you so you revitalize yourself. It may even seem much like dropping off to sleep, as you drift deeper and deeper into hypnosis, using this powerful mesmerism."**

Then grip your client's hands in yours, so the balls of each other's thumbs touch, and establish a close eye-to-eye contact.

Start the energy flowing from you to your client. Think it, and you will experience the force start flowing. Along with the flow of energy, think (visualize, affirm and project) what the client is to experience. In other words, via the bio-energy you send think them into hypnosis and project thoughts of well-being and the correction of their problem.

As you proceed, you will feel the energy flowing down your arms and out your hands into his hands (especially at the points where the balls of your thumbs meet). Not only will you feel the energy flowing, so will the client. Throughout the process, keep projecting, flowing your energy, and thinking about the thought pattern of behavior you wish to establish in your client.

As you think, **"Your eyes become tired and heavy and will close;"** the client's body relaxes. As you energetically project the thought **"your breathing deepens"**; you will note a shift in their breathing. As you think, **"you drop into profound hypnosis;"** it will happen for them. Mentally suggest what would be verbal suggestions in a conventional hypnosis. You flow your energy and your thoughts to your client.

Your fascinated client will respond to your thoughts: their eyes will close, breath will deepen, and they will drop down into a sleep-like state. And the deeper they go, the more you will feel your energy passing into them. But, you will not feel tired or drained because it is not a physical energy you transmit. It is psychic/animal magnetism and the more you give, the more you get. It is a beautiful experience.

After the client's eyes have closed and they have passed into a tranquil state, release their hands and place them in their lap. Now stand before them, and make long sweeping passes (without contact) over their body– beginning at the top of their head, and ending at the knees. When you reach the knees, forcefully shake your hands as though throwing off a sticky fluid, turn your palms outward, lift your hands up again to the top of his head, turn palms inwards, and again make the long sweeping pass from his head to his knees, as you stand before the person. Make these passes slowly, and you will note the flow of energy from your hands passing into the body of the client.

At the same time, along with this energy flow, keep thinking of the client going deeper and

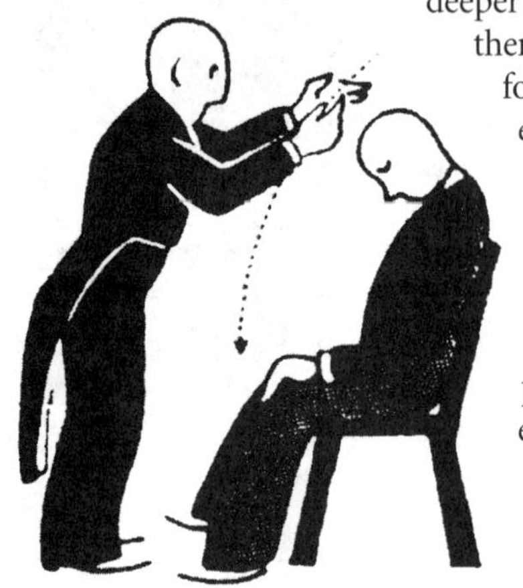

Down Sweep

deeper into hypnosis. Perform these passes a number of times, and then you can vary them by making short passes over the forehead and face, circular passes about the region of the heart, etc. Occasionally you can even make gentle contact on the body with your hands, as you make the passes.

Observe your client. Their body language tells you hypnosis is occurring. Note their breath deepening. Their eyelids may flutter or move back and forth under closed eyelids. And then there will occur a most remarkable phenomenon; you will sense a "kickback" of the flow of energy from the subject to yourself. This energy will seem to build up, and they will become aglow with their own energy. It's as if the energy flow you first sent triggers the production of their own energy, and literally transforms them into a living generator of their own magnetic energy. A stimulation of their aura appears to take place and they become powerfully charged, like a battery of animal magnetism! It is a striking effect.

As you sweep your hands past your client's head, you will sense their energy tingling in your hands from them to you. When this happens, you can stop your own mesmerizing process, as they now have become their own generator of energy. This wonderful exhilarating experience is most beneficial to the subject. Their entire body becomes alive with the force. What was low vitality is now changed into a source of vitality.

If you wish, at this point, you can speak softly to the client:

"The energy I have given is yours to use in any way beneficial way your subconscious feels it needs to be used. Now your entire body has become its own battery of energy, which you draw in surges of energy from the Cosmos. Let this surging energy go into the parts of your body in which it is most needed, to heal your body, and make it perfect in every way."

When you feel that the hypnosis/mesmerism session has gone on long enough, you can suggest quietly, **"Rest a few moments now, and then I will bring you back, and you will return to full wakefulness charged with energy, filled with vitality, aglow with life."**

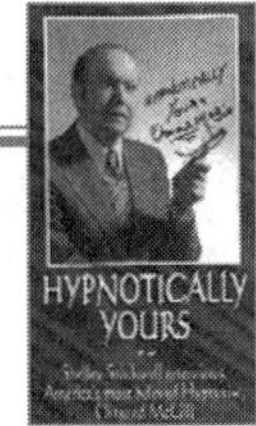

Hypno-Helper

"Hypnotically Yours, Ormond McGill" video does a fine job of Ormond actually demonstrating the use of Mesmerism. It is available on line at www.hypnosisfederation.com or at the back of this book.

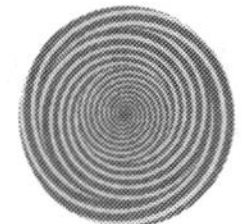

~ *Chapter 129* ~
MESMER ON MESMERISM

Includes
Mesmer's Five-step Clinical Procedure
      Rapport
      Bringing in Cosmic Energy
Mesmeric Sitting Technique
Hand Passes And Thought Projection
Bring Them Home

You learned about Human Energy Hypnosis in the foregoing chapter. Now, let Master Mesmer advance your skills.

Every so often, in the unfolding of history, there comes a great artist whose talents raise the consciousness of humankind. We have great painters, great musicians, great singers, and great scientists (Nikola Tesla for example). Sometimes they are appreciated while they are living but, more often, when they are dead. Some are feared and others try to destroy their credibility.

Dr. Mesmer was a great mental healer and virtuoso psychotherapist. He was the greatest mesmerist; after all they named this form of mental healing after him. He practiced what he preached upon himself. Every true artist practices, practices, practices. Mesmer daily went through the process of generating Human Energies. It was his daily workout.

A person coming to Mesmer's clinic for treatment was usually ill. An ill person is very low on self-esteem. Mesmer's first procedure was to raise the person's self-esteem. He had an ingenious way of doing this:

MODUS OPERANDI: MESMER'S FIVE-STEP CLINICAL PROCEDURE
1. Rapport

Mesmer had the client sit in a throne-like chair so they sat tall and were raised high. Mesmer himself took a seat on a low stool before them. Thus, he was in a low position to the client's high position. The healing began right there. Instead of feeling intimidated by Mesmer, the client felt his (or her) own self-worth commence to rise, just by this body positioning. Instead of becoming a master, Mesmer had become a friend. Friendship is rapport, and rapport between client and the hypnotherapist is the backbone of good therapy.

When comfortably ready, the consultation between client and physician began. What was the condition to be treated? The client confidentially told the doctor their need, and what they wanted in the way of healing.

A good hypnotherapist is a good listener. Mesmer was a good listener, and what he learned during the consultation allowed him to form the mental picture of the cure they desired. This mental picture would be visualized back into the person's mind during the session. It was an early form of mental biofeedback.

The consultation complete, Mesmer had a planned mental projection established in his own mind. He then had his client perform a unique process before any mesmerizing began. He brought to them cosmic energy. It contributed greatly to his results and his reputation and prestige as a healer. Here's how he did it:

2. Bringing In Cosmic Energy

The client was told **"Stand, with your feet approximately eighteen inches apart, and allow your hands rest at your sides. Hold them out about six inches from your body dangling in the air."**

The positioning arranged, the mesmerist stood before the client so they had direct eye-to-eye contact. The client is now told **"Relax and take a deep breath, and affirm out loud, 'I open myself to the guidance of Dr. Mesmer to bring his magnetic energy into my body while asking for Strength, Guidance, and Protection. He will make me well.'"** This process was performed three times. You'll recognize this as a personalized variation of the method for bringing in the Cosmic Force.

What will your client feel if you have them do this? Something like electricity, perhaps a somewhat new sensation. It will be a definite experience for them. They will now be open and ready for being mesmerized.

3. Mesmerizing Sitting Technique

Sit opposite the client. Use two chairs facing each other, so that you, the mesmerist, and your client are at the same level, facing each other eye-to-eye or you can kneel before them. Take the client's right hand in your left, and their left hand in your right. Firmly grip hands allowing balls of thumbs to meet. Lean forward in chair until knees touch, and your face is about twelve inches from them.

Tell them:

"Gaze steadily into my eyes as I gaze back. You will experience an electric-like sensation passing between your hands. And soon you will feel a tingling in your hands as I send my curing energy into you to make you well and healthy, exactly as you wish to be. This tingling sensation will gradually extend up your arms to the shoulders, and a sort of numbness will creep over your body. Enjoy any sensations that may occur, just be passive and calm, and open to receive the healing energy I send you. You are the recipient. I am the giver. Just make yourself receptive to the magnetism that I shall project into your mind and body. As the numbness proceeds and you find you can no longer bear to keep your eyes open and fasten upon mine, close them. You will then pass into a profound trance-like state; down into the abyss of the realm of sleep. Your whole body will feel warm, and you will feel a gentle current, which will seem to you like a surge of body electricity, and the pulse in your thumbs will throb."

Illustration by Ormond McGill

As these instructions are given, think each thought as if it as occurring to the client.

Continue: **"When your eyes are closed, I will make passes over you, which will fill you with bio-energy, animal magnetism which will feel like a pleasurable warmth coming into your body, and you will drop down in Mesmeric Sleep as the healing force comes to you and heals you as you have requested."**

With the initial mesmeric induction completed (the outward signs of trance are very similar to conventional hypnosis), you are now ready to perform the next process in mesmerizing, which is to bring Magnetic Force to the client.

4. Hand Passes And Thought Projection

Go silent now. Further suggestions are given mentally not verbally.

To do this, breathe deeply while centering your mind on yourself becoming an open channel for the slowing in of the energy.

Now, stand in front of your client, and make long sweeping passes in front of and around their body. Think of the force flowing out of your hands into their body. You will experience the flow yourself, like an electrical tingling in your fingers, as you make the passes. The passes are made with palms turned in towards them, starting at top of head and moving slowly downward. Make the passes in slow sweeps terminating at the knees. At the end of each pass, throw your hands outward and shake them. Turn your palms inward again and continue the downward passes over and around the body.

Make the passes with hands held about six inches from surface of body, all the while concentrating on the flow of magnetic energy coming out of your fingertips into them, as the downward passes proceed. You will experience the flow of energy yourself, as you continue. The very air about them will seem to become alive with energy. (Mesmer would often continue these passes about them for a full hour –saturating the energy).

All the while, simultaneously, hold centered in your mind the mental picture (visualization) of the end result they want to accomplish. No verbal comment is needed. Just hold the visualization firmly and it will pass into them with the vital energy focused upon the benefit envisioned for the finalized healing.

A mental picture of complete healing infused into a person who is energized by the building flow of Animal Magnetism is unique to Mesmerism.

When you have completed enough downward passes, you will sense a subtle resistance to more energy being given… stop and allow the client to rest in silence. This lets the energy soak in. Five minutes for this is sufficient. You are now ready to conclude the session.

5. Bring Them Home

To conclude the session, arouse the client by a reversing the downward passes. Make these upward passes brisk and they will arouse and throw off the energy. As you do think, "awaken!" Blow on their forehead if you like and Mesmer's method of mesmerizing is complete.

"Practice by looking fixedly and pertinaciously into the subject's eyes at a distance of a few inches, and at the same time, holding the hands. In a few minutes, all expression goes out of the face and the subject sees nothing but the operator's eyes, which shine with intense brilliancy."
—Dr. Tuckey on Mesmerism, 1800's

HERE IS THE 5-STEP PROCESS IN BRIEF SUMMATION:

1. Rapport

A high chair for the client and a lower one for you gives the client a sense of empowerment as they tell you what benefit they want to accomplish.

2. Bringing In Cosmic Energy

Bring in cosmic energy (animal magnetism) as you stand facing each other. Allow it to flow through you, via hand passes, into their body. Centered in your mind, hold the mental-picture (visualization) of them having achieved well-being perfection at the conclusion of the session.

3. Mesmeric Sitting Technique

Then, sitting at the same level, eye-to-eye, thumb-to-thumb and knee-to-knee, send energy through your thumbs. You tell them what to expect.

4. Hand Passes And Thought Projection

5. Bring Them Home

Allow the energy to sink home for some minutes before the arousal from mesmeric trance. Arouse the client from mesmeric trance by upward passes.

Mesmerism plus cosmic energy plus your knowledge of hypnotherapy equals profound mental healing of the 21st century. Thank you, Mesmer.

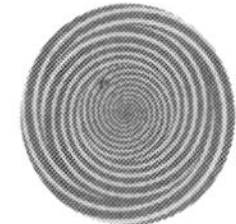

~ *Chapter 130* ~
MESMER'S FANTASY AND FACTS

In the realm of mind, what is fact and what is fantasy?

After all, out of fantasy frequently comes fact.

A couple of hundred years ago, Mesmer watched a mountebank, or magician, perform an act with lodestones (the magnets of the time). The magician declared he could make a spectator do his bidding by touching him with a magnet, and that the person would move in the direction the magnet was moved. He proceeded to demonstrate that he could do it.

Mesmer took it literally. He was interested in magnets to cure disease. If a magnet could exert an invisible influence to attract iron filings, maybe it could exert similar power in attracting and pulling disease from the sick.

Mesmer believed that good health depended on properly directing magnetic fluid energy within the body in an harmonious ebb and flow and that illness was a blockage of this energy. Initially he gave "magnetic treatments" by applying physical magnets to patients. Later, he did the same thing just using his hands. He then called his hand approach, "animal magnetism" and the use of magnets "organic magnatism."

Mesmer's writings on "Animal Magnetism" (or "gravitas") appeared in a little monograph entitled, "Memoir sur la decouverte du Magetism Animal," printed in Geneva in 1779, and published in Paris by the Deuphin's Libraire-Imprimeur, F.Fr. Didot le jeune.

His success was outstanding. The aristocracy acknowledged him.

At one time, more than three thousand patients a week sought his services. To meet the demand he dug up an antiquated medical instrument from the past century, the "baquet." It was a tub full of bottles of "magnitized water" and bits of broken glass, tree roots and various chemicals. The tub was placed in the center of the room. Music played as patients stood in a circle around it touching the ropes and iron rods coming from the fermenting solution. The rods were said to give healing benefits. It worked well to treat so many patients. He took on assistant "magnitizers," opened a clinic in Creteil and bought the Hotel Bullion where he set up four baquets.

Mesmer was so famous in Paris that Marie Antoinette offered him a life pension and money to set up a clinic.

Mesmer's use of the old "baquet" (and probably his success and his refusal to let government representatives supervise his work) eventually led to his downfall as the medical profession regarded his work as an "abomination." Later, psychology explained Mesmer's success with healing as the mental power of suggestion and disregarded his physiological explanation. It was just the fodder rival physicians needed to discredit Mesmer's work. In spite of his problems, the French granted him a pension in 1802 and he still continued practicing animal magnatism into his 80's.

Lack of adequate scientific knowledge caused these people to overlook the fact that the body affects the mind and the mind affects the body, and that all human behavior is basically an energy phenomenon. They had missed what all hypnotherapists know; the creative power of mind creates everything in our life!

Knowledge has an interesting way of going around in a full circle: a belief is held, then it is discarded and a new belief installed in its place. Then, in time, the old belief is revived again. In our contemporary times, a careful study of "human energies" is being conducted in scientific laboratories and the formula for hypnosis is Human Energy + Suggestion = Hypnotherapy.

In spite of past harsh judgments, Mesmer's "animal magnetism," became known simply as "mesmerism." The adjective "mesmeric," the noun "mesmerism," and the verb "mesmerize" have not changed their meaning since they became current in his day. The fact that they are still included in modern dictionaries speaks volumes for Mesmer's continuing influence upon society.

Mesmer is known as "The Father of Hypnotherapy."

Hypnotism/mesmerism is actually a mutual mental/physical process, each augmenting the other. In other words, a psychological process is likewise a physiological process. A thought produces a bio/energy discharge within the brain (possibly like a micro-radio wave) that produces a thought.

Two types of human energies are involved in the hypnotism/mesmerism: "animal magnetism," and "telepathic energy." Animal magnetism is "raw human magnetic energy" while telepathic energy is "magnetic energy directed via the mind or brain."

I like to think of animal magnetism as a racehorse and directive telepathic energy as the jockey that rides piggyback upon it– steering it to its goal.

Hypnotism and mesmerism overlap and yet are divergent: hypnotism is currently thought of as a psychological methodology while mesmerism is via a physiological methodology.

More Fantastic Facts

Prominent physicians, as Elliotson and Esdaile, continued Mesmer's theories and work. Esdaile wrote a book about his surgical work titled "Mesmerism In India."

Out of mesmerism came hypnotism. Creation moves like the flowing of a river.

The Nancy School founded by Drs. Bernheim and Liebault, based their work upon THE POWER OF SUGGESTION, another fact that grew out of fantasy.

Dr. Charcot hypnotized neurotic and psychotic patients in his hospital. Hysterics responded best to hypnosis, he said because hypnosis puts the disturbed mind under control. Charcot's and Bernheim's work influenced the work of Dr. Freud, out of which Psychoanalysis grew.

Early 20th century movies depicted a Victorian parlor with a waistcoat clad man swinging his pocket watch before a seated woman and monotoning, "you are getting sleeeepy..."

We rapidly move from one fad to another and call it progress.

Out of historical fantasy came contemporary fact:

Hypnosis is now a mainstream cognitive science. In 1955, the American Medical Association approved hypnosis sanctioning its medical uses. Medical doctors jumped on the bandwagon to learn "hypnotherapy," the new "legal" profession.

Many of these early enthusiasts, believed that hypnosis was too time consuming. Based on their limited training, they thought that a litany of time-consuming susceptibility tests was required to get the job done. So professional hypnotherapists like Dave Elman, schooled with hundreds of hours in their specialty, demonstrated how to induce hypnosis somnambulism in less that three minutes! How's that!

Today, papers on hypnosis are published regularly in reputable scientific, medical and hypnosis journals and in magazines like Scientific American. Hypnosis is used by law enforcement, the FBI, in sports, medicine, in schools, business, as entertainment and by Hypnotherapists. Television and radio programs feature hypnosis. Hypnosis books are best sellers, and people worldwide benefit from hypnosis at work, at play and in their personal lives.

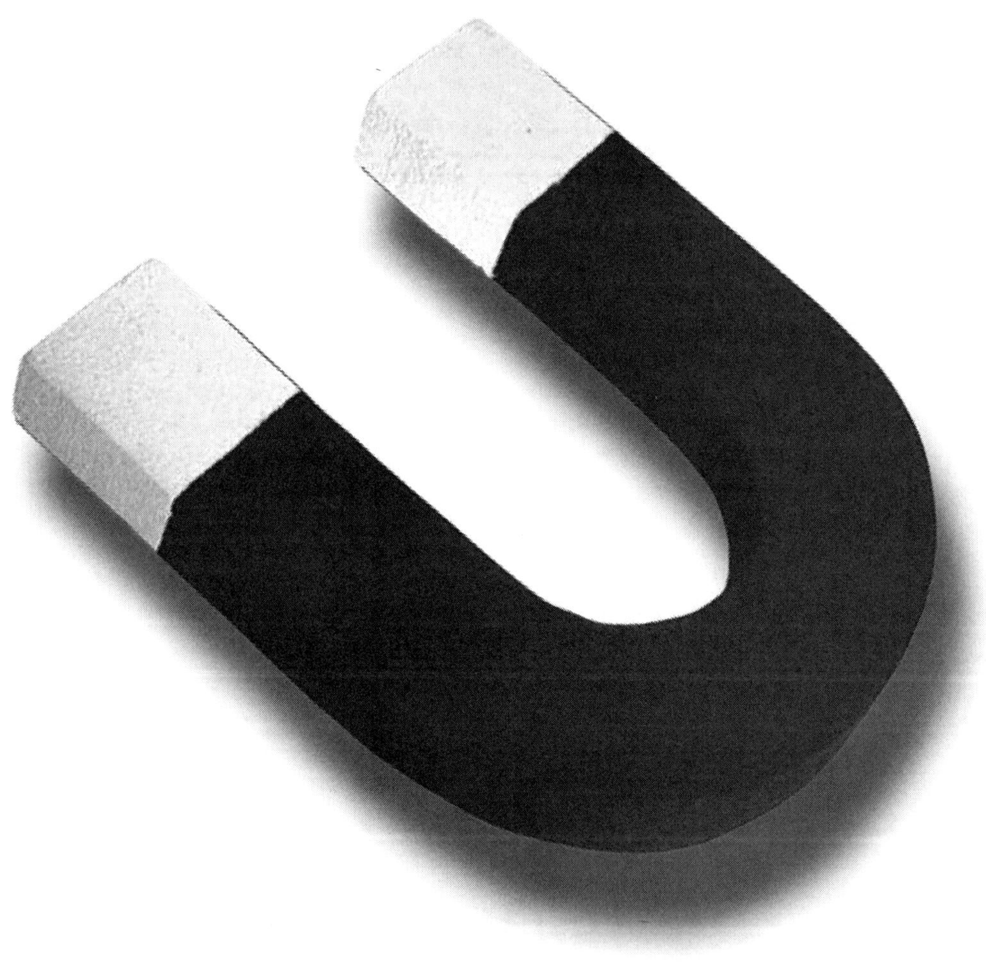

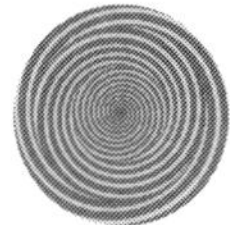

~ *Chapter 131* ~
BIO-MAGNETIC HYPNOTHERAPY:
BARON VON REICHENBACH

In the mid 19th century, following Mesmer's animal magnetism work, scientist Baron Charles Von Reichenbach advanced the theory of a universal form of magnetic healing energy that he named the "Odic Vital Force." The Baron thought the Aurora Borealis was the source of the force. Reichenbach tested the curative and physiological effects of magnetic energy with hospital patients. He insisted that hospital patients healed faster when their head faced towards the North Pole (the positive polarity of the planet) and their feet towards the South Pole (the negative polarity of the planet.) (Every 10,000 years the polarity of the earth shifts and so do the poles but that is another story.)

His one book, "The Dynamics Of Magnetism, Electricity, Heat, Light, Crystallization And Chemistry In Their Relation To Vital Force" was written in 1846. John Ashburner, M.D. performed the Herculean task of translating the original book from German into English in 1855 and arranged to have it published by Partridge & Britain, of the Shekimah & Spiritual Telegraph, in Great Britain the following year. This ageless book today is a priceless collectable.

All living things depend on electromagnetism as we are all composted of atoms, which are in part small magnets. Scientists confirm that specific nutrition affects the magnetic activity of each individual organ in the body and of the auric field outside of the body. Could this be the Baron's Odic Force at work?

Both Mesmer and the Baron believed in the healing virtue of magnetic energy.

Is it real or just belief?

After all, belief has been responsible for many healing miracles. Scientific research seeks knowledge of "cause and effect." The Hypnotherapist is rarely a researcher. Mostly, hypnotherapy focuses upon effect. That is to say, if it works, it works! Cause is a conscious mind activity. Effect is subconscious mind activity. Whatever your sentiments, a consideration of the healing energy of physical magnets deserves a place in an Encyclopedia Of Hypnotherapy. Bio-magnetic hypnotherapy produces curative effects. Is it the Bio-magnetic Energy or The Power of Suggestion? Little difference: in hypnotherapy the beneficial effect is of major importance.

Experiments revealed that the North Pole of the magnet (which is opposite of the actual north pole or the negative side of the magnet) placed over an afflicted part of the patient has a very different influence from that of the South Pole (or positive side). In testing, he noted that the negative position of the magnet tended to control inflammation in human joints and aided in more rapid healing of injuries while exerting an antibiotic effect on bacteria and a sedating effect on nerves. According to the Baron, the North Pole actually causes an alkaline reaction that works like an astringent, hardens tissue, attracts oxygen, stops hemorrhage and diminishes congestion.

Recent studies reported by Dr Robert R. Holcomb at Vanderbilt University claim that four magnets together arranged alternating as positive and negative poles can stop the transmission of pain at the cellular level.

Bio-magnetic Hypnosis applies a magnet to the meridian centers related to the affliction being treated. It is related to acupuncture; only in this case, a magnet is used rather than needles to produce a balancing of the meridians for healing and return to good health.

MODUS OPERANDI: MAGNETIC HYPNOTHERAPY

During bio-magnetic hypnotherapy, the client lies prone upon their back. They remain fully clothed, as energy from the magnet penetrates cloth material. A rod magnet is used as the healing instrument and left in place for as long as 15 minutes.

Have your client close their eyes and then induce hypnosis using a relaxing method. It is then suggested, **"Magnets will be placed over** _________(the afflicted area or meridian). **I place it in this location to heal your** _____________**."**

Explain the healing purpose of the magnet and its placement, then hold the North Pole, or negative side of the magnet upon the place that needs healing. Unquestionably your verbal suggestions are a factor in amplifying the healing. Silence is maintained for the remainder of the period of procedure. When complete, the client is aroused from hypnosis.

Be sure to tell them how well it went.

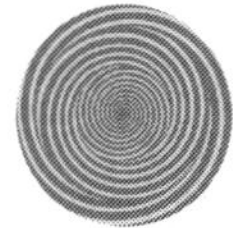

~ *Chapter 132* ~
MAGNETIC HEALING

Includes
Magnetic Healing Rules
Magnetic Healing
Magnetizing Water
Magnetically Treat A Headache
Magnetically Treat Neuralgia
Magnetically Treat A Toothache
Magnetically Treat Arthritis
Magnetically Treat An Earache
Magnetically Treat Heart Trouble
Magnetically Treat A General Debility
Magnetically Treat Eye Trouble
Magnetically Treat A Fever
Magnetically Treat Paralysis
Magnetically Treat Indigestion
General Instructions For Successful Magnetic Healing

Magnetic Healing is an early form of hypnotherapy. That belongs to the realm of speculation; as some say it works and others say it is "hooey." You decide.

Magnetic Healing has been defined as physiological/psychological energies operating in artful combination. Everything takes energy to do everything. Magnetic Healing directs healing energy to their to the client. Call it Personal Magnetism, if you wish. Call it you charisma. Call it your presence, whatever. In this chapter, we simply call it MAGNETIC HEALING and consider it along with some historical applications.

What is presented in this chapter is speculation, however it is speculation that millions believe in. You will find it interesting giving it a good ol' college try. Results are astounding.

MAGNETIC HEALING RULES
Make it your rule when you perform MAGNETIC HEALING to give full attention to the operation, under the direction of your "will power." In other words, put your heart and soul into the procedure. Will directs your Magnetic Energy wherever it is desired to benefit your client, where healing is needed. Use your will power to keep your mind on what you are doing and do not let your mind wander. This applies to all work. Think always of what you are doing, and concentrate your mind on it.

To facilitate the concentration of your will and induce a receptive condition in the client, perform the treatment in a quiet room. It is best be alone with the person you are healing (one close relative of friend is acceptable). Others can prove a distraction.

There is no set time for the special treating of any ailment. Some persons will have an immediate healing, while others may take several sessions. The moral is: NEVER GIVE UP.

Hot breath is very beneficial where pain exists. Instructions will be given how to use it.

Passes over the body are always made in a downward fashion…that is from head down toward the feet. Start a pass about eight to ten inches above the seat of pain and draw your hands downward over the affected part throwing in your energy as you make the pass, and flip it off your fingertips as you conclude the making of the long pass. In making healing passes, use both hands when possible, and spread the fingers slightly. Make the passes with an even stroking motion, not too fast and not too slow. As you make these passes you will experience a tingling electric-like current flowing out of your fingertips into the body of your client. It is a distinct sensation. It is a very tangible force, and the more you use it the more powerful it will become. As the energy flows out of your hands, concentrate your thoughts of healing, and project them along with your Personal Magnetism, into the client, especially to the place where healing is needed.

Your hands must not be cold when you make the passes. Never have cold hands when giving any form of Magnetic Healing treatment. Rub them briskly for a few moments and get them warm before ever touching the skin of a client. Some like a basin of warm water nearby, and whenever they finish a pass, they dip their fingers in it after throwing off the "force," and leave them wet before making another pass.

Start by charging yourself with Cosmic Force. Then MAKE UP YOUR MIND that you will aid/cure your client by sending healing energy telepathically along with verbal suggestions.

Have the ill person take a seat in a chair, or if very ill, lie upon a couch or bed. Never work on contagious diseases. That is not your domain. Properly used in a conscientious manner, Magnetic Healing has great value, and many wonderful cures have been reported to make sure you fell personally well. Never attempt Magnetic Healing if you are not personally feeling up to par.

MODUS OPERANDI: MAGNETIC HEALING

Have the client take a comfortable position so they can relax, and you can easily reach the affected part.

Tell them **"Relax all your muscles as much as you can and close your eyes. You are not to open your eyes again until I give you permission to do so. It is important to the treatment that you not open your eyes until the treatment is completed.** *Insist on this point strongly.*

In performing this kind of hypnotherapy (healing) have the client drink a glass of Magnetized Water before commencing external operations.

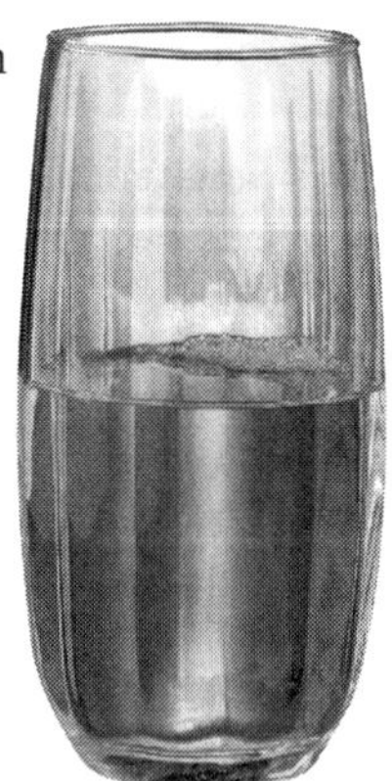

MODUS OPERANDI: MAGNETIZING WATER

You Will Need:
A Glass Of Room Temperature Water
A Table To Rest Your Hand

Come to appreciate the value of Magnetized Water. In this form of magnetic hypnotherapy, a healing energy actually passes from the therapist to the client, and invigorates and regenerates them by exterior manipulation and mental influence. Magnetized Water introduces this "force" internally. It will prove to be "good medicine."

Give a person a glass of Magnetized Water to drink, if possible, before actual treatment and impress on their mind its objective value to their healing. It is always well to tell a person to drink more water, as that is a great help in cleansing the body of any illness. Have them drink slowly, while thinking of it bringing good health into his body.

To Magnetize Water:
Take a glass of fresh water of normal temperature (not iced) and set it on your left hand, closing the hand around it much as possible while resting the hand and class of water upon a table.

Now, using your right hand, press the thumb against the first three fingers, in the manner of taking a pinch of salt, and hold the hand in this position over the glass to within an eight of an inch above the surface of the water in the glass. Now "will" with all your power that the force of Magnetism shall pass into the water. Hold the hand in this manner and perform this operation for about several minutes.

So prepared, instruct your client to **"Drink the water slowly"** and as you watch them drink it, mentally "will" it to invigorate and cure them.

Magnetized water usually gets crystal clear like water from a spring. In magnetizing the water never hold your left hand over the glass, unless you are left-handed. If you are naturally right handed, consider your right hand as being your positive pole and your left hand the negative. If you should try to magnetize the water with your left hand, it will get flat and stale, and will have a queer taste…it will act negative instead of positive upon the person drinking it. Here is an experiment using this principle that you can try:

Delicious Water Experiment
Take two glasses of water filled to the brim and place the palms of your hands over each so as to exclude all air for five minutes. Then remove your hands and taste the water in each glass. You will find that the water in the glass which has been covered by your left hand (if you are right handed) has become lukewarm and has a flat taste, while the water in the other glass is sparkling and fresh, and invigorating to drink.

MODUS OPERANDI:
MAGNETICALLY TREAT A HEADACHE
You Will Need:
A Fan Or Something To Fan With
A Glass of Water
A Table
A Fan of Some Kind

Headaches respond readily to the treatment, and provide good first experience for you in working with Magnetic Healing. Once you have learned how to relieve a headache, you will be able to relieve most any kind of pain.

Seat the client in a chair with a low back, so the person's head is free for you to work on. Magnetize a glass of water and have them slowly drink it. Instruct them to **"Drink the water slowly"** and as you watch them drink it, mentally "will" it to invigorate and cure them.

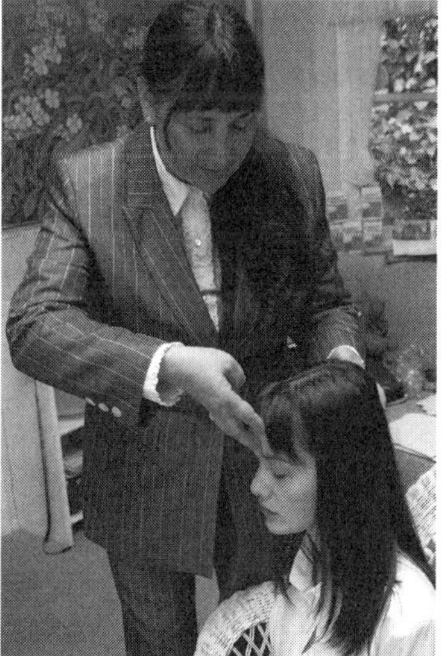

Headache

Ask the client to **"Relax your muscles and sit comfortably as possible with your hands lying on your thighs, and now close your eyes. Don't open them until you are through with the treatment, and when I give you permission to open them."**

All the while when giving the treatment, use your will power and concentrate your thoughts "willing" that the headache shall leave.

If the headache is in the forehead, place your left hand firmly across the back of the head near the base of the brain and your right hand across their forehead. If the client has their hair in a rubber band, take the hair down so you can work closer to the scalp.

If the headache is on top of the head, press as before, but make passes down the back of head to shoulders and throw it off, and proceed as instructed.

In this handclasp, press in on the head firmly in an upward direction. Hold this pressure for a full minute. Then stand behind the person, and using both your hands, make passes from the center of the forehead over the temples. At the end of each pass, throw off the collected energy. "Throw off" means to fling or snap your hands outward in such manner as if you had some sticky substance you wanted to get rid of; as though you had drops of honey on your fingertips and desired to shake it off. One fling at the end of each pass is sufficient. This "throwing off" applies to all cases where you use passes. Look upon it as a disposing of old and unwanted magnetic energy so your hands are clear to bring in the fresh and new.

After you have made passes for about three minutes, use the pressure again and then make further passes for a couple of more minutes, as described. Then stand behind the person and tell them to **"Inhale a deep breath through the nose and exhale it through the mouth."** Perform this breathing about four times.

While they are thus breathing, "will" powerfully that their headache has disappeared. All pain is gone!

Wave a fan of any kind, up and down the heart side of their body to make a slight breeze. Them say to them, **"When I count to four, I want you to open your eyes and you will find that your headache is gone and you feel fine. One…two…three…four…now you are all right!"**

As a rule, the client will feel their head and exclaim, "The pain is gone!"

Avoid talking further on the subject if the person feels all right. If there should be some residue of pain remaining, give another treatment at once. The time for headache removal treatment should not exceed ten minutes.

Sometimes when making passes over the head, while directing the magnetic energy, the client will fall almost asleep. If this should happen, simply clap your hands close to his ear, and say: **"All right! Your headache is gone. Wake up!"** Make a few upward passes without touching the person, starting from the waist up to over the head, which will dispel any sleepiness.

MODUS OPERANDI: MAGNETICALLY TREAT NEURALGIA
Use same method as applied to headaches.

MODUS OPERANDI: MAGNETICALLY TREAT A TOOTHACHE
You will need:
A Glass Of Water
A Table
A Cloth Handkerchief

To remove a toothache, have the client sit comfortably. Magnetize and give them this glass of magnetized water to drink slowly. Then tell them **"Close your eyes and tell me the location of the tooth that aches so I may remove the pain."**

Make passes about the bad tooth in the jaw downward along the side of the jawbone, and throw it off. Make about a dozen of these passes, then take a cloth handkerchief (never use silk cloth) and fold it into a pad, and place it over the spot where the aching tooth is…then blow your hot breath in the center of the cloth pad as it rests upon the cheek.

In blowing hot breath inhale through your nose and exhale through your mouth slowly. It produces a warm current of air. Place your lips on the cloth and force this breath through the cloth. It produces warmth upon the cheek, which passes the magnetic influence through the cheek, and it will reach the tooth or the seat of pain.

Inhale and exhale the warm breath upon the cloth ten times and then remove the cloth pad. Make passes for a minute or two over the painful spot, use hot breath again, and then verbalize these suggestions: **"When I count to four, open your eyes and you will find your toothache is gone and you are feeling fine. One…two…three…four. Now you are all right."**

You will find that hot breath into a folded handkerchief pad is helpful to use in removing all types of pain, in special spots upon the body. The breath is an excellent conveyor of healing energy.

MODUS OPERANDI: MAGNETICALLY TREAT ARTHRITIS
You Will Need:
A Glass Of Water
A Table
A Cloth Handkerchief

This is the Magnetic Healing way of helping arthritis and rheumatic related maladies.

Seat the person or have them lie on a bed, all-depending on where the trouble is. Give them a glass of magnetized water, and proceed to make passes over the area of his trouble, while concentrating your thoughts on the healing taking place. For instance, if the pain is in the elbow, start your passes from the shoulder down to the fingertips and throw it off. If in the knee, start eight or ten inches above and throw it off at the toes. When it is possible and appropriate, remove any clothing necessary so you can get as close to the skin as you can.

Then use hot breath on a handkerchief the seat of pain, using passes again and terminate with the suggestion formula **"The pain is gone, and you are healing."**

Further, instruct the person **"Drink a half glass of this magnetized water every day. It is an additional aid in affecting a cure."**

This treatment for rheumatic type disorders should be frequently performed until the swelling is reduced.

MODUS OPERANDI: MAGNETICALLY TREAT AN EARACHE
You will need:
A Cloth Handkerchief

Place a folded cloth pad over the person's ear and blow hot breath. Make passes over the ear and around it, and draw it off at the shoulder point. Always have the person take a few deep breaths at the conclusion of treatment.

MODUS OPERANDI: MAGNETICALLY TREAT HEART TROUBLE
Hypnotize client and blow hot breath over the heart. Make passes over the heart and draw it off to left side of body. Make the passes over heart for a full ten minutes. Follow the general direction you have learned for this treatment, and treat heart trouble every other day.

MODUS OPERANDI: MAGNETICALLY TREAT A GENERAL DEBILITY
Have the client lie their stomach and make passes from the crown of the head down the full length of spine; then draw the hands across the kidneys and down along each leg to the toes, and draw off. Make passes for ten minutes and increase the speed of them gradually. Use no hot breath.

Turn the client over on their back and make passes from the shoulders down first over the body to toes then over arms to fingertips. Then shake off fully. Perform treatment for ten minutes at each session, which is best when given when the person is in bed and ready to go to sleep. After the treatment, let sleep come in naturally. The following morning the client will be much improved.

MODUS OPERANDI: MAGNETICALLY TREAT EYE TROUBLE
You will need:
A Cloth Handkerchief

Blow hot breath on eyes and gently stroke the eyelids towards the nose for some minutes, then use hot breath again. The blowing of breath upon the cloth pad placed on eyes is very restful to the eyes. In many instances, Magnetic Healing has improved vision.

MODUS OPERANDI: MAGNETICALLY TREAT A FEVER
Fever of any kind responds well to Magnetic Healing. Place your hand on the client's forehead for a few minutes, then make passes down the body to toes and throw it off. Continue this for ten or fifteen minutes. Tell them **"When you open your eyes the fever has left you and you feel much better."**

MODUS OPERANDI: MAGNETICALLY TREAT PARALYSIS
When working on paralysis use hypnotic trance in combination with your magnetic healing processes. Remove necessary clothing to expose the paralyzed part. Make passes over the area and increase the speed of passes for ten to fifteen minutes. Then gently slap the area until color commences to show and a better circulation of blood is produced. Suggest firmly that **"You will get better and better."** If, for example, you have been working on a paralyzed leg, have them try to use the leg after treatment. Paralysis responds well to hypnotic suggestion.

MODUS OPERANDI: MAGNETICALLY TREAT INDIGESTION
You will need:
A Cloth Handkerchief

Make passes from the neck down over chest and stomach of client. Use hot breath and manipulate stomach thoroughly for fifteen minutes. Instruct the client **"Drink plenty of water, and restrain from eating too much meat. Substitute fruit for meat."** Several treatments will often bring about a permanent cure.

GENERAL INSTRUCTIONS FOR SUCCESSFUL MAGNETIC HEALING
Here are ten rules to follow:

1. Know that you can help. Be confident of your ability to heal
2. Be cheerful in your work. Let the person know you have helped people with a condition far worse than his own.
3. Seat the client comfortably so they can relax and start the session by giving them a glass of "magnetized water" to slowly drink.
4. Have the client **"Close your eyes at the beginning of session and do not to open them until I give you permission to do so at end of session."**
5. Except for close relatives or friends, dismiss all other people from the room when working with a client. Magnetic healing is largely a private matter between operator and client.

6. Have your hands warm when making passes. When convenient soak your hands in warm water for ten minutes prior to making passes over body. Then dry hands and shake both hands vigorously to get the circulation flowing strongly.
7. In the throwing off process, at end of passes, dip your hands in warm water for a moment, before commencing another pass.
8. Become conscious of the flow of magnetic energy in your hands. Experience it fully as an electrical tingling in your fingers. When you lay a hand on an affected part, sense the energy passing into the patient from your hands. Same with breath: experience the "force."
9. Develop a rapport with your client, and when a cure is achieved, instruct them to tell no one. Magnetic Healing is a private affair.
10. Combine the use of suggestive therapeutics with magnetic healing. The combination is very powerful.

Is magnetic healing real or just imagination? Just imagination! How we do tend to run down imagination; never full appreciating that imagination is the creative function of the mind, and that everything created starts in the imagination. Imagination! Use it fully in all forms of hypnotic work.

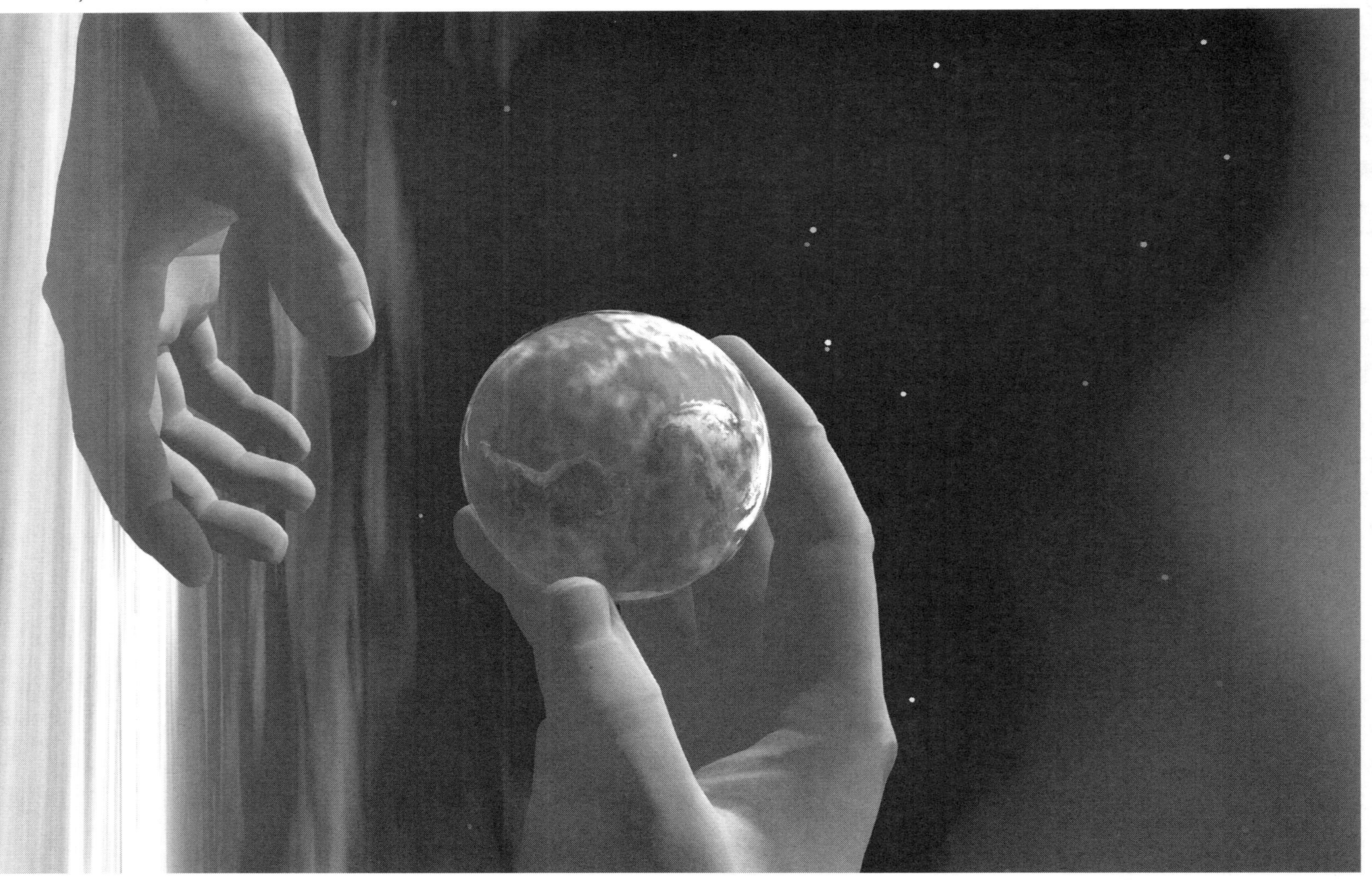

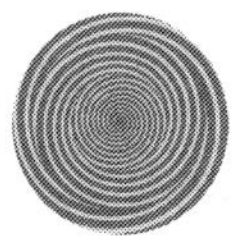

~ *Chapter 133* ~
HYPNO-REIKI:
ENERGY HYPNOSIS

By Shelley Stockwell-Nicholas, PhD

Remember, *"a rose is a rose and by whatever name still smells as sweet."*

It's amusing that when one process is given a different name and looked upon as being a different process. Energy shifting and healing through vibration is reminiscent of Mesmerism isn't it? Reiki is a current popular form of energy healing hypnotherapy. Here is what Editor, Shelley Stockwell has to say about it:

REIKI
By Shelley Stockwell-Nicholas

Reiki the soil of the mind, open your thoughts to air.
Human warmth and angels view melt away your cares.
Reiki the soil of mind: heighten your vibration
Awaken your true essence in spiritual restoration.

With planted feet upon the earth, and tongue at the roof of the mouth.
Visualize pure violet light east, west, north and south.
Place your dominant hand upon them, as the other in mid air
draws a Chinese symbol as you silently declare:
"CHO•KU•REI" (a word you say) for the power of the sword
to carve the universe light to tap the sacred chord.

Sacred geometry for enlightenment has been used by every recorded civilization. Ancient Egyptians used it in initiation rites in their sleep temples and as hieroglyphics. Cave drawings, the Kabala, and Sanskrit are loaded with these teachings. Hebraic language and our own alphabet are outgrowths of these ancient systems. For thousands of years, ancient Tibetan Buddhists (the "Great White Brotherhood"), lamas or holy ones, meditated on some three hundred drawn symbols as they chanted associated sacred sounds. Today, practitioners "pass attunements" by getting centered, imaging and silently sounding one of five symbols and sending it through their hand. Only these five symbols and sounds are said to remain from ancient times (want Tibet)!

Reiki practitioners are quite secretive about the symbols and sounds unless you study the system with them.

To become "certified" as a Reiki Practitioner, you are "attuned" during your own Reiki sessions by a Certified Master Teacher. This "prepares you" to channel the frequencies needed for each level. Once you've been attuned you are said to have opened your own energy to heal others.

First degree Reiki teaches a series of hand positions that run energy and balance meridians. Each advanced "degree" incorporates different symbols and sounds. Second Degree or Reiki Two combines Reiki one hand placements with in-visioning and in-toning sacred symbols, sounds and the color violet or purple. It teaches mental/emotional healing and long distant healing. And Third degree Reiki Master attunement teaches you to open the crown chakra of others.

You can Reiki a person. object, plant or animal. Cats love Reiki energy. To Reiki a fish, place your hands around an aquarium for 15 to 20 minutes: the cat may love that, too. To Reiki a plant, focus your energy at the root system.

Studies show that prayer before you eat and blessing your food gives you more nutritional benefit. Reiki your food, it can't hurt. You can also Reiki gifts before giving them and letters before mailing them.

The Word "Reiki" Has Its Ups And Downs

Named in the mid 1800's by Japanese physician, Mikao Usui, the word "reiki" comes from the Japanese language.

Rei is the Japanese equivalent of "universal transcendent power, spirit, ghost and soul." The corresponding Chinese word *lei* means "subtle ethereal influences." Tibetans say it means a "clever, supernatural spirit entity that acts on others."

Ki means "vital life force" similar to the Chinese Chi (pronounced "Chee"), Qi, or Qi Gong. In Japanese, *Raku-Kei* translates as Raku meaning vertical energy flow and Kei meaning horizontal energy flow. So loosely translated, Reiki means "divinely guided multidirectional universal life force energy."

Like all hands-on energy-directed healing Reiki is used to promote positivity, integrate mind and body and spirit and to heal and revitalize. It is an excellent adjunct to hypnosis. You can easily "reiki" your client as an induction technique or for the whole session. A Hypno-Reiki session can be any length. It usually take about forty-five minutes to an hour. You can run energy for a few minutes or for the entire session.

Hypnosis combined with hands-on healing Reiki is called "Hypno-Reiki." Here's how you do it.

MODUS OPERANDI: SHELLEY STOCKWELL'S HYPNOSIS/REIKI PROCESS

Preparation: A Native American will sage a room to cleanse it, a Reiki practitioner will Reiki it. You can *Reiki* your office before your client arrives

1. **Get Permission**
    Explain to your client that you will be respectful of their person and mean it. It goes without saying that you would indeed be appropriate. **"We are going to do an energetic session today. It will be non-verbal. Hypno-Reiki uses gently and respectful touch and, of course, I will not violate your trust in any way. Is it ok with you if I gently lay hands upon your _______________** (afflicted area) **head, shoulders, throat, heart, stomach?"**

    If they say "yes" proceed. If they have an objection say, **"Fine. Will it be ok if I send the energy without physically touching you?"**

    After you get the ok, proceed.

Legal Note: Because of ridiculously litigious society, always know the laws of your state and town. Get verbal or written approval. The State of California requires an "Alternative/Complimentary Health Provider Disclosure Form" to be signed by all clients at their first visit. A copy of their signed form is to be kept in your records for three years so you avoid being charged with "practicing medicine without a license." It's a good idea to use such a form wherever you practice. The International Hypnosis Federation has preprinted disclosure forms available by calling (800) 366-7908 or you can order them at the back of this book.

The law in some states allows you to "lay hands" on someone (appropriately of course), but if you move your hand along the body, you are considered "massaging them" and you can't do without a massage therapist's license. Some Hypnotists and Reiki workers get certified as a minister to sanction the "laying of hands" as a religious rite. The Universal Light Church, on the internet, can help you do that. Another person present during the session is always welcome.

2. **Make Your Client Comfortable**
   Have your client remove their shoes and relax while sitting in a chair or resting upon a message table.

3. **Briskly Rub Your Hands Together**

4. **Give a Prayer or Blessing**
   Bless yourself and the one you choose to heal. Here is the prayer that I use:
   "Dear God, all great healers who have gone before,
   and all great healers who are yet to come here in the future,
   Bless us both on all levels;
   Physically with radiant health,
   Mentally with clear thinking,
   Emotionally with unconditional love,
   And spiritually so that we may take the path of higher consciousness.
   Let me be a pure conduit of live and light.
   I now open myself to channel your love.
   Let this session be for the welfare of the planet and all living things
   Amen. Awomen. Ah Life."

5. **Rest Your Tongue and Tighten Your Pelvis**
   Touch your tongue to the little piece of skin behind your two front teeth and then let it rest comfortably on the roof of the mouth. Contract your pelvic muscles (called hui yin in Japan and kagle in the United States) and then relax. This activates your Kundalini energy.

6. **Placement of the Hands**
   Your hands rest in a series of hand placements for about five minutes per position before moving to the next position. Meanwhile, you intone and focus light and energy from outside of yourself through your hands. You'll find that the process is quite relaxing and energy boosting for you as well. About ten minutes into the session your client may feel the Reiki flow as a tingling sensation, particularly over the part of the body or organ that is in poor health. You'll feel it too.

Chair Hypno-Reiki Placements

Your client (fully clothed) is seated in a chair. Move your hand placements to the head, eye, forehead (or ears), base of head (or chin), shoulders, throat, heart (etheric heart), stomach, hips, hands and elbows, knees and ankles, hand and back, thigh, knees, calf to ankle, lower back (for adrenals and kidneys), and to the spine top and bottom. When complete stroke over the head, heart and back.

Massage Table Hypno-Reiki Placements:

If your client is reclining on a massage table, do the hand placements for the back of the head, neck and upper, mid and lower back while they lay on their stomach.

7. Create a Mental Image And Lay Your Hands

If you don't know a formal Reiki visualization, simply envision a violet flame through your third eye as you hold your dominant hand one-inch above your client. When you feel that you have energetic permission, lay your other hand upon the afflicted spot.

It is also perfectly ok to send energy without touching by holding your hand above the region in need of energy. Let your intuition be your guide as you replace your hands where they need to go to "run energy." You'll notice subtle energy if you pass over any weak part of their body. If that happens linger there and say to yourself, "balanced and well."

6. Let Energy Flow As You Intone

You may recite a mantra like TM's "Sha Ring" or the Tibetan "Hon Sah" or simply intone "Ohm" and visualize any sacred symbol that appeals to you.

7. Complete The Session

As you sense an energy shift or temperature change you'll intuit that you are complete. When you get that sense, stroke upward over their head, heart and back. Shake out your hands and let the energy drain from your palms into the earth, smile and say "Yes!"

After your session, expect your client to feel deeply relaxed.

Hypno-Helper

"Essential Reiki: A Complete Guide to an Ancient Healing Art" by Diane Stein (Crossing Press) reveals the "secret" symbols and attunements for the three degrees of Reiki.

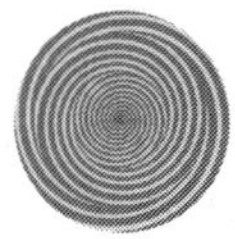

~ *Chapter 134* ~
TAPPING TECHNIQUES
By Shelley Stockwell

Includes
Tapping
Tapping Sequences

Tapping, Emotional Freedom Technique or EFT uses a repeated phrase as you tap on special body spots. It is based on channeled material that claims acupressure, acupuncture and meridians for its usefulness. EFT aficionados say it busts fears in minutes and that results are long lasting or permanent.

This technique is touted to be very successful for people with post-traumatic stress disorder and addictive cravings. It is a popular hypnotherapy adjunct. As you tap each of the "spots" you say and have the client repeat a negative affirmation like; **"Even though I have this fear (problem, issue, challenge),** (e.g. "even though I'm afraid of dogs") **I deeply and completely accept and love myself."** This is said to build self-esteem and eliminate self-condemnation. I prefer positive affirmations myself. See what you think.

MODUS OPERANDI: TAPPING

Put your client into a trance and speak slowly and clearly as you instruct them:

"I am speaking to your subconscious mind, the part of you that is wise beyond wise. This part of you knows exactly what you need to do to let go of this negative pattern once and for your highest good."

1. DEFINE THIS ISSUE TO BE RELEASED

"Subconscious mind, what is the issue that you want to permanently release?" Pause and let them answer. Focus on one aspect or emotion at a time. (Some fears or issues have many emotions attached to them. If so, use one tapping sequence for each aspect.) **"Are you willing to support _____________ (person's name) in letting this go once and for good? Excellent."**

If they do not say exactly what they want to accomplish say, **"In our conversations before entering trance, you said that you wanted to _____________. Is it in your best interest to do that at this time? Very well, let's make that happen now. Repeat this to yourself or out loud. 'I choose to be free to _________ (e.g. walk past a dog). I am open to any and all changes that occur.'"**

2. CLARIFY THE DESIRED OUTCOME

Tell your subconscious mind what you would like the result to be from tapping. Or ask your subconscious mind, **"Subconscious mind, when you let go of this pattern of thinking or action, how will _____ (the person's name) benefit?**

3a. NEGATIVE TAPS

Instruct them to tap each of the "spots," or you do the tapping, by saying; **"As I** (or you) **tap each spot, repeat this phrase inside yourself, 'even though I have this fear** (problem, issue, challenge e.g. even though I'm afraid of dogs), **I deeply and completely accept and love myself.'"**

Or

3b. POSITIVE TAPS

"Give me a word or phase to describe the positive outcome, that _____________ (client's name) **gets to have when they release this pattern once and for good."**

Words like, "peace" "harmony," "joy" or "love" usually comes forth.

"(Their special word) _____________. From this moment forward, _____________ (their special word) **becomes your reality. As I** (or you) **tap each spot, repeat this phrase inside yourself, 'Peace. I deeply and completely accept and love myself.'**

With each tap, you will permanently release, once and for your highest good, any and every thing that needs to be let go so that you are entirely free of this issue. You let go of any unhealthy benefits, physical manifestations, patterns, trauma or upset that have interfered with your full energy and happiness. And you instantly replace it with (their special word) **_____________. You will feel the healing effects immediately"**

4. RELEASEMENT

When tapping is complete **"Let's begin, 'I now permanently release this issue and any related issues and I am _________** (their word).

5. PERMANENTLY ACCEPT THE DESIRED OUTCOME.

"You are now completely comfortable physically, mentally, emotionally and spiritually. You completely and deeply accept and love yourself. You are happy inside yourself while you are asleep and while you are awake. It is safe in your world."

6. BRING IT ON HOME

"Take a deep breath and notice on a scale of one to ten how much better you feel. It is gone! When this is so, mentally tap each point saying to yourself; 'I am completely at ease and the problem is solved." As you rub the top of the head and all points.

If your client still has a charge on the initial problem, negative tapping would have you repeat the process again, this time saying: **"Even though I still have SOME remaining _________** (ie fear), **I deeply and completely accept myself."** Positive tapping would have you tap again instructing, **"I let it go naturally in the next hour. By tomorrow it is completely gone."**

TAPPING SEQUENCES:
The Ear Tap

A simple tapping sequence is around the ear starting at the temple and moving to the bottom of the ear. Start with the left ear tapping 5-7 times and repeat the sequence for five rounds repeating your affirmation as you do. Then do the same with the right ear. Acupuncturists might say that you have activated calming/sedating meridians that help relieve stress, fear, and trauma.

The Body Tap

1. **The OUTSIDE OF the HAND**
   Tap the tender place on the side of your hand, above your wrist and below your little finger. Rub or karate chop this place seven to ten times and say with feeling: **"Even though I _______________, (or their word) I deeply and completely accept myself."**

2. **TOP OF HEAD (TH)**
   Seven to ten taps on what was the soft spot of fontanel top and slightly back.

3. **EYEBROW (EB)**

4. **SIDE OF EYE (SE)**

5. **UNDER EYE (UE)**

7. **UNDER THE NOSE (UN)**

8. **CHIN (CH)**

9. **COLLAR BONE (CB)** One inch down from the center of the clavicle and one inch to the right and then to the left.

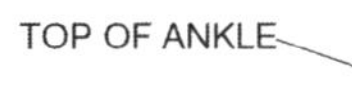

10. **UNDER YOUR ARM (UA)**
    Tap four inches down from the armpit or in the middle of the bra for women. For men, tap on the side in line with your nipple.

11. **WRIST (W)**

12. **TOP OF ANKLE (TA)**
    Tap both inside and outside about four inches above the anklebone.

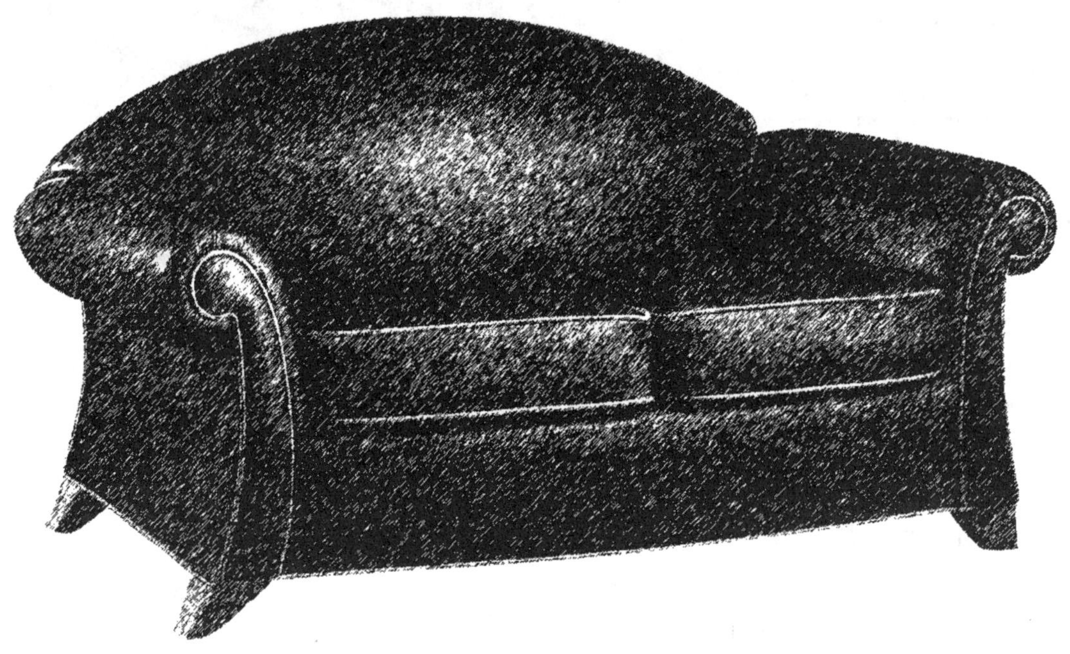

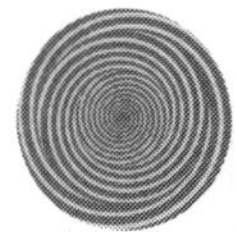

~ *Chapter 135* ~
VOGEL'S ENERGIZED HYPNOTHERAPY COUCH

Electrical Induction Field + Crystal Directed Energy
toward a reclining client/patient.

More and more, technology infiltrates hypnotherapy. IBM Senior Scientist Dr. Marcel Vogel is credited with this innovative hypnosis. Prior to his death, he was deeply interested in how low-voltage energies, amplified through quartz crystal, affected the body. He directed an electrically-energized crystal toward the client. If you are into this sort of thing, it is worthy of experimentation. If you try it, I recommend that you add the Serenity Resonance Sound in the background to further deepen the trance.

Vogel's device uses electrical alternating current (AC). An energized large coil, placed on the floor, surrounds the hypnotherapeutic couch, to produce a field that is transmitted to a smaller coil above the couch. This energy is then amplified and directed downwards via a crystal towards the third eye of a reclining client. A straight-line molecular structure of the quartz crystal amplifies and directs energy out through its apex. Vogel's experiments directly connect technology and psychology.

You are amplifying the natural power of the crystal with an electrical field.

Disclaimer: Consult a professional electrician when working with such powerful and potentially dangerous electricity.

MODUS OPERANDI: VOGEL'S ENERGIZED HYPNOTHERAPY COUCH

I include his approach based on Dr. Vogel's notes:

1. Place a comfortable couch for your client to recline upon in the center of the hypnotherapy session room.

2. Take a coil made of 30 turns of insulated Bell Telephone Wire under the couch. Use a length large enough to circumvent your hypnosis couch and place it on the floor. Energize the coil with a low voltage AC current. I suggest using a small transformer for this. Transform 110 AC to around 12 volts DC. You can use a battery for this purpose too. The exact voltage requires experimentation.

3. Wrap the inner end of a similar smaller wire coil, with about 20 turns, around a clear quartz crystal with the apex pointed the 3rd eye of the client. Suspend this coil above the couch (near ceiling of session room).

4. Operation:
   The reclining person, will be bathed in a continuous field of low voltage inductive energy, passing from the energized large coil on floor– through space –via induction and picked up by the suspended smaller coil above. The AC electrical energy is amplified and directed back towards the person on the couch by the down-pointed crystal.

5. The device produces a continuous circling of energy surrounding the client/patient.

"Further experimentation is needed, but advance study seems to offer an increasing of effective responses to suggestions given subject during sessions. The Energized Hypnotherapeutic Couch seems to intensify hypnotic depth," said Dr. Vogel.

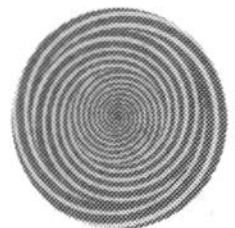

~ *Chapter 136* ~
LIGHT AND SOUND HYPNOTHERAPY

Includes
Historic Observations
Contemporary Observations
Light & Sound Hypnotherapy

In this text, I've commented on how to increase a hypnotic state of mind using vibrational brain wave frequencies. Now, I'm experimenting with physical (kinetic) vibration combined with rhythmic sound and flickering light. This combination is a powerful trance inducer. Thanks to Hypnotherapist, Joseph Berg for sharing with me his ideas on using Light and Sound for hypnotic induction.

HISTORIC OBSERVATIONS
The intrigue of rhythmic sounds for producing hypnotic states of mind is ancient history. Frequencies of sound were and are used by indigenous peoples in rites and ceremonies. Sound is a basic tool for entering the Shamanic State of Consciousness. Drums, rattle, hand clapping and chanting alter mind state. Drumbeats during tribal rituals often create theta frequency.

Ancient scientists were fascinated by the phenomenon of flickering lights. Apuleius, experimenting with them in 125 A.D., produced flickering light by rotating a light source on a potter's wheel. He observed that if you concentrated on it, it could produce a "type of epilepsy."

Ptolemy, in 200 A.D. studied the flickering lights of sunlight observed through the spokes of a spinning wheel. He noted that when patterns and colors appeared in the eyes of the observer, a feeling of "euphoria developed."

Early French psychologist, Pierre Janet, noticed that patients at Salpetriere Hospital in Paris experienced reduction in hysteria and increased relaxation when exposed to flickering lights.

CONTEMPORARY OBSERVATIONS
In the 1930's and 1940's, scientists like W. Gray Walter used powerful electronic strobe lights and the new Electro-Encephalogram (EEG) equipment to alter and measure brainwave activity. He correlated light with trance-like states of profound relaxation and vivid imagery. Walter's research aroused the attention of numerous artists including William Burroughs. A flicker device called the "Dream Machine" caused subjects to report "dazzling lights of unearthly brilliance and color." And "geometric mandalas appearing like brightly colored dreams."

During the 1960's and 1970's, drumming became a popular way to produce altered states.

Dr. Joe Kamiya, with his EEG feedback device at Langley-Porter Neuropsychiatry Institute in San Francisco, launched the age of biofeedback.

Others embraced the psychedelic effects in rhythmic strobe lights and sound in rock and roll nightclubs.

Scientific research examined hemispheric synchronization. Jack Schwarz, best known for his demonstrations of subconscious mind control over automatic responses, developed the "ISIS", a device which used rhythmic sounds and variable frequencies of light in goggles (worn by the client) to produce hypnotic states.

Computer expert Joseph Worrell, sound technician, Rolf Wyler, and I are experimented with kinetic vibration, using a recliner chair arranged to vibrate the person relaxing in it. This proved effective to increase the depth and intensity of relaxation…intense relaxation is hypnosis.

The combination of sound, light, and kinetic frequencies, when applied in conjunction with hypnotherapeutic techniques produces profound hypnosis (somnambulism).

MODUS OPERANDI: LIGHT & SOUND HYPNOTHERAPY
You will need:
Light Blinking Goggles
Stereo Headphones
Microphone Connected To The Headphones
A Reclining Chair (one that vibrates if available)
Serenity Resonance Sound (available at the back of this book)

Have your client recline on a vibrating chair . Place the light flickering goggles on them and have them close their eyes. The flickering will appear through their closed eyelids. Play the Serenity Resonance Sound tape through the earphones.

"Take three deep breaths (inhale…hold…exhale."
(Pause)

"Take a fourth breath and exhale through your nose in sync with the light and sound frequency. Do this synchronized breath as long as you like until you slack off and relax."

At this time, turn on the vibration in the reclining chair and offer your suggestions. The client will drift into profound hypnosis.

Do not rush to arouse them. Allow time for the subconscious to bring them back. When they return to their regular state of mind discuss the experience, their thoughts, the music, the colors, and the lights. Above all else, listen carefully to what they say.

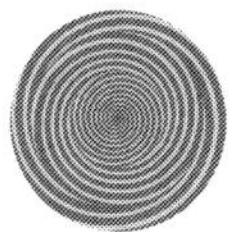

~ *Chapter 137* ~
PSYCHO ACOUSTIC HYPNOTHERAPY

By Shelley Stockwell-Nicholas
Sound comes from vibration - everything vibrates - how often it does is called "frequency."

Includes
Biological Follow Response
Jeffrey Thompson's Bio Tuning And Sonic Induction
Four Session Bio Tuning And Sonic Induction

Meditation gongs, bells, cymbals, drums, singing bowls, horns, whistles, flutes and chanting have been used throughout history to enhance states of consciousness. Sound creates bodily responses in pulse rate, respiration, pupillary dilation, body temperature, brain wave frequencies and how you feel. Hearing ranges are frequencies you detect.

When you were a fetus, floating in your own private flotation tank of mother's amniotic fluid, your ear canals filled with sound. After all, sound travels five times more efficiently in water than in air. This intense sound offered you deep mental relaxation. That is why the "Entrancing Music" tape I produced has a woven thread of womb sounds among the alpha-theta brain wave patterns and serene classical-like music.

BIOLOGICAL FOLLOW RESPONSE
The "follow response" or "entrainment" from our environment is something we take for granted. Menstrual cycles coincide with the cycles of the moon. Your sleep and circadian rhythms are influenced by the length of the day. Some people exhibit depression called seasonal affective disorder when deprived of sunlight. Atmospheric disturbances can disturb. Barometric pressure effects your cerebral capillaries.

Visual stimulation induces trance. Your internal rhythms follow the strongest external pulse patterns. 1950's U.S. Navy experiments confirmed that brain waves could be controlled by strobe light stimulation.

Sounds themselves can induce trance. Electronically disguised primordial nature sounds like the ocean, waves, water, wind, animals, heartbeat and breath, not recognized by conscious awareness, evoke specific brain wave patterns impacting emotion and make us open and receptive to both internal and external suggestion.

Space sounds recorded by NASA on the Voyager I and II missions when slowed 64 times are similar to human voice, animal and nature sounds. Jupiter sounds like dolphins, the small moon of Uranus (Miranda) sounds like a choir of voices and rings of Uranus resonate like a giant Tibetan bowl with bells. Those who listen to these recordings often report profound enlightenment experiences.

Dr's Jeffrey Thompson and Richard Stamper, along with dozens of space agencies like NASA, major universities and institutions, conducted a research project to explore the effects of these space recordings on the subconscious mind. They mixed space sounds and sound pulse patterns using "binaural holophonic integration," 3-D surround sound processing, and "Bedini audio special environment (B.A.S.E.), via a high powered computer system. These CD's are currently being used in a government sponsored program at the Neuropsychiatry Division of UCLA with those addicted to opiates with the hope that they will tap "deeper levels of the subconscious mind for accelerated positive inner change."

JEFFREY THOMPSON'S BIO TUNING & SONIC INDUCTION

"In actuality there is nothing solid in the universe at all. Consciousness itself is a vibrational pattern."
　　　—Jeffrey Thompson

Imagine chanting, dancing and watching yourself all at the same time!

Jeffrey D Thompson a Chiropractor and musician from Encinitas, California uses a person's own voice as a template for sound therapy. Speakers built into a massage table play a person's unique voice tone harmonics and overtones in a 3-D recording. The sound table has electronic "tuning fork" transducers making it a giant vibrational sounding board. Blinking lights cause closed eyes to "dance" to vibrations and sound. "For physical, emotional and mental balance and healing." This "melting into the vibration is what a mantra truly is" says Thompson.

The theory goes that your biological system, that created your vocal cords, recognizes and resonates with your own voice print. Like homeopathy, where a remedy is made from drop of your own tissue, sonics bring you home to yourself. You will need a high-tech computer system.

MODUS OPERANDI: FOUR SESSION BIO TUNING AND SONIC INDUCTION

First determine the client's optimum brain wave frequency patterns in a process that accurately divides between notes by 100 steps- or 100 divisions of sharp or flat between two notes on a piano keyboard.

Here is how Dr. Thompson conducts his following four-session approach:

Session One

The client lays upon the table wearing headphones playing specific brainwave entrainment frequencies and noting your responses.

Session Two

The client is retested with the frequencies they best responded to during the first session. Then the client "sings" favored frequencies aloud to be recorded using special 3D microphones. This recording is then processed and slowed by being dropped it a number of octaves so the sound will be recognized and the client will not awaken.

"Light goggles" are emplaced and flash tiny light bulbs in sync with the sound frequencies. This allows them to "see, hear and feel their own tonality.

Session Three & Four

The client "listens" to the 3-D sound as they did in the last session and is then instructed after session 4 to "listen to the audio taped version of their signature sounds for the next 30 days and then to return for a booster table session to retest the systems.

Hypno-Helper
Dr. Thompson's NASA space sounds are available in stores on compact disc or audio tape.

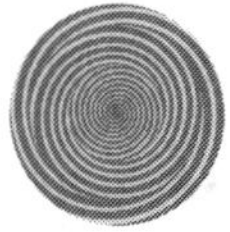

~ *Chapter 138* ~
VITALITY HYPNOSIS

Use this process both for yourself and to benefit your clients. Increasing vitality is important to everything you do in life. Enough vitality lets you handle a stressful and highly demanding life. The process starts by visualizing a mass of energy, the size of a glowing light bulb, forming in the base of the spine and glowing within your SELF. Present the process in a personal manner. Use it often for yourself…then you can pass it on to others.

Visualizing is directed imagination, and imagination is the Creative Power of the mind.

MODUS OPERANDI: VITALITY HYPNOSIS
You Will Need:
Soft Music

Present this in a personal manner:
"Close your eyes, relax and drift into the privacy of yourself. This is your own personal space. Allow your mind to enter into this space and become silent. Become quiet and enter the silence of your inner self. Silence. Silence. Silence."

Play some soft music as they relax. The Serenity Resonance sound may be played very quietly in the background as well. About three minutes is enough.

"Visualize a mass of energy, the size of a glowing light bulb, forming in the base of your spine. Visualizing is directed imagination, and imagination is the creative power of the mind. Develop this ability to powerfully VISUALIZE and see that glowing ball of light brightly in your mind's eye glowing within your SELF. See it shining. Now feel it also. Feel it as a vibrating source of energy, as you mentally move it about your body. Feel it as an experience of WARMTH; feel it fully as bringing life-giving vitality into your Being. Move the light throughout your body in the following steps:"

STEP ONE:
"Now visualize the energy from the base of your spine moving up your spine to the top of your head. Experience it. Relax."

STEP TWO:
"Now visualize the energy glowing at the top of your head, and move it down between your eyes clear down to the top of your nose. Experience it. Relax."

STEP THREE:
"Now take a deep breath and draw the light into your nose, visualize it going down in to your throat and into your lungs. Strongly with your mind see your lungs as alive with light. Experience it. Relax."

STEP FOUR:
"Imagine the energy permeating your lungs – filling all space between your armpits. Your lungs are alive with light. Your lungs are alive with energy. Experience it. Relax."

STEP FIVE:
"Now with your mind move the energy from your armpits down your arms to the thumbs of your hands. Feel your thumbs become warm and commence to tingle. Then, from your thumbs visualize the energy in your thumbs sparking across to your forefingers, and spark on to other fingers, as a living electric current, until your hands are alive with energy. Experience it. Relax."

STEP SIX:
"Now move the energy from your hands on back up your arms to your shoulders. (Pause there a moment) then move across your shoulders to your neck to the points where your jaws meet your cheeks. Feel your cheeks flush and glow with warmth. Experience it. Relax."

STEP SEVEN:
"Now move the energy from your face down the front of your body to your navel – to a point in the area of your appendix just right of your navel. Experience it. Relax."

STEP EIGHT:
"Now move the energy up the right side of your abdomen, and move it into the colon…bathing any obstruction therein in the light and healing. Experience it. Relax."

STEP NINE:
"Now move the energy from your colon on out of the rectum. Experience it. Relax."

STEP TEN:
"Now imagine the warm tingling energy flowing over your sex organs causing teasing sexual feelings. (Experience it.) Now from your sex organs move the energy straight up the front of your body– up and up until it covers your chin…now let it divide and move over each cheek just below the bottom of each eye. Experience it. Relax."

STEP ELEVEN:
"Now from your cheeks visualize the energy flowing down your cheeks over the sides of your jaws, and again descending clear down to your stomach. Bathe your stomach in the energy, aiding every digestive and assimilation process. Feel your stomach glow…filling the entire center of your Being with vitality. Experience it. Relax."

STEP TWELVE:
"Now move the energy down either side of your abdomen and on across your groin… continue on and move it on down the front of your legs letting it find its way to your feet and moving across to the second toe. Take your time. There is no hurry. Experience it fully. Experience it. Relax."

STEP THIRTEEN:
"Now let the energy leap from toe to toe until your toes are tingling with the energy. Think it and you will feel it. Finally let the energy leap to your big toe on each foot. Experience it. Relax."

STEP FOURTEEN:
"Now move the energy up the inside of your feet to your ankles, and on up the inside of each leg. Experience it. Relax."

STEP FIFTEEN:
"Now let the energy move into the inside of your thighs. Experience it. Relax."

STEP SIXTEEN:
"Now move the energy again across your groin and then divide it so it passes up each side of the center of your body moving on up to reach beneath each armpit. Experience it. Relax."

STEP SEVENTEEN:
"Now let the energy move to the area of your pancreas which is located on the left side of your abdomen just below the bottom of the ribcage. Feel this entire area become warm and filled with light. Feel a freedom from all tension in this area of your body. Experience it. Relax."

STEP EIGHTEEN:
"Now let the energy, which is your life-force, move to the center of your body on to your heart. Feel your heart become filled with the energy…healing the heart in every way and opening it up to loving emotion for everyone and everything. Let the energy bathe your heart. Experience it. Relax."

STEP NINETEEN:
"Now move the energy again back into your armpits…then move it on down the inside of each arm…and across the palms of your hands to the fingers. Feel your fingers tingle. Experience it. Relax."

STEP TWENTY:
"Now move the energy up the back of your arms…to the outside of your elbows…and again on up to the armpits and on across your shoulders. Experience it. Relax."

STEP TWENTY ONE:
"Now move the energy across your jawbone and bury it in either cheek. Now imagine the energy manifesting itself deep in the center of each ear. Experience it. Relax."

STEP TWENTY TWO:

"Now move the energy to your third eye center at a point between the eyebrows. Imagine a glowing in the center like the bursting of a star. Let the glow from that center move on to the top of your head and let your entire head become hot with force. Then see it in your mind's eye as sending the generated force as a searchlight of energy from the top of your head far out into the space of the very universe itself. Your entire head is aglow with energy. Your brain is filled with energy...the energy brings in KNOWING of truth to you, and activates your powers of intuition. Experience it. Relax."

STEP TWENTY THREE:

"Know you have benefited your body and mind in every way. You have charged yourself with vitality. YOU ARE FULL OF LIFE! Experience it. Relax."

STEP TWENTY FOUR:

"Now rest. Feel your entire body alive with vitality– aglow with energy. Breathe deeply and fully, as you relax and allow the energy of life to surge through you from head to toe.

When you feel like it, come back to the here and now ready to go on. YOU ARE IN HIGH GEAR."

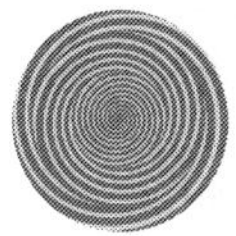

~ *Chapter 139* ~
STOCKWELL'S BIOCHEMISTRY
OF WHAT YOU FEEL

By Shelley Stockwell, PhD

What makes you think, say and do what you think, say and do? What makes you feel emotion? The following is my synthesis and speculation of conventional research in the Neur-Chemistry of Emotion.

Includes:
Cybernetic Bio-Feedback
Your Brain
Wisdom Weighs Heavy On The Mind
Your Abdominal Brain
The Mind/Body Connection
Neurons
Sensory Receptors
>**Hypnotically Soothe Your Neurons**
>**Hypnotic Spinal Tap Exercise**
>**Breathe To Relieve**

The Sex Life Of Your Cells: Chemical Messengers
Five Ligands To Know & Love
The Psychosomatic Illusion
>**Descartes Before De Hearse**
>**The New Paradigm**
>**Biology Is Big Business**
>**Pull Down Your Genes Theory**
>**Proteomics**
>**Glycomics**

Emotional Molecules: Candace Pert's High Challenge
Stockwell's Conclusions

Hypnotherapists know that your body IS your mind! Everything you create begins as a conscious or subconscious thought manifested in your neurology. Your biological self recognizes, processes, remembers, learns and creates every behavior and then decides if you will consciously notice and if it will remain unconscious.

You were born instinctively knowing how to lift your head, roll over or walk. It was hard-wired into your thoughts and neurology. So was your ability to speak. Your ear canals filled with sound amplified amniotic fluid were so finely tuned that from birth to four months you could distinguish some 150 sounds that make up human speech. These miracles came with you as pre-programmed behavioral instructions.

As you evolved and grew, you learned and honed additional behaviors that dramatically sculpted your molecules, neurons and structural development. Each biological adjustment in turn affected who you are and what you feel, think, say and do.

CYBERNETIC BIO-FEEDBACK

Emotions and body responses are the same. Jumping when startled or "chilling out" when you hear good news is an almost instantaneous response. Yogis control heart rate and blood flow with thoughts; so do you. But to do it consciously, you need to learn to control your thoughts. Hypnosis is a perfect way to do this.

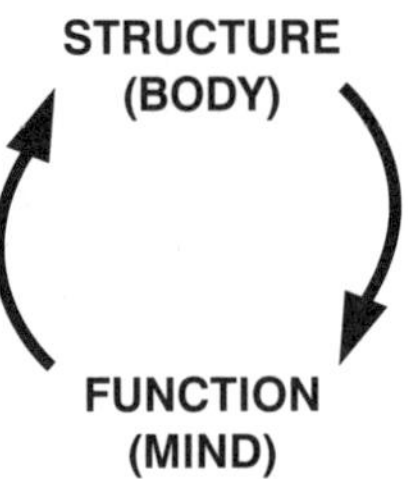

Every physical change creates an emotional change and every emotional change creates a physical change. Receptors interactively give and receive messages with other receptors.

YOUR BRAIN

"Did you ever stop to think and forget to start again?"

The awesome brain in your skull is primarily made of water, fat, carbohydrates and protein. No two brains are the same, and your brain is not the same moment to moment. Your brain hemispheres differ in size and distribution of gray and white matter, chemistry and structure.

The very structure of your brain is influenced by how you use it.

Every instant, your brain electrochemically alters neurons and their countless links. Puberty, pregnancy, aging, past events and memory may cause helpful structural brain function changes. Your internal and external environment sends a message to your cells, which then are changed according to the information received and every modification affects your emotions and physiology. A cell and its modifications influence other cells.

WISDOM WEIGHS HEAVY ON THE MIND

"The mind, once expanded by a new idea, never returns to its original size."
—Oliver Wendell Holmes

The visual cortex in the brain of someone with a photographic mind is twice the thickness of a brain without this attribute. The average brain weighs about three pounds, or 51 ounces. You can approximate the weight of your brain by multiplying your weight by .01. We lose, I've read, about 4% of brain weight per decade. However, the smarter you are, the more elaborate the network between cells and the more your brain weighs. A University of California study of 11 gifted peoples' brains, reported Albert Einstein with four times more brain cells (oligodendroglia-glial cells) than any other and structural "childlike" smoothness not usually seen in adults!

YOUR ABDOMINAL BRAIN

"Everything is of course a product of the brain…but identify the seat of emotive element as the viscera, where nervous change based on each emotional thought takes place."
—1866, Ambroise-August Liebeault, MD

"There is a brain in your bowel, however inappropriate that concept might seem to be, that ugly gut is more intellectual than the heart and may have a greater capacity for feeling."
—1998, Michael Gurshon, MD
"The Second Brain"

Have you ever wondered why you get "butterflies in your stomach" or a "sinking feeling" in your solar plexus? A latticework of receptors in your gut neurologically link, monitor, maintain and regulate every major organ, and most endocrine glands, to your mind. Perhaps we turn our back on stressful occurrence or cross our arms to protect these neural receptors and feel less vulnerable.

THE MIND/BODY CONNECTION

Ever notice how your heart beats rapidly and your breathing changes when you are excited, angry or in love? Or how your thoughts turn you on or off sexually?

A baby cries and a woman's milk starts flowing.

Emotions effect your blood pressure, heart, lungs, liver and digestion.

Emotion is "e-motion" or "energy in motion." Each conscious or subconscious emotion results from an intricate biochemical action inside yourself that then inspires the next thing you feel. What you think emanates from inside your bio-computer. So does what you choose to do. Your biology determines what you do and how you feel and what you do and how you feel influences your biology.

What you see, hear, smell, taste, feel and intuit is received within a millisecond and placed into your memory. This, in turn, along with past imprints affects your decisions, feelings and imagination and colors what next you see, hear, smell, taste, feel and intuit.

"The first symptoms of poor blood circulation" says Dr. H.A. Parkyn "appear in your head as poor memory, the inability to concentrate, sleeplessness, nervousness, headaches and then reduced circulation."

Physical environment can affect your energy. Breathing stale air in a poorly ventilated room can make you mentally sluggish.

The color and your expectation of food determines your perception of its taste, smell and how well you digest it. My grandfather was repulsed by his favorite strawberry jam when we colored it green with food coloring. A 1970's experiment gave people blue colored steak and green french fries that looked normal under colored lights. The lighting went to normal and some people actually got sick!

Depression makes you feel physically rotten, super sensitive, or numb and happiness makes you free, easy and more vital. Depression over time can cause illness and chronic illness can cause depression. Arthritis-like symptoms, digestive problems, (gastric ulcers, irritable bowel syndrome, colitis, constipation, diarrhea, sinus problems) headaches (migraines) difficult breathing (upper respiratory infections, asthma), heart palpitations, dizziness, arthritis, fibromyalgia, shingles and chronic fatigue result from, contribute to and activate depressing changes in chemistry.

NEURONS (also called brain cells or nerve cells)

The number of possible nerve cell interactions exceeds the number of particles of matter in the universe!"

—Richard M. Restak, Neurologist

Neurons are the basic unit of your nervous system and transmit billions of messages per second. These messages allow you to collect, integrate, send and store data and enhance or inhibit thoughts, feelings, behavior and bodily function. Neurons communicate electrically and chemically and constantly change and modify themselves. Neuro-peptide receptors (of your nucleus-of-barrington) process, filter, switch and modify sensory input (in-formation)

Dark in color, neurons cluster and appear gray. That's where we get the notion of *gray matter.*

To date, science has counted more than one hundred billion neurons. The quantity is so vast that new numbers bigger than a zillion like petabytes, exabytes, yottabytes and zenabytes have been invented. To get idea of how vast these numbers are; an exabytes would be all the words ever uttered by everyone who ever lived!

You were born with twice as many neurons than you had at age three. With maturity, neuron loss is more gradual and as an adult, you have about fifty thousand, to one hundred thousand (50,000 to 100,000) less then when you arrived. MSG, drugs or alcohol, can cause you to lose more than that. But don't despair, your brain likes to "clone around" and throughout your life it can generate new brain cells and bio-chemicals.

A neuron is composed of a central cell body with branches, called dendrites. Dendrites receive information aided by receptor "ligands" that determine and fingerprint your behavior, activity, mood, and emotion.

Neurons also have long tendrils, called axons. Axons are thought to communicate by electrically pulsing and releasing small packets of chemicals throughout the body. These chemicals are called "information substances" or "IS." From the time you initially formed, your brain produced these chemical-bioelectrical impulses as communication links from one neuron to another.

Synapses are a sort of telephone line that communicates and stores information. If a synapse is destroyed, usually the information it stored slips your mind. In-formation that neurons send and receive travel long distances and form complex networks. Networks of brain cells and synapses are called a neural web.

A single neuron can receive more than fifteen thousand connections from other cells. Over 100 trillion neural connections have been counted; more than the number of galaxies in the known universe. As you age and neuron numbers dwindle, remaining neurons send out more dendrites, axons and bio chemical messengers. As you get older, it's good to have connections.

SENSORY RECEPTORS

Someone gives you a pat on the back and you feel a rush of pride and confidence. You feel timid about speaking in front of an audience and you break out in a cold sweat. Someone attractive comes into the room and you flush as excitement surges through you. How in the world do these things happen?

Your sensory receptors take and give "in-formation" to determine how you feel, act and react. And how you feel act and react determines the structure and function of your sensory receptors. How your sensory receptors take and give "in-formation" also determines what remains unconscious, and what is moved to conscious priority.

Why do you get a chill up your spine when you are surprised, startled or thrilled? Your spinal cord is loaded with receptors and millions (or perhaps billions) of neuropeptides in the rows of nerve ganglia. They instantly receive and return your brain messages.

These amazing sensory receptors aren't only in your brain; your whole body receives information via the ends of your organs (where you see, hear, taste, smell and touch) and your abdomen, which sports the highest concentration of receptors.

MODUS OPERANDI: HYPNOTICALLY SOOTHE YOUR NEURONS

You know how important touch is. Without it a baby dies. Your skin is highly concentrated with receptors. Touch and acupuncture activates your touch receptors. So do verbal suggestions like, **"Focus your attention on your stomach and soothe that place with a pleasant glow of relaxation."**

Or

"Imagine someone gently tickling and stroking your skin moving gently up your arms and face and over your entire body."

MODUS OPERANDI: HYPNOTIC SPINAL TAP EXERCISE

Have someone stand up and gently tap the bones of the spine, up and down and down and up.

"Stand up, close your eyes and imagine that you or someone else is gently tapping your spine up and down and down and up. Notice what that is like for you." (Pause to give time to process this thought)

"You have used the power of suggestion to activate the receptors and ligands that make you healthy, happy and full of pep. This powerful mind/body suggestion changes you emotionally, can stop discomfort and heal ailments. Activate a receptive nodal point and your body's intricate neural network influences all parts of self.

Now, for fun, have someone gently tap the bones of your spine, up and down and down and up and notice how quickly it affects your emotional tone. Or, just think about someone gently tapping the bones of your spine, up and down and down and up. How does that feel?"

MODUS OPERANDI: BREATHE TO RELIEVE

Biofeedback, yoga, hypnosis, holding your breath, or breathing rapidly, causes peptides to diffuse throughout your cerebrospinal fluid. Many of the peptides that disperse are endorphins—natural opiates that relieve pain. **"Breathe from the top of your spine down to the bottom of…hold it…and let it out…good. Now breathe from the bottom of your feet to the top of your head…hold it and let it out…good. Now, breathe gently up and down your spine all the way into the spinal cord and bathe it with white light."**

THE SEX LIFE OF YOUR CELLS: CHEMICAL MESSENGERS

ODE TO A TRUE LIVING LIGAND

Shape shifter, activator; you command my show
You direct the course of cells, you tell them where to go.
You can cause a merger or split up any cell.
You control my channels when I'm not feeling well.
You can tell a phosphate to show up or take a hike.
You can keep me humming or destroy me if you like.
You reinvent each molecule, fiber and tissue
commanding vitally; I really want to kiss you.

Receptors on the surface of your cells act like little satellite dishes that scan and sense just as your eyes and ears do. Receptors scan or sense the right chemical messenger (neurotransmitters, hormones and tropic factors) that swim up to them. When the perfect chemical messenger "key" fits into their special keyhole, they bind. This binding adds energy to the receptor molecule causing it to fidget, wriggle, wiggle, shimmy, bend and purr as it dances and modifies back and forth between two or three favorite shapes or arrangements.

This chemical key that turns on your receptors is called the *ligand*. The word comes from the Latin *ligare* meaning, "that which binds." Ligands are molecules on the surface of a protein that enter and tickle the molecule to rearrange until, SNAP! It opens information into the cell and dramatically shape shifts changes. The entire life of your cells is determined by the receptors and ligands upon it. If a cell was a computer, the receptor would be the keyboard and the ligand would be the fingers that get things going.

What's a Ligand to Do?
A ligand directs your cells to:
1. Manufacture a new protein
2. Divide
3. Open or close channels to itself or another cell
4. Add or subtract chemical groups like phosphates.

Ligand messenger molecules come in five chemical groups:
1. Peptides, Neuropeptides, Polypeptides, Proteins
2. Small-Molecular Chemical Neurotransmitters
3. Hormones and steroids
4. Factors

Ligand 1. Peptides, Neuropeptides, Polypeptides and Proteins
"Peptides are the sheet music containing the notes, phrases and rhythms that allow your orchestra (the body) to play like an integrated entity the music that results in the tone or feeling that you subjectively experience as emotions."
—Candace Pert, Neuropharmacologist

Biofeedback, yoga and hypnosis, breathing rapidly or holding your breath cause your brain's naturally occurring painkilling peptide opiate endorphins to disperse throughout your cerebrospinal fluid.

Peptides
Peptides act upon brain receptors to pep you up and represent 95% of all ligands. The Scottish research team, who isolated the ligend for opium produced within the body called it an enkaphalin (Greek for "from the head"). An American research team renamed it "endorphin." Endorphines/enkaphalins are a great example of a peptide.

Peptides like endorphins can be made in the brain or by white blood cells. Interferon is a peptide made by blood that releases mood altering endorphins as well as ACTH, a stress hormone once thought only to be made by the pituitary gland.

Nueropeptides
Nueropeptides can alter blood flow from one part of the body to another.

Polypeptides
Polypeptides are larger (usually comprised of 200 or more amino acids) yet still smaller than proteins. They protect your nerve endings with swelling if you are injured. That is why a hypnotic suggestion, **"Let your body's chemical messengers, your polypeptides, subside so that the tissue remains in its normal state as you heal"** is very effective.

Proteins

A cell's behavior; respiration, digestion, excretion and movement are coordinated by proteins. Like an orchestra proteins play your song of life.

Angiotensin, both a hormone and peptide, mediates thirst. Even if you are well-watered, apply a drop of it to the receptors of your lungs or kidney and within ten seconds you'll crave water and your whole system will work together to conserve water. Immediately, your lungs exhale less water vapor and your kidneys hold back urine.

Ligand 2. Neurotransmitters

These small units generally carry information across the synapses or gaps between neurons. Neurotransmitters are simple amino acids, acetylcholine, nerepinephrine, dopamine, histamine, glycine, GABA, and seratonin.

Ligand 3. Steroids

Steroids start out as cholesterol and transform into the sex hormones testosterone, progesterone and estrogen, and steroid hormones like cortisol, which is secreted by the outer layer of the adrenal glands when you are under stress. One of the reasons we find high sugar/fat foods comforting according to a study published in the September 30, 2003 issue of the *Los Angeles Times* is that they are part of "a complex feedback system that turns off the release of stress hormones like cortisol."

Ligand 4. Factors

Science is still deciding how these factor in.

THE PSYCHOSOMATIC ILLUSION

"What's love got to do with it?"

Ancient people honored the mind/body/environment connection. Chinese medical and indigenous traditions still correlate organs and illness with specific mental/emotional states. The idea is to return one to holistic balance.

Western medical doctors too often ask about symptoms and then prescribe drugs. They often assume that mind influencing body is *"unscientific"* or *"psychosomatic."* Psyche means the mind or soul, and soma, means body. "The brain and body are separate entities" is a most prevalent and, in my opinion, peculiar paradigm.

How did this happen?

Go back to 17th century, Frenchman, philosopher and highly touted "father of modern medicine", Rene Descartes. He's the fellow who wrote: *'I think therefore I am.'* Descartes wanted to dissect dead human bodies. To get the powerful Pope to agree, he made this deal: "Anything to do with the soul, mind or emotions, I leave to the clergy. I will only claim the realm of the body."

Because of this, the medical Cartesian Construct regarded the body as physical matter, and the mind (or spirit) as immaterial...two distinct, separate and unrelated substances. "Your body is a mechanical, reactive machine; a predictable mass of matter and energy. Thoughts and behavior are just hardwired reflexes caused by electrical stimulation across synapses," "pathogens cause disease," and "either your illness can be physically determined or it's all in your head" said that antiquated paradigm. To understand a human all you had to do is take one apart and study its physical components.

DESCARTES BEFORE DE HEARSE
"I think, therefore I am" came first
before you changed it to something worse.
So tell me why you said, Descartes,
"Forget the head, forget the heart."
Was it the Pope that caused the issue?
saying "keep mind separate from physical tissue?"
And you replied, "Cognito ergo sum:"
"Without a thought, life begins and is done."
Mind as church and body state
is a myth-illogical church mandate
that keeps us like powerless segmented worms
drug invested with poor returns
and views my body as just a machine
without mind or spirit on my wellness team.
Pharmaceuticals abound and medicine kills
when you seek outside cures to heal your ills

So goodbye Descartes, hello awareness
I embrace good thoughts and won't be careless.
If since your "I think, therefore I am" rings true
Descartes you never existed unless I think of you.
                    —Shelley Stockwell

In the 17th century, the "father of modern science," Sir Isaac Newton, said the universe too is a "matter" machine. His "Newtonian construct" said matter is real and all that really mattered.

The New Western Medicine

In the 1920's Dr. Walter Cannon, a physiology professor at Harvard University, coined the phrase "homeostasis" from the Greek word "homoios" meaning "similar" and "stasis" meaning "position." His studies revealed a relationship between emotions and perceptions and the physical fight, flight, fright response. A new paradigm was emerging: the brain is hooked up to the body and the body is hooked up to the brain! About the same time, Hans Selye noted that animals under stress had weakened immune responses. These ideas led to the modern science we call psycho-neuro immunology, which studies the inter-relationship of mind, and body wellness.

Biology Is Big Business

Pharmaceutical manufacturers, with their well-controlled medical industry, happily keep the old "body-machine" attitude. "If you hurt, take this pill then come back next month so we can sell you the perfect drug or implant the perfectly engineered mechanical part or gene and make you as good as new" is their message.

Genes separated from a living organism can be legally patented by the US Patent Office. Of the thirty-to-forty thousand genes isolated by the multi-billion-dollar congress funded genome projects, twenty thousand genes (and related molecules) are now patented. The idea is that if you own the gene and drugs that influence that gene, you can introduce it into the body to generate the right instructions to the protein receptors. What if the underlying belief that disease is caused on the cell level is untrue?

Pull Down Your Genes Theory

"When a gene product is needed, a signal from its environment, not an emergent property of the gene itself, activates expression of that gene."
　　　　—H.F. Nijhout, BioEssayist

Your brain is the control center for your body, right?

So what happens if we remove your brain from your body?

You'd die of course.

Genetic theory implies that DNA and genes in the cell nucleus, is the control central of your emotion/thought. So what happens if we remove the nucleus (de-nucleate) the DNA and genes from a cell?

No, it doesn't die…it lives.

How can that be?

Genes are *not* the master controller of your cell!

Scientist, Bruce Lipton, says that if you remove receptors from your cell, the cell *dies*. Are receptors the control center of your mind/body; not genes? And where do the receptors get their information? They get their information from the environment (your interior environment and the environment of the everything else in the universe.) And armed with these environmental signals, the receptors regulatory proteins control the expression of the genes. All genes are controlled by signals from the environment via receptors. Receptors alter genes, not the other way around. It is the proteins receptors that turn genes on and off. Cancer may correlate to a specific gene but a specific gene does not cause it. So much for the genetic determination theory.

Proteomics

A cell is only alive because protein pathways regulate and integrate its function. Proteins structure, move and coordinate all cell behavior; respiration, digestion, excretion and movement. They control the firing of neurotransmitters that allow you to think, your muscles to move, they switch your genes on and off and bind your DNA.

Marc Wilkins of Australia coined the word "proteome" at a scientific conference in Italy in 1994 to describe "all proteins expressed by genome, cell or tissue." Proteins are composed of some 20 different amino acids (as apposed to just 4 building blocks of the DNA of your genes). And we are clueless as to their astronomical numbers. At this time, there is no simple way to identify, or characterize them. The "proteome project" is now attempting this feat. Between June of 2000 to October of 2001 more than $700 million poured into "proteomics" companies from venture capitalists and IPO's.

Proteins generally look like a "pop-it" bead necklace. Each bead contains twenty different amino acids in specific sequences. These beads, along with electromagnetic charges, determine its shape. The charged molecules resemble magnets! Mesmer was right! We do have a natural "animal magnetism." Dr Mark George, Neurologist at London Hospital confirms that magnets applied at first about two inches above the left ear (making the thumb jerk) and, then moved forward three inches of so along the skull to the frontal cortex, helps depressed folks sleep better, cry less and eat more.

Thousands of times a second, charged proteins bind to molecules and other proteins and alter their electrical charge distribution as their bead-like "backbones" adapt with specific movement. When the bind is severed, a protein usually re-expresses itself back to its original shape and configuration.

Glycomics

In October of 2001, the U.S. National Institute of Health (NIH) awarded a five-year, $34-million "glue" grant to a 54-member Consortium for Functional Glycomics to identify carbohydrates (simple and complex sugars) that are known to combine with proteins and fats on cell surfaces and "influence" cell-to-cell communication. Next to bring in the big bucks bid will most likely be a study to categorize fats (lipids).

EMOTIONAL MOLECULES: CANDACE PERT'S HIGH CHALLENGE

In the 1970's, neuro-biology student, Candace Pert was laid up in a hospital bed enjoying regular shots of Talwin (a morphine derivative). She so liked the opiate's "wonderful feeling of being deeply nourished and satisfied" she considered taking the drug with her when she was discharged from the hospital. Though she resisted that urge, her intense, physical and emotional experience fascinated her. She wasn't alone in her intrigue. Hippies and scientists wanted to know why heroin, marijuana, Librium and PCP (angel dust) elicited such radical emotional changes.

Candace wanted to identify the biochemical ligand behind her feel good reaction to drugs. A ligand she surmised, only binds with a receptor that is perfect for it. This is called receptor *specificity.* A Valium receptor ligand would then only attach to a Valium or Valium-like peptide. An opiate receptor ligand, would then only attach to the perfect opiate group, like endorphins, morphine or heroine. The thesis; opium excites a specific ligand that binds to a receptor and changes the neuron.

She knew that when opium enters the body, it generates a ligand that binds to a receptor for only a brief time before it exits as urine. How could Candace identify such a small unit that comes and goes so quickly? British scientist, W.D.M. Patton's "ping-pong" theory gave her the solution. His approach explained how two similar drugs bind with the same receptor: one drug, the agonist, enters the receptor and creates cell changes, while the other drug, the antagonist, blocks the receptor by occupying it. The magnitude of a drug reaction is proportional to how many times a drug hits (or pings) the receptor, and therefore remains on the receptor.

This idea gave her more time to observe the process. She knew that a few injected milligrams of the drug Naloxone reversed heroin overdose effects, so she used Naloxone, (labeled with a radioactive isotope) to act as the antagonist to bump up the heroin from the receptor. And on October 25, 1972, the brilliant Candace Pert measured a cell's opiate receptor ligand, in a test tube! This put opium receptors into the realm of science for the first time. Her book, *Molecules of Emotions,* tells of Pert's personal challenges in trapping the morphine molecule on its receptor.

It is now known that you don't have to take a drug to get high. Your brain naturally manufactures its own endogenous, (from within) morphine. How and why we do this goes back to how we receive and interpret energetic input from the inside and from the vast universe.

STOCKWELL'S CONCLUSIONS
What we know so far about the biochemistry of what you think, say, and do.

1. **Everything you create begins as a conscious or subconscious thought manifested in your neurology.**

2. **Physical and emotional change is inseparable and interactive. There is a direct relationship between emotional states and the physical body. A physical change creates an emotional change and an emotional change creates a physical change.**

3. **Neurons and their receptors create billions of messages per second that allow you to collect, integrate, send and store data and enhance or inhibit thoughts, feelings, behavior and bodily function.**

4. **Environment and your reaction to it (without mastering your consciousness), creates your biological actions and reactions.**

5. **Survival requires effective and accurate receiving and interpreting of environmental signals.**

6. **How your receptors take and give "in-formation" determines what remains unconscious, and what is moved to conscious priority.**

7. **Hypnosis taps the holistic nature self and the integration of though, intention, biochemistry and common sense.**

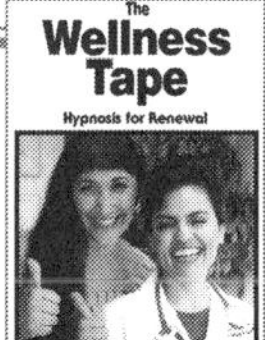

Hypno-Helper
"The Wellness Tape" by Shelley Stockwell-Nicholas, PhD, and Dr. Lilia Prado, D.O.
"Magnetic Mind Toning" by Ormond McGill, PhD teaches you to control conscious awareness and are both audio tapes are available at the back of this book.

The awesome power of hypnosis helps people of all ages:

Feel Well
Address Individual Needs
Promote Healthy Thought & Action
Accelerate Healing & Recovery
Program A Positive Outcome
Relieve Temporary, Chronic & Phantom Limb Pain
Calm Fears
De-Stress & Relax
Build Confidence
Sleep Soundly
Lose Weight
Encourage An Appetite
Quit Harmful Habits
Improve Memory & Concentration
Boost Self-Esteem & Self-Image
Strengthen The Immune Response
Birth Babies Without Pain
Better Treatment Results
Get The Most From Medical Procedures
Communicate Better With The Doctor
Minimize Drugs
Reduce Bleeding
Balance Body During & After Surgery & Tests
Keep Vital Signs Steady In ER & ICU
Reduce Nausea & Side Effects Of Chemotherapy
Druglessly Anesthetize
Rapid Rehabilitation
Be In The Driver's Seat Of Yourself

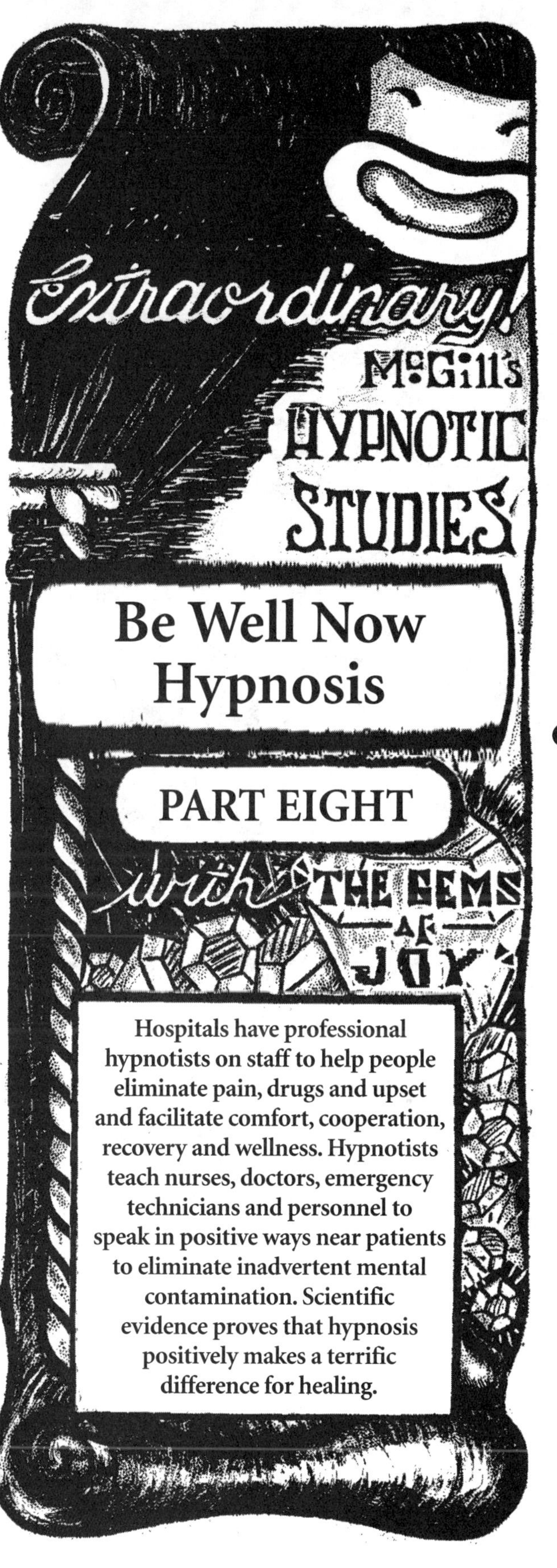

Hospitals have professional hypnotists on staff to help people eliminate pain, drugs and upset and facilitate comfort, cooperation, recovery and wellness. Hypnotists teach nurses, doctors, emergency technicians and personnel to speak in positive ways near patients to eliminate inadvertent mental contamination. Scientific evidence proves that hypnosis positively makes a terrific difference for healing.

CHAPTERS IN PART EIGHT

140. Mental Anesthesia: Esdaile And Munro ....page 531
141. Suggestive Therapeutics 533
142. Suggestive Therapeutics For Habits....537
143. Waking Anesthesia 539
144. Mulder's Glove Anesthesia 543
145. Stockwell's Hypno-Anesthesia 545
146. Stockwell's Pain Management..............551
147. Good Bye Headache 559

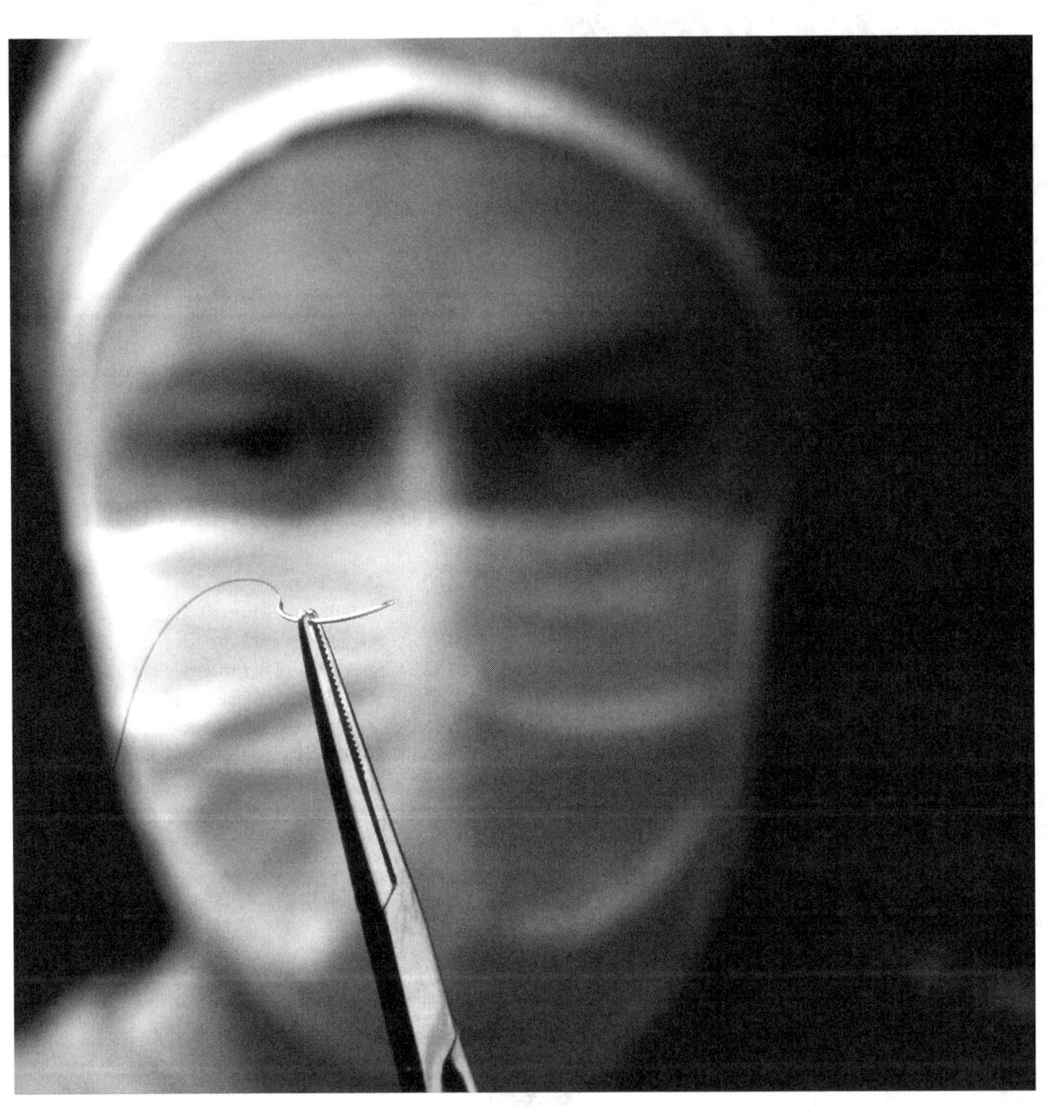

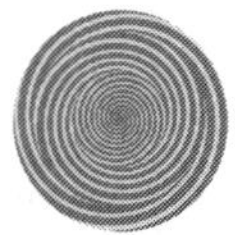

~ *Chapter 140* ~
MENTAL ANESTHESIA:
ESDAILE & MUNRO

Includes
James Esdaile
Henry Munro

Mesmerists proved that a person was hypnotized by showing a subject impervious to pain. Abby de Farria, a Portuguese priest, in pain control demonstrations, stood in flowing colorful robes, looking deeply into a person's eyes, yelling, "Sleep." Like magic, any pain was gone.

Modern tent revivalists and faith healers use this same approach to hypnosis. Expectation and the induction techniques of loss of equilibrium combined with a startling tap or push on the forehead causes the subject to "swoon" into the loving arms of helpers. When the person is back on their feet, they experience miracles from the "holy spirit." Their pain is gone!

Two great doctors advanced a more clinical approach to hypnotherapy and pain management.

JAMES ESDAILE

Drugs of many kinds, from opium poppies to snakeroot, found anesthetic employment. But while chemical anesthesia is of great importance in the history of healing, it lacks many of the advantages of hypnotic or mental anesthesia.

The first in modern times to rediscover the power of mental anesthesia to remove pain was an English surgeon by the name of James Esdaile. He became interested in mesmerism before the word hypnotism was even known. Esdaile went to India in 1845 and combined the techniques of Mesmer with his surgical practice. As was customary in this early period, approximately an hour and a half was required to induce the state. It was a slow process.

These were the days before chemical anesthetics had been discovered, and something was desperately needed to subdue pain. Esdaile had the inspiration to try eliminating pain during his surgeries, and told his patients that he could do so using mesmerism. It worked. Patients were desperate for this mental anesthesia. Esdaile, himself, was amazed. India was elated. It is reported that Dr. Esdaile performed major surgical operations of all kinds using the mental process of the patient as the only pain remover. His reputation for "pain-free surgery" spread like wildfire throughout the country.

Belief! Inadvertently the power of suggestion had set in, and even the doctor did not know why. He just knew it worked and he was scientist enough to allow results to speak for themselves. At the time, mortality in surgery, in Esdaile's day, was fifty percent. Using his technique, the surgeon was able to reduce this mortality rate to eight percent, and his patients recovered more rapidly.

Esdaile returned to England elated with his discovery. Unfortunately, it was at the very time when the chemical forms of anesthetics, ether and chloroform, had been discovered. These drugs were easy to use and unfortunately frequently fatal. Drug use swept the medical profession and Esdaile's discovery that mind alone could do the same thing and better went unheeded. Had this not been so, mental medicine might have taken a quantum leap.

HENRY MUNRO

By the 1900's one in four hundred patients died on the operating table as a result of the anesthesia not the surgery. Ether was most commonly used. Facing a surgical operation is always a cause for anxiety. Possibly more so in those early times, but most assuredly the fear is still there today.

Dr. Henry Munro, M.D. had devoted his work to medical hypnosis. He lived and practiced in Omaha, Nebraska. He called hypnosis, "Suggestive Therapeutics" and used it to alleviate fear. It proved a master method, and it remarkably reduced fatalities as well.

Prior to an operation, he used hypnosis to give affirmative suggestions that the patient would come through the operation successfully. Dr. Munro found that only about ten percent of the usually required amount of ether was necessary to obtain perfect pain free surgical anesthesia. Dr. Munro noted that all his patients using the combination of hypnosis with chemical anesthesia did not experience the excitement state of ether and recovered more quickly. The postoperative recovery was almost miraculous.

A series of lectures took Munro to Rochester, Minnesota. Among the doctors attending were the Mayo brothers who were working at St. Mary's Hospital. This was prior to starting their own clinic. The Mayo's decided to test Munro's process. Thus began deep abdominal surgery Case Number One and the prelude of some seventeen thousand cases that followed; each without a single death occurring. With Dr. Munro's hypnotic method, there was no longer a danger of a patient dying from anesthesia.

The eyes of the world focused upon the Mayo Brothers, and their Mayo Clinic became legendary. They became known as the only "safe" hospital where one had an excellent chance of surviving. Strangely, the Mayo Brothers never said that they used hypnosis, even though an article on this was written about it in the May 1906 Obstetrical Journal. That Journal was not widely circulated so the story remained obscure.

Old ideas are tenacious and new ideas take time to blossom. Though Dr. Munro's discovery saved many lives humanity was timid about receiving his "breakthrough" wisdom.

Munro's process was simple. He merely hypnotized the patient prior to the operation and suggested: **"We are in the operating room and you are going in for surgery. It will be very easy for you, and you will recover fine."** The power of the mind is wonderful and its full potential for miraculous healing has but barely been scratched (and healed).

Fortunately, both doctors left a legacy of this pioneer work in hypnotherapy in detailed texts. Esdaile's "Mesmerism in India" was originally published at the close of the 19th Century. Munro's "Suggestive Therapeutics" was published early in the 20th Century. Both books were way ahead of their time. They have been long out-of-print, and are now valuable collector's items.

The pioneer work of James Esdaile and Henry Munro became a searchlight of truth for the innovative work of Dave Elman who carried the torch of hypnotherapy onward. It flooded his work. Go you, and do likewise.

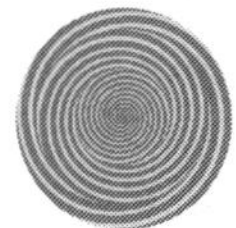

~ *Chapter 141* ~
SUGGESTIVE THERAPEUTICS

Suggestive Therapeutics = Hypnotherapy for Dealing with Physical Health Problems

Includes
For General Disability
For Arthritis
Neuralgia
Earache
Heart Conditions

Four major objectives are effectively obtained when using Suggestive Therapeutic Hypnosis:
1. Perfect patient cooperation during surgery
2. Removal of pain during procedures frequently causes the body to provide its own pain control and lessens the amount of required anesthesia.
3. Bleeding is controlled
4. The patient recovers rapidly

Be bold in your use of hypnosis to help heal the body. Have no fear of going where others have seldom gone. Results can be astonishing. Expect miracles of healing and miracles occur. Moving on to Suggestive Therapeutics you will be moving into the realm of the physician to help heal physical ailments. You can erase the pain, but always remember that pain is nature's warning system that says something is wrong which is in need of healing. Such work is best done in cooperation and with the recommendation of the physician. This cooperation is much needed in this the 21st century. Respect the trust from the physician as you enter their domain as a healer and aid. Suggestive Therapeutics has been reported by medical authority to assist:

Appetite	Dyspareunia	Hoarseness	Pains	Tics
Arthritis	Eczema	Hysteria	Palpitations	Tumors
Asthma	Ears	Impotence	Paralysis	Twitches
Allergies	Enuresis	Indigestion	Perspiration	Ulcers
Colds	Epilepsy	Itches	Psoriasis	Urination
Cold Hands	Erotomania	Labor Pains	Rheumatism	Uticaria
Cold Feet	Eye Strain	Lumbago	Sciatica	Voice
Colitis	Fears	Manias	Sex Problems	Vomiting
Constipation	Frigidity	MS	Snoring	Varicose Veins
Diabetes	Gall Bladder	Neuralgia	Stammering	Warts
Digestion	Glands	Nervous Stomach	Stomach	
Diarrhea	Hallucinations	Nose	Stuttering	
Dysmenorrhea	Headaches	Obesity	Throat	

Since you may have little opportunity to work with the client/patient, induce as profound hypnosis as possible and be willing to work with whatever depth of hypnosis is achieved. Suggestions given should be straight from the shoulder, right on target and pull no punches. Do not hold back. State exactly what you want to occur. Expect the cure to be effective. So be it!

Tell the subconscious exactly what you want the client/patient to do to be healed. Then get a subjective affirmation that the hypnotic suggestions have been accepted and that healing will be the case.

Before inducing trance, find out the exact nature of the trouble the client is facing and the places where pain exists. Have them describe the symptoms several times so as to learn them by heart. Then centralize your suggestions on those pain canters. Repeat suggestions eight to ten times. The repetition of suggestions has a compounding effect. Present the suggestions in an earnest and convincing manner. Hold thoughts of the expected healing as you verbalize the suggestions. Put your heart and soul into your work.

In treating all body pains stroke over the seat of the pain while sending healing energies into the affected part and suggest: **"Going, going, GONE!"** This is remarkably powerful as the words are triggers to action that direct the subconscious.

When dealing with body functions that are naturally continual, day after day, like bowel movements, heart action, breathing, suggest that the operation functions perfectly in a regular fashion. There is no need to be specific as the subconscious is the automatic regulator of such functions.

All "dis-ease" causes stress and stress makes it more difficult to handle a situation. Suggestive therapeutics controls stress, whenever un-wellness is present. No matter what the disease it can be strengthened or weakened by the action of the subconscious mind. It is simply impossible for anyone to take a neutral position. Either we aid the disease to harm us by allowing the inner mind to destructively dwell on it, or we oppose it and help the subconscious destroy it by the use of healthful selective directed suggestions for good health.

A study of hypnosis to help patients at the Syracuse Medical Pediatric/Pulmonary Center, with children ages 6–18, reported the following results. The presenting ailments were pulmonary, gastro-intestinal, psychological, iatrogenic (embracing medical help) and personal requests for school and sports performance:

81% of patents who used hypnosis improved psychologically

80% had marked physical improvement

None had worsening of symptoms.

MODUS OPERANDI: FOR GENERAL DISABILITY

Have the client lie down and induce hypnosis. Then suggest:

"________________ (Client's name) **When I awaken you today you will feel very much improved. You will feel stronger. Your appetite will be healthy and you will enjoy three good square healthy meals a day. Your bowels will mover regularly every day. Your strength will increase every hour. You are becoming stronger and better in every way. In fact, when you arouse from hypnosis now your will feel wonderful and fine."**

MODUS OPERANDI: FOR ARTHRITIS

Hypnotize your client and directly suggest

"_______________ (Client's name) **When I arouse you from hypnosis, you will find that the pain in your arms** (or whatever part of the body is ailing) **has entirely disappeared. You will not be troubled with arthritis any longer. The blood flow in your arms will be strong. The circulation is becoming perfect. It will cause the arthritis to disappear. All pain is GONE! From now on, you can use your arms perfectly; free from pain. When you complete this session with me you will never be bothered with arthritis again.**

Subconscious mind if these suggestions are agreeable and are accepted, nod your head. Understand."

Wait for the subconscious nodding of the head. It indicates an affirmation that all will be dealt with. Wait for the affirmation. If there is any resistance, be insistent. Then wait again for the affirmation.

Continue…

"**Go deeper into hypnosis now and allow these healing suggestions to become your reality. Your ARTHRITIS IS NO MORE. When you know that the healing is underway, arouse yourself from the hypnosis. Take your time; there is no hurry. When the healing is underway, come back and join me in the here and now feeling much, much better in every way."**

MODUS OPERANDI: FOR NEURALGIA

Hypnotize your client Induce as deep a trance as possible and then stroke your hand over the affected area while giving these suggestions.:

"**You are relaxing more and more…so just go ahead and drop down into the realm of sleep. When you arouse from the hypnosis your neuralgia will be gone. Every trace of neuralgic pain is no more. It is GONE! Gone! Gone! In every way you are well and fine."**

Then arouse them slowly. So simple, it's almost hard to believe. Just a few words given in the hypnotic state and pain is gone. Simple? Not really. The subconscious phase of mind is beyond doubt one of the most remarkable mechanisms we possess.

MODUS OPERANDI: FOR EARACHE

Hypnotize your client. Induce as deep a trance as possible and then place your hand over the aching ear while giving these suggestions.:

"**This ache in your ear is vanishing. When you arouse from hypnosis your earache will be GONE! You will feel fine."**

Then arouse them slowly. So simple, it's almost hard to believe. Just a few words given in the hypnotic state and pain is gone. Simple? Not really. The subconscious phase of mind is beyond doubt one of the most remarkable mechanisms we possess.

MODUS OPERANDI: FOR A TOOTHACHE

Hypnotize your client. Induce as deep a trance as possible and then place your hand over the client/patient's jaw and suggest:

"**The pain is GONE! You feel well and fine."**

Then arouse them slowly.

MODUS OPERANDI: FOR TREATING HEART CONDITIONS

Use a gentle progressive relaxation method for hypnotizing someone with a heart condition. A mesmeric approach is also effective. In every way make your client calm and serene. Work slowly. Take your time in hypnotizing. Place your hand over their heart when repeating these suggestions eight to ten times and then suggest:

"You are becoming calm and relaxed all over. Your heartbeat is perfectly normal, as is your blood pressure. Your heart functions perfectly. Every time I treat you, you will steadily get better and better. You improve every day. You are well and fine. When you arouse from hypnosis your heart will be benefited in every way."

Arouse the client slowly and gently. In treating heart conditions avoid any shock techniques.

MODUS OPERANDI: FOR CONSTIPATION

Functions such as bowel movements respond well to a subconscious setting of a schedule for operation.

It is a medical fact that constipation may be a base trouble for many illnesses. Special attention should be given to its treatment. In the consultation, find out as much detail as you can from the person. Hypnotize your client and always speak plainly so they will know precisely what is meant. Directly suggest:

"_______________ (Client's name)**you will from now on every morning go to the bathroom at the same time and have a movement. You will also drink a glass of water before breakfast every morning. Remember this. Every morning before breakfast, you will drink a glass of water. In a few days, your bowels will be in a normal condition again. And easily throw off all poisons from your system and you will commence to feel better in every way."**

Repeat these suggestions for ten minutes before arousing the client/patient.

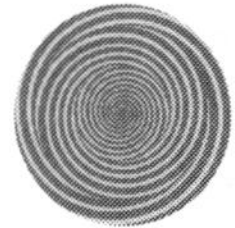

~ *Chapter 142* ~
SUGGESTIVE THERAPEUTICS
FOR MASTERING UNWANTED HABITS

Includes
Mastering A Drinking Habit

Habits can be good or bad. We want the good ones without the bad ones. Habits are usually based on bringing pleasure to the user. Once habits become solidly established as a way of behavior, they enter the realm of the subconscious and operate beyond critical thought. Hence, since hypnosis provides a direct means of controlling the subconscious, it obviously provides an excellent means to rid someone of unwanted habits. And, since habits are plainly based on a pleasure response, all that is needed is to reverse them from pleasure to displeasure. With this understanding, here are some Suggestive Therapeutics that control habits. Suggestions relate to the particular habit. The essential thing is to repeat the anti-habit suggestions many times to counter a mental set. Mentally set non-pleasant responses to the habit.

Habits become ingrained into an individual's behavior, thus patience and not haste is the essential requirement to successfully treat an unwanted habit.

MODUS OPERANDI: MASTERING THE DRINKING HABIT

Use this method when working with any client who wants to master a drinking habit. To begin find out how much alcohol your client consumes. Then hypnotize them and suggest:

"________________ (Client's name) **From now on you only drink half of what you have been used to drinking. If you try to drink one glass more than that, it will taste like vinegar to you. You cannot drink any more than that. Every day you will care less and less for whiskey, beer, wine and liqueur of any kind. Any drink with alcohol in it is losing its appeal for you. You will learn to hate it. It will make you sick. All craving for alcoholic drinks of any kind is leaving you. You have no desire for it anymore and the habit is leaving you. You will sleep well at night and you have no desire at all for alcohol when you awaken."**

Repeat these suggestions for twenty minutes. Do not tell them to stop at once altogether. Reduce their allowance every day for three or four days and then you tell them that they positively do not care to drink any more. Then underscore how proud they are that they have kicked their old drinking habit and how happy it has made everyone that they love. Tell them what a credit they will be to their family, friends, and all those for and with whom they work. Spread a bright future before them as a non-drinker and appeal to their pride and ambition.

MODUS OPERANDI: FOR MASTERING ADDICTIVE DRUGS

Use this method when working with any client who wants to stop drugs like cocaine, heroin, etc. Deeply hypnotize them and suggest:

"________________ (Client's name) **When I awaken you from deep hypnosis, you will say NO to drugs forever. You know that drugs are dangerous for you. You will positively abhor all dangerous drugs. All cravings for them are completely gone. It is easy for you now to stop the habit of taking any kind of vicious drug and you are so glad you have.**

And understand this…there is never any need for you to take outside drugs as your body itself can manufacture whatever you need in the proper proportions for your health and well-being."

Repeat these suggestions over and over. Their attitude towards dangerous drugs will drastically alter. Sometimes habits become mastered immediately. With others, a suggestion to gradually cut down will prove most effective. Use your intuition as to how best to apply Suggestive Therapeutics to handle specific situations. The key to success is that the more pleasure for living a good life you instill the less likely your client will be to cater to their hurtful habits.

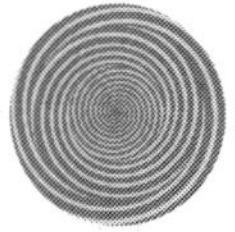

~ *Chapter 143* ~
WAKING ANESTHESIA

Includes
"New" Anesthesia
Krasner's Bogus Chemicals
Anesthetic Tapping
Wake Up Well Anesthesia
Medical Touch Anesthesia

The absence of pain is easily suggested in the waking state. Medical doctors, dentists, nurses, hypnotists and wellness practitioners use these hypnosis approaches to evoke the placebo affect. Suggest it in an even-toned, positive voice and what you say will be believed:

MODUS OPERANDI: "NEW" ANESTHESIA

Medical personnel, especially a doctor must learn to give positive suggestions using an even tone of voice and knowing that the patient will believe whatever they say:

"________________ (Client's name) **I have here a new kind of anesthesia that was just recently developed. It works very rapidly and will completely remove any discomfort from this place that will have a procedure done to it. It will make this place completely, absolutely numb."** Rub a little imaginary anesthetic on the spot that hurts or on their finger and then have them transfer it to the spot. After waiting just a few moments the job is done. The physician may proceed with the surgery. This is an excellent suggestion to give to someone afraid of being given a shot.

He can add his own suggestions by stroking a spot and saying:

"You have no feeling here at all. See even when I pinch you here you feel nothing at all."
Or
"Just turn the blood flow off. Turn it off like a faucet and stop any bleeding. Good."

MODUS OPERANDI: KRASNER'S BOGUS CHEMICALS

Dr. Al Krasner uses this wonderful waking placebo approach:

"I will drop 'sensodine 7', a standard chemical used by doctors to irritate the skin for tests here to the back of your hand. This will make your hand very sensitive to the touch…so sensitive that the slightest touch will feel painful and you will want to move your hand from me." (Put a drop of water on their hand.) **"How powerful that chemical is."**

Wait a minute and gently touch the hand and when they react say, "Now I will replace this with an amazing and even more powerful drop called 'topical anesthesia 8' used by doctors to numb an area completely. This will make your hand so completely numb that nothing bothers it in the least." (Another little drop of water) **"This completely numbs your hand now."**

MODUS OPERANDI: ANESTHETIC TAPPING

"There is a center of numbness on your body through which you can increase your comfort. It is a powerful form of hypnotherapy as it helps you master pain in the body and emotional pain and mental disturbances as well.

The center of numbness is located high on your chest on the left side, in the region of your collarbone at its termination point, where it forms a socket for the top bone of your left arm. Move down from this area slightly and you will find a little valley that you press. This is your center of numbness.

To activate it, take a deep breath, hold the breath while you tap with your fingertip three times on this valley area."

Then…

"Inhale, and as you exhale, speak forcefully out loud the word, 'Anesthetic. Anesthetic. Anesthetic.' As you say the word think 'numbness' to yourself. Perform this process twenty times in sequence and you will gain control over pain in any part of your body or mind upon which you focus your attention."

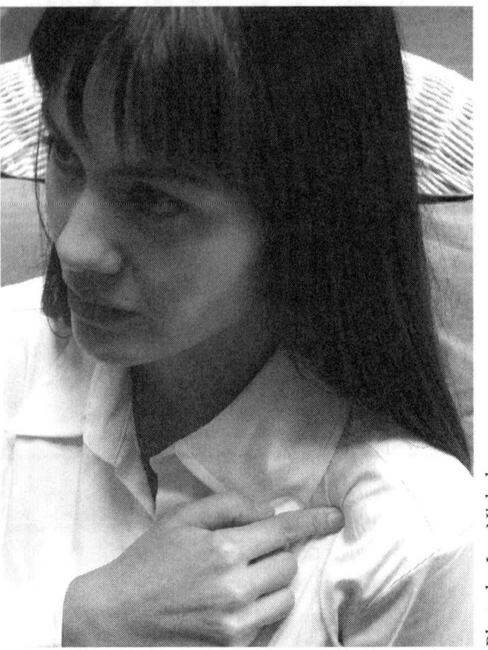

Anesthesia

MODUS OPERANDI: WAKE UP WELL ANESTHESIA

Induce a deep state of hypnosis and suggest:

"You are relaxing more and more, so just drop down into the realm of sleep. When you awaken, the pain in your _______ (name the location) will be entirely gone. You will feel well and fine. You will easily walk and move with no discomfort whatsoever. Your muscles, nerves and ligaments are comfortable and easy. You feel terrific."

You can place your hand on the place where the reported pain was (i.e. the jaw or back)

"The trouble you had here is leaving you. When you awaken you feel fine. The trouble is gone forever."

Repeat these suggestions 8-10 times before bringing them to room awareness. Repeat this session often for best results.

MODUS OPERANDI: MEDICAL TOUCH ANESTHESIA

In your pre-hypnotic talk, inspire your client to have faith and confidence in your ability to positively assist them and you have already advanced them toward a cure.

Put your subject into a deep trance and make energetic hand passes over the spot to be anesthetized. Then press your hands firmly on the spot until they complain. As soon as they do, release the pressure with your hand still resting on the spot.

"The place where I am laying my hands is becoming numb and insensitive. All sensations in this spot, even when I pinch it, feels nothing at all. It is insensitive. It is completely numb and anesthetized."

Repeat this three times and then give the skin a pinch over the spot that is being desensitized. If nothing is felt you have done the job. Avoid the word "pain" in your suggestion formula.

"You will do whatever your __________ (Medical helper i.e. surgeon, dentist, nurse doctor…) **tells you to do perfectly. It feels completely numb your teeth and gums and cheeks (or whatever) completely numb as you have a peaceful sleep and your mind drifts off while your dentist makes your mouth perfect in every way."**

You or your dentist can chime in now and again with, **"you are snoozing pleasantly and feel nothing. Your mouth remains numb until your dentist or I tell you to awaken. When you come back you will feel fine and heal immediately and recall nothing but pleasant thoughts about your experience."**

If you were to anesthetize more than the mouth you would want to suggest anesthesia separately to each part of the body rather than saying "your whole body is relaxed' which is too general.

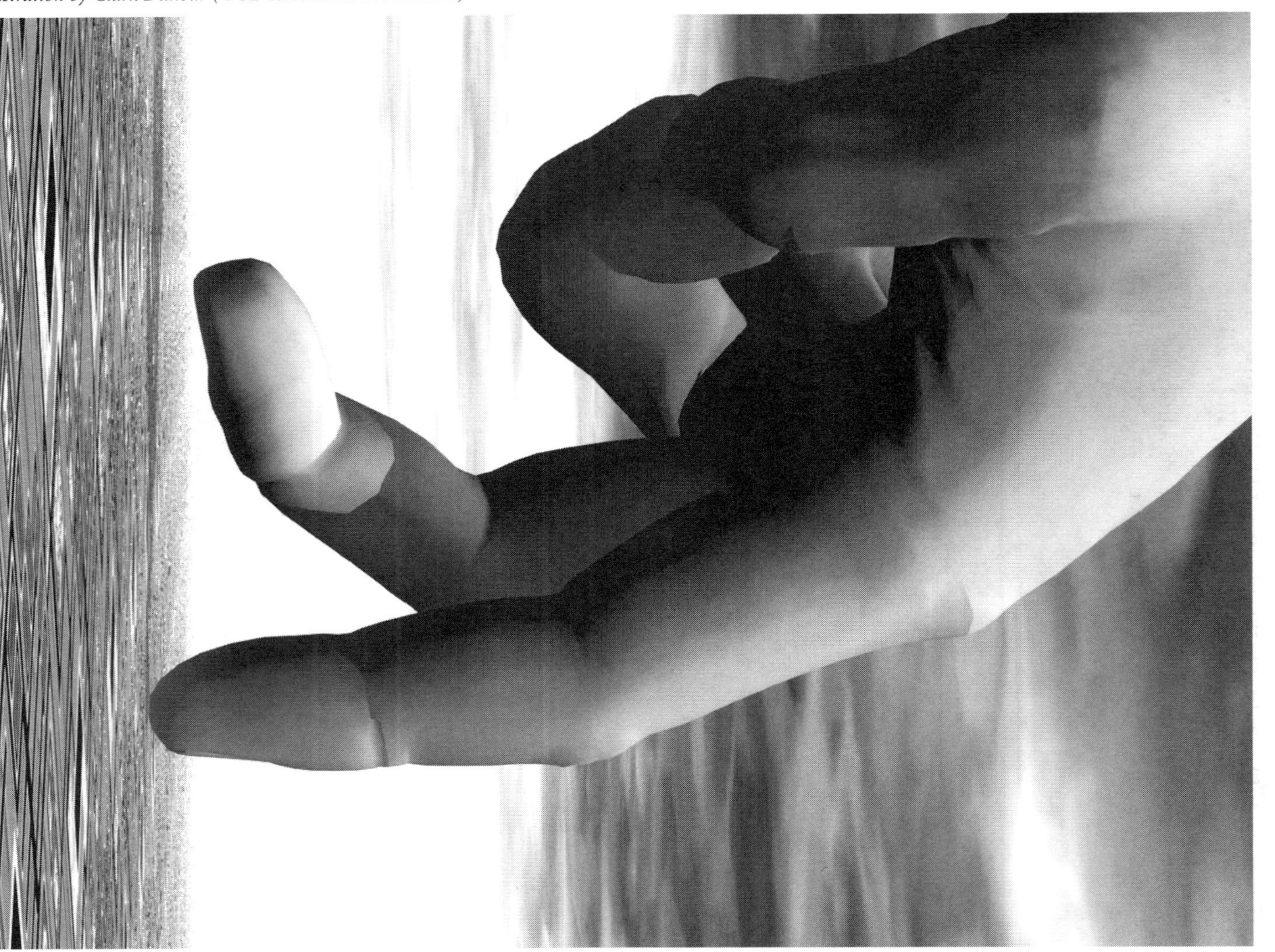

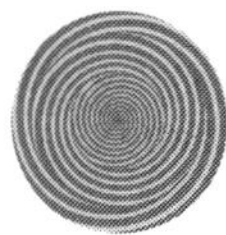

~ *Chapter 144* ~
MULDER'S GLOVE ANESTHESIA

Hypnotherapy instructor, Marleen Mulder expertly teaches glove anesthesia in this chapter. It leads to hypnotic pain control, which is an important aspect of hypnotherapy.

MODUS OPERANDI: MULDER'S GLOVE ANESTHESIA

1. Induce Trance

2. Have your client **"Focus on a pleasant scene from your life experience. Something that brings you a peaceful, happy feeling."**

3. Anchor this scene by touching the left shoulder of the client and saying **"As I touch your shoulder or arm and hand you easily think of this scene and are aware of the pleasant feelings that go with it."**

4. Establish band numbness. Tell the client, **"I am placing a band of numbness across the right shoulder by touching and tracing a band across the shoulder."** Continue giving suggestions of numbness in the right arm from the "band" on down.

5. Request an ideomotor response signal from the subconscious that the suggestion of numbness is being accepted. This can be any spontaneous indication you arrange, such as lifting a forefinger of the right hand or a nod of the head.

6. Establish a second "band of numbness" around the wrist. Continue the suggestions of numbness as you stroke hands toward the wrist. A variation of this procedure can be to suggest that the healing energy is **"spreading through the hand,"'** then place your hand on their shoulder.

7. To transport numbness to wherever the client wishes on the body, you can help by placing a "healing hand" upon the desired place and stroking that part of the body while continuing to give suggestions of numbness. Numbness is a more or less ambiguous suggestion and carries differing "feelings" to different clients. Generally speaking, it means sensation dullness.

8. Request another ideomotor signal that the **"Numbness is being accepted by the subconscious."**

9. In giving glove anesthesia suggestions it is often well to transport the numbness first and then the healing second via hand stroking. To transport numbness to a place on the body that is difficult to reach, place the client's hand in front of the body and instruct them to **"send the numbness (or healing) through the body to the place where it is needed."**

10. In each session have the client **"select a place inside themselves where they sense the feeling of numbness and healing is most needed."** Once in place, it can be suggested that the "bands" are removed and just the numbness and healing remain.

11. Request the subconscious to give ideomotor signals when the session has been successfully completed.

12. Arouse from hypnosis.

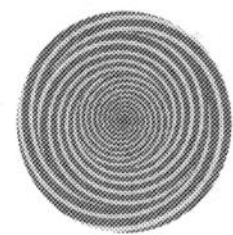

~ *Chapter 145* ~
STOCKWELL'S HYPNO-ANESTHESIA
(nonpharmacologic anesthesia)

By Shelley Stockwell-Nicholas, PhD
with special thanks to Hypnotherapists Norbert Bakas, Gaye Wilson,
Del Hunter Morrill and Al Krasner for their great ideas!

---

*"**Anesthesia**: a loss of sensitivity to pain in all or a part of the body for medical reasons induced by drugs, acupuncture and hypnosis."*

Includes:
Norbert Bakas' Surgery Preparation
Gaye Wilson's Surgery Preparation
Disappearing Touch
Bucket of Ice Glove Anesthesia
Hand In the Snow Glove Anesthesia
Transferring Glove Anesthesia short and long versions
Glove Anesthesia Return

Some 63 billion people a year in the United States deal with pain. Hypnosis eases pain and anxiety associated with it. Hypnosis is popularly used to help those undergoing painful exams, heart, kidney, facial surgery, biopsies, dental procedures, childbirth and more invasive surgery. With hypnosis, panic and fear depart, the body is more relaxed, drugs are minimized or eliminated, and healing is faster.

> **Hypnosis Proven Safer and More Cost Saving For Hospital Procedures**
> *April 29, 2000*
>
> Elvira Long, M.D., the Director of Interventional Radiology, and her colleagues at Beth Israel Deaconess Hospital in Boston, reported in Lancet Magazine, that hypnosis reduces pain, anxiety and I.V. sedation during invasive surgery. The surgical procedures included angiograms, angioplasties, naphrostomies (kidney drainage), and liver biopsies. Researchers randomly assigned 241 invasive surgical patients into three groups:
>
> 1. One group received standard treatment.
>
> 2. Another group had someone in the room attentively responding to the patient's concerns that avoided upsetting responses like "How bad is your pain." Or, "You'll feel a sting now."
>
> 3. The third group employed the same attentive positive strategy as the second group and also used hypnosis. The patient read a script that instructed them to *"close your eyes and roll the eyes upwards, breathe deeply and concentrate on the sensation of floating."* They were then verbally guided to move away from any pain or discomfort to a *"safe and comfortable place."*
>
> What were the results of the separate data analysis?
>
> The hypnosis group's procedures were 17 minutes shorter (even though the hypnosis itself took up 10 minutes),
>
> Each required less than 1/2 the amount of drugs, reducing the IV drug costs $130 per patient.
>
> Stunningly, *only* the hypnosis group maintained stable blood pressure and heart rate during the procedure!
>
> And an hour and four hours after the procedure, hypnotized individuals had the least pain or anxiety (regardless of the amount of drugs given).

Comprehensive reports and studies by the National Institute of Health, the New England Journal of Medicine, and others say that people of all ages and backgrounds prefer and receive health care services from "alternative" health care providers. In California alone, over five million people currently use the services of hypnotherapists and other client-centered disciplines.

The following preparations for surgery greatly help your clients avoid pain, fear and stress: before, during and after surgery and enhance healing.

MODUS OPERANDI: NORBERT BAKAS' SURGERY PREPARATION

"You have a positive attitude and a positive experience during this special time of wellness. You produce a healing feeling now inside yourself. You have a positive attitude toward those who are helping you and a positive experience during the important and helpful procedures that they do with you."

546

MODUS OPERANDI: GAYE WILSON'S, SURGERY PREPARATION

"Put yourself in a trance so that you will need very little anesthesia. Those who are with you during surgery have hands aglow with divine love and compassion. Your healing starts at the beginning of the surgery. With each stitch you are mending and healing. Your breathing gives you great relief and comfort. You require very little recovery time because the anesthesia leaves your body rapidly. Every hand that touches you brings you more comfort and release. The IV fluid flushes away any drugs. You are being healed. God watches over you...'Thy will, not mine.'"

MODUS OPERANDI: SHELLEY STOCKWELL'S, SURGERY PREPARATION

Induce trance and then suggest:

"**Ask yourself, 'is it in my highest good to have this surgery?'**" (If they respond 'no' seriously consider having them reconsider the surgery)...**good.**

Because you know it is in your best interest to have this procedure, what do you need to say to yourself to make it easy and a perfect healing experience?" (Pause for answer. If they do not answer continue...).

"Visualize and imagine yourself the night before your procedure. You sleep soundly and awaken refreshed and blessed with white light. Your doctor, nurses and team are blessed with white light. They lovingly take over your care and as they do there is a sense of calm that comes over you. You easily communicate with your team.

Think of a perfect place to be in your imagination. A place you have visited, read about, seen on television, a place you create in your imagination, or it could be your own back yard. Make it a most happy and peaceful place. Somewhere made to your specifications...somewhere that brings you joy and serenity. This place makes you smile all over. Your job now, during the procedure and after the procedure is to imagine yourself in this peaceful, happy place. Your vital signs are perfect. Your bleeding is minimal. Your body responds perfectly. You are calm and comfortable before, during, and after the procedure.

Now in this perfect place, imagine a bubble of white light surrounding you. Only good enters into your body and mind. Should anyone say anything negative during this healing procedure it will have no effect and will just fade away as if it was spoken in a foreign language. You only accept good, positive and healing suggestions into your perfect body and mind. It is safe in your world.

You think of your surgery as a fascinating adventure and when it is over you will be amazed at how good and comfortable you feel and how quickly you heal. The creative force within you heals you. Your blood pressure is normal and your blood count perfect. Any sensations you feel are the feeling of healing taking place. Any discomfort is instantly vaporized and leaves quickly. It reminds you that you are as good as new. You are doing just fine ___________ (Call your client by name.)

When you awaken from the procedure you are quiet and comfortable feeling as if you have just awakened from a full refreshing slumber. You heal quickly and rapidly in no time at all.

Now take a deep and gentle breath and relax more deeply realizing that everything has been done exactly as it was planned and you are relaxed, comfortable, safe and secure in every way."

MODUS OPERANDI: DISAPPEARING TOUCH

"All sound disappears except my voice. You will not feel a thing as I talk to you and rub your arm. When I bring you back, your body will return to full feeling except your arm."

MODUS OPERANDI: BUCKET OF ICE VERSION GLOVE ANESTHESIA

Induce trance and create imagery for what is pleasurable for the client. Then bring to them an image like this **"You are embarking on a wonderful journey of body and mind so that you feel so very comfortable in your body."** (Or, "so you enjoy the healing work of your dentist, doctor, healer…")

"Use the power of your imagination now and call in your senses. At the count of three, I will gently touch your hand as you think and imagine that your hand is being submerged into a bucket of icy cold water. It is so cold. Your hand becomes numb, cold and numb. The tingly icy water soaks into every muscle, nerve, ligament and molecule of your precious hand as it goes completely and entirely numb…very good."

MODUS OPERANDI: HAND IN THE SNOW GLOVE ANESTHESIA

Induce trance and create imagery for what is pleasurable for the client. Then present this suggestion formula…

"Relax more with each beat of your heart. Imagine a beautiful snowy place. You are comfortably and warm. Choose a perfect scene in the snow. It is completely up to you. This glorious place brings you a special happiness. Be there 100%.

See it, hear it, smell it, taste it, feel it. As you exhale, imagine your breath misting in the chilly air. It feels so good to breathe. When you are in the scene 100%, nod you head…very good.

Slide your hand into the soft snow ever so slowly and feel the icy cold blanket each finger with a tingly chill. At first, this icy sensation may be surprisingly cold to your fingers but instantly this sensation gives way to a numb, wooden leather-like feeling. It is similar to the way your hand goes entirely numb when you sit or lie upon it for a very long time. Notice as the tips of your fingers just fade away into the icy coolness. (Pause)

Like a numb leather glove, your fingers, your thumb and even the palm of your hand enjoy wonderful numbness. Your fingers and hand disappear into the ice cold. It's impossible to know where your fingers begin and end.

Keep your hand in the snow and notice now that your fingers, thumb and hand are totally numb, totally numb, totally numb, it's impossible to say where your fingers begin and end. Enjoy the sensations of your snowy hand being completely numb. You are having a sensational experience. The icy cold sensation penetrates the bones of your hand… totally numb, totally numb… as you lose contact with your hand. It is as if your hand has a calm numb separate life of its own. Your hand is totally numb."

MODUS OPERANDI: TRANSFERRING GLOVE ANESTHESIA SHORT VERSION

"A river of numbness travels now from your hand to any part of the body you touch."

MODUS OPERANDI: TRANSFERRING GLOVE ANESTHESIA LONG VERSION

"Very good. You go even deeper and relax even more now as I take your hand and place it upon your cheek (or whatever needs numbing). **Notice how the numbness now flows and moves from your hand into your cheek** (or wherever). **Your cheek and now your jaw become completely numb as if Novocain was administered to that spot…completely numb and insensitive to anything that happens there. Take a few moments as the numbing coldness moves all the way into the bones and you feel completely numb…perfectly numb: your cheek, teeth and face** (wherever) **is numb, wooden, and leathery. Take your time and now I will lower your hand.**

In a moment I will touch your cheek (make sure that you are ethical and appropriate in the place you touch. If it is an awkward or inappropriate place say "You and I and your angels and guides now send numbing energy to that place and, as we do, it becomes completely and totally numb and you will not feel a thing.") **As I count from 10 down to 1 and touch your cheek with my numbing touch...10...you may feel my touch as you become even more numb...nine...you can feel my touch like a sensation as you become even more numb...eight...deeper and deeper relaxed...numb and insensitive everything is just fine and comfortable...seven...number and more relaxed...six...five...even if I were to pinch you, it wouldn't bother you in the least...four...three...completely numb and as we go to even more numb...two and on one...completely numb, every molecule happy and comfortable.**

MODUS OPERANDI: GLOVE ANESTHESIA RETURN
"Take a deep breath and you will notice that your hand is coming back to a warm and deliciously sensitive state.

MODUS OPERANDI: POST-HYPNOTIC GLOVE ANESTHESIA
"Any time you need to, you will easily take a deep breath and your hand will relax and become like a healing cold glove that you can place on any part of your body so you instantly transfer a river of anesthesia from your hand right there."

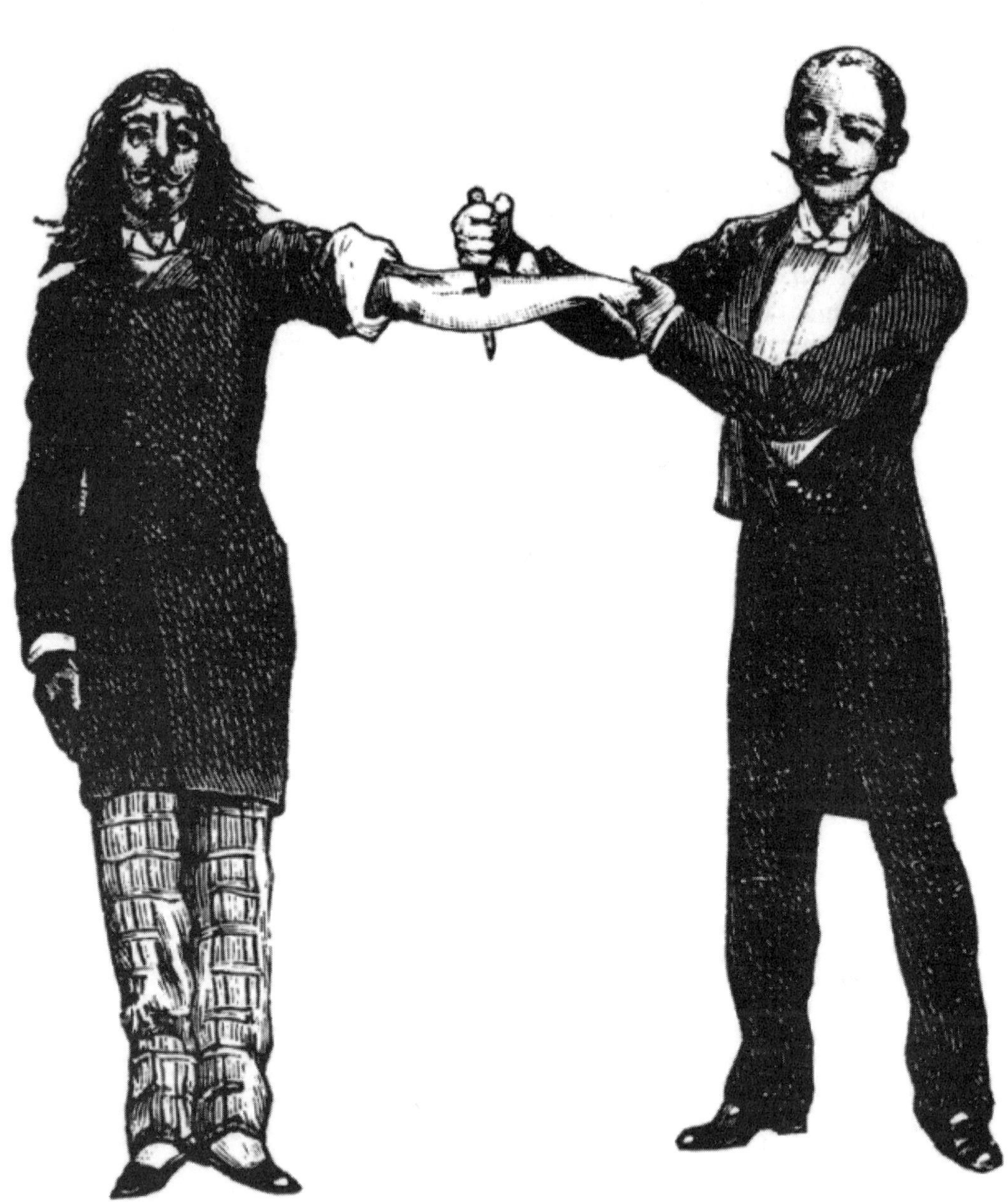

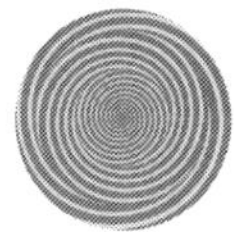

~ *Chapter 146* ~
STOCKWELL'S PAIN MANAGEMENT

By Shelley Stockwell-Nicholas, PhD

Includes
Pain & the Brain
Pain Management Strategies:
 1. **Discover Pain's Purpose**
        Dialog With Pain
        Dialog With Symptoms
        Dialog With Needs
        Dialog With Pain's Punishment
 2. **Dissociate**
        The Still-Point Approach
        Burmese Pain Control
        Control Room Magic
        Tunnel As A Funnel
 3. **Direct Suggestion Approach**
 4. **Utilizing the Environment**
 5. **Future Pacing**
 6. **The Feel Good Overlay**
 7. **Mental Rehearsal**
 8. **Running Hot And Cold**
 9. **Up/Down/Turn It Off**
        Control Room Kick It Up A Notch
10. **Laugh It Off**
11. **Touch & Away**
12. **The Lavender Oil Approach**

"Pain is only a telephone message. It is not the hurt. If someone stomps on your toe, it isn't your toe that says "ouch," it's your mind. A nerve impulse goes up your spine to the perfect receptor in the brain and tells the foot to jump and say "ouch." Nobody knows exactly how this happens."

—Norbert Bakas, CHt

Pain is like an avalanche
It puts you in a trauma trance.
First discover what your pain is for,
then drop it like a coat at the door.
Pain hurts, alerts and emits analgesia
so you can live a life to please ya'.
For the pain and worry of a trauma trance
hypnosis gives your mind the chance
to chill with the power of suggestion
and take yourself in a new direction.
Hypnosis transforms agitation
And replaces it with jubilation.
                              —Shelley Stockwell, PhD

Hypnosis is a holistic mind/body/spirit approach to fitness. It is meta-fitness. The byproduct of trance, deep relaxation, naturally evokes ease from pain and dis-ease. You eliminate pain by enlisting endogenous opiates, the naturally occurring biochemistry within you, to calm and heal. You can cut to the chase and chase pain away or discover its purpose and work or play with it so it subsides. Nobody really knows exactly what causes a pain response but we do know for sure that hypnosis helps people feel better. Use it and you contribute something priceless to a life.

PAIN & THE BRAIN
"There is no illness of the body apart from the mind."
                    —Socrates, 6 Century BC

Pain is a physical sensation that causes suffering. Pain is not the issue but rather how we interpret what pain is and our reaction to it. Distressing emotions can cause pain and pain can cause distressing emotions.

Pain and pleasure are cross-wired. Tickling can cross over into agony. Masochists find pleasure in pain. If we associate pain with something pleasant it almost "hurts good." Have you ever repetitively touched a sore tooth with your tongue or crossed the finish line with a delicious muscle burn?

Herta Flor of the University of Heidelberg's Central Institute of Mental Health studied the social element to pain. 20 couples with one partner suffering from severe chronic back pain showed that a solicitous spouse, who clucks most lovingly over their partner's discomfort, triggers pain and alters the way their partner's brain responds to pain. "When we forget to reinforce things that are not pain-related, like when a person smiles, and instead pay too much attention to another's pain, we reinforce pain and influence the brain's response to pain." She concluded.

When something goes astray kinesthetically your whole body registers it. Sometimes it's a message to immobilize or relax. Always ask the person while in trance "Higher self since you know this person's body very well do you think that it is in their best interest to see a medical doctor regarding this pain?"

Placebo Effect
Mommy kisses a booboo and junior runs off smiling…the placebo effect in action. This natural outcome turns something neutral; a kiss, a word, a thought, a sugar pill, a hypnotic suggestion into something beneficial. The word "placebo is Latin meaning "I shall please."

Positive belief is the foundation of the placebos given at clinical drug trials that evoke actual changes in the body. Hypnosis and the power of suggestion offer equally effective placebo effects. The expectation that hypnosis changes pain makes hypnosis change pain.

Nocebo Effect

The reverse of a placebo is the nocebo that negatively influences your pain perception and anatomy. If you are "hypnotized" to believe that you have only one month to live, it can be severely emotionally painful. With every "diagnosed" and professionally labeled "medical problem" comes a painful overlay of anxiety and stress. Have you seen those lovely TV drug commercials showing happy smiling users and then when they list the disgusting side effects you feel grossed out? That is the nocebo effect in action.

PAIN MANAGEMENT STRATEGIES

Here are some of my favorite suggestion processes that increase the natural soothing effectiveness of trance:

1. DISCOVER PAIN'S PURPOSE

If you would like to explore the underlying causes ask when in trance. You can address your questions to their higher self, subconscious mind or actually talk to the part of the body where the pain lives.

"What is going on here?"

"What are you trying to tell us?"

"How does this pain benefit you?"

"In other words, what are the secondary gains; the payoffs? Is it an emotional reaction to stress? Is it a way to get attention from yourself or another? Is it fear? Is it a way to identify with someone else? Don't be concerned if it makes sense, just tell us what is going on."

When you get the answers, work with the person's internal wisdom to find a better way to satisfy the payoffs and reinforce these with positive suggestions.

MODUS OPERANDI: DIALOG WITH PAIN

"Pain often serves a purpose. You now listen 100% to what it is trying to tell you. I am speaking directly to the pain, 'exactly what does _________ (client's name) need to do to be well and balanced and comfortable?' (Listen to what the body speaks)

What simple positive steps can they take to not speak so loudly or work so hard to get their attention? (Listen to what the body speaks.) **As you think of a step you can take to solve the problem that you have been speaking up about, either nod your head or say the solution out loud…good.** (Wait for the acknowledgement)

Now another action step so that you can have a vacation…excellent!

Thank your precious body for speaking up loudly to get your attention. Your body did a wonderful job, and its purpose has been fulfilled so it is time to let it go. We hear you. (Pause)

MODUS OPERANDI: DIALOG WITH SYMPTOMS

"Thank your dear _________ (symptom) for getting _________ (your client's name) attention. What is it you would like to tell them? Exactly what do you need to do to simmer down and not get their attention anymore? Since _________ (client's name) is committed and willing to do that thing, you can go away and let them feel terrific."

MODUS OPERANDI: DIALOG WITH NEEDS

"Sometimes we choose to pay for things in life with pain. In which case pain takes the place of a pleasant way to get what you need, want or desire. This is very easy to change once and for good. Was your discomfort being used to take the place of something you really need? If so, let me know with a nod of your head…very good.

Or the verbal approach: Just report the first thing that comes to your mind, don't think, analyze, edit or judge, just pay attention to any payoff or any reason that you may have manifested the discomfort in your _______ (name the place). If any comes to mind, just let the idea come from your sweet lips. It doesn't matter if it makes sense…just report…very good.

This is easy to change hurtful behavior for loving feelings once and for good. Let's do it right now. Take a deep breath and when you let it out pledge to yourself that you are ready, willing and able to give yourself what you need and feel terrific in your body. As you let it go, instantly your body and any place that needs extra attention is flooded with a flow of joy and peace. Say to yourself 'I give myself what I need and want. I choose joy.'"

MODUS OPERANDI: DIALOG WITH PAIN'S PUNISHMENT

"Sometimes we choose discomfort to hurt or punish ourselves or someone else for being insensitive. If your discomfort is being used to punish…let me know with a nod of your head…very good. This too is very easy to change once and for good. We always forgive for ourselves. Let's do it right now. Take a deep breath and, when you let it out, forgive anyone who has harmed you with insensitivity. Just let them go…take as long as you need and when you are complete let me know…very good!

Now that you have let it go, take a deep breath and pledge to yourself that you are ready, willing and able to give yourself what you need and feel terrific in your body. As you let it go, instantly your body and any place that needs extra attention is flooded with a flow of joy and peace. Your body is now renewed and restored in comfort and ease and you feel terrific. You now focus your energies on feeling terrific. You do good, kind and loving things for your precious body."

2. DISSOCIATE

You can block the perception of pain in the brain/mind so they don't feel it. This can be done via age regression, a mental vacation to a favorite place, or suggestion.

Detaching from discomfort is a good strategy to use if pain flares up. You can imagine that the painful part of the body is engaged in anther position or place:

"As soon as the hand that is being repaired is touched, you will imagine that it is floating on a beautiful lily pad and enjoying a vacation in Bali." (Or "…resting comfortably on your lap.")

You can view discomfort from afar or rise above it:

"Imagine yourself floating out of your body and traveling to a part of the universe that makes you so very comfortable and immediately you will feel a flow of comfort throughout your body and mind."

MODUS OPERANDI: THE STILL POINT APPROACH

"To be comfortable with any pain or anxiety you 'move into it' and notice the 'still point' above and beyond it. Here's how; breathe. Good. If a sensation of discomfort is present, notice and feel it as it comes and goes. Ride the sensation as it comes and goes. Observe thoughts as they shift and change always escorting the mind back to mindful breathing. If your thoughts are like a jumpy monkey, chattering and jumping from thought to thought, look at them and say, 'Oh that was just a thought.' And return to your breath. Good.

Notice the still point within or below any discomfort and let it go. You now deliciously savor each moment of your life and feel great from top to bottom.

Let these ideas become your very own; 'my nerve cells, neurons and neural circuits are constantly remodeling themselves to accommodate my comfort and ease. My response to what I experience outside and inside myself makes me more and more comfortable. I allow myself new ways to respond with comfort and ease. I am comfortable in my body. I enjoy the still point of ease whether I am with others or by myself. I only reinforce positive attention from myself and others. I celebrate and invite positive happy attention. I create a comfortable psychological environment. I create a comfortable physical environment. I am comfortable on all levels.'

Very good ______________ (Say your client's name.)

In just a moment, when you return to the room awareness, you will discover how much better you feel and with each passing moment, you feel better and better in every way."

MODUS OPERANDI: BURMESE PAIN CONTROL

"Take a deep breath, and notice the part of your body or mind that is uncomfortable. Notice the size, shape, color, texture, and areas that surround this problem spot. Now call in the carpenter, who sands, slices, planes, and shrinks this uncomfortable place from your awareness. Continue to breathe and relax."

MODUS OPERANDI: CONTROL ROOM MAGIC

"You are taking a journey into your self to release, once and for good, any discomfort in your _________ (name the place). Are you ready? Good, let's begin.

Take a deep breath, get into center and relax just the way you do when you are at peace as you do when you are deep and sound in slumber. Excellent. Think of your body as a fantastic factory or palace with your brain operating the 'control room.' Your control room has passages and messengers that easily extend to every part of your body and mind.

Picture and imagine yourself in this extraordinary control center with all its dials and buttons. It looks, feels, and sounds just the way you like it. It has your favorite colors and smells and tastes. What a fine control room you have…very good.

All right, let's journey now from the control room down into ____________ (A painful or absent leg or the part of the body that you are addressing). We are here to learn what's going on in this place. You can actually go there or scan it on a screen in your control room. You are in charge. Just be there…good.

When you have keyed into this place let me know with a nod of your head…excellent.

Activate this spot's communication system. What does it want to communicate? What does it want you to know? Listen carefully and hear what it has to say. Take your time…it doesn't have to make sense…just listen. When you get the message, let me know with a nod of your head. Good.

OK, now find out why it's not working properly. (Pause)

When it communicates the answer, thank it for getting your attention and telling you its message and let me know with a nod…good. Make sure that it has told you everything it wants you to hear. When that is complete let me know.

It's time to reach an agreement…one that results in a new, comfortable pattern or sensation. What can you both do to let your body be comfortable, renewed, restored and in harmony? Listen and learn. Let me know when this communication is complete. (Pause)

Good. Are you willing to do what is necessary to take on this new comfortable pattern? (Wait for an affirmation). **Good. Now that agreement has been accepted let that place in your body stop getting your attention and it now eases and releases. You feel good."**

MODUS OPERANDI: TUNNEL AS A FUNNEL
"Imagine your pain as a tunnel that you can enter or exit. With the next breath go to the light at the end of the tunnel to end your pain. With the next breath exit the tunnel."

3. DIRECT SUGGESTION APPROACH

Often pain is just a matter of semantics. The right words change your perception and perception is what pain is all about. Exchanging the word "pain" for "pressure," "interesting" or "sensation" can often work miracles.

"It doesn't bother you a bit."
"Any discomfort is gone entirely. That's the end of that."
"You listen well to your body and feel only that which is very important for you to feel."
"You now relax entirely."
"Let any tightness drain out of your fingertips into the earth. It soaks into the earth, the way the earth soaks rain…very good. It's all gone."

Sip a glass of water:
"As I drink from this water, each sip improves my health and by the time I finish any discomfort (sickness) will be gone…" and repeat with each sip **"I will feel just fine."**

Post-hypnotic suggestions alleviate pain if it returns and encourages the client to change their daily dialogue.

4. UTILIZING THE ENVIRONMENT

Casually incorporate whatever is gong on in the environment with the desired results.
"With every click of the machine you go deeper into relaxation."
"Whenever you see the beautiful blue color you love so much you will notice how relaxed your body becomes."
"The fact that you are sitting where you are sitting, hearing my voice means your sincere desire to positively satisfy the heartfelt desires of your __________ (The part of body that hurts) **to feel terrific and move with ease."**

5. FUTURE PACING

"If ever you hear yourself saying 'my stupid back is killing me' (Use their phrase) **you'll immediately shift it to 'my healthy back is feeling better and better.'"**
"When you enter the MRI machine for your test (Or "when the tube goes down your throat for the procedure") **it will not bother you in the least. Your entire body will relax, and you'll feel secure just like you were in your mother's womb and so relaxed. You'll have plenty of space and lots of air and with each beat of your heart you will feel more and more relaxed. So relaxed that the whole experience of the procedure will seem like a far away dream."**

6. THE FEEL GOOD OVERLAY

Bringing to mind a past "feel good" experience revitalizes happiness and comfort.
"Recall a time when you felt intensely good and very, very happy."
"Recall a time when you had a pleasant feeling under anesthesia and you will notice that the part of your body that needs to calm down begins to feel numb just like it did then."

7. MENTAL REHEARSAL

Have them mentally rehearse their day-to-day activities as if they were feeling perfect. **"Now, when you leave here and actually do these activities you will notice how comfortable you feel. Exactly as you mentally rehearsed it."** When they imagine what it is like without the pain it becomes less painful.

8. RUNNING HOT AND COLD

For backaches think warm: **"It is as if you have a warm heating pad on your back for 15 or 20 minutes and you are soothed and healed."**

For headaches think cold: **"Imagine that I am placing a nice ice pack on your forehead. As I do, the cold tightens blood vessels and you are soothed and comfortable."**

9. UP/DOWN/TURN IT OFF

This is an excellent approach to use with phantom limb pain.

"Think back and remember a time when your pain _________ (Describe the location as they told you in the interview) **was very strong. Be there. On a scale of one to ten how strong is the discomfort? One… it is gone entirely and 10 … it is the worst possible. When you have your number tell me…excellent. You might imagine that you are looking at a gauge and you can see feel or intuit at that number… good.**

Now let's crank it up a little more. Go ahead and make the pain stronger yet and when you have brought it up a number or two let me know… very good.

Now that you know that you can turn up the pain…turn it down. What number are you now? Ok turn it off entirely."

If the client doesn't dramatically reduce the pain at this point (by at least 50%) address the issue of secondary gains or unconscious payoffs.

MODUS OPERANDI: CONTROL ROOM KICK IT UP/DOWN A NOTCH

"Go into the control room of your body and mind and find a gauge, switch or volume control that shows any discomfort or hurt level for that specific place. On a scale of one to ten what does it read? (Pause for answer). **Good. Now kick it up a notch. Just for a minute so that it will never bother you again. OK. If it was at a 5** (for instance) **bring it up to a 7. Good.**

Now that you know how to turn up the gauge you understand that you can easily turn it down. Bring the level down to a lower number (three for example): **Good. Now turn it off entirely. Let me know when this is complete. Excellent.**

If for any reason the signal tries to get your attention again in the future you easily and quickly say 'God bless you' and you go into the control room and turn off the volume and gauges and you stop the signals entirely. You feel great!

When the surgery is complete, you go into the control room and gently tap the 'healing button' and your systems automatically and easily bring you back better than new. Like a computer, your amazing control panel now upgrades all programs for radiant wellness, comfort and letting go of any limits and keeping all of the good and up-to-date vitality that is yours."

10. LAUGH IT OFF

Instruct them to literally laugh. This emits feel good endorphins that are the antithesis of pain and illness.

11. TOUCH & AWAY

"In a moment, and with your permission, I will respectfully lay my hands upon your _______ ('head, arm, foot' … be appropriate) **to assist it to feel terrific. Is that all right with you?** (If they say, yes, proceed. If not, have them imagine the "healing hands of God" touching them there.)

Tension centered, where I am placing my hands is there to tell you that it is now time for you to relax and let it go. Relax these muscles now and notice every nerve and ligament relaxing too. It may feel as if my hand is actually drawing away any tension. I just take it from you. You don't need it any more…and you go deeper 5-4-3-2-1 all the way down. Excellent job!

Your _______ (head, arm, foot…) **feels perfect in every way. All is well. You are renewed, restored and reinvigorated. Feeling comfortable and happy. Every day in every way you feel better and better."**

12. THE LAVENDER OIL APPROACH

In 1937 Rene-Maurice Gottefosse put his seriously burned hand into the lavender oil he was distilling. The pain stopped immediately and his hand healed without a scar. Is it the lavender or the healing placebo effect? Try it yourself and decide. Here's how:

First induce trance and then suggest, **"Since the time of the Ancient Egyptians, lavender essences have been proven to bring comfort, eliminate discomfort, heal and boost immunity. As you breath, imagine yourself in a beautiful place in nature with a field luscious with lavender plants.'** (If you actually have some natural lavender essence, you can waft it under their nose) **"You smell its healing fragrance now as the lavender wraps its aroma around your** ___________, (Place in need of comfort) **entering each cell and molecule and making you radiantly healthy and comfortable."**

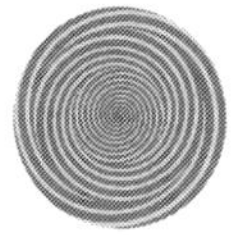

~ *Chapter 147* ~
GOOD-BYE HEADACHE

By Shelley Stockwell-Nicholas, PhD

Includes
Six Headache Remedies
Tell The Truce
Magnetic Magic
Hocus Focus
Mental Cold Pack
McGill's Gone, Gone, Gone
McGill's Handkerchief Relief

Headaches result from blood vessel changes and muscle spasms. Certain behaviors can depress the autonomic nervous system and in turn affect your blood pressure and muscles.

It is a good idea to first find out about a person's intake when dealing with headaches. Headaches can result from dehydration. Ask if they drink sufficient water.

Headaches can also result from withdrawal from addictions, eating processed foods (which often contain additives like nitrites, sulfites, hormones, and bug spray), meat (tenderizer and steroids are the culprit), MSG (mono sodium glutamate, also labeled natural flavorings, plant protein among other things. Chinese food is loaded with MSG), salty, pickled, smoked, aged and marinated foods, cheese (especially yellow cheese), wine (especially red), alcohol, caffeine, chocolate, soups, nuts, sour cream, powdered coffee creamers and soy protein powders.

If the headache is a reaction to these things, give your client a glass of water and then hypnotize saying "This water is now cleansing and purifying you. And you feel better and better in every way. From this moment on you take in healthy things for your body and drink six to eight glasses of water a day to flush your system."

HEADACHE CAUSES

Aspartame	Processed foods with nitrites, sulfites, hormones
Alcohol	
Bug spray	Meat with hidden tenderizers and steroids.
Caffeine	MSG (mono sodium glutamate)
Cheese (especially yellow cheese)	Salty, pickled, smoked, aged and marinated foods
Chocolate	
Dehydration	Soy protein powders
Withdrawal from addictions	Wine (especially red)
Powdered coffee creamers	

If a client suffers from chronic headaches not related to the above behaviors, be sure to ask them if they have seen a doctor. If not, recommend that they do so. In the meantime, use one of these remedies:

MODUS OPERANDI: SIX HEADACHE REMEDIES

HEADACHE REMEDY ONE: TELL THE TRUCE
"Imagine a war going on in your head with guns, cannons, warriors and bombs...focus your attention on your feet and imagine the soldiers marching...and running...count from 1 to 3 and the war is over."

HEADACHE REMEDY TWO: MAGNETIC MAGIC
Have your client sit in a chair.
"My hands are giant magnets and as I pull them from your head all pain and tension will move from your head to my hands."
Draw hands away and say:
"Notice how much better you feel!" or **"Feeling fine...how do you feel?"**

HEADACHE REMEDY THREE: HOCUS FOCUS
"Describe the feeling in your head.
What color is it?
How much does it weigh?
Where is it located?
Is it transparent, translucent or opaque?
It's moving. Where is it now?
What color is it? How much does it weigh now?
Is it transparent, translucent or opaque?"
Keep going asking more and more detailed questions as you interject suggestions like:
"It's getting smaller. What size is it now?"

And, finally as it shifts, say,
"I'll take it now" and sweep hands upward from the crown of the subject
"It's gone now. Excellent."

HEADACHE REMEDY FOUR: MENTAL COLD PACK
For headaches think cold: **"Think of a nice ice pack on your forehead. The cold tightens your blood vessels and your head is relieved and comfortable."**

HEADACHE REMEDY FIVE: McGILL'S GONE, GONE, GONE

Hypnotize your client and stroke their forehead from the center to the temples as you directly suggest:

"With every stroke of my fingers your headache becomes less and less. Soon all aching will be gone. When you arouse from this hypnosis session, your headache will have disappeared. You will feel fine. You will even have forgotten you had a headache. It is GONE, GONE, GONE!"

Repeat these suggestions eight or ten times. Obtain subconscious affirmation that the suggestions have been accepted and allow the client to arouse him or herself when they wish. Most will find that they have forgotten all about their headache.

HEADACHE REMEDY SIX: McGILL'S HANDKERCHIEF RELIEF

Another method for treating headaches that is effective and easy to apply is to take a clean pocket-handkerchief and fold it over a number of times forming a pad. Place this pad over the spot where the headache is felt. Then place your open mouth in the center of the pad and blow warm air upon the folded cloth. It will become heated in the process. Ten minutes of such treatment often cures even pronounced headaches.

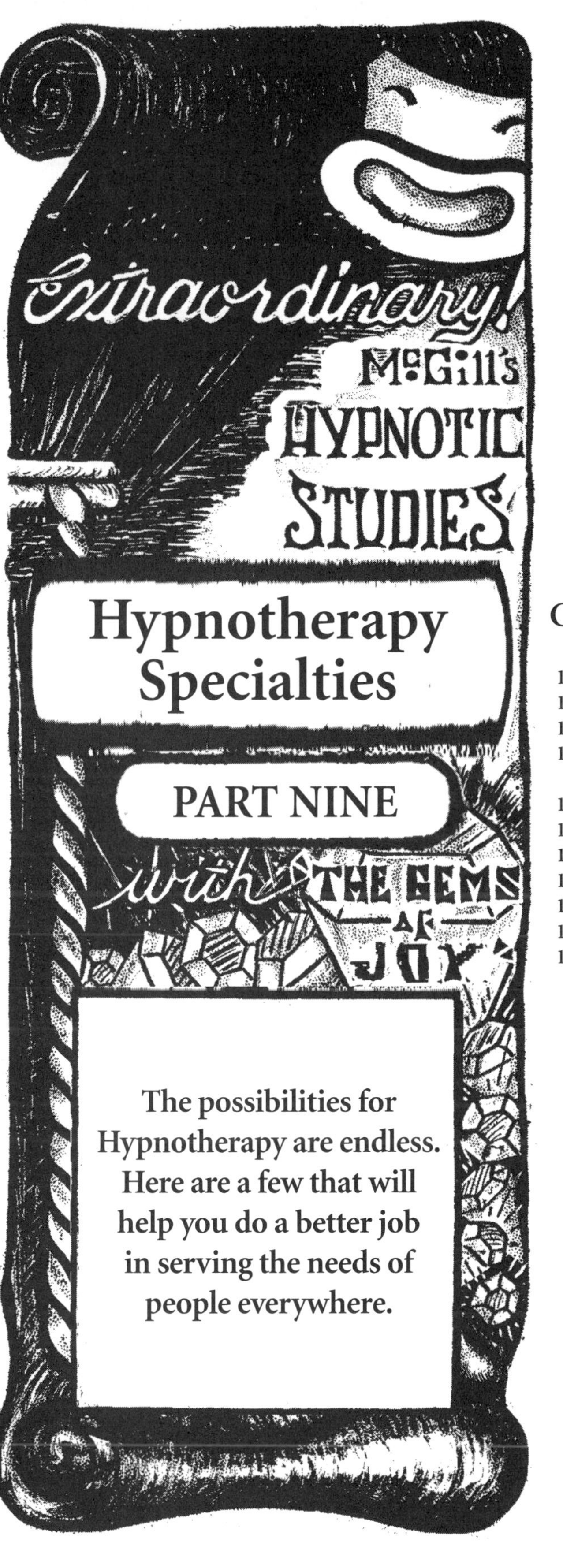

CHAPTERS IN PART NINE

148. Pre-Birth Hypnotherapy ....page 565
149. Stockwell's Happy HypnoBirthday 567
150. Hypnotherapy Of Immortality............573
151. Thompson's Hypnosis For ADD & ADHD 579
152. Hypno-Creativity 583
153. International Hypnotherapy 587
154. Oates' Reverse Speech 589
155. Talent Hypnotherapy 593
156. The Long Hypnotic Sleep 595
157. Demonstrational & Stage Hypnosis....597
158. The Guardian Angel Hypnosis Show ..607

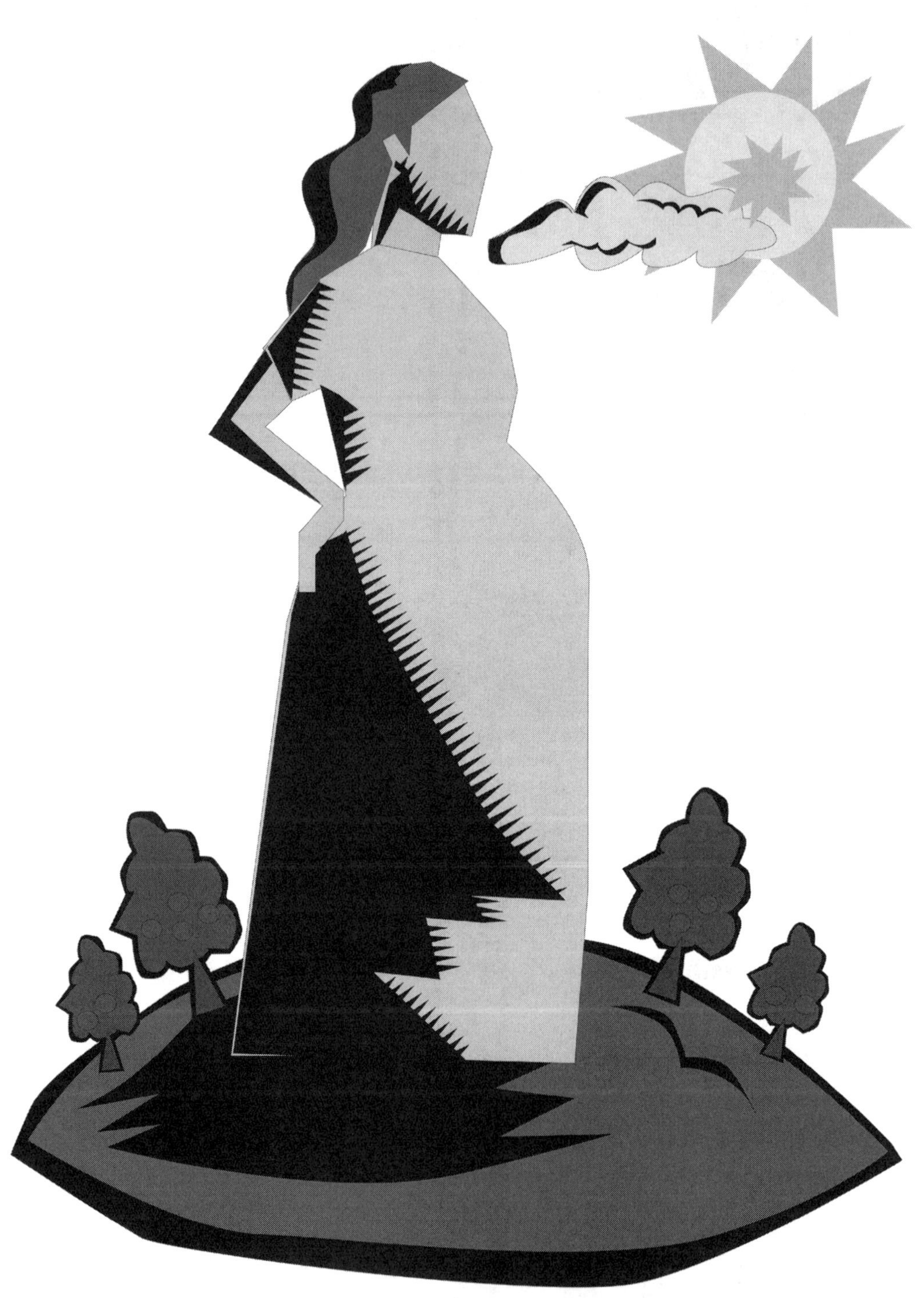

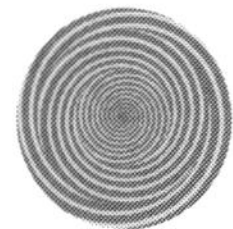

~ *Chapter 148* ~
PRE-BIRTH HYPNOTHERAPY

"You and I have lived many lives, Arjuna. I remember them all but thou do not."
—Lord Krishna

This form of hypnotherapy has been largely overlooked, yet it holds tremendous potential. It may well prove a most important form of hypnotherapy in the 21st Century.

A baby once conceived develops within their mother. Through her brain-computer, via her nervous system, the mother has direct contact with the fetus within her womb. That developing soul may be ages old, holding the wisdom of many past lifetimes. Who knows, that child may be a sage, a genius…

How seldom is such potential appreciated. A baby is looked upon as "knowing nothing" until it gradually obtains maturity in the world. Parents see to it that their child "knows nothing," until they teach it what to know. How could their child possibly know more than they do, when it has just commenced?

Quite impossible!

Ego can be quite a game. On first entering the fetus, the memories are clear, but when the mother/child connection discourages or puts down such wisdom, it recedes back into the subconscious, and is bypassed. In other words, no opportunity is provided for child expressiveness.

What a waste.

Give the infant, recently entering their new body, encouragement to remember and express what they know and the results can be astounding. You reach, develop, and recall the inner wisdom of the developing child and provide an opportunity for lifetimes of experience to be expressed. You also help the mother to encourage the wisdom of her child. Pre-birth Hypnotherapy with its appreciation of developing genius could advance the human race from homosapien to homosuperior.

Speculation:

The mother, using hypnosis, reaches the growing child within. That child then comes in with remarkable remembering and knowing gleaned from previous, and interim lifetimes.

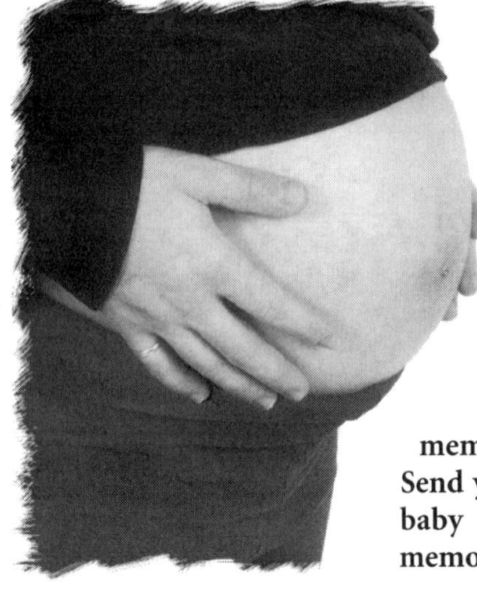

**MODUS OPERANDI:
FOR PRE-BIRTH HYPNOTHERAPY**

Hypnotize the mother. Produce deep trance. Give direct suggestions to her subconscious:

"Mother to be, within you grows a child with the memories of many lifetimes. There is much wisdom there. Send your love, understanding and energy to that precious baby of yours so they easily hold on and recall those memories. There is much wisdom there."

Such will suffice. You have given the mother's subconscious a needed directive to aid her baby to hold on to for ready recall the memories that are there pre-birth, at birth, and after birth. The child will not forget.

Impossible? Nothing is impossible within the amazing realm of mind.

When the child is born, again hypnotize the mother and suggest:

"You encourage your child to express what comes out to be expressed. You listen with respect."

When the mother encourages the newborn is such regard remarkable results are achieved.

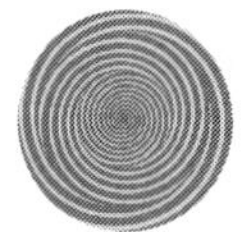

~ *Chapter 149* ~
STOCKWELL'S HAPPY HYPNOBIRTHDAY™

By Shelley Stockwell-Nicholas, PhD

Includes
Can Hypnosis Help You Get Pregnant?
Hypnosis For Conception
Shift the Fear Gear
The Delivery Warm Up
Hello Baby
The Contraction Giggle
Stockwell's, Happy HypnoBirthday™ Preparation
Trouble Shooting
Overcoming Morning Sickness
Mom's Teddy Bear Meditation

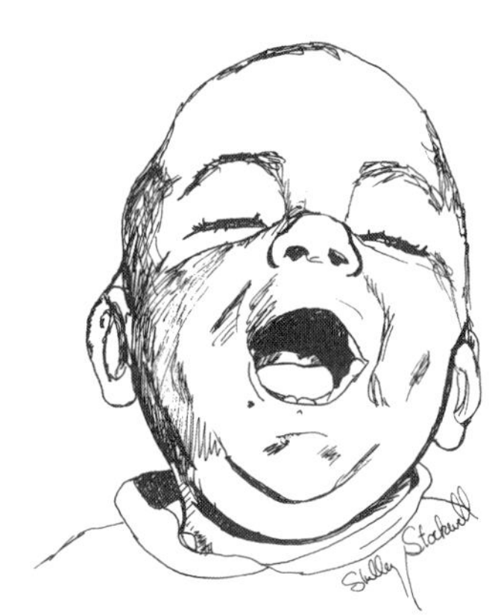

Hypnosis suggestions give you and your baby a positive attitude, behavior and internal data bank.

Hypnosis is a rite of passage that lets you:
Get pregnant and feel great
Be in the driver's seat and celebrate your pregnancy, birth & life
Be totally relaxed and totally in control
Push the right buttons to activate your natural anesthesia
Have a blissful delivery
Focus upon your truth
Identify and communicate what you need
Get you high with your higher self
Re-member and bring forth positive experiences
Be more intuitive

Hypnosis works!

Giving birth is the greatest privilege women have.'
        —Golda Meir

In Spanish, to birth is called *dar la luz* or *to give light*. Throughout time women give light and bring forth life to miracle babies from their miraculous bodies. Birthing is naturally pain free when you learn to honor your innate instincts to relax, anesthetize, and do what it is intended to do. During pregnancy mom gives her body over to the small person inside of her.

As a natural childbirth method, hypnosis lets mom and baby profoundly relax during labor, between uterine surges and during delivery. Any discomfort is experienced as sensation; making birth sensational. Because hypnosis birthing requires little or no invasive drugs or medical procedures, mom is aware and completely in control. A Happy HypnoBirthday™ can be done at home, in a birthing center, or medical facility.

Natural Happy Hypnosis Birthdays do not require stoic bravery. Instead mom is in a calm state of ultra-relaxation. With each surge a laboring mom enters into trance and takes a long slow breath enjoying the ebb and flow of nature's most wonderful experience.

Studies published in the American Journal of Clinical Hypnosis in 1998 report that hypnosis during labor reduces pain and needed analgesics, shortens labor, lessens complications and evokes a speedier recovery. Higher APGAR scores demonstrate the baby's overall good health. Breech babies easily turn over when given hypnotic instruction and hypnotists report that even the time of birth can be negotiated.

What a valuable and personally profitable specialty this is! You can offer weekly classes for moms and coaches, work one on one, receive referrals from doctors and hospitals and even attend the birth. Providing hypnosis tapes are a great idea too.

Sessions include mental rehearsal, guided journeys and post hypnotic cues to trigger relaxation and emotional protection from the environment. If any of the students deliver, invite them to come to class with their baby to share their experience with all. You could take a field trip to the hospital or birthing center if you like. Sessions can go like this:

Session 1. Introduction and About Hypnosis

Attendees introduce themselves and share a little about their pregnancy. Explain what is hypnosis and hypnotize everyone to relax. Show a video of a Happy HypnoBirthday if available.

Session 2. Sharing and Teaching Hypnosis

Educate mom and coach about what to expect during pregnancy, labor and delivery. Hypnotize mom to look forward to each contraction. Teach the coach to hypnotize the moms. Question and answer session.

Session 3. Sharing, Practicing and Making Plans

Practice hypnosis with moms and coaches, make a plan for the day of the birth. Write a list of expectations to give to the doctor or midwife. End with a question and answer period.

Session 4. Sharing, Rapid Inductions and Troubleshooting

Teach rapid induction techniques; offer music selections to play at the birth. Discuss troubleshooting and any possible complications so that they will be easy to cope with if they arise.

Session 5. Sharing, Glove Anesthesia and Mental Rehearsal

Include sharing, then teach glove anesthesia, turning off the discomfort switch techniques (see the section on anesthesia) and do a mental rehearsal for a perfect birthday. Question and answer period finishes up the session.

CAN HYPNOSIS HELP YOU GET PREGNANT?

There is anecdotal proof that hypnosis influences fertility. It for sure helps one enjoy the process. Confidence and positive expectations make more sex more fun.

Trying to get pregnant can cause anxiety and anxiety can change biochemistry. For sure your attitude affects nerve excitation, muscle contraction, hormone secretion, gastric activity, cell reparation and changes in your immune activity. Hypnosis takes stress away and may change the necessary balance needed for conception. If you are undergoing infertility treatments or medically aided conception, hypnosis definitely helps. Hypnosis can help motivate you to make healthy food choices and avoid hurtful habits and this in itself can enhance the chance of pregnancy.

MODUS OPERANDI: HYPNOSIS FOR CONCEPTION

Induce trance and then offer the following suggestion formula:

"Think about a time when you were filled with sexual desire and yearning for your sweetheart and let those feelings flood your whole being. Now take a deep breath and imagine that you are in the arms of your mate right now. Mating with them is a wonderful experience. It is fun for you.

Now imagine that little egg inside you easily moving down to greet and meet his sperm with the very same enthusiasm. The egg and sperm meet and the little one travels comfortably and easily down the tube and soon becomes snugly nestled and grows perfectly into a healthy embryo. You are making a baby. You will soon have your baby."

MODUS OPERANDI: SHIFT THE FEAR GEAR

"Go into the mental room of fright and instruct your body to create hormones that shut down the blood supply to the uterus. The uterus is birth's natural instrument. It is made up of circular and vertical muscles that naturally work together to push the baby out. Natural anesthesia swirls over body and mind. With your body's natural hormones let your baby arrive with ease."

MODUS OPERANDI: THE DELIVERY WARM UP

"Imagine yourself walking down a country path. Begin at a slight incline and let your path wend its way to a beautiful place in nature. Imagine yourself becoming more and more relaxed as you walk. When you reach the bottom you think to yourself, 'birthing my beautiful baby is easy for me. I am comfortable, safe, secure and peaceful. I am blessed.' After enjoying this lovely mental vacation, you can walk back up the path feeling refreshed and invigorated.

Anytime you choose you can take your thoughts far away to this serene place and you will feel peaceful, comfortable and full of divine light. Because you are in this beautiful place any contractions seem like a brief annoyance and nothing more."

MODUS OPERANDI: HELLO BABY

"I am speaking to the little one inside you. Sweet child, I know that you can hear me. Very soon you will get to leave the place you are now so that you can see your mommy and daddy as they look from the outside. This will be very special for you. You will help your mommy to birth you. You and your mommy will work together and you will be in her arms in no time at all. How happy you are to come out into the world for a fine earth walk. Welcome. We've been waiting a long time just for you.

MODUS OPERANDI: THE CONTRACTION GIGGLE

"Each time your uterus contracts, it brings you closer to your baby. Each contraction is a comfortable easy feeling just like you have when your heart contracts with every beat. You don't even think about it.

Make a fist. The tighter your hand the more you want to giggle. Now tighten the muscles in your leg and it makes you giggle. When your muscles tighten you are going to giggle. In the future, the tighter your contraction the more you giggle."

MODUS OPERANDI: STOCKWELL'S HAPPY HYPNOBIRTHDAY PREPARATION

Here is a lovely script in preparation for the lovely event:

"This session will prepare you for your most blessed event. You look forward to birthing your sweet baby with eager anticipation. Pregnancy and delivery is such an interesting experience that just thinking about it puts you in a terrific mood. You are an excellent mother.

You have fun while you are in labor and delivery. Your body knows exactly what to do to get things going and brings your sweet one to the light of your loving arms. You are flooded with the tremendous love you have for your baby and your own perfect body. You work as a team. You are thrilled that you are bringing forth a product of love.

You naturally relax when you need to relax and you are alert when you need to be alert. Your labor is mild and relaxed. It will seem only like a vague distraction before you hold your little love. You do everything just right. You know when to laugh, breathe, smile, push or not push. Everything is natural, easy and automatic.

You turn your birthing over to nature. You are easy and calm. Your body sways with relaxation and easily supports and nurtures your healthy baby. Every part of your body, mind and guidance and your baby's body, mind and guidance are in harmony and play together to create a perfect environment for your perfect miracle. Your baby develops perfectly. Your body lovingly supports your sweet baby's growth. Your uterus is strong and easily supports your healthy baby. Listen well to your body and it tells you exactly what it needs to do good, kind and loving things for yourself and your baby.

When your baby is fully formed and ready to be born, you work together as a team. You are familiar with opening your body, you open your mouth and your eyes and you easily open and close your fists (which delights you). Now is the time for you to become completely relaxed and open your body like a beautiful unfolding rose. Your hormones flow perfectly and help you to begin labor and open for your perfect little one.

Together you move gently with each surge to the glorious moment of life outside of your healthy, radiant womb. Your body is completely at ease. Birthing is a natural and easy experience. Your healthy baby is born quickly and easily. Your birthing is successful in every way.

White light surrounds you and your baby and lets you know that you are doing everything just right. You are happy, proud and a new mother.

Now that you know that you are completely comfortable and happy during this special event you take a gentle breath and return to your special place in nature as white light soothes you and your sweet baby. Everything we have talked about has made a deep permanent and lasting impression on your mind and body and when you leave hypnosis and return to your wakeful state at the count of five my words will be there and you know just what to do. It is as natural for you as breathing.

Slowly now at your own pace: One coming back,...two feeling refreshed and invigorated...three perfect in every way...four coming back now wide awake and ready to stretch and open your eyes and five come back now. Excellent job, your childbirth is easy for you and welcome back."

MODUS OPERANDI: TROUBLE SHOOTING

Go to the part of your brain that controls all functions of your body: your endocrine system, muscles, nerves, ligaments, organs, breath, blood flow, elimination and rejuvenation. Take a gentle breath and let your brain bring you to the part of itself that controls your particular challenge or condition of _______________ (morning sickness, swelling, constipation, discomfort).

Ask this part of your brain what you need to do to make yourself feel perfect in every way. Pause and listen, feel, see and intuit what your inner wisdom communicates. What information do you find there? Is there something that you need to do right now in this very moment to solve the problem of _______________ (morning sickness, swelling, constipation, discomfort)? **Very good, Mommy!**

Discover now a gauge, a fuse, or a control panel…one that gives you a read-out of your responses to _______ (morning sickness, swelling, constipation, discomfort). **It doesn't have to make sense. Just report whatever pops into your head.**

Good.

There is a switch that controls your feeling great. Flick that switch to influence the place that needs correction and renewal. If it's been turned off turn it on right now. That's right.

Now, check the gauge, fuse or control panel and make sure that every system in your body is now in balance as you have reset the system. Your whole body is working together in harmony. Every muscle nerve, ligament, organ and tissue is working from a blueprint of excellent wellness.

MODUS OPERANDI: OVERCOMING MORNING SICKNESS

Nausea is a very unpleasant symptom of pregnancy for some. It usually subsides after the first trimester for most. Hypnosis is very effective for reducing or eliminating mom being a halfway house for food. A session for nausea or vomiting consists of the interview, induction and then reverse any negative imprints and add these suggestions:

"An upset digestive system is one of the ways your body tells you that you are pregnant. This is a terrific thing. Thank your body for doing a perfect job of cluing you in. You are a little baby factory and are proud of it.

Now that you know that you are with child, it is time to stop those signals and to feel comfortable. Tell your body that you will take excellent care of yourself and your baby by eating whole foods, walking, moving your body and taking vitamins. Therefore, any signals can be forgotten and released. Your body feels normal and fit. You digest healthy foods and enjoy water. You are thoroughly enjoying your pregnancy.

If for any reason you have an upset feeling in your mind or body, you take a deep breath and touch your thumb to your forefinger in the "ok sign' and say to yourself I feel great."

MODUS OPERANDI: MOM'S TEDDY BEAR HYPNOTHERAPY
You Will Need:
A Teddy Bear

Try Ormond's lovely process:
Get a cuddly little teddy bear. You are ready to use this method for mom's and dad's when feeling tired, blue or lonely.

"Sit in a comfortable chair or lie on a couch. Hold the teddy bear in your arms while relaxing and getting sleepy. Let the mind run wild…if it seems silly for an adult to do such a childish thing as to cuddle a bear, don't worry, do it anyway…just cuddle the bear for ten minutes while relaxing. Mind will eventually become quiet and will refresh itself via this simple loving act."

When the session is over…arouse your client. Surprisingly, all tiredness, depression and loneliness will have vanished. Your client will feel refreshed all over. Try this technique for yourself. The results are remarkable.

Hypno-Helper

Child Birthing specialist certification courses are available through the International Hypnosis Federation. They include pregnancy, labor, birth, pain management, relaxation, medical and legal concerns, coaching, and marketing strategies.

Kerry Tuschhoff's "HypnoBabies Home Study Course" for birthing mothers

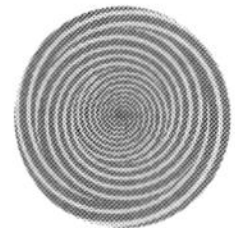

~ *Chapter 150* ~
HYPNOTHERAPY OF IMMORTALITY

"It is quite impossible for YOU to die. Your body can but your soul, never. Your soul is your real SELF. Your SELF has no other possibility than to exist."
  —Buddha

Fear of something frequently lies at the root of the mental disturbance that your client would like you to help calm. Fear of death and dying is the base cause of all fears. Remove the fear of death and you remove the basic cause of the disturbance. Mastery over the fear of death is "Great Mystery."

To exist eternally is immortality. This hypnotherapy form brings in an appreciation of your immortality as you experience and review life-beyond-death. Upon this mapping you superimpose your own life-beyond-death experiences and then you KNOW. One has scant fear of the familiar.

Every person has actually been through the death experience many times, although for most the memories are tucked away in their subconscious and not recalled. Really this is to be expected as a curtain of forgetfulness drops upon each lifetime to make way for a fully new experience of living. Each lifetime provides lessons to be mastered in the soul's steady upward path towards increased pinnacles of consciousness.

All memories are there. Hypnosis provides a method to bring them forth from the subconscious. The experience will be much like a dream while basking in hypnotic reverie. Your client will use these patterns of life-beyond-death to associate with their own recalled experiences.

As in life sit it is in life-beyond-death, the experience is personal and individual. In the Universe there is no other BEING precisely like oneself.

MODUS OPERANDI: THE HYPNOTHERAPY OF IMMORTALITY

Darken the room, no light is needed.

Have your client lie prone if possible. It is best to have them assume the position of death. You instruct them.

"In this position of death let your mind drift as though drifting through a stream. It is the flow. Relax in the reverie of your subconscious memory banks. A most fascinating experience is about to unfold in exploring life beyond death.

As life-beyond-death experiences are very personal, this journey will show you the way to your own personal description. It is easy to let your mind flow free of pre-conceived notions. Allow this hypnotherapy session to refresh your memory so you will recognize the true nature of death and the immortal being you truly are. It is an enlightening adventure.

First accept the concept of reincarnation. The entire universe follows that pattern; every minute something dies and is reborn. Humans are a miniature of the universe and eternal

like the stars. You have been through the dying experience many times and you know them intimately. They are all there for you to review.

Using hypnosis will relax your mind and body so the normal wakeful phase of your mind can be moved to one side and your subconscious memories will be allowed to flow forth. The experience will be much like daydreaming and the daydreams you will have will bring forth the knowledge of your immortality. It is a wonderful experience to review and refresh these memories that bubble forth from deep inside yourself.

Your senses now begin to swirl as if you are sinking into a black pit. If fear grips you for a brief moment feel yourself caught up in a gust of wind and your body will feel almost like a feather with the wind sweeping you into a dark tunnel. There is a roaring in your ears as though you are in the center of a storm. You are calm for you see a white light at the end of the tunnel and know that you will soon be out of the tunnel and into that white light. It gives you a wonderful sense of assurance as you come to know there is a destination and purpose of this mystical trip.

You are filled with anticipation and wonderment as you allow yourself to be swept through this tunnel of light. As suddenly as it started what felt like a windstorm subsides and you are now out of the tunnel into what seems like the light of day. You feel good all over and know that you are safe wherever you are as the scene fades away. You must have gone to sleep.

The next scene that appears on your screen of mind is yourself seated upon a bench in a beautiful garden. Look down upon your body and it no longer feels light as a feather, it now seems solid.

A figure of a sage-like person approaches and sits beside you. You know them well and they look at you and say 'Of course you know me well, for I have been your guide for your past lives on earth.'

As they look into your eyes, visions of past lifetimes arise before you.

In some you may notice how many mistakes you have made and ways you could have made life better. In others, it is easy to recall many things you did quite well. Take your time.

(Pause)

Your guide just smiles and explains that these are lessons you have learned. You have been to school and where you made mistakes you do better next time. That is exactly how you feel. You have learned much and know that you will do better next time.

A group of people approach and greet you in a joyous reunion. These people love you very much. They have made the transition from the earth before you depart. How happy you are to meet these people again. They tell you that they will help you adjust to your new life, beyond the life you have just left behind.

(Pause)

As your subconscious opens wide its memory banks, you recognize life as a continuum you intimately know. You remember. You recall. The group tells you of the experiences of dying, life-after-death and rebirth as you drop down ever deeper and deeper into hypnosis and what they tell you blends with your own recalled experiences of dying, life-after-death and rebirth and becomes your very own. Everyone's death, life-after-death and rebirth experiences are individual yet follow a general pattern.

As they tell you, and you recall, you witness these experiences as though watching a motion picture on the screen. Your eyes are closed as you see before yourself on the screen of your mind, scenes of your dying, your life beyond death and your rebirth again into physical life in the world. You witness these with great interest but you are not personally involved in the happening. They are memories you look upon from out to the past from your subconscious mind.

You body is incased in an aura of white light and you are safe and protected…snug in your cocoon of light as you witness and learn from each death and transition and rebirth. You are deathless. Only your body can die and that is not you at all…for you are an immortal consciousness who exists eternally.

You recognize yourself as a consciousness of yourself that dwells within your body. Your body is like a suit of clothes that you wear in this current space and time. You experience the real YOU inside your body looking out through your eyes as if you are looking out a window at the world.

With this realization you are a witness to life and simultaneously a witness to death and you recognize that life and death are but polarities of the same. In truth, one cannot be without the other. What is called birth is merely the reverse of death and what is called death is the reverse of life. They are two sides of the coin or a door marked entrance on one side and exit on the other.

The scenes you now view on the screen of your mind take you ever more deeply into hypnosis and free you to map and reactivate your personal experiences. They are said in the first person and so you more easily take yourself along the past of time.

The journey begins…

I remember the experience of dying and all pain is now gone and I feel very light, like I am floating up near the ceiling. From this levitated position see what is beneath you the scene of someone lifeless and prone covered perhaps with a white sheet. Around the form may be others who are grief stricken and sad. I recognize these people as ones I know well. Some are very dead to me. Why are they sad?

I recognize that the still figure is myself. That is my dead body. I am dead but goodness gracious I do not feel dead at all. I recall the last minutes of my life when I dwelt in that body…the body that now has no meaning to me a t all. I make no further demands upon that body and it makes no further demands upon me.

The people leave the room. I want to tell them to stop the dying nonsense as I am still very much alive but they do not hear me. I am left here in this place in time looking upon this vacated body with this indestructible part of myself soaring onward.

I wonder what comes next?

A special guide takes me by the hand and we walk through a beautiful garden and I am led to a wall of luminous mist. A sense of anticipation mounts within me as I realize that I stand before the VEIL. I must past through this VEIL with my guide. My guide beside me we enter the mist and it is positively amazing. I sense myself as though I am walking on clouds in a place without dimensions. And I become almost at one with the mist…the mists of time and forever. I hear voices that encourage me to stay but my guide says 'hurry on' and the mists thin as I pass out into what I know as the Bardo. The Bardo is a gray flat plain which is not a place of being but a state of being. My guides says '________ (their name) soon you must decide what your next adventure into reality will be here in this after life' and things fade as that which seems like sleep engulfs me.

The next scene on the screen of mind is me in the Bardo standing before the Primary Clear Light, the Secondary Light and possibly the mind world in preparation for rebirth and return again to the earth plain and physical form. Before me blazes the Clear Light so dazzling it makes my senses swirl and I find myself drawn towards it like bits of iron filings attracted to a magnet. I am drawn, engulfed completely in the light. Bright as it is my eyes are comfortable and see perfectly. I come to know the true nature of myself. I am an immortal soul I come to recognize that I am the judge of myself and what my personal reality will be next.

I ask myself 'what is this clear light that surrounds me and fills me with awe? Is it the radiance of God, Christ, Buddha or the other great masters? Or is it the brilliant essence of my own soul that I recognize?' What can I do to elevate the quality of Existence?

There are two paths I can choose an upward path that advances my consciousness to higher spiritual realms or I can take the path toward a dim light. The light attracts me as I take the high road and my senses swirl around and around, as things just seem to fade away.

In the next scene, I find myself standing before the Secondary light. It is not as bright as the Primary Light but in its way it is even more amazing. It makes me dizzy and opens vista upon vista of past experiences. Somehow that Secondary Light penetrates right through me as everything about myself is now known to me. It reveals every one of my inner secrets about myself

This Secondary light brings a kaleidoscope of experiences from my lifetime after lifetime none are there to hurt me all are there to help me learn for it is my time to graduate.

I am now offered two choices again. Do I move into the Mind World for a time or return immediately to the Physical World and rebirth? My guide helps me choose the to enter the Mind World.

I go blank.

The next scene now appears before me that is much like the Physical World I left behind but somehow it is very different. Somehow it does not seem so set in limitations. It is a mental realm in which whatever is imagined as reality becomes reality. It is much like ling in a dream where everything you dream you want is granted. If you want great wealth, you have great wealth. If you want to travel you can instantly travel to any place you with to be. It is a world of direct creativity with just a whim of thought.

It may seem a wonderful world where you humor yourself in every way. But that is the lesson it has to teach foe when you have everything you want with just a thought and a whim you miss the striving to achieve it and live may become astonishingly boring. Nothing is more deadly than being bored.

There is one special quality about the mind world…it affords time to free your creative genius. If you use it as an artist, musician, inventor, or writer breakthroughs occur. I am glad to pay a visit to the Mind World as it taught me many things but now I am being pulled to return to the Physical World of striving and I am looking forward to being born afresh.

This new scene is a panorama appears again as the gray world of the Bardo and this time I know that it is not a place but a state that is devoted to forming the formless back into form.

I look down upon my body and it has lost its solidity. It is almost like the void the energy center and the crucible of creation. It seems that I have become somehow pure consciousness I scan for the perfect womb of my new mother. I seek my parents for my lifetime to come and I find myself slipping from one dimension to another as I respond to the Bardo's force of rebirth.

Finally I find a womb to my liking and enter meshing myself into every fiber of my newly forming body. Inside the war, and comfortable womb I sleep a lot and each time I awaken, I see my body growing until it is time for me to emerge in full form of my rebirth. I will remember all this well and will not allow a curtain of forgetfulness to fall. I now remember the experiences of life beyond death. Remember it well.

It is time to come back to the here and now. As I count from one to five, you will come back. When I reach the count of five, you will awaken fully, feeling well and fine in every way and vow that this time when you return to form that you will not allow the curtain of forgetfulness to fall. You remember vividly your experiences of living in life-after-death.

It is time to come back to the here and now. I will gradually bring you back....One...Two...Three...Four...Five! Feeling well and fine in every way. You are back, fully alert and knowing that there is no death. There is only a continuum of eternal life. It has been a wonderful experience you have enjoyed.

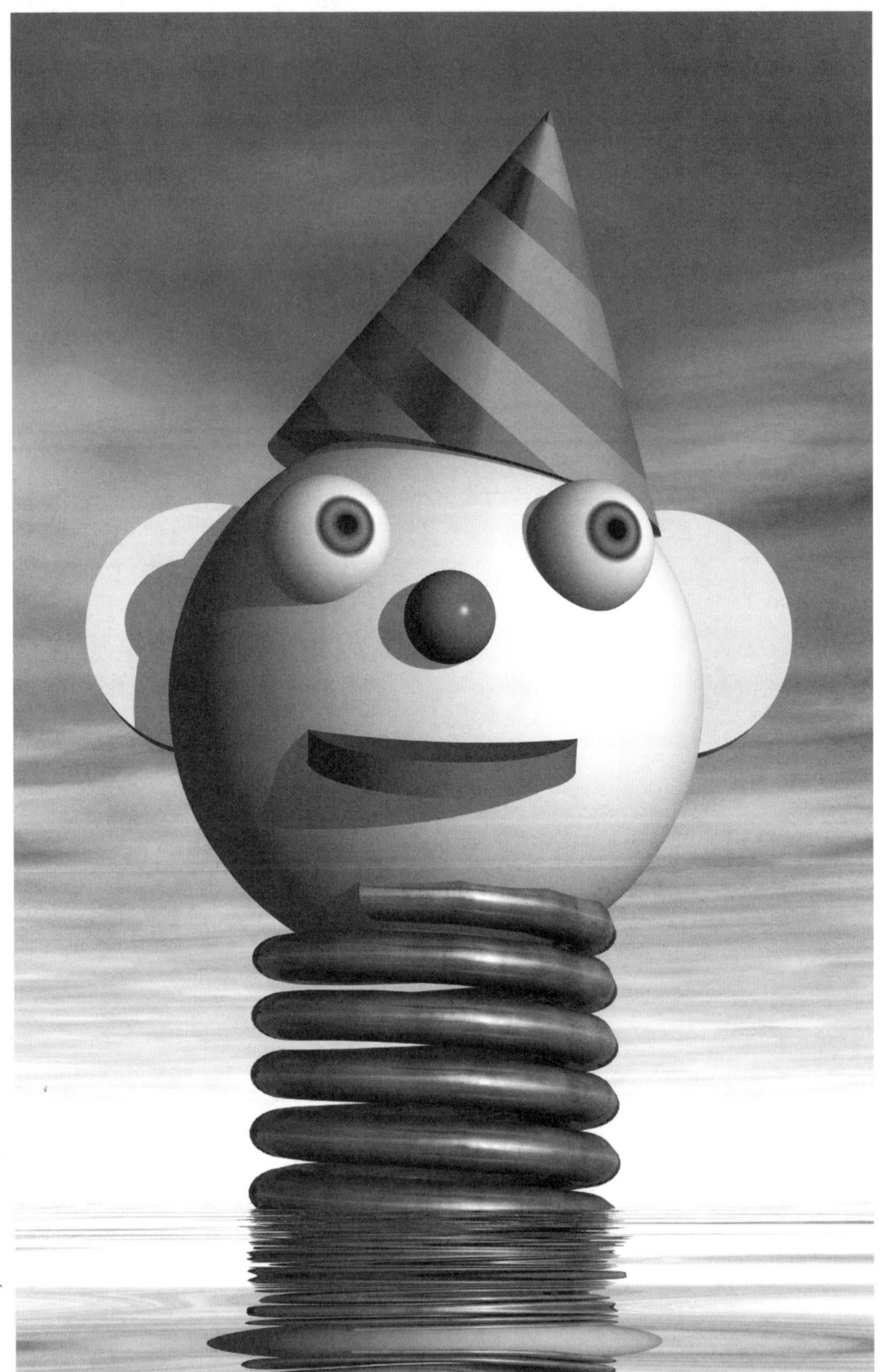

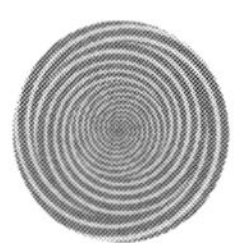

~ *Chapter 151* ~
THOMPSON'S HYPNOSIS FOR ADD & ADHD
By Niccolous Thompson, PhD
Excerpted from the "Hypnotherapy for Children"

Includes
Active Induction and ADD/ADHD Children

Imagine information that comes to you as a large volume of water and picture the brain's ability to process information as a large pipe, like a storm drainpipe. If the brain lacks something to process incoming information (like not enough neural connections or neural density) then the pipe would be too small to funnel a large volume of water.

It will take in some, but the rest will be stopped and won't go down the pipe rapidly. Learning may take place but the time that it takes to process information will be slowed significantly. Information from the outside would, the touch of the clothes on the skin, the buzz of lights overhead, the sound of kids playing outside, new information the teacher is talking about and the thoughts of the person, are included as input.

An ADD or ADHD child needs lots of time to process ideas. When working with one, it is important to keep their attention directed toward you. Never do a long induction and use a story format.

Hypnotherapy sessions vary and are usually 4 to 6 a weeks, one week apart and after that, monthly follow-up sessions. I have had fantastic results with every child with ADD/ADHD I have ever worked with using this method. I'm sure you will too. Your goal is to enhance memory, concentration, self-confidence, success, comprehension and study skills.

MODUS OPERANDI: ACTIVE INDUCTION & ADD/ADHD CHILDREN

This script is geared toward boys between 9-14 years old.

"_______ (Child's Name) **Close your eyes and pretend that you can't open them. Now as soon as you are sure that they can't open, go ahead and try to open them and you will see that they don't want to open. Good.**

_______(Child's Name) **your eyes stay closed now as you listen to this story. It is OK for you to wiggle and move as long as your eyes remain closed, but if you wiggle or move too much you will not remember any of the story and since this story is very important to you, you want to remain as still as possible."**

(By saying this you will notice a child will move and wiggle for a few minutes as the story begins but will settle down once their mind experiences the fun and excitement in your voice. Wiggling is common even while in trance with these children.)

"You are in a very warm, snug comfortable bed. It is very early in the morning. The covers feel so good. You are in a farmhouse in Kansas. It is late August. You hear a rooster crow. It is 5:30 in the morning. You drift off back to sleep. Suddenly you are awakened by the

shrill sound of an alarm clock. **It is 6:00 in the morning. You get out of bed and go to the window. The sun is just beginning to rise. The sky is turning scarlet, crimson, gold, amber and blue; beautiful colors.** (These words require them to pay attention as they try to decipher the colors. Notice their eye movements as a cue that they are responding well.)

With every breath you take, the sky gets bluer and bluer. (Blue for boys) **You go into the kitchen. There is a blue platter of bacon hot from the frying pan. Next to it on a white platter are piping hot squares of cornbread with rich melted butter.** (You may notice them licking their chops or swallowing the food. This is a great cue that they are responding well.)

[Editor's note: be sensitive if the child is a vegetarian or on a special diet that would preclude these foods and substitute something else more appropriate if necessary].

You sink your teeth into the delicious bacon and feel it crunch between your teeth. Taste the smoky flavor. You take your time and enjoy each bite. Now eat the cornbread, feel the course texture of the bread and creamy taste of the butter. You are deliciously calm. It is 6:30 in the morning. (You are tabbing to slow time down a bit. This assists them to model this behavior in their normal state.)

You go out on the porch and sit down in a rocking chair and rock back and forth, to and fro, listening to the creaking of the porch boards beneath the rocker. You look out over the farmyard. You see the mud yard with ruts from a tractor, a white henhouse, a red barn, a garden with cucumbers, tomatoes, lettuce, squash, pumpkins, radishes, peas and carrots. There is a ditch, a gravel road, bright green cornfields and a brilliant blue sky. Suddenly, off to your left you hear the voices of children. You turn your head and see three 8 year-old boys (switch the age or gender for the client you are working with) **hurrying off to school. It is five minutes to nine and they are late. They rush down the gravel road, up the hill to your right and disappear into a white schoolhouse.**

You continue rocking. (Many ADD/ADHD are late for school and/or have schedules that differ from other children.)

You are getting hungry again it is now 10 o'clock. You go back to the kitchen. There on the table is a blue platter with a piping hot stack of blueberry muffins fresh from the oven. You sink your teeth into a muffin and the ripe blueberries burst in your mouth. Taste the sweet blueberry juice. Taste the nutty flavor of the muffin. You take the time to completely enjoy the flavor.

You go back to the porch and continue to rock. Now you get up, walk down the porch steps, across the farmyard, down the ditch, onto the gravel road and make your way up a small hill to the old white schoolhouse. You notice your seat empty in the room and sit down. The boys you saw earlier are paying careful attention to the teacher. You can tell that they love what they are learning. Immediately your attention too is directed from the boys to the teacher. You are excited to learn too.

While you sit in the classroom you realize that your concentration is growing and expanding. You now find in school your confidence is growing, other students like you because you are such a good listener. (Make sure to watch the facial reactions of the child. These suggestions are vitally important. Eye movement and small smile tell you that the suggestion is exciting them, If not, compound or repeat suggestions for a reaction.)

As you sit in the class you notice how the rest of the classroom has faded to black.

Now your complete attention is directed to the teacher. You notice how everything the teacher says is being recorded like a recorder and your mind is able to play back everything the teacher is saying to you. This makes you feel so good about yourself. You are proud to be in control of your life. You feel your mind expanding, growing, memorizing, focusing and you get a feeling of mental power and pride. You are now one of the vast majority of students

who are strong enough and smart enough to allow yourself to become the best at focusing. In fact, everyday in school brings your mind more in tune with your teachers.

As class ends, you feel a smile growing on your face. It feels so good to be so much smarter, so much more focused. Notice how in the classroom your mind stays on the teacher and what they are teaching you. It has a single focus to learn what you need to be your best and you have a lot of fun learning from your teacher. You feel better than you have ever felt before.

It is 3:30 and school is finished for the day. You had a terrific time at school and learned so much! As you walk out of the school house and begin to make your way down the hill, you notice that you feel confident, you walk tall and are very proud of yourself. You are sure that tomorrow in school you will be even more focused and have fun because your mind is expanding and it holds your attention for longer periods of time now.

As you make it back to the gravel road and onto the porch of the old farmhouse you sit in the rocker and smile as you look up at the old school house. You are excited about being in class tomorrow.

Now when you are ready and you know that you can pay attention in school tomorrow even better. Open your eyes. How do you feel?

You did fantastic! What did you notice? Isn't it amazing how you saw and heard and learned everything the teacher was teaching.

How was the food did you enjoy it?"

Various brain functions are suspect with behavior we call ADD (Attention Deficit Disorder) or ADHD (Attention Deficit Hyperactivity Disorder). The frontal lobes that help us pay attention, focus, concentrate, make good decisions, plan ahead, learn and remember what we learned is said to malfunction. The cortex, a natural inhibiter that keeps us from being overactive, saying things out of turn and getting mad at inappropriate time seems out of kilter. And finally, a malfunctioning limbic system may evoke over active wide mood swings or quick temper outbursts, and sleep problems associated with ADD/ADHD. What causes these brain systems to get out of balance?

The goal of working with someone struggling with these problems is to harness the attention center of the brain- the reticular activating system - and motivate it to balance itself and all the other systems so they function normally. If the reticular activating system is inactive, difficulty learning, poor memory and little self-control result. If it failed all together we would be comatose. If the reticular activating system is over-active and too excited we get restless and hyperactive.

Ritalin is given to children to increase levels of norepinephrine and increases dopamine levels. This stimulant drug strategy may work for some inattentive or over aroused kids. Of course, there are side effects from this and other stimulants and they should always be used with caution and closely monitored. These medications only work for a short term. Ritalin begins to work about 20 minutes after ingestion, peaks in effectiveness at about 90 minutes, and is used up and supposedly gone in 3 1/2 to 4 hours. Then the person returns right back to where they started and the underlying problem has not been addressed.

Hypnosis works wonders.

[Editor's note: Why the rash of such diagnosed problems in our culture. Could it be dietary? Too much caffeine and "de-cocain-ized" coca leaves from soft drinks? Prescription medicines? Is it inherited? Is it modeled-behavior or simple old-fashioned high energy? This is the subject of a much longer article. Prescription drugs for these "problems" are given like candy and this is a huge problem]

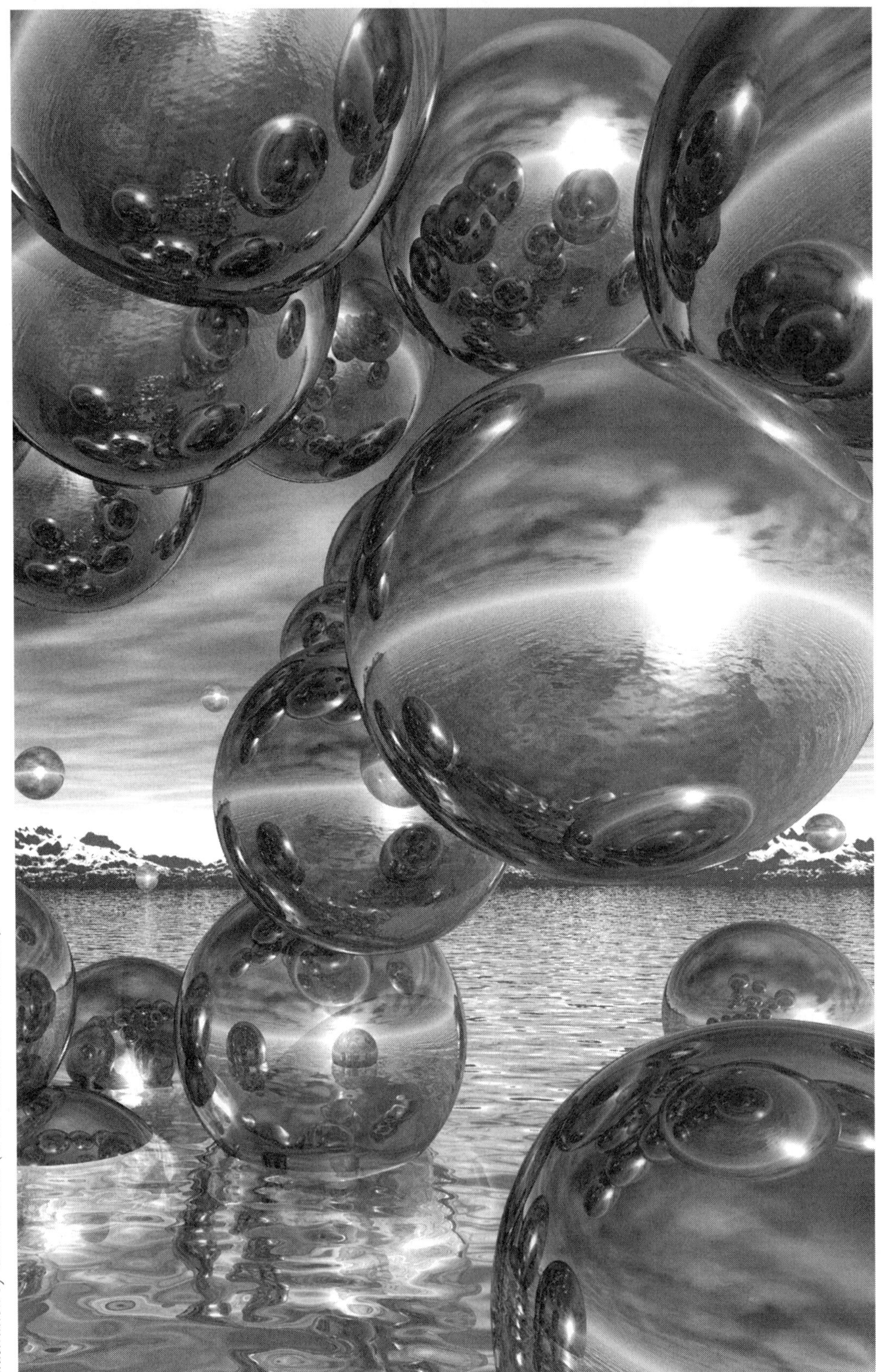

Illustration by Clark Dunbar (© RF RubberBall Productions)

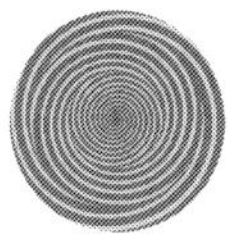

~ *Chapter 152* ~
HYPNO-CREATIVITY

Includes
Hypnosis For Creativity
Hypnotically Structure Creative Writing
Unleash Your Creative Writing Genius

CREATIVITY
Dehydrated thoughts,
saltine crackers in the desert,
ideas gone dry,
scattered, spinning in lost wind and settling like dust.
And each is a seed that any
instant, blooms tender in the
wastelands.
What a wonderful idea!
(It grows on you.)
—Shelley Stockwell, PhD

Hypnocreativity is fun and easy and the results outstanding. It helps your clients harness unlimited creative answers that let them reach their potentials, master unwanted habits, overcome stress, conquer pain, improve concentration, cultivate talents and sports performance, and appreciate themselves.

Everyone is awed that their profound inner wisdom and creativity so easily springs forth from altered states of mind. Hypnocreativity stokes the fires of that innate wisdom.

In Russia, a special institution hypnotically trains artists to paint. The subject first researches all information about a famous artist they most admire; studying every masterpiece. After that—then and then only— is hypnosis used to motivate the budding artist in creating his own masterpiece.

This approach works perfectly with any creativity. If a writer, dancer, musician, or sculptor first consciously studies the style of one they most admire, they prepare to unleash their own creative genius. Imitating the master is not the purpose; allowing another's expression to resonate within our own expression is. After studying or using regression to embrace the teachings of the master, use this hypnosis to enhance creativity.

MODUS OPERANDI: HYPNOSIS FOR CREATIVITY

Hypnosis allows your subconscious to be programmed to accept suggestions you place within it to increase your creative talents. Here's how to do it....

Go into a place where you will not be disturbed. Darken the room, take a seat in a comfortable chair and just relax. Mind works best when your body is relaxed, for body affects mind just as mind affects body.

"The process we are going to use employs the ideomotor response idea, meaning that every thought held in the mind produces an accompanying subjective response in the body. That is to say, if we consciously think an idea we subconscious move in that direction.

Now, while relaxing THINK about yawning and actually yawn. As you do this, you'll find yourself really yawning, and yawning is very relaxing to the body. It moves you in the direction of sleep. Deliberately think of going to sleep and you move yourself into sleep. Continue on, relaxing, and think sleep. Think going to sleep. Think sleep.

You will find yourself becoming very sleepy, but just let your mind drift and don't allow yourself to actually go to sleep. You are close to sleep, yet still not asleep. You are placing yourself into a hypnotic type of sleep, where suggestions modify and enhance behavior.

Think about the master you have studied. This provides an excellent example how you can develop of your own creative skills. This Master has shown you how to develop your own talents. You now appreciate your own creative ability. The Master has shown you the way. So on we go now together for a trip into the infinite with a Master who wonderfully tells you how to enjoy to the utmost every moment of creativity that you are."

Creative Writing Hypnosis

If you to want to write a book on some subject that interests you, begin by cramming into the memory banks of your personal biocomputer, all the knowledge you can get your hands on about your subject. Your writing is based on a subtle combining of the objective (conscious) and subjective (subconscious) talents of this biocomputer. All creativity is a combined expression of both your conscious mind and subconscious mind.

Hypnosis then applied becomes the ultimate writing tool. In trance, there is no writer's block; only creative genius. And, because you relive each scene through your senses, your words transmit full flavor to your reader.

Hypnotize yourself or your client into this marvelous state of creative genius and then record what is said and then type these words exactly as they flow from subconscious memory banks. Or while still in trance sit down before paper and pencil, or computer. Whole novels have been "written" using this automatic writing technique. So extraordinary is your mind that United States president James Garfield (1881) could easily write in two languages at the same time. He was ambidextrous and wrote Greek with one hand while his other scribed in Latin.

Where Do These Stories Come From?

The true source of the tales your subconscious weaves is fodder for much discussion. Are they based upon stories we have been told or read? Stories stored long ago and retrieved by the inner mind? Are they new? Are stories imprinted in your genetic coding, inherited like her beautiful eyes or the way you dimple your right cheek? Are these tales a product of a creative imagination that pieces together snippets of fantasy into a rare quilt? Is it proof of reincarnation that you turn and return from form into formless and back to form again? The source of your personal re-membering will be for you to decide.

Regression As A Writing Tool

Hypno-regression allows your client to "re-call" forgotten memories of other places, other times, and, unlimited perhaps, adventures of deaths, births and rebirths and hypnocreativity allows them to record these memories. A plot spirals from your mind's fathomless memory banks. Buried subconscious treasures awaiting discovery.

MODUS OPERANDI: UNLEASH YOUR CREATIVE WRITING GENIUS

Have your client sit back and relax. Induce trance and begin:

"In this receptive and passive state of mind, place the palms of your hands over your ears and press in a little. Now, SPEAKING OUT LOUD TO YOURSELF repeat these suggestions. They will seem to ring inside your head as you program your biocomputer.

'Writing is as easy as breathing. My mind and body are perfectly relaxed. My subconscious is ready and open to receive and accept what I put into it. My subconscious puts into action every positive suggestion I give myself.

Writing skills belong to me…and are mine to use as I wish. My Creative Writing talent increases by leaps and bounds. Every breath I take automatically increases my creative writing skills. Writing just flows out of me.

I write freely and effortlessly. I am inspired and become a creative master of whatever subject I choose. I consciously and unconsciously tap unlimited information. I am a master crafter of creative writing. I perfectly capture the full and beautiful meaning of my ideas. I am a perfect author of all I write. I write with ease.'

Repeat these ideas to yourself while you relaxing and before you drift to sleep…and when you awaken you start writing. Or you can begin right away. It is up to you.

You're amazed and delighted at the creativity that comes from you. You do not censor edit or judge as you write. Just write. Simple. Easy. It's really very pleasant.

The effects of these hypnotic suggestions compound. The more you use this process the more you develop of your creativity and writing. And in seemingly no time at all, your writing skills become so mentally set within you, you will know that this training has turned you into an expert writer."

MODUS OPERANDI: HYPNOTICALLY STRUCTURE CREATIVE WRITING

Put your client in a trance and ask these questions. The answers may be spoken and recorded or the client may simply be placed before a computer to type their answers.

1. **"What do you want to write about? Write down a one or two paragraph statement of purpose or message."**

2. **"How are we going to introduce the subject upon which the book is written? Introductions tell the reader what you are going to tell them. Tell me, the reader, an advanced idea of what the book is all about. Tell me some interesting information that will make me want to know more."**

3. **"Who are you writing for? Are you writing this book for yourself or for a specifically targeted audience?"**

4. **"A good title captures the imagination of the reader before they even dip into what you write. What title will you use?"**

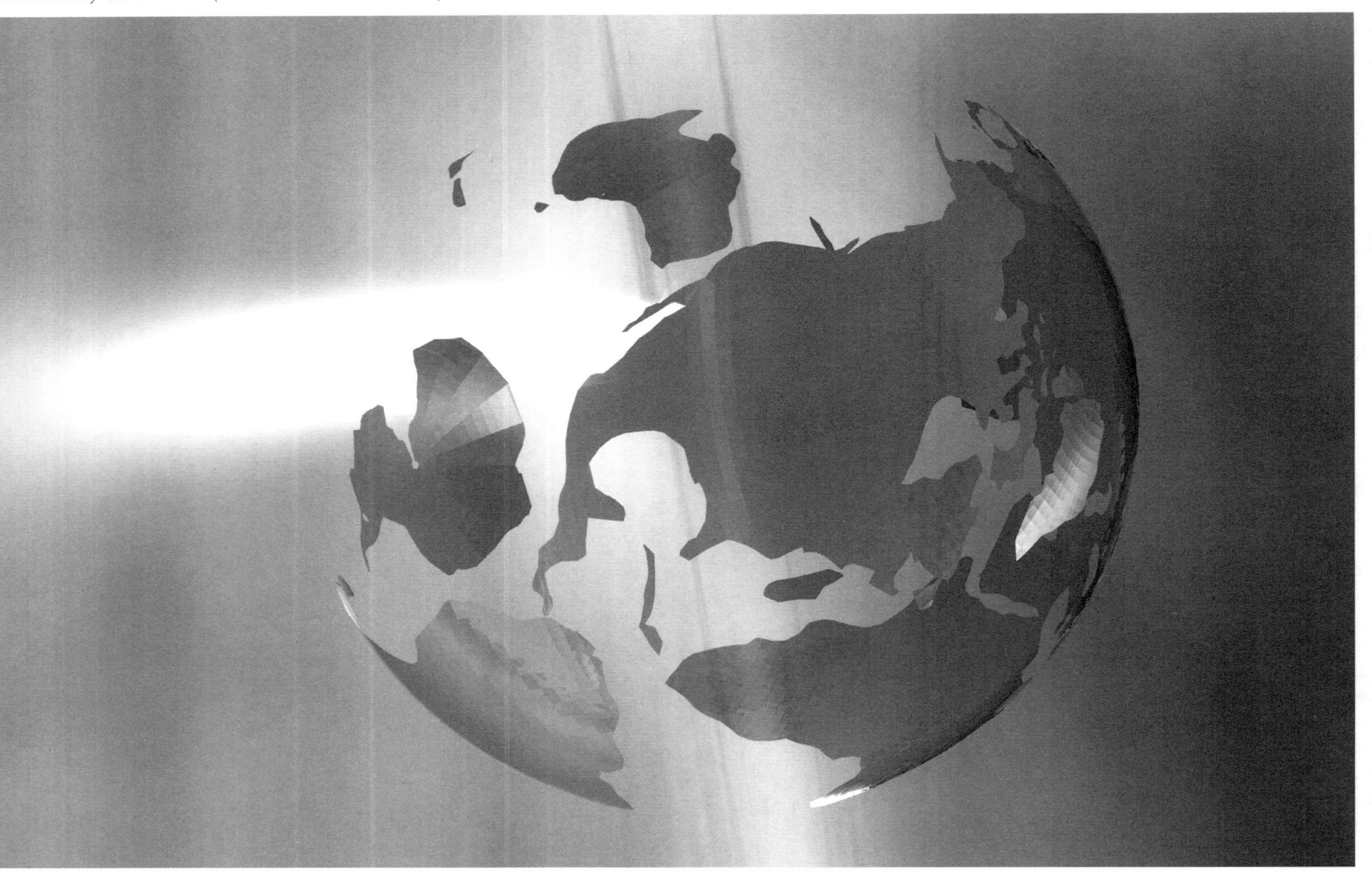

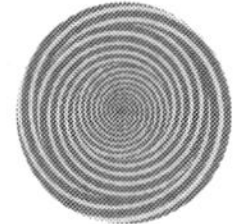

~ *Chapter 153* ~
INTERNATIONAL HYPNOSIS
By Shelley Stockwell-Nicholas, PhD

Includes
Inter-Lingual Hypnosis

It's fun to do hypnotherapy in a language other than your own and our cross-cultural society makes it a very viable source of clients. All you need is a good translator and the desire.

Many of my English speaking friends have been wildly successful doing hypnosis in countries like Japan, China, Taiwan, Holland, France, Bali, Sweden, and Egypt without knowing the native tongue. All report being warmly received and celebrated.

When I teach hypnosis, past life regression or spiritual counseling in Egypt, Japan and Bali groups of thousands and private clients alike are entranced and delighted. People everywhere are hungry to explore consciousness and master their own mind.

American Hypnotherapist and author Charlene Ackerman, who teaches at major universities, colleges of psychology and psychiatric hospitals in Taiwan agrees, "Be ready and willing to accept any opportunity to teach in foreign countries. It is a phenomenal gift. People everywhere are interested in helping each other to overcome challenges and victimization. One of my students wrote a book in Chinese about my classes called 'Setting Your Mind At Ease,' teaching others to put their mind at ease makes you a most effective instructor in any language."

MODUS OPERANDI: INTER-LANGUAGE HYPNOSIS
The following helpful hints let you succeed with inter-lingual hypnosis:

1. Choose A Good Translator
Usually the organization that invites you to come over finds this important helper.
If you choose one on your own, look for a simultaneous interpreter if possible. Then you don't have to wait so long for your words to be conveyed. Simultaneous translators are not always easy to find. I was lucky to have two who worked for the United Nations. Also make sure that your translator is fluent in the dialect of the audience as well as your language.

It is helpful in Japan to have someone with "new age" savvy so they easily use hypnosis terms. Before you begin, request that your translator 1. Quote you directly and not embellish your words with their own ideas and 2. Tell you to slow down if you are going too fast for them.

2. Check Out Important Words and Phrases Before You Begin
Make sure that your interpreter understands the same meaning you wish to convey with key phrases and concepts. The word "hypnosis" needs to be clearly identified for its meaning. Words have different meaning in different languages. "Sleep" and "relax" may convey different ideas in different countries. For example "Coca Cola" in Chinese means, "bite the wax tadpole."

3. Keep It Simple and Literal
It is important to speak slowly, enunciate clearly, and use short sentences so that your translator can stay with you. Unless you have a simultaneous translator you will need to speak a few words and than wait for the translation. Some languages like Japanese have to reverse the beginning and end of English to translate it properly. Be patient. Literal, exact and clear transmissions are the ones that translate.
"You feel fine."
"You move your finger easily"
"You sleep all night."
"All tension is gone! You relax."
"You easily pass your exam."

Especially avoid slang and jokes that are puns, or your translator will look at you like you are speaking Swahili.

4. Set It Up First
Tell Your Audience or Client exactly what you are going to do before you do it. Give simple instructions **"In a moment I will snap my fingers like this and you will close your eyes. (Wait for translation). When I do, let your eyelids relax completely…**(Wait for translation). **Then I will ask you to take a deep breath and relax even more.** (Wait for translation) **Then I will ask you to open your eyes and when I snap my finger a second time you close your eyes and relax even more.** (Wait for translation) **When you are ready say yes?** (Wait for translation and affirmation) **Let's begin."** (Wait for translation)

5. Do Cultural Research
Every society has rules. Knowing the rules keeps you from an embarrassing faux pas. In Japan for example you need to keep a greater distance from your client or subject than you would in the United States or Britain because the Japanese are trained to bow to each other. Being too close makes for discomfort. Having business cards printed in the native language is very important in many countries and especially the orient. Always hand your card with two hands and never write on their card. Simple education about the people you address lets you be yourself and establish the necessary rapport to let others comfortable become entranced.

6. Be Friendly ALL The Time
A smile or laugh is the best bridge between all people. Your friendly and sincere warmth makes it safe to trust you and the hypnosis process. Non-verbal communication is very important as the translation is going on. Your clients or students are watching you as they hear your words translate. Always stay attentive, centered and kindly. When you speak your foreign language the client is still reading your energy. Telepathy and empathy are always operative.

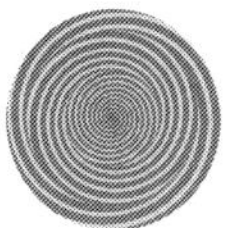

~ *Chapter 154* ~
OATES' REVERSE SPEECH:
THE LANGUAGE OF THE SUBCONSCIOUS

Includes
Reverse Speech Hypnosis
Clinical Reverse Speech Hypnotherapy

"Once every five to ten seconds, very clear and precise phrases are heard mixed within the normal gibberish of reversed audio. These phrases are usually one to two seconds long and normally consist of four or five words. They are quite plain with little room for doubt and are mostly grammatically correct."
> —David John Oates
> Beyond Backward Masking:
> Reverse Speech and the Language of the Inner Mind

Reverse Speech= Voices from the Subconscious

A client can hide behind ordinary speech. Reverse speech is said to reveal true information to the hypnotherapist.

In 1984, Australian researcher David John Oates, (who now lives in the US) believing that he would disprove that covert language was hidden in rock and roll recordings, verified that not only did backward phrases exist in song lyrics but they also occur in all human speech. Thanks to his efforts the US Department of Labor has approved Reverse Speech Analysts and Practitioners as legitimate occupational fields. Reverse Speech specialists record a consultation, review the resulting backwards transmissions and analyze what is said.

Imbedded in spoken language is a second language that is constructed and heard unconsciously. It becomes audible when spoken language is recorded and played backwards. Blunt, abrupt and to the point, reverse speech can be beautiful, poetic or coarse. Each verbal picture, image and metaphor is a powerful hologram of the motives, facts and distortions of forward conversation. Reverse speech unconsciously edits, encapsulates and holds the emotions of inner programming and thoughts. To present the pure, uncut version of your inner truth and Universal Mind into cognition.

Since Reverse Speech speaks in the language of your personal subconscious it can give more correct counsel, feedback and direction from self and a most perfect success formula.

Subconscious information, presented as hidden coded messages within the texture of "objective" language, is called "subjective" language. Its raw, unedited truth is not manipulated or directed by the conscious mind so advocates say it reflects a purer viewpoint for "infinite intelligence and boundless knowledge of your Universe Mind." As future technology helps us to more and more accurately capture inner dialogue, reverse speech may offer an exciting path to the internal and higher self.

The messages may come in full every-day sentences like "I love my son, Bryce" or in action statements like "get me a pillow." Mostly they are metaphorical sentences like "The horse can't move" and "Joe is lost at sea" or singular words like "eagle" or "bear" or mythological universal references to ancient gods, goddesses, heroes, sheroes, and dragons. Action verbs like *heal, attack, happy,* send and love are commonly heard.

To discover reverse messages you'll need a reversing tape recorder. A child's toy called *Yak Backwards,* manufactured by *Yes! Entertainment Corporation* is fine for deciphering a short phrase. It also is a lot of fun to play with. It can take a bit of time to hone your hearing into clear reverse messages so this toy is a good practice tool. To record longer interviews, a tape recorder with headphones, microphone and a variable speed control with an instant forward reverse function is required.

MODUS OPERANDI: REVERSE SPEECH HYPNOSIS

1. Record your conventional consultation.

2. Afterward, play back the consultation recording backwards. Listen to it with great care. Mainly what will be heard will be a garble of sounds, but here and there amidst the garble will be heard clearly spoken understandable words and even phrases that tell what is truly needed for the personal benefit of the client. It is like the subconscious speaking to itself, and directing the session.

Listen. Listen. Listen to the secondary language that comes forth. It provides greatest guidance for the greatest benefit of the particular client involved. It is very personal. As you listen to the "language of the subconscious," incorporate relevant "suggestion formulas" to the client while in hypnosis.

3. Make notations of the voices from the subconscious.

4. Then hypnotize the client using the insights gleaned from the reverse speech.

MODUS OPERANDI: CLINICAL REVERSE SPEECH HYPNOTHERAPY

Oates recommends a lengthy process of ten client visits and an additional ten hours of analysis time.

1. **Session One With Client: Record a Consultation**

   Record a half hour consultation with your client. The discussion should concern who the client is and the history and nature of a problem or challenge they want to rise above.

2. **Hypnotist's Homework: Review the Recording Backwards**

   When the client is gone, review and analyze the recording in reverse and prepare a written transcript. Listen. Listen. Listen to the secondary language that comes forth. It will be heard in the high tones of speech and are fast and melodious. If charged with emotion the speech reversals may appear every 2-3 seconds. During normal conversation a reverse message is heard about every 15 seconds and in written speeches there are as few as one every 5-10 minutes. The reverse messages are very personal and provide greatest guidance for the greatest benefit of the particular client involved. With the current technology this process is time consuming and takes about five hours!

3. **Session Two With Client: Discuss Your Observations and Solutions**
   Share examples of your observations with your client, i.e. a verbalized problems spoken and the reverse message below those words. Oates gives an example of a woman who falls instantly in love, gets scared and then instigates arguments. The reversed word "goddess" came from her talk about falling in love and "wolf" from her verbalized perceived threat that she protects with an argument.

   Some clients may be startled or uneasy with such in-their-face mirror of the unconscious. Be kind and loving and explain that the idea is to solve their problem and alter unsatisfactory patterns. Discuss their reactions to the speech reversals and ask them to tell you ways that they think will alter any unsatisfactory patterns. Record their comments. This will reveal their unconscious reverse speech reaction to change.

   In the example of our love-struck woman when asked, "How can we heal the goddess?" and a reversal may come back as "Let the goddess go to the garden and soak up the Sun." And regarding the wolf, "How can the wolf be more comfortable?" the reversal said "Take the wolf to the stream and have it drink."

   Make an appointment for their next hypnosis session.

4. **Hypnotist's Homework: Review The Solutions Interview Backwards**
   Incorporate a client's reverse solutions into their "suggestion formula." Decoded covert "language of the subconscious," suggests to the hypnotized client the metaphor for transformation and resolution. The lady, "takes the wolf to the stream and lets him drink." "The goddess goes to the garden and soaks up the sun."

Oates claims that astounding long-term behavioral shifts result.

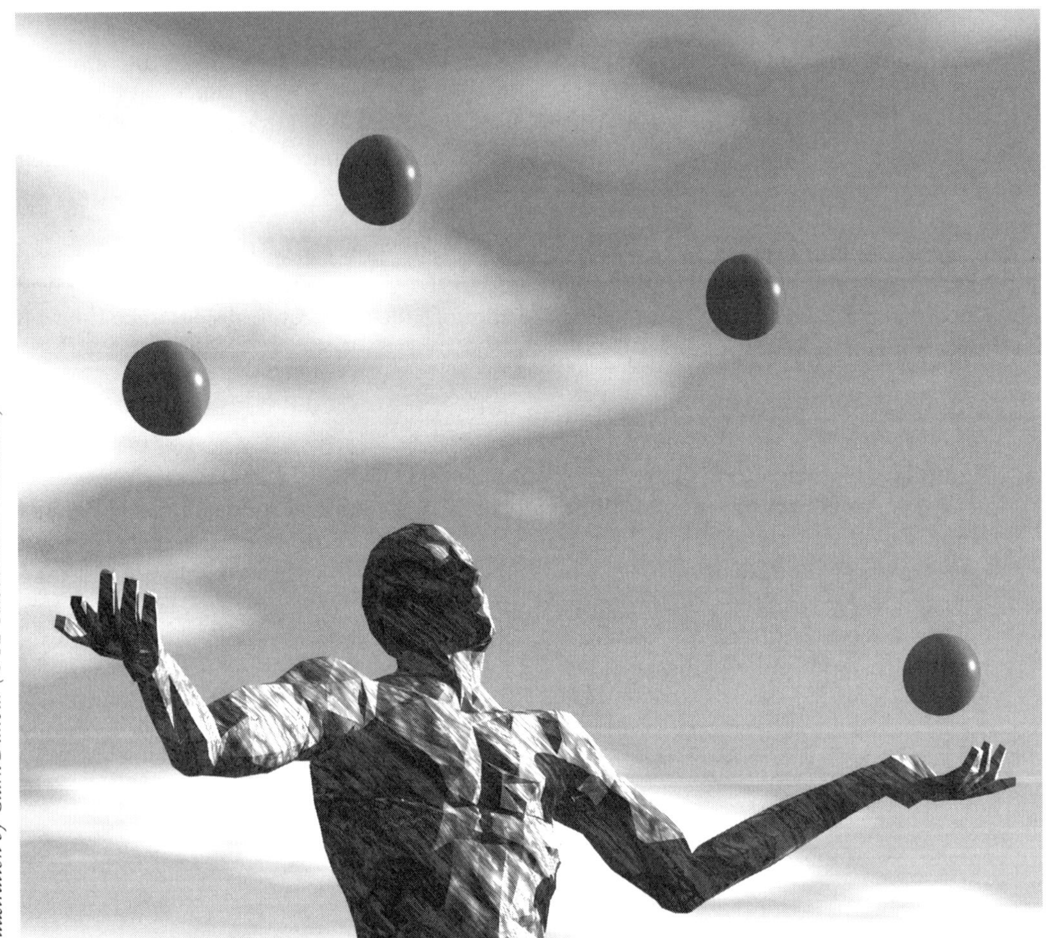

Illustration by Clark Dunbar (© RF RubberBall Productions)

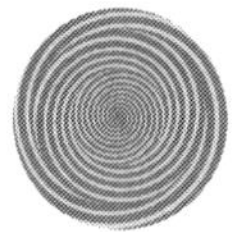

~ *Chapter 155* ~
TALENT HYPNOTHERAPY

Talent Hypnotherapy is a positive application of hypnosis. Of course, at its roots all hypnotherapy is positive, however most often hypnosis is used to remove what is not wanted. Talent Hypnosis is used to improve what is wanted. When you help talented people advance in many creative fields such as art, music, writing, dance, and inventiveness talent hypnotherapy can become a specialty of your office.

To be most successful, select clients who show some talent already; not with those who express desire to be given a talent. With talented clients, hypnotherapy increases their motivation to advance the talent they have, gives permission to polish their craft and energizes breathing new life into their talent.

Talent is something you are born with and can be developed further. Talent is not something you learn how to do (at least not in this lifetime). Talents also offer objective evidence for the reality of past lifetime gifts. A famous historic example is the boy musician, Mozart, who while just a child, began writing advanced musical scores for which he had no objective training at all. Classical examples of talented persons showing early evidence of their talent can be found throughout history.

The main purpose of talent hypnotherapy is to advance already existing talent of the client. This is accomplished by energizing the "brain computer" by submerging the client's mind in Serenity Resonance Sound, while he or she thinks of their talent.

THE MODUS OPERANDI: TALENT HYPNOTHERAPY
   You Will Need:
   The *Serenity Resonance Sound*

1. Consult with the client to ascertain the extent of their talent. Obtain a demonstration of their talent already existing when possible.

2. Formal hypnosis is employed only to relax the client to afford subjective/objective motivation to advance existing talent. There is little purpose in repeating suggestions such as, "You will develop the talent." Of course, there is no harm in this, but it has slight purpose as the talent is already established in the subconscious. However, such subjective "pep talks" are pleasant to hear, and may have some limited motivational value.

3. With client in relaxed/subjective state, tell them to **"Relax your mind along with your body and center attention on your talent.** (Serenity Resonance Sound commences) **Submerge the thoughts of your talent into the sound. Its purpose is to energize your talent, and the increase of energy advances your talent surprisingly rapidly.**

    In centering the mind on your talent, it is to be expected that, from time to time, mind will wander from its center of purpose. There is no harm in this, and mind can easily be recalled by thought in that direction. The whole process of talent advancement is to make the effort without effort, in this directing of mind. Make it as a game one plays. There is an ancient proverb from India: 'Mind is like a restless monkey. If you try with effort to control the monkey, it only becomes more restless. Just let the monkey alone, and it will control itself.' Mind is like that. It controls best when allowed to do without being forced to do."

4. With the thoughts of the specific talent being worked with centered in the mind, submerge it in the Serenity Resonance Sound for fifteen minutes. Then turn off the sound. Tell the client **"Rest and arouse from this reverie state when you desire."**

5. As desired, client will arouse and return to full wakefulness. No comment is made…one way or the other…as to how client feels about the process. The entire experience has been a pleasant relaxing one.

6. The client is dismissed.

What results of advancing current talent has been obtained by this process?
Results will speak for themselves!

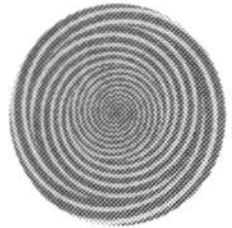

~ *Chapter 156* ~
THE LONG HYPNOTIC SLEEP

Includes
The Therapeutic Value Of The Long Hypnotic Sleep
The Long Hypnotic Sleep

THE THERAPEUTIC VALUE OF THE LONG HYPNOTIC SLEEP
1. Affords the client the opportunity to get away from it all.
2. Affords the client's body an opportunity for a concentrated period of rest.
3. Affords the client's mind freedom from constant "mental chattering." Allows room for internal silence.
4. Affords the client's subconscious the opportunity to be its own physician. That is to say, the source of "healing" comes directly from the client to himself or herself.

Outwardly the long hypnotic sleep may seem the most elementary of clinical hypnotic procedures. The client simply remains in hypnosis for a period of from twenty-four to forty-eight hours. After the initial hypnosis is induced with the suggestions for what will transpire, the client continues in hypnosis without any specific suggestions being given. An attendant must be continuously on hand for handling such an extended hypnotic session. The hypnotized client needs to be comfortable.

Inwardly it is an exceeding complex state, as it provides an extended cleansing (catharsis) of both mind and body.

Because of the long hours and logistics, the long hypnotic sleep is seldom conducted. The average hypnotherapist does not have the facility to handle it. If you are interested in doing this approach and have the facility for such handling, the business opportunity is great; its need far exceeds the supply. This technique is used most successfully when dealing with a mentally disturbed person.

MODUS OPERANDI: THE LONG HYPNOTIC SLEEP
The session begins by client going to bed and becoming at ease. Then they are profoundly hypnotized. The room used for this session should be private and dark. Having a sense of being left alone is the <u>key</u> to success with this form of hypnotherapy. The bed used must be comfortable and room temperature should be at the right and comfortable level.

Have the client eat and drink a little something prior to the commencement of the extended "sleep" session.

During the session you will suggest that **"Your body will make little demands for food and drink, and whatever is required you will take in without arousing from hypnosis. In fact, any needful body movements will serve to deepen the hypnosis. The same is true with elimination.**

It is suggested, **"Any bodily requirements will be minimal. Whatever is required is asked for without arousing from hypnosis with someone standing by to assist you."**

The client must be *conditioned* for profound hypnosis in advance of the long hypnotic sleep. The Long Hypnotic Sleep uses a physical response of the body that is designed to amplify these suggestions with the deepening association that **"Every breath taken throughout the session will produce a continual deepening of the Long Hypnotic Sleep."** Breathing being a continual process, such functions as a continual suggestion to the subconscious of going ever deeper and deeper into hypnosis.

A hypnotic contract is arranged between hypnotherapist and client where each agrees to have cooperation and confidence in each other. The length of time the extended session is to last and the exact time of arousal is agreed upon and this is presented as a posthypnotic suggestion. Once the arousal time is "mentally set" no further attention is given to it. The arousal will occur right on the conditioned schedule.

"You enter into complete privacy and undisturbed aloneness of mind/body connection as you sleep soundly and completely until the time we have agreed upon that you will arouse."

Further, the hypnotic contract expresses that **"while in hypnosis, you will just allow your mind and body to coast. Everything is placed in neutral gear."**

No attempt is made to instruct behavior. The subconscious is allowed absolute freedom to tend to its own healing, for whatever the inner requirements of the patient may be.

On "cue" the patient will arouse from the hypnosis. Sometimes the patient will feel disoriented for a short time on coming out of such an extended hypnosis. An attendant can handle this and reorient the person. There is no need for hurry.

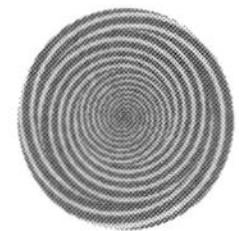

~ *Chapter 157* ~
DEMONSTRATIONAL & STAGE HYPNOSIS

Includes
Stockwell On Demonstrational And Stage Hypnosis
Why Do a Demonstration or Show?
Rules For Success
The Structure of a Demonstration or Show
Tell 'Em. Tell 'Em. Tell 'Em Formula
How To Do A Demonstration or Show
The Pre Talk
For The Volunteers
Induction And Deepening Techniques
McGill's Crystal Ball Induction
Show Ideas And Routines
Hypno-Helpers

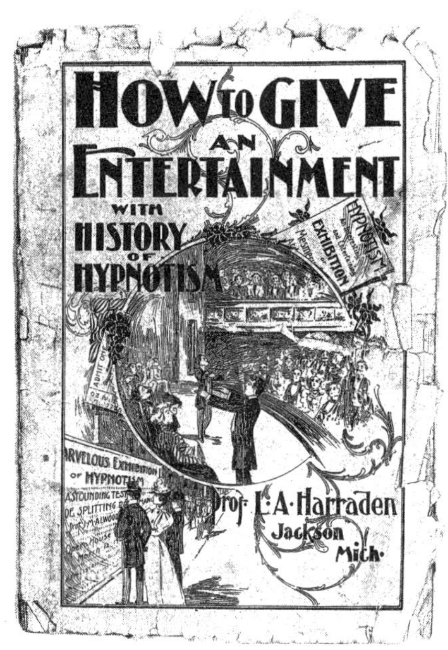

1900's Book

Some hypnotherapists grumble that stage hypnotism or hypnotism used for entertainment defames the serious use of hypnotherapy. With this I disagree. Naturally, I am prejudice as I have been a stage hypnotist for over half a century. However I can present some arguments:

Entertainment is one of the most effective ways to learn anything. In entertainment is found the principle of making the effort to learn without need to make an effort to learn.

Entertainment can make people laugh and have a good time. It is the antithesis of seriousness. Taking life too seriously is a major reason people get screwed up. Stage hypnosis reduces stress and tension. Laughter helps people unwind. It is a great form of hypnotherapy.

No form of entertainment is more basically appealing than hypnotic exhibitions. It is one of the very few types of shows, which may be seen over and over and never lose its fascination.

Hypnotism shows and demonstrations are warmly human and demonstrate the magic of the mind. Properly presented, they provide quality entertainment that emphasizes academic and clinical hypnotherapy. Two skills are needed to successfully perform a great demonstration or show:

1. Knowledge of Hypnotism and

2. Being an Entertainer

Mix these two ingredients together, stir well and you will turn out a concoction that is a GREAT HYPNOTISM SHOW.

Demonstrational or Stage hypnotism entertains people with people. There is nothing more interesting in the world to people than people. People like people and as stage hypnotism is devoted entirely to audience participation, it represents "human interest' at its best. Combine this with the fact that the human mind is the greatest gift you have and you create wonder-full entertainment. The human mind is the greatest wonder of all.

Stage Hypnotism demonstrates the MAGIC OF THE MIND, is a lot of fun and produces much laughter. But always present your demonstrations with the dignity and respect mind deserves. Hypnosis demonstrations and shows are very popular and many have developed them into successful careers.

Of course depending on the presenter, it can be silly or provide an educational opportunity to bring people to hypnosis who otherwise would have no chance to know about it.

Presented with dignity, stage and demonstrational hypnosis provides the hypnotherapist with the best advertising for a bonanza one-on-one business.

If you are going to be a thriving stage hypnotist, you must develop a good business sense and know the ropes. Editor, Shelley Stockwell wrote this chapter to show you the ropes:

STOCKWELL ON DEMONSTRATIONAL AND STAGE HYPNOSIS

By Shelley Stockwell, PhD

(©Excerpts from "Stockwell's Stage Hypnosis Made Easy" available at the back of this book)

You'll be dazzled
You'll be jazzed
You'll love the hypnosis razzmatazz
My show tonight is starring you
The way you smile and the things you do.
My volunteers have so much fun
They always say when the show is done
"You had me spellbound, charmed, entranced;
I laughed and played and sang and danced
And had more fun since I don't know when.
'Please Doctor Shelley hypnotize me again!'l"
   —Shelley Stockwell-Nicholas
   The First Lady Of Stage Hypnosis

Entertaining with hypnosis isn't magic; it just seem to be!

It entertains and educates as people do what they love best: to look upon other people. That's what makes it so compelling. A demonstration or stage show is actually two shows in one. You entertain and amaze your audience as you entertain and exhilarate your volunteers: the real stars of your show.

Entertainment hypnosis greatly advances hypnotherapy by demonstrating the truly remarkable nature of the human mind. You can easily teach an entire audience self-hypnosis so that each leaves with a practical tool that they can easily use to take charge or their thoughts and better their life. And, of course, performance hypnosis brings you an avalanche of new clients who already like and enjoy your fine work.

Old and young, male and female, sales people, business people, domestic engineers, students and retirees all love a great demonstration or stage hypnosis show.

WHY DO A DEMONSTRATION OR SHOW?
Let's count the ways:

1. RAISE THE CONSCIOUSNESS OF OTHERS
   Your audience leaves feeling confident, relaxed and good. You've given them a laugh and a message that they are a winner. They leave loving hypnosis, themselves and you!

2. BUILD A CAREER Performances bring in scads of private hypnotherapy clients.

3. HAVE FUN Stage Shows are fun and make you the life of the party.

4. LET YOUR HAIR DOWN Performing develops your charisma and makes you a more confident and competent.

5. BRING JOY Everyone feels terrific during the show and when your show is done.

6. MAKE A FORTUNE Stage shows are BIG business paying as much as $3000 an hour plus expenses. You can travel for FREE! Companies and meeting planners pay big money for entertainment and solutions to their problems. When you mention how hypnosis improves their work performance, alleviates stress and stops bad habits, you open the door to coach employees on hypno-sales techniques or up-sell the public on a stress or quit smoking seminar.

Stage hypnosis is booked every day for corporate conferences, meetings, conventions, trade shows, cruises, night clubs, resorts, fairs, television, radio, sporting event half times, grad nights, proms, parties and top-notch casinos from Vegas to Europe and Asia. Someone has to fill these slots. Why not you?

You can create and present your seminars in a theater, office, hotel, motel, school, office building with training facility, bookstore, fair, libraries, company, club, church and private home. Many offer you a free space to make it more convenient for their friends, employees or patients to attend.

RULES FOR SUCCESS
ONE. Learn to Entertain
Play with your audience and volunteers.
Take your time. Let laughter linger; laughter builds on laughter.
Use the power of group dynamics.
Develop a deep connection with your audience.
Use wholesome language- no swearing or ethnic humor.
Rehearsals are a great way to hear yourself. Use a tape recorder and capture your show on cassette so you can decide if you sound good.

TWO. Have a Great Attitude

Celebrate People: People are interested and fascinated with people.

The stage is your domain; those who come up are your guests.

Direct applause to your performers: they are the stars. Don't block what they do.

Get rave reviews in writing: testimonials help sell you.

Don't expect to please everyone. A good critique is worth a million bucks.

Be physically fit: traveling and speaking can be taxing.

Be respectful of your volunteers and the environment. Don't trash your subjects or the venue.

THREE. Build Financial Skills

Stage hypnosis is a business. Because the money is not constant you need to be organized. Track sales and marketing. Document agreements.

FOUR. Stage Presence

The audience feels what you feel inside. Consider the stage your home; your domain. When you walk out, think to yourself "I love you" to your audience. They will feel your acceptance and like you. This is very important, for then they will trust you and volunteer.

Give the audience time to look you over. Ormond tells of an old time stage Danish performer, Danny who started his U.S. show with dancing girls and stage lighting, a blackout and then fanfare music, stage lights and the curtain opening to reveal himself. He walked forward and said NOTHING. He just looked at his audience. Finally, after some time he speaks…in Danish! "Oh I forgot. Am I in San Francisco?" he says with a twinkle in his eye.

Find a friendly looking person in the audience who smiles and befriend them. When you befriend one person you befriend the entire audience.

FIVE. Debts to Society

Be sensitive to the laws for businesses in your community. Most cities want you to have a business license so that they can take their slice of your pie. Find out what your city requires first and then decide. Give yourself a title that satisfies the requirements of your state and community: "Hypnocounselor," "Hypnotist," "Trainer," or "Entertainer." Do whatever your local laws require for you to help local citizens. They need you. Don't let legislation get in the way, work with it. Insurance is available for stage shows. In some places the disclosure statement on your table tent might be wise.

THE STRUCTURE OF A DEMONSTRATION OR SHOW

Have easy to use routines and equipment. Structure your presentation for 20 minutes to two hours depending on the venue. Be sensitive to time frames. You'll need to know how much time that you'll be given for this show. Stay within the time limit.

To plan your banter, take a moment and think about what you want to tell them. Put your statement of purpose into key words or one or two sentences. If it interests you, it's sure to interest the audience. If you're talking to a special interest group be sensitive to their interests and feelings.

You don't have to have an earth-shattering theme. Chat about hypnosis, like you might with your mate at breakfast, makes for a fascinating talk. The show speaks for itself.

After you've written down your central theme, write down an outline. What routines would you like to include? This roughs out the structure of your talk and clarifies for yourself where you're going. If you take a trip, it's a good idea to look at the map first.

Introduction: Use an interest grabber or hook. Tell 'em what you are going to tell them.

Body: Tell 'em. Use two or three basic points and any related "stories" that go with these points.

Volunteers and induction

Routines: Give clear and logical instructions to the subjects. Tell what is going to happen before they do it. Give them space to do it. Hold the mike near them so they can talk and be heard. Hypnotized people are funny. When the bit is over, tell them what they just did.

Conclusion: Tell the audience what you showed 'em. Review the point you are making. Always bring them back feeling terrific.

TELL 'EM. TELL 'EM. TELL 'EM FORMULA

Make sure your talk flows in a logical progression. To shine, follow this simple formula:

1. Tell Everyone What You're Going to Tell Them
"In the next 45 minutes you going to witness a demonstration of hypnosis, what it is and how you can use it as a delightful and powerful tool for yourself, your family and your friends..."

2. Tell Them
What you say is important to them…make it so. Be interested, enthusiastic and energetic in your message and your audience will be interested. If you use visual aids, make them BIG.

3. Tell Them What You Told Them
"So now, you've learned what hypnosis is and how much fun it is. Stay Mesmerized until the next time we meet and you are again the star of the Shelley Show!"

MODUS OPERANDI: HOW TO DO A SHOW OR DEMONSTRATION

When it's time to perform, make sure you arrive early to check out the sound system and room logistics. The best routine in the world will be meaningless if no one can hear you or your volume hurts ears.

THE PRE-TALK

Your pre-talk actually hypnotizes before you formally hypnotize. Everything you say and behave is being accepted. Stay positive. Think the meaning of your words. Music sets the tone.

Introduce Yourself

Give a brief background of your credentials. It is best to have a written introduction that someone else reads. Your introduction should sell the benefits and build expectation and trust.

Explain Hypnosis

Talk about hypnosis just like you would do with any new client that came to see you. Answer questions if you like. Be lighthearted and playful. After all, they are there for fun.

Remember that you are beginning to hypnotize the audience with your introduction and the first words you utter. A powerful way to get things moving is to tell the audience (and, of course, your soon-to-be clients among them) what is going to happen here tonight:
"You are going to witness and experience the remarkable power of hypnosis."
"I am about to show you some very scientific demonstrations of the power of suggestion."

"**You are about to have the second best experience you have ever had in your life.**"

"**Hypnosis gives you the chance to witness your mind self. A demonstration** (or stage show) **celebrates that mind self.**"

Or quote someone like Ormond does:

"**The famous Dave Ellman explained it this way to Medical Doctors; 'Hypnosis bypasses the critical mind and establishes critical thinking.'**"

And you continue;

"**As you listen carefully, you will learn how you can use the power of your mind to focus on exactly what you want for yourself. For those of you who have the opportunity to come on stage, you will learn simple tools that will permanently enhance your life and you'll have a terrific time doing it!**"

"**You'll feel better than you have ever felt. You'll feel marvelous like you had a long restful nap.**"

"**Use your mind to be happy, to chill out**"

"**A hypnosis show is full of laughter and surprises. The volunteers are the stars. If you are one of my volunteers, you'll learn the power of hypnosis.**"

"**The trance state is like being glued to the television set or missing the exits on the freeway, day dreaming.**"

If you are going to videotape, now is a good time to mention, "**Those who volunteer will be video taped. If you come up you are agreeing to do so.**"

Imagine The Perfect Introduction

When you call upon the audience's imagination, their subconscious mind works overtime to fill in the blanks. This makes for a fascinating and exhilarating demonstration/show. The language you use triggers the response. You need to engage a person's creativity, imagination and concentration.

When you use the word "IF" or "IMAGINE" you stoke the imagination:

"**The more imaginative and creative you are, the more fun you'll have.**"

"**Lend me the use of your imagination.**"

"**Don't resist just imagine and go deeper.**"

"**What would it be like if you won the lottery?**"

"**Imagine that you are watching television and they have just announced your name. You just won SIX Million dollars.**"

A disclaimer eliminates those who want to jerk your chain. Martin St James, from Australia, says in his act:

"**There are only four types of people that cannot be hypnotized tonight:**

1. Children

2. Those who are mentally defective

3. Alcoholics

4. Those who say; I can't be hypnotized"

Other Key Phrases that Work Well:

"**No one gets embarrassed. We just have a lot of fun as we explore our minds together.**"

"**Later when you hear about what happened...you'll feel so good.**"

"**Volunteers must be sincere and willing to go for it.**"

"What my volunteers do will be very special to them."

"You will love the feeling."

"Everyone of us will have a blast. Everyone is a good subject. If I ask one of my volunteers to sit down, don't take it personally. Just take your seat and enjoy the show."

"Let's have fun!"

FOR THE VOLUNTEERS

Always remember that you are conducting two shows: your volunteers and your audience both are waiting to be entertained:

"Dear audience, I am going to turn my back to you for a few minutes as I address my committee."

Welcome your volunteers as personal guests. Greet and speak to each personally. As your volunteers come up, a nametag is helpful. Greet each volunteer. Go to each volunteer. Take their hand, look them in the eye and thank them for coming up. Say something like:

"Welcome Henry. Hypnosis is going to be great for you. You'll become the master of your mind."

Separate friends from each other so that they do not distract each other. Once they are on stage, explain hypnosis again in a short, precise manner to let them know what to expect from their experience.

"Hypnosis is like a dream. In this vivid sleep, all the others just slip away."

"Hypnosis is a gift that makes you feel wonderful."

"You'll find that you are able to easily concentrate on everything I say and the rest of the world just drifts away."

"Hypnosis is based on concentration; not mine but yours. You are allowing yourself to concentrate and this gives your mind and body the ability to control itself perfectly. I'm going to select those who concentrate the best to stay here on stage. You'll find that you will easily respond to every suggestion that I give for the rest of the show. (If you think you won't concentrate just go back to your seat and you'll thoroughly enjoy watching the show.)"

As you begin your hypnosis or actually your "re-induction" of your volunteers use these phrases:

"Lend me the use of your imagination."

"It makes no difference to you what the audience is saying and doing, it doesn't matter if you are on stage or in the audience. You notice only my voice and you follow my suggestions fully with a lot of animation and facial expression."

"It is as if we are in a special circle of light."

"You go deeper with each thing that happens."

"We are friends."

"Pretend…"

"Act as if."

"It's as if you are an actor doing an Academy award performance. You play your roll fully. So well you win an Oscar!"

"In this scene, we are going to pretend…"

"Use your voice to the maximum."

"Be animated."

"Interact and have a ball."

INDUCTION & DEEPENING TECHNIQUES

Use rapid inductions so as to not take too long. All inductions can be layered to serve as a deepening technique and all deepening techniques can be considered an induction. Don't make deepening a big deal. Let each subject do their own deepening…it's more fun. Here are some of my favorite deepening techniques:

"With each and every beat of your heart, you go deeper and deeper."
"With each and every breath you take, you go deeper and deeper."
"With each and every sound you hear, you go deeper and deeper."

"Every thought in your mind takes you deeper."
"Every sound that you hear takes you deeper."
"Everything that you do takes you deeper."

"Every time I say 'sleep' (or snap my finger, or touch your hand) you go deeper."

MCGILL'S CRYSTAL BALL INDUCTION

"Hypnosis is like meditation, an East Indian term used when we turn our attention inward to the mind. In India, they use a crystal ball to send the mind to the abyss of your inner self. This is a crystal ball used in India. As I hold it in my hand, look at it and you will start to see lights and images. Watch the flickering lights within the crystal. Hypnosis and meditation are the same.

You will notice that the flickering of lights causes you to relax. You notice a slight tingling sensation as you put your feet on the floor and your hands in your lap. Confusion takes you into the realm of speculation and you move your mind into the abyss of your inner self.

Your head begins to feel heavy and just drops gently to your chest. Mr. Jones I'm glad to see that your head is resting on your chest as you go deeper and deeper into your inner mind."

MCGILL'S HAND ABOVE HEAD INDUCTION

"Spread your fingers apart and bring your hands together with fingers interlocking. Rotate your hands above your head so you can see the back of your hands. Now, stretch them upward as far as they will go. Your arms stiffen and your hands are locked so tightly. One, two, three, they cannot unlock no matter how hard you try."

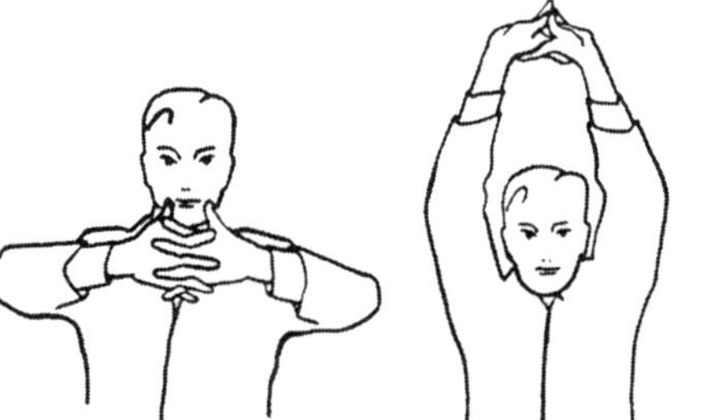

Illustrations by Ormond McGill

Rapid Inductions prove to the subject that they are hypnotized (testing) and are built into these inductions. They are ridiculously easy to learn and there are more of them than you or I could possibly imagine.

SHOW IDEAS & ROUTINES

Play with your volunteers and make them feel great about themselves and laugh. Make your show playful. Celebrate each volunteer. Here are some suggestions for a mini hypnosis show:

"You are watching the funniest movie you've ever seen."

"Everything I say is funny." (What did you do today?)

"A huge helium balloon is pulling your arm up, up, up, lifting you up off your chair, up, up, up."

"It's the hottest day of your life. Oops a blizzard just rolled into town."

"You're seven years old and your best friend is sitting next to you. You both have a case of the sillies."

"You can speak moon talk. And this guy here next to you will translate for us."

"You are now your favorite singing star. Belt out a song."

"You are driving the winning car in the Grand Prix."

"You can fly."

"You have just been elected President of the World. Give your acceptance speech."

"You are the world's greatest hypnotist. Hypnotize another subject on stage."

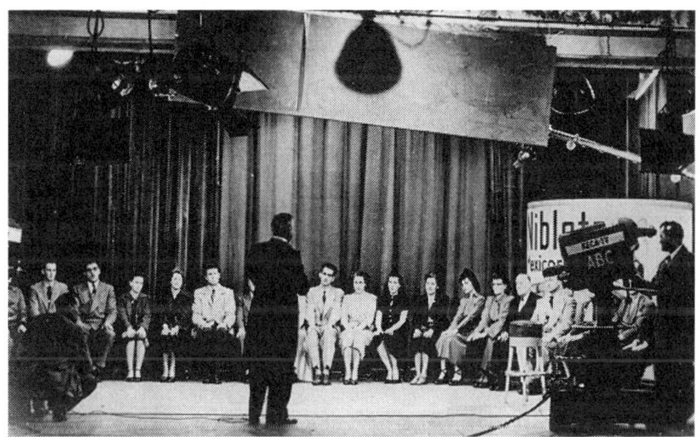

Ormond McGill on The Art Linkletter Show 1955

Hypno-Helpers

"The Complete Encyclopedia of Stage Hypnosis" by Ormond McGill is the bible of stage hypnosis

"Stockwell's Stage Hypnosis Made Easy" loaded with routines, forms and marketing plans for demonstrational and stage hypnosis.

"How to Hypnotize in 30 Seconds- The ZAP" with Shelley Stockwell-Nicholas. This video demonstrates numerous rapid inductions.

"Hypnotically Yours, Ormond McGill" by Ormond McGill. This video discusses hypnosis and demonstrates inductions and techniques.

"McGill's Secrets of Magic and Stage Hypnosis" by Ormond McGill. This v ideo demonstrates a stage show, inductions and discusses techniques.

"Hypnosis How To Put A Smile On Your Face and Money In Your Pocket" by Shelley Stockwell. This book has many helpful hypnosis ideas and techniques.

All are available at the back of this book or by going on line at hypnosisfederation.com

---

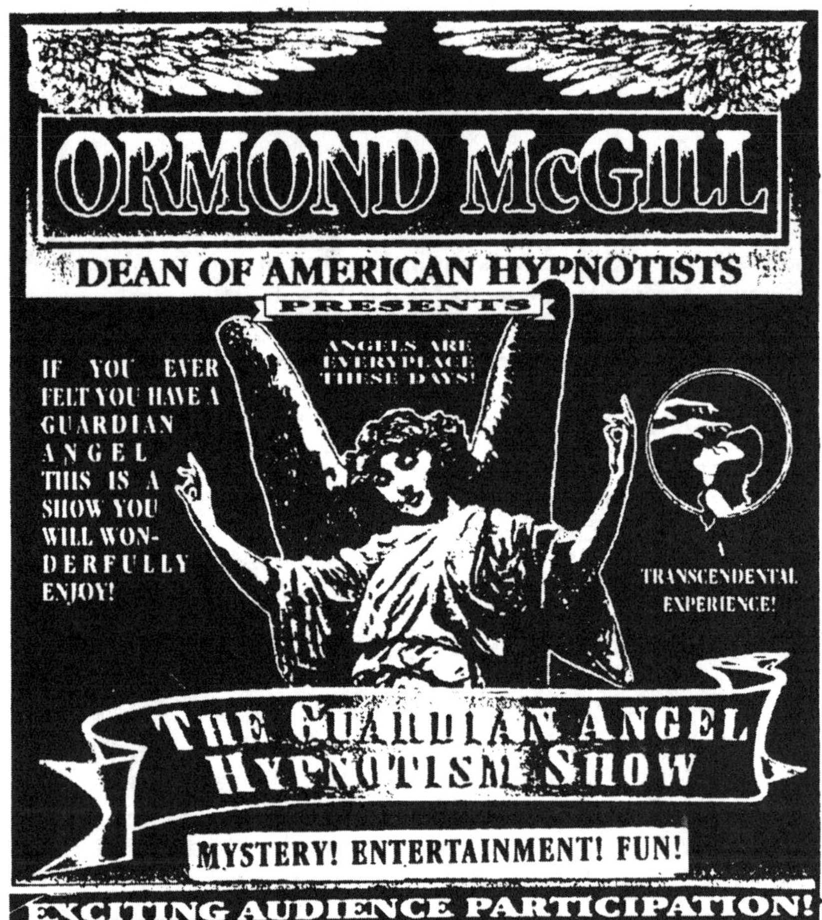

ORMOND McGILL
STAGE SCRIPT

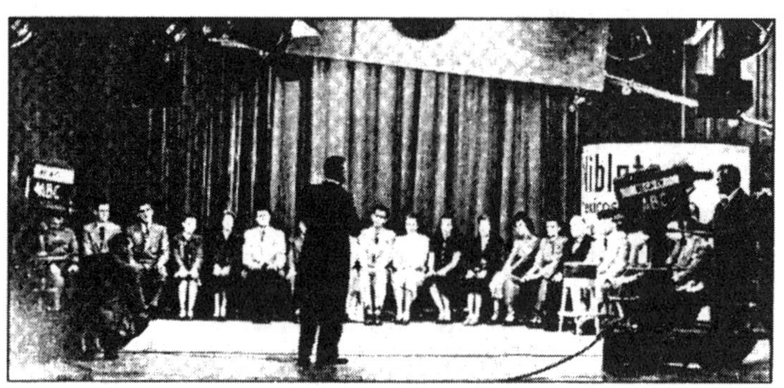

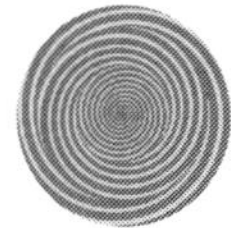

~ *Chapter 158* ~
THE GUARDIAN ANGEL HYPNOSIS SHOW

Includes
Guardian Angel Show Version One
Guardian Angel Show Version Two

The current popularity in angels prompted me to develop the Guardian Angel Hypnotism Show. Hypnotherapy is hypnosis directed towards therapeutic purpose. It is directed towards belief in Guardian Angels. It is spiritual. It is beautiful. It has great depth.

Presenting Hypnosis Shows is an extra source of income plus excellent publicity for your Clinical practice and good for business. Service Clubs such as Lions, Rotary, Kiwanis, and others are constantly on the lookout for interesting speakers at their weekly luncheons. A hypnotism lecture and demonstration is most welcomed. Many of the experiences can be used in your office as proof positive that hypnosis is a profound altered state.

MODUS OPERANDI: THE GUARDIAN ANGEL HYPNOTISM SHOW: Version One

You Will Need:
A Row Of Chairs For The Volunteers (However many the room allows.)
A Piece Of Paper At Each Seat In The Audience Explaining The Premise Of The Show
Music To Play Before The Show
    Like "Divine Lullaby," "I'll String Along With You," Or "I'm Looking For An Angel"
    (Sung by Nat King Cole)
A Small Crystal Ball
A Candle and something to light it
A Small Table

This show follows this routine:

1. PRE-SHOW GUARDIAN ANGEL PREMISE SHEET
Before the show begins, a "Guardian Angel Explanation Sheet' is placed on every seat in the auditorium and music is played. That way the guests have read about what to expect before the show and established an expectation for what is to follow. The paper gives an explanation of the premise of the show and also lets people know how to get in touch with me in the future.

The performer is introduced, takes a seat up front in the center of the stage and then gives a few moments of silence as they look upon the audience.

AUDIENCE TALK AND VOLUNTEERS VERSION 1

A brief dissertation explains things about angels, soothes the audience more fully to appreciate the show. This advanced understanding saves a lot of patter later. I begin by saying:

"Good evening Ladies and Gentlemen. As a professional internationally stage hypnotist for close to three quarters of a century, my shows were designed for entertainment fun and instructional information about hypnosis. In 1995, I created a hypnotism show around the theme of The Force, which concept was made popular by George Lukas' Star Wars trilogy. Two years following, it dawned on me to give attention to developing The Guardian Angel Hypnotism Show.

At no time in history have angels been more in public awareness than they are today. A recent survey affirmed that fully 65% of the American public believes in the existence of Guardian Angels, and 50% of these feel they had personal experiences of a Guardian Angel having intervened to help and even saved their life.

Angels seems to be a separate creation from humans. Apparently they live in a universe of higher vibration. We exist in a three dimensional universe bounded by length, breath, and height within a range of lower frequencies; the realm of angels appears as being multidimensional, and, as such, of higher frequencies. Thus being close to the God-Source and spiritual. Possibly that is why artists have portrayed them as having wings and halos.

The wall between the universe of angels and that of humankind is paper thin– only a matter of vibration. Higher vibrations can easily enter the lower, which possibly is why angels are so often felt by humans, and even occasionally seen in physical form. Their vibrational frequencies are very healing.

Love is the strongest force in the universe. Angels have been referred to as 'God's Messengers of Love.' Angels seem to have a love affair with human beings, and they elect to act as guide and guardian, helpful and protective. But their influence is never intrusive—often requested and allowed, and strongly founded in belief and faith.

Ask, **'How many in the audience believe in Guardian Angels?'**

(Dozens of hands go up.)

Those who believe that they have a Guardian Angel and who would like to have their Guardian Angel assist them now to achieve a remarkable hypnotic experience may join me on stage, to form a committee.

And so I invite upon my stage those who know they have a Guardian Angel to help them to use hypnosis to become masters of their mind and thus become a Mastermind…then miracles occur."

As volunteers come up and take their seats on stage play some Marching Music and a soft background of the Serenity Resonance Sound, which will be used throughout the show.

Turn to the volunteers and conduct your first instruction.

INDUCTION OF TRANCE FOR VOLUNTEERS

"Everyone relax and look at me. Those seated, place your feet flat on the floor and rest your hands in your lap. Those standing stand firm and erect while you relax.

Now grip hands and form a chain amongst yourselves. Everyone is clasping the hand of your neighbor and forming a chain. Now close your eyes and feel the force pass through you from hand to hand along the chain. Feel it strongly pass through you all.

Now, keep your eyes closed and release all hands and rest your hands in your lap or by your sides as we learn 'let's pretend hypnosis.'"

PRETENDING INDUCTION WITH A CRYSTAL BALL FIXATION

(Plays soft music) **Go back to a time when you were a playful child and loved to pretend. Possibly you pretended that you were Peter Pan or Wendy and could fly, or you were a super hero or cops and robbers or cowboys and Indians. You pretended so hard that what your pretended actually seemed real to you. Picture yourself in your mind's eye pretending strongly as the music plays.**

How wonderful and pleasant you feel. Those in the audience can try the experience along with those on stage, as you drop down into the abyss of your inner self. Drop into your subconscious now and go deep into the realm of hypnotic sleep. Sleep, sleep, sleep…go down sound asleep now in profound hypnosis…as you go deeper and deeper give a sigh of contentment and pleasure."

Observe the subjects sink into hypnosis and pick up a burning candle and hold it before you. As you talk to the audience:

"Ladies and gentlemen, when we think of consciousness, we tend to think of it as something inside your head but actually consciousness is wherever we wish to place it. I will show you."

Blow out the candle and put it aside as you address the committee of volunteers;

"Everyone continue going deeper and deeper into hypnosis as you become conscious of your hands. Lift your hands six inches up in the air and become conscious of the air around your hands.

Pause a moment to allow this suggestion to sink in.

Pretend that your hands are becoming very light and they rise up and up and up until your hands are straight out in front of yourself. Now experience a pulling on your extended hands as your guardian angel grips them and pulls you out of your seat…if you are one of those who are seated…until you are standing upright with your hands extended. And follow your guardian angel and walk forward a few feet."

As this is happening this is a subtle time to whisper to any unresponsive volunteers "Return to your seat in the audience to enjoy the show from there."

"You will find that your extended hands and arms have become so rigid that you cannot bend or lower them. They have become like steel. Try…try to bend or lower them and you will find it is impossible. Don't be concerned about it, just let your arms remain extended and I will relax them in a moment but for now their immobility is your reality."

(Subjects attempt to move their arms and this objective awareness of a subjective response to suggestion deepens hypnosis.)

"I will soon return you to being alert in the here and now, but first allow this suggestion to become rooted in your subconscious; every time I touch you in the center of your forehead…on the spot between your eyebrows…the sacred spot known in India as the Eye Of Shiva, you will instantly return to hypnosis going ten times deeper than you are now. You will drop into the abyss of your subconscious in profound hypnosis.

I will bring you back to the here and now and when you return you will be fully awake in every way except for your extended arms and hands which will still be fast asleep and even though the rest of yourself is wide awake, your hands and arms remain asleep until I personally come to you and blow upon them at which time they will awaken and you will find that they are normal in every way.

Get ready to arouse and come back awake and feeling fine ad you will find that your arms and hands are still asleep in the here and now, as your guardian angel guides you. One…two…three…four…five come on back. You find yourself fully aroused and your arms are still asleep and you cannot move them at all."

You can go to subjects and discuss this with them they talk and their arms are extended. Then blow on the arms and they drop down.

"Take your seats."

Talk to the audience:

"Ladies and gentlemen, give the members of this committee a rousing applause for their fine efforts in concentration and achieving hypnosis under the guidance of their guardian angel."

Watch your audience when you perform this induction. If any person in the audience is seen standing with their hands outstretched, bring them on stage to join the committee. They will willingly join in with the committee.

"We will now demonstrate instantaneous hypnosis, which is rarely seen. You may well remember it as long as you live. I will demonstrate the profound depth of hypnosis guardian angel hypnotism produces."

Place a chair in the center of the stage and select a responsive male subject and have them take this seat.

"Ladies and gentlemen, observe instantaneous hypnosis!"

Tap the person on their forehead and they instantly fall into the chair. Say to the man:

"In a moment I will arouse you from profound hypnosis and you will immediately run from this stage back to your seat in the audience and go fast asleep in your seat out there. Ready? One…two…three…four…five you are fully awake…

The subject will do as you have instructed.

Will two strong men from the audience please lift the hypnotized man from his chair and carry the body back to the stage and replace him in his chair here.

Thank them when they have completed the task and have them remain on stage, as you will need them for the next test. And say to the man who was returned to the stage.

I am going to bring you out of hypnosis now and your guardian angel has made it possible for you to achieve such a depth of hypnosis that you have no memory whatsoever of this exhilarating experience. When your friends tell you about what occurred you will not believe them. As far as your conscious recall is concerned, you were hypnotized in this chair on stage and awoke from the trance still sitting in this same chair. At the count of five you come back with me here on this stage together. One…two…three…four…five…

And to the audience **"After the show ladies and gentlemen, you can speak to this man and ask him about this experience and his answers will confirm how profound the depth of hypnosis that he achieved tonight as guided by his guardian angel."**

And now talk to all the volunteers:

"What you now witness is transcendental. Step forward in a row and these two gentlemen who are assisting me from the audience you will stand behind each one of the people on this committee as I stand before them and I will instantly hypnotize them. As they fall backward in a trance you will catch them and gently outstretch them to the floor. All ready."

Go to each in turn and tap their eye of Shiva as they fall back into the helper's arms and are laid in a line upon the floor. Suggest to the group on the floor when completed:

"You look and it seems as though you are dead, but of course you are not for you are fully protected by your guardian angel. However you cannot move in any way. You just lie there upon the floor immobile. What a wonderful opportunity you have now to marvel at a personal out of body experience for yourself. Allow it to happen and it will…you will seem to rise out of your physical body in invisible form and you will view it from an elevated position as it lies beneath you, as though in death and you marvel and are completely joyous and calm as you realize the truly divine and deathless being you are and that the body you

see lying before you on this stage is but the shell in which you dwell as you roam about the planet in 3-D.

As you do this, members of the audience are invited to walk around and over your outstretched bodies and without touching you or talking to you or trying to arouse you, you will find that you are not the least bit bothered."

Audience members can do just that as can your two male assistants.

"**Come back into your physical body now everyone.**"

Allow some moments for this to happen and play celestial music that fills the room.

"**Each of your guardian angels will arouse you now and you will awaken as though coming back from a deep sleep. You will arise, stand up and stretch yourself, feeling fine and well in every way. And as you leave the stage, you will see the dazzling rainbow colors that fill this room and note that every person in the audience has a golden halo resting on their head.**

Everyone now open your eyes and enjoy hearing about the wonderful transcendental experiences that the committee has had. Perchance their angel will touch you have seen this demonstration. And for my volunteers all that has happened here is just an exquisite dream.

Ladies and gentlemen, you come to appreciate that everything is a miracle and you are the greatest miracle of all. Good night I take leave now as the celestial guidance rules this room."

You exit

GUARDIAN ANGEL SHOW VERSION 2

AUDIENCE TALK AND VOLUNTEERS: THE FORCE

"**Good evening Ladies and Gentlemen and welcome to the Guardian Angel Hypnosis Show. In a few moments, I will invite a committee of volunteers from this audience who would like to experience and experiment with the wonderful science of hypnotism. As this is a very special kind of hypnotism show, I would like the members of this committee to consist of those of you who personally and sincerely feel that you have a guardian angel who helps you live a protected and productive life. We will ask each one's guardian angel to assist them on this stage to achieve a profound state of hypnosis to advance your talents.**

But first, I will show you how to bring the great cosmic force into yourself, which will be of great value to you in advancing your subconscious talents and strengthening your closeness to your guardian angel.

The force is cosmic in origin and is not something you create but is the power of the universe you can channel into yourself. George Lucas called it 'the Force' in his Star Wars Trilogy. My personal attention to the cosmic power was directed by the work of David St. Clair. He tells of first learning of it from a medium in the jungles of Brazil. A psychic in the States later confirmed this technique. I'll show you haw to use it for yourself. We will all do it together.

Everyone in the audience stand up. Put your feet slightly apart, your hands at your sides but not touching your body. Also make sure that you do not touch another person while performing this for yourself. I don't want your body to have any outside sensations. The incoming force alone is what I want you to experience.

Now, while standing, close your eyes and take a deep breath. We will say this affirmation out loud all together: 'I BRING THE COSMIC FORCE INTO MY BODY. INHALE AND HOLD YOUR BREATH… (Audibly inhale and hold your breath) **ASKING FOR STRENGTH, GUIDANCE, PROTECTION AND CLOSENESS TO MY GUARDIAN ANGEL…AND EXHALE. Now repeat this process three times.** (repeat the same three times).

Open your eyes. What do you feel? Did you feel something running into your body like electricity…some new sensation? Did you get a tingling in your spine…your face…your hands?

I now invite a selected group of persons upon the stage to occupy these chairs and form a committee to experience profound hypnosis. If you felt the force come into your hands and cause your fingers to tingle…if you feel that you have a personal guardian angel…if you wish to achieve profound hypnosis and advance your subconscious talents…I invite you to come on stage now in this space and time. Come and have a seat up here with me."

(After they have been seated, play soft music) **I will show you how to do 'let's pretend' hypnosis now. Start by going back to a time when you were a playful child and loved to pretend. Possibly you pretended that you were Peter Pan or Wendy and could fly, or you were a super hero or cops and robbers or cowboys and Indians. You pretended so hard that what your pretended actually seemed real to you. Picture yourself in your mind's eye pretending strongly as the music plays.**

Pretend, pretend, pretend! Pretend that your eyelids are stuck together so tightly that you cannot open them. You cannot open your eyes as hard as you try. As long as you keep pretending it is impossible to open your eyes as pretending becomes your reality.

Your eyes are closed. Squeeze them tightly together and pretend that they are stuck so tightly together that you cannot open them as hard as you try."

(Another version: "Pretend that your eyes are completely relaxed as you stare now at my crystal ball. Eventually your eyelids will just close and pretend that they are even more relaxed. Pretend that the relaxation you brought into your eyes now moves through your entire body. And notice how pretending becomes reality.")

"Now relax all over and sink down into your chair or, if you are standing, grip the back of the chair in front of you so you can easily stand and relax.

Know this: everything that you pretend to do upon this stage becomes that which you actually do. When I tell you to stop pretending and open your eyes, your eyes will open and I will show you some wonderful experiments in the power of pretending. Open your eyes now and come back here with me in the here and now."

Subjects eyes open.

OPTIONAL EXPERIENCES
Many of the following tests are covered in the hypnosis induction and convincers chapter 24 in more detail.

PROOF THEIR GUARDIAN ANGEL IS THERE
Have the seated volunteers stand in front of their chair with their eyes closed. Suggest, **"Guardian Angels, place your hands on each person's shoulders and push them back into their seat."**
(All fall backwards into their chairs.)

EXPERIENCE: FINGERS ARE STUCK TOGETHER
The volunteer's eyes will open and you are ready to proceed.
"Relax and look closely at me. Now place the tips of your fingers together and pretend that they are stuck together so tightly that you cannot pull them apart, try as hard as you will. The tips of your fingers have become welded together and you cannot separate your hands try as hard as you will. Try. Try hard. You cannot release your fingertips from each other. Pretending makes it so.

One by one I will go to each of you and blow upon your fingers and the welding will be removed and your hands will separate."

Blow upon each set of glued fingertips and they will come apart. When you come to the last person bring them forward to center front stage and you are ready to perform the topper of this test.

"To prove to you how firmly your fingertips are welded together, will a strong man kindly step forward and test the power as the guardian angel guards the grip." And to the man quietly, **"As you try to pull them apart do not jerk but exert a steady pull."**

The man comes forward as you instruct them to grasp the volunteer's wrists and instruct them to **"Pull and you will see how powerful is mind over body."**

A secret process is employed. While the person with the fastened fingertips is brought center stage, you move their hands close to their chest. To prove how firmly they are stuck the man comes up to grip the wrists and pull the hands apart as you explain that he is **"Not to jerk but is to exert a steady pull."**

The leverage is such that that even a child can resist a man.

After the strength of the welding has been tested, blow on the "welded" hands and they separate then send them to their seat on the stage and thank the strong man for coming up.

You then blow on their hands and they easily come apart.

EXPERIENCE: HAND STUCK ON YOUR HEAD

You can now try a similar experiment Bring one subject up from the group and instruct them, **"Close your eyes and pretend that you hand is stuck firmly on the top of your head. You cannot remove it as hard as you try."** To prove how stuck the hand is have a strong man come forward and stand behind the subject and grip the wrist to prove how stuck the hand is.

"You cannot remove their hand as hard as you try."

EXPERIENCE: THE MIRACLE OF THE MIND

You can now try an experiment to show the power of the strong man from the audience to **"Place your one fist stacked upon the other fist and clasp them together as strongly as you possibly can."** And say to the hypnotized person.

"Your forefingers as so strong and empowered that you can knock those clamped fists apart no matter how firmly they are clamped together." You clasp the subject's forefingers as if to energize them. The result is that they become so powerful that a mere sweep of their fingers knocks the clasped hands of the strong man apart. It surprises everyone.

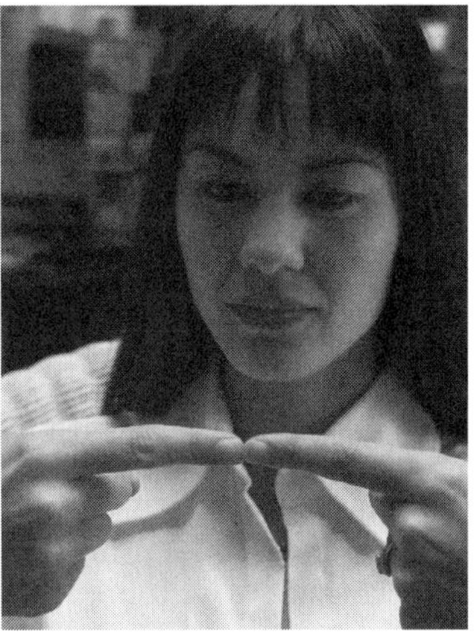

Fingers Stuck

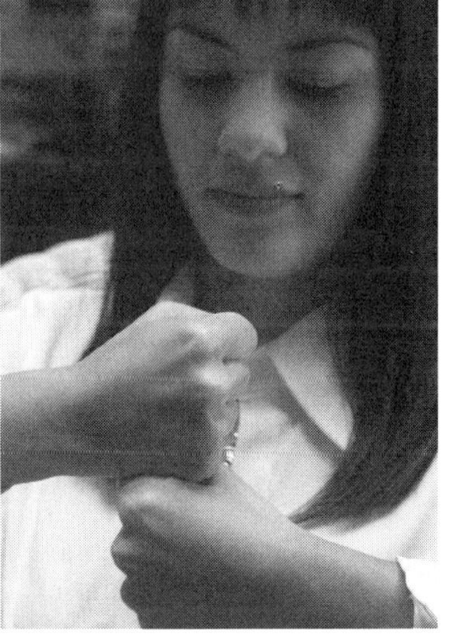

Should anyone challenge you and say that they can easily do the same, make a demonstration with yourself and use a little secret; at you clamp your clenched fists together you secretly grip your left thumb into the right fist. Do this so that it is unnoticed by the challenger. I will be impossible for them to pull apart.

EXPERIENCE: ANTIGRAVITY BODY LIFT.

Seat a hypnotized person in a chair center stage and have them close their eyes and think of their body becoming very heave. Heavy as lead or marble. Have four volunteers stand around the hypnotic subject and have them place their hands with pointer fingers extended side by side.

One of the four puts their two extended fingers under the persons left armpit, the second person places theirs under the right armpit and a third person under the left knee and the forth under the right knee. Tell them **"It is impossible to lift the seated person with your finger only because the person is using the power of their mind with hypnosis to be very heavy. Try to lift them and see for yourself."**

Now tell the group **"Now let me show you the hypnotic way to lose weight with antigravity. You'll notice that this next time the person will seem to float up in the air and it will seem like levitation. Arrange the group of lifters around the seated person. Everyone take a deep breath and now another and another three in unison. Okay, let's go. At the third breath held in your lungs when I say 'Go' you will make the lift all together and up goes the hypnotized person light as a feather. All right breathing in unison one, two, three hold it and 'go' light as a feather."**
The effect is astonishing.

EXPERIENCE: HANDS SHAKING

"Everyone would like to know how not to be self conscious and have complete abandon. Here is how to do that.

Everyone, all together, sit up straight in your chairs and hold your hands on each side of your head. Now start shaking them…shake them anyway they want to go…shake…shake…shake.

Now pretend that they won't stop shaking. Shake…shake…shake…and the more you try not to shake them the more they automatically shake."
(Play some bouncy music)
Now run down the line of volunteers and touch each on the knee and say, **"Just like your hands, your legs are shaking…they go up and down. Legs shake…legs shake…legs shake.**

As you shake, it prepares your mind and body to drop down into the wonderful 'let's pretend' relaxation that is next to come…as you drop far away…way down into profound hypnosis.

All right now, gradually simmer down…slow down…stop shaking and you are ready for the fun of 'let's pretend' being hypnotized."
To the audience you say, **"If there are those in the audience who would like to enjoy the experience of let's pretend, you can perform the process right along with those on the stage."**
Back to the volunteers, **"Gradually the shaking subsides. What a lot of fun that was and believe me after doing that, you will never be self-conscious again!**

You now have the energy to plunge into the depth of profound hypnosis as you come to know your subconscious talents and experience the divine nature of yourself."
(Soft music plays. A candle on a small table is placed before your subjects in the center of the stage.)

"Sit upright in your chairs. Place your feet flat on the floor and rest your hands in your lap so your fingers do not touch. Those standing behind hold on to the top of the chair in front to you. I light the candle. Now close your eyes for moment and visualize that your guardian angel stands beside you and gives you strength, guidance and protection of the power of the universe to be with you and aid you as you now enter the depth of your subconscious in profound hypnosis.

(Music drops off and silence prevails for a few moments. Then the music comes up again.)

"Open your eyes now and relax completely as you direct your attention fixedly upon the flickering candle flame that burns before you. Pretend that you are becoming that candle flame.

Keep staring, staring…staring into the candle flame and you will experience yourself drifting and dreamy, as you commence to enter the inner world of mind as you pass into the realm of sleep. At the count of three…take a deep breath with me now…

(All inhale deeply.)

Hold your breath deep in your lungs for a few moments. Exhale now and experience how sleepy you are becoming. Your eyes feel heavy and they want to close. But don't close your eyes yet, keep on staring at the candle flame and take one more deep, deep breath…

(All inhale deeply.)

Exhale now and get ready for the third and last deep breath just before your eyes close and you enter the realm of sleep and dreams.

All right breathing one, two, three…inhale now…hold the breath for a minute now exhale and your eyes will close as I count slowly from one to ten and slip down into the realm of sleep and pass into profound hypnosis under the loving guidance of your guardian angel.

(Count slowly from one to ten and all the eyes will close as your volunteers relax.)

Now everyone continue breathing slowly in and out and every breath you take takes sends you deeper and deeper into profound hypnosis. How pleasant and wonderful you feel. Those in the audience trying the experiences along with those on the stage fell it too as you drop down into the abyss of your inner self. Drop into your subconscious now and go deep into the realm of hypnotic sleep."

At this point the show goes pretty much like version #1.

Observe the audience and say to them:

"Ladies and gentlemen, when we think of consciousness, we tend to think of it as something inside your head but actually consciousness is wherever we wish to place it. I will show you."

(Blow out the candle and put it aside as you address the committee of volunteers;)

"Everyone continue going deeper and deeper into hypnosis as you become conscious of your hands. Lift your hands six inches up in the air and become conscious of the air around your hands.

Pause a moment to allow this suggestion to sink in.

Pretend that your hands are becoming very light and they rise up and up and up until your hands are straight out in front of yourself. Now experience a pulling on your extended hands as your guardian angel grips them and pulls you out of your seat…if you are one of those who are seated…until you are standing upright with your hands extended. And follow your guardian angel and walk forward a few feet."

As this is happening this is a subtle time to whisper to any unresponsive volunteers "Return to your seat in the audience to enjoy the show from there."

"You will find that your extended hands and arms have become so rigid that you cannot bend or lower them. They have become like steel. Try…try to bend or lower them and you will find it is impossible. Don't be concerned about it, just let your arms remain extended and I will relax them in a moment but for now their immobility is your reality."

(Subjects attempt to move their arms and this objective awareness of a subjective response to suggestion deepens hypnosis.)

"I will soon return you to being alert in the here and now, but first allow this suggestion to become rooted in your subconscious; every time I touch you in the center of your forehead…on the spot between your eyebrows…the sacred spot known in India as the Eye Of Shiva, you will instantly return to hypnosis going ten times deeper than you are now. You will drop into the abyss of your subconscious in profound hypnosis.

I will bring you back to the here and now and when you return you will be fully awake in every way except for your extended arms and hands which will still be fast asleep and even though the rest of yourself is wide awake, your hands and arms remain asleep until I personally come to you and blow upon them at which time they will awaken and you will find that they are normal in every way.

Get ready to arouse and come back awake and feeling fine ad you will find that your arms and hands are still asleep in the here and now, as your guardian angel guides you. One…two…three…four…five come on back. You find yourself fully aroused and your arms are still asleep and you cannot move them at all."

You can go to subjects and discuss this with them they talk and their arms are extended. Then blow on the arms and they drop down.

"Take your seats."

Talk to the audience:

"Ladies and gentlemen, let's give the members of this committee a rousing applause for their fine efforts in concentration and achieving hypnosis under the guidance of their guardian angel."

Watch your audience when you perform this induction. If any person in the audience is seen standing with their hands outstretched, bring them on stage to join the committee. They will willingly join in with the committee.

"We will now demonstrate instantaneously hypnosis, which is rarely seen You may well remember it as long as you live. I will demonstrate the profound depth of hypnosis guardian angel hypnotism produces."

Place a chair in the center of the stage and select a responsive male subject and have them take this seat.

"Ladies and gentlemen observe instantaneous hypnosis!"

Tap the person on their forehead and they instantly fall into the chair. Say to the man:

"In a moment I will arouse you from profound hypnosis and you will immediately run from this stage back to your seat in the audience and go fast asleep in your seat out there. Ready? One…two…three…four…five you are fully awake…

The subject will do as you have instructed.

"Will two strong men from the audience please lift the hypnotized man from his chair and carry the body back to the stage and replace him in his chair here."

Thank them when they have completed the task and have them remain on stage, as you will need them for the next test. And say to the man who was returned to the stage

"I am going to bring you out of hypnosis now and your guardian angel has made it possible for you to achieve such a depth of hypnosis that you have no memory whatsoever of this exhilarating experience. When your friends tell you about what occurred you will not believe them. As far as your conscious recall is concerned, you were hypnotized in this chair on stage and awoke from the trance still sitting in this same chair. At the count of five you come back with me here on this stage together. One…two…three…four…five…"

And to the audience **"After the show ladies and gentlemen, you can speak to this man and ask him about this experience and his answers will confirm how profound the depth of hypnosis that he achieved tonight as guided by his guardian angel.**

And now talk to all the volunteers:

"What you now witness is transcendental. Step forward in a row and these two gentlemen who are assisting me from the audience you will stand behind each one of the people on this committee as I stand before them and I will instantly hypnotize them. As they fall backward in a trance you will catch them and gently outstretch them to the floor. All ready."

Go to each in turn and tap their eye of Shiva as they fall back into the helper's arms and are laid in a line upon the floor. Suggest to the group on the floor when completed:

"You look and it seems as though you are dead, but of course you are not for you are fully protected by your guardian angel. However you cannot move in any way. You just lie there upon the floor immobile. What a wonderful opportunity you have now to marvel at a personal out of body experience for yourself. Allow it to happen and it will…you will seem to rise out of your physical body in invisible form and you will view it from an elevated position as it lied beneath you, as though in death and you marvel and are completely joyous and calm as you realize the truly divine and deathless being you are and that the body you see lying before you on this stage is but the shell in which you dwell as you roam about the planet in 3-D.

As you do this members of the audience are invited to walk around and over your outstretched bodies and without touching you or talking to you or trying to arouse you, you will find that you are not the least bit bothered."

Audience members can do just that as can your two male assistants.

"Come back into your physical body now everyone."

Allow some moments for this to happen and play celestial music that fills the room.

"Each of your guardian angels will arouse you now and you will awaken as though coming back from a deep sleep. You will arise, stand up and stretch yourself, feeling fine and will in every way. And as you leave the stage, you will see the dazzling rainbow colors that fill this room and note that every person in the audience has a golden halo resting on their head.

Everyone now open your eyes and enjoy hearing about the wonderful transcendental experiences that the committee has had. Perchance their angel will touch you have seen this demonstration. And for my volunteers all that has happened here is just an exquisite dream.

Ladies and gentlemen you come to appreciate that everything is a miracle and you are the greatest miracle of all. Good night I take leave now as the celestial guidance rules this room."

You exit.

OVERVIEW OF EXPERIMENTS:
Fingertips Locking:
Pretend you can't pull them apart and releasing when you blow upon their fingers. One person shows a "test of strength" demonstration with a strong guy from the audience.

Hand Stuck On Your Head:
Suggest that their hand is stuck on the top of their head. And as a test of strength have someone else try to lift it off.

Antigravity Body Lift
Four persons surround hypnotized person and perform the lift.

Hand Shaking Experience

Candle Flame Profound Hypnotic Induction

Placement Of Consciousness
Standing… Moving Forward
Post-Hypnotic Arms Rigidity
Post Hypnotic Return To Trance. Release.
Instantaneous Hypnosis On Subjects One By One

OPTIONS FOR MORE FUN

Angels allow some fun.
"You are at an Hawaii luau and having so much fun laughing."

 "Let your angel take you on a trip to Hawaii."
(Play "Lovely Hula hands" **"As the music plays you are a beautiful hula dancer
and when the music stops you freeze. The music makes you move again."**
(Music resumes as they dance again.)

Bounce In Chair

Whirling Arms

Invisible Hypnotist

Taking The Cherubs On A Trip To Mars

Awaken

Back To Sleep

Lying Down On Floor

Dance With Your Angel (Blue Danube Waltz)

Stuck To Floor

Back To Seat And Seeing Auras

Sit With Your Angel And Go To Sleep

Personal Awakening Of Each Person In Audience

Background Music Divine Lullaby

End Of Show

Finale Music

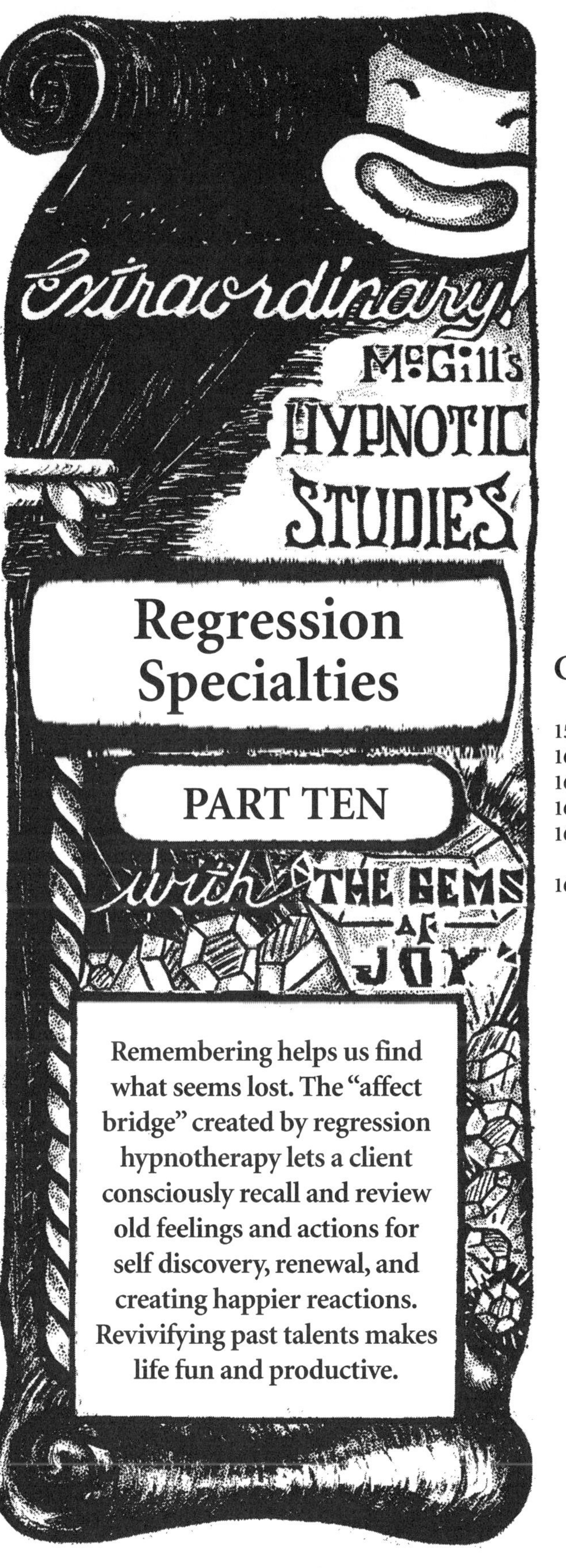

Remembering helps us find what seems lost. The "affect bridge" created by regression hypnotherapy lets a client consciously recall and review old feelings and actions for self discovery, renewal, and creating happier reactions. Revivifying past talents makes life fun and productive.

CHAPTERS IN PART TEN

159. Regression & Hypnoanalysis ......page 623
160. Fantasy Hypnoanalysis 625
161. Stop Stuttering 629
162. Evidence of Previous Life Times..........633
163. Previous Life
       Regression Hypnotherapy....................641
164. The Question Of Karma 649

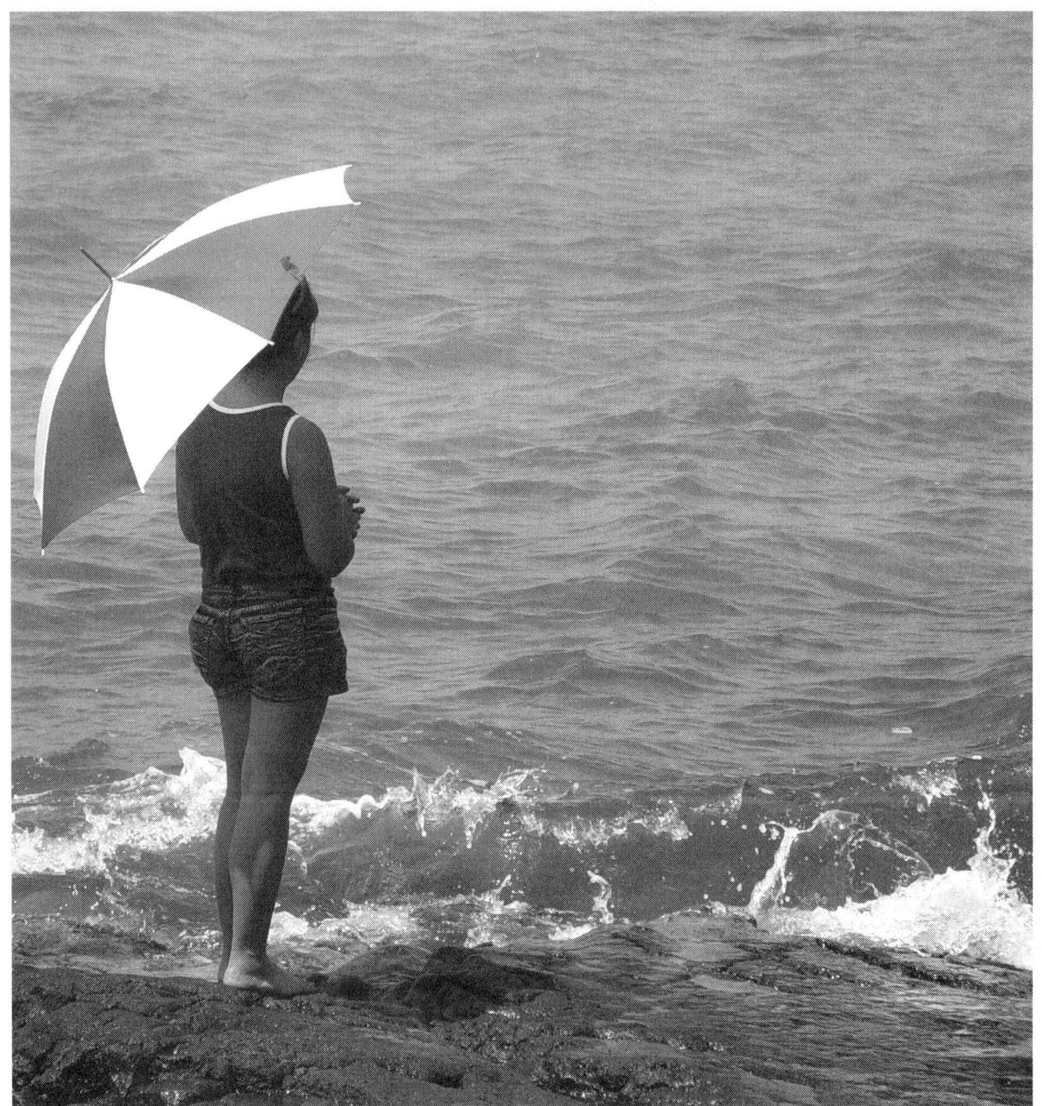

Photo by Jon Nicholas

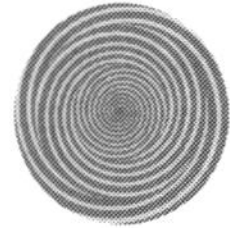

~ *Chapter 159* ~
REGRESSION & HYPNOANALYSIS

Includes
How To Be A Terrific Regression Hypnotherapist
Meet Your Inner Child

HYPNOANALYSIS

Hypnoanalysis regresses the client to earlier periods in this lifetime to uncover any buried subconscious experiences that produce neurotic behavior in the here and now. It is delightful to regress a client back to subconscious imprints that enhance beneficial behavior. Many re-experience their gestation and birth as well as every minute of their lives. The goal of current lifetime regression is commonplace. It teaches more about who you are in the here and now, heals past hurts, releases current pain, and renews or forgives old acquaintances.

1. Encourage any hurtful experiences to be witnessed as a spectator in an impersonal manner.
2. Let the client know that you are with them every moment as a supportive friend.
3. Suggest that in the discovering and telling of the experience it will lessen and remove any negative influence of the event.
4. Allow the subject to probe their own subconscious memory and discover for themself the original source of their trouble. When they make such a personal discovery they recite it to you, and you record it.
5. Finally, upon awakening, offer a post-hypnotic suggestion that if they listen to the recording of their past memory, which is the source of his current problem, that the very listening will lessen any problems. And when they listen to memories that positively enhance their lives those gifts will grow stronger within them.

This is wonderful hypnotherapy. The client gently and pleasantly awakens from the hypnosis feeling fine. The tape is played for them, and with the playing, the post-hypnotic suggestion of his being cured of the neurosis goes into effect. Just allow the subconscious to be its own healer. Give the tape to the client; every time he plays it, it is helpful to him, until the removal of the neurosis is complete. This is the general pattern for safely dealing with Previous Life Regressions as well.

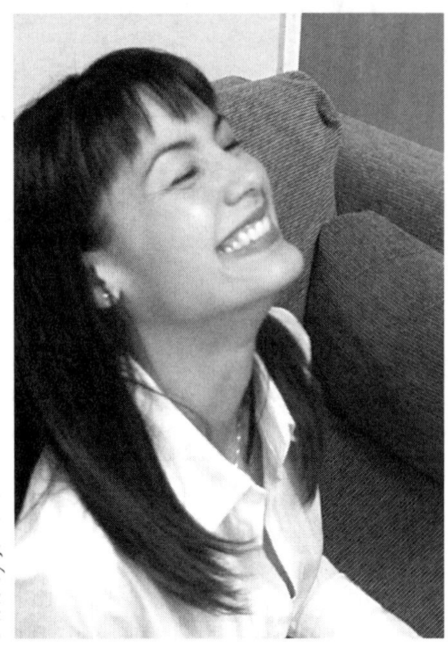

MODUS OPERANDI:
MEET YOUR INNER CHILD

A beautiful thing about regression hypnotherapy is the reconnection with your instinctual feelings of fun, fulfillment and your desires. Your inner child is your essential natural self just waiting to be greeted. Regression can bring forth that vital self who then becomes a valuable ally. Hypnotize your client and suggest,

"Create for yourselves a perfect sanctuary. A place enjoyed by all your senses. Created just to your specifications; just the way you like it, made perfectly for you.

Now in your own time and way notice the presence of the little you; the one who came here to this earth perfect in every way. Very good. (You could actually give your client a pillow or doll to hold during this entire process.)

Now from your heart ask the little you what they would like to tell you.

Ask them what they do for fun.

What would they like to do when they grow up?

Do they have any complaints? If so, let them tell you and answer them. Very good.

How can you support your inner child to be in their full energy and joy?

How can they support you?

Tell each other how much you love one another.

You and your inner child now work as a perfect team. Each teaches the other, new ways to be happy, healthy creative, and joyous. Very good. And then when the time is right you will come back to the here and now knowing that you are and always have been perfectly you and feeling so glad to be alive.

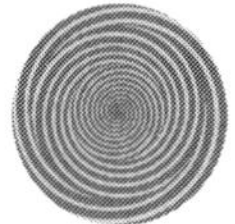

~ *Chapter 160* ~
FANTASY HYPNOANALYSIS

Includes
The Structure of Hypnoanalysis
Overcoming Fear (Of Cats)

Fantasy Hypnoanalysis is closely associated with Previous Life Regression. It, too, must be handled correctly or revived traumatic memory may cause anguish. This method can be safely used in dealing with all forms of regression hypnotherapy.

Most neurosis stems from hurtful past experiences. The original cause is long past yet its unconscious memory still unreasonably disturbs us. The mind hides painful memory by burying them deeply in the subconscious. That's why hypnosis is such an effective approach to bring it into open conscious awareness. Your client's subconscious mind knows the suppressed source of a fear, and simply and safely guides them through painful key sensitizing events, to remove negative energy and reframe the neurotic response.

Let's say that a fellow with an unreasonable fear (phobia) of enclosed places comes to see you. He may be unconsciously reacting to a buried childhood memory. As a child, for example, he may recall being locked in a dark closet and nearly suffocating. Though the original trauma is long forgotten consciously, it manifests in an automatic response fear to closed spaces now. This is similar to a posthypnotic suggestion, where an idea given in the past manifests spontaneously in the present.

The entire session is a "remedy" for the client. Rather than an upsetting re-experience, they became a neutral witness to a scene from the past. There is no emotional disturbance. The client is relieved and helped.

THE STRUCTURE OF HYPNOANALYSIS
A session has the following structure:
1. **Regress the Client**
   Take the person back to the source of their problem

2. **Reframe the Problem**
   The safest way to heal a revived traumatic memory is to suggest that the client rise above or detach from the experience. A disagreeable experience viewed in an impersonal and even entertaining manner loses its emotional power.
   Suggest: **"Rise above the image or thoughts of you __________ (in the closet for example)"** or **"Witness the event as a motion picture upon the screen"** or
   "Review it like a storybook incident."
   You can further add to this detached fantasy effect by suggesting that: **"Whatever you observe will be taken lightly and you see the humor in it."** Laughter gives the subject a release mechanism. The association of humor with the phobia, causes fear to vanish.

MODUS OPERANDI: FANTASY HYPNOANALYSIS TO OVERCOME FEAR (of cats)

Observe carefully how the suggestions are handled in the entire process:

Suppose that during the client interview, the person reveals an unreasonable fear of cats. Place the subject in a deep state of hypnosis and, when possible, in profound hypnosis. This produces stronger posthypnotic effects and amnesia upon awakening.

Study this "suggestion formula" carefully.

"We are going to play a game together and you will have some fun. You say you have a fear of cats (or whatever). **That means that sometime back in your past, you must have experienced something with cats that produced fear. By facing that fear and bringing it to the surface, the fear will vanish completely.**

What makes this so interesting is that you are going to probe your mind to find the cause of your fear, and when you find that cause, you will be completely impersonal about it. You'll see the happening as though you are witnessing an event upon a motion picture screen.

No matter what you see, it will seem to be happening outside of yourself, and you watch it happening as a fun adventure. In fact, you'll laugh that you have been uncomfortable about cats. This is just a game we play together that is enjoyable and fun. You will be absolutely impersonal about whatever you bring from out of your memory, and will enjoy observing it.

Go back in your memory now, seeing the humor in the situation. Discover for yourself the origin of your feelings about cats (or whatever). What happened that caused your phobia. Remember always, the past is but a memory of things that will never happen again. You live your life in the here and now."

A phobia is a fearful memory from the past that you have taken seriously in the present. Now that you can witness your memory in this way you can keep it where it belongs in the past and will never happen again."

The client journeys back inside of himself to locate the experience that caused his phobia. When discovered, it is again suggested that the incident will be as though viewed as a "funny motion picture."

Do not tell your client where or what time to go back into. Allow the subconscious freedom to drift there by itself.

The "suggestion formula" continues…

"What you see or remember is now before you as a motion picture. A motion picture of an event which happened years ago and has no purpose in your current living."

Next, suggest that the client speak up and relate the story of the scene as they observe it. Report it in a detached and calm way.

"This very telling of this story recalled and told from memory will remove any traumatic effects from further affecting your life. Speak up now and tell me the story of how you see the scene enacted before you in this motion picture, and as you tell the story to me, its effects upon you all drop away and vanish."

Finally, you repeat the suggestion, **"Tell me the story now of what you see."**

The subject recounts the story of the happening of what caused his original trauma, but it comes through to him as a witnessed experience and not a disturbing one, while, at the same time, the telling removes the "power" of the traumatic experience that has for so long been locked in his subconscious. The precise story the subject tells depends upon the particular case.

"You may remove yourself from hypnosis anytime you desire by raising your right forefinger a fraction of an inch. If you do you will immediately come out of the hypnosis feeling well and fine."

The story told is of a real traumatic incident, which happened in the past, but is hypnotically transformed from being personal to being impersonal. This phobia of cats continues:

"What an interesting story you have told me of how your fear of cats developed; you have told it to me as you have witnessed it upon your mental picture screen."

Now comes an important series of suggestions which associates the impersonal viewing of the event with a "tying-in" of the event as an actual experience in the subject's life from out of the past, incorporating in it a "healing" of the trauma at the same time.

"It has been impersonal to you, and yet you know that it is your story based upon an incident in your life which occurred long ago. An incident that affected you deeply at that time and which you buried away in the depth of your memory, but now that you see it in this time and space, and observe it objectively, it has lost its emotional impact over you, and you simply see it now as an event that occurred long ago and is no more. All these years, because of that incident, you have had an unreasoning fear of cats, but now that you see it objectively, that fear is gone, and a cat is just a cat to you now – no more, no less."

You now go into the awaking from hypnosis process which process is combined with suggestions of happiness of being freed from the phobia.

"In a moment, I will awaken you from this deep hypnosis, and you will awaken feeling well and fine, feeling so glad that that which has disturbed you for so long is all gone now, and you are so happy to be freed of this phobia."

Finally, the session is concluded with some direct suggestions of removing the trauma, such as, **"From this time on, your fear of cats is gone, Gone, GONE!"** The client is pleasantly aroused. The posthypnotic goes into effect, and the phobia has been healed.

You will observe in this the "compounding of suggestions"– the awakening from hypnosis reinforcing the suggestions of the removal of the phobia. These suggestions are then reemphasized, and finally the posthypnotic suggestion is given the subject to say, "Here kitty, kitty, kitty," combined with ending the session on a good laugh. There is powerful impact in this handling: a phobia is a serious thing; in reversing it into humor, it loses its power to further cause neurotic disturbance.

The subject awakens, following these suggestions, gently and pleasantly, and feeling fine. The posthypnotic goes into effect, and he says impulsively, and possibly even to his own surprise, **"Here kitty, kitty, kitty."** You both get a good laugh from it, and the session is over. The entire session has been a "therapy" for the subject, but handled in this manner as a witnessing of the traumatic experience from out of the past rather than as a re-experiencing of the experience. There is no disturbance, and yet the subject has been helped tremendously. Through the proper use of this technique, the "power of the incident" has been taken away from unduly further disturbing the person.

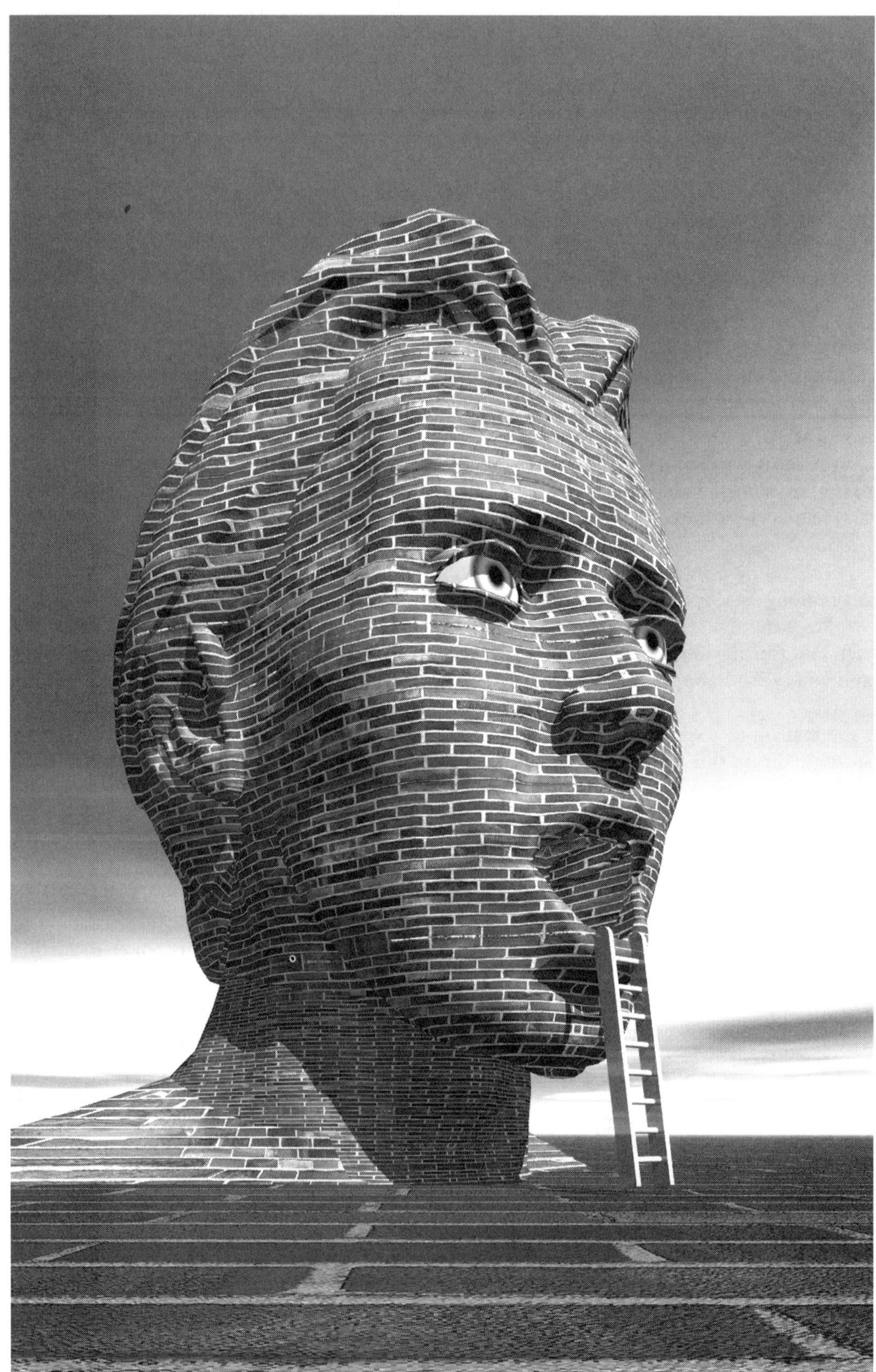

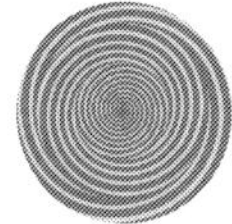

~ *Chapter 161* ~
STOP STUTTERING

Includes
Regression Therapy For Stuttering
Thompson's Stop Children From Stuttering

Regression hypnotherapy seeks out mental causes for various current complaints. Often these are of a physical nature and the cause seems unexplainable. Generally speaking, such are caused by traumatic experiences suffered by the person at an early age in this current lifetime. Some may be traced to previous lifetime (more on that in the next chapter).

As time moves on, the memory of the unhappy event slips from conscious memory and becomes established in the subconscious mind causing disturbing behavior patterns that continue in current space and time.

In general when using regression hypnotherapy as a healing method the client is hypnotized and it is suggested that the buried memory or event of the past be recalled and surfaced to conscious awareness. This is sometimes results in reliving and re-experiencing the past trauma or defining moment that is manifest in the present. Locating subconscious material is easy for your biocomputer. Memory is easily retrieved and called forth by a direct request. As long as the affect is known the cause will surface.

Tars are frequent when recalling, remembering and reliving early trauma and well worth it as it produces a cure. You handle effects to find causes. Once the cause becomes consciously known and the hidden hurt is removed, healing is on its way…sometimes in an instant.

MODUS OPERANDI: REGRESSION THERAPY FOR STUTTERING

Stuttering is a familiar form of human difficulty. There is no such thing as a congenital stutterer. No one is born a stutterer. It is something learned. Usually it starts when a person is very young and it grows from a variety of causes. A psychic wound can be caused by adults hushing them and rejecting their ability to speak.

Dave Elman empathized with "the deep anguish and frustration the stutterer goes through… the difficulty expressing what they want to say, makes it so hard to speak with freedom. The more they try the worse they get. Few who do not stutter understand the turmoil within the heart of those who do. Some even think it's funny."

Dave did not think it funny and worked out hypnotic methods to help them. "When someone tells you 'be quiet, no one wants to hear you speak' long enough" he said, "the subconscious gets the idea and sure enough stuttering starts. The child speaks in a way that nobody wants to hear."

Stuttering may also start as an imitation of someone the child respects who stutters…a mother, father, or close friend. Most, but not all, stuttering begins in childhood and subsides as a person matures.

Begin by having an intimate conversation with the client and ask the person why they think they stutter. Then hypnotize them and ask the subconscious to tell their story. No need to tell the stutterer to stop stuttering that creates resistance. Instead suggest

"Now that you have gotten to the reason why you stutter, it will bring you a great relief and you will notice an inner calm within you. It had taken a burden off your heart and now gradually you will find that you stutter less and less. So gradually that you will scarcely know that you have stopped stuttering. Suddenly it will dawn on your inner self, 'I'll be darned, I'm not stuttering anymore.'"

THOMPSON'S STOP CHILDREN FROM STUTTERING

Hypnotherapist Niccolous Thompson uses this script for children who stutter it is excerpted from his book "Hypnotherapy For Children"

"I know for a while _________ (child's name) **that you have had some trouble saying a few words and that there are other words you say perfectly, and I know how you must feel when those other words do not come out right, so I am going to help you to speak perfectly. Is that okay with you?** (Wait for approval).

Great, then listen closely to me and you will see you will be able to speak perfectly in just a few minutes, and I know you must be excited, so here we go…(pause…wait for anticipation to build in the child…)

Okay, Imagine that there are two huge chalkboards in front of you, one on the left and one on the right. Do you know which is your right? Very good!

The chalkboard on the right is filled with all the words that seem to be jumbled, those are the words you USE-to have trouble with, the ones on the left are all the words you say perfectly, so we do not want to bother the ones on the left. What we want to do is to move the words you USE-to have trouble with on the right, and move them to the left. After we move one word, we will test to make sure it went into the right place on the left, understand everything so far?

(Again…wait for a nod, or a child might say "yes", then proceed)

Okay, think of a word that you have had trouble saying that you see on the right…Do you see it? (Wait for a yes)

What is the word? (Wait for the word…they may stutter it and that is just fine at this moment, however, most DO NOT stutter when in hypnosis)

Let's move the word to the board on the left now…good…is it in the right spot? (Wait for response) **Great…now say the word and you will notice you will not stutter, or have problem with this word again. Cool huh? Let's do another word…**

(Do a few more words, having them say the words and then proceed)

Good, now over the next few days __________ (Child's name) **practice any other words we may have not noticed before, so if find that there is a word that is hard to say…close your eyes and move it to the left board, and it will never bother you again, you will be able to say it anytime you want with no problems. And in school you will feel so proud to be able to speak with others with no problems at all, in fact you will even find you will be able to be a better student because of how well you speak."** (This last suggestions has nothing to do with intellect, it has to do with confidence…now…do a simple wake up procedure…)

"At the count of three open your eyes, and notice how big your smile gets with each count…one…it is getting bigger…two…big smile…and…three open your eyes, what a great smile…"

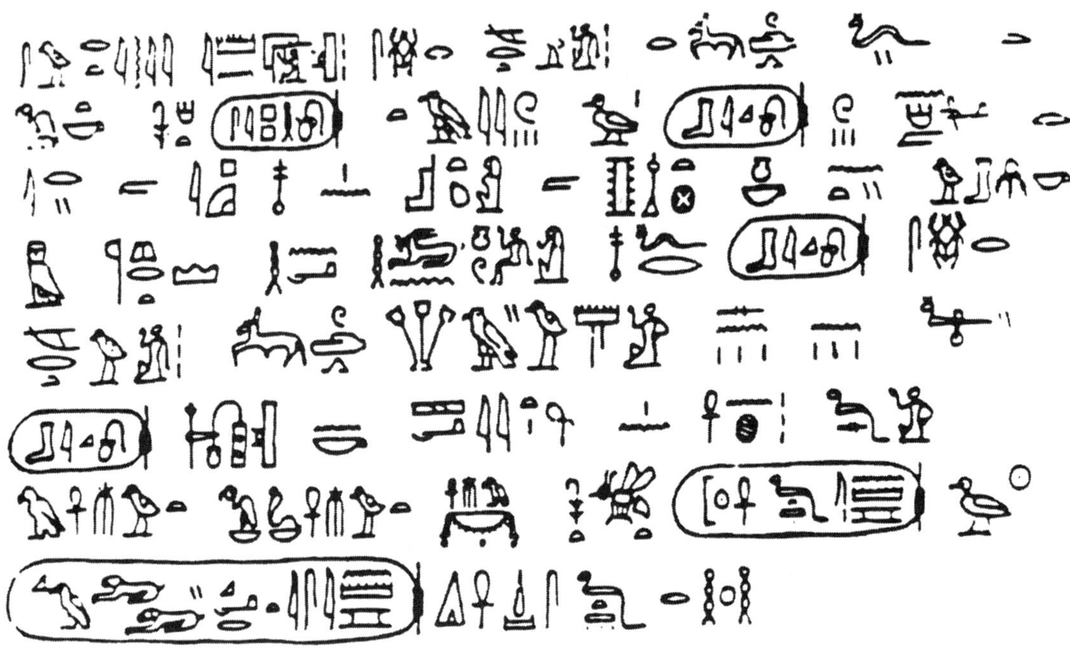

Hieroglyphs written during hypnosis regression.

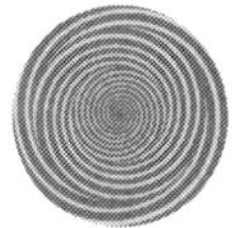

~ *Chapter 162* ~
EVIDENCE OF PREVIOUS LIFETIMES

Excerpted from "The Many Lives Of Alan Lee" by Ormond McGill with Irvin Mordes

Includes
The Alan Lee Regressions

Do you believe in reincarnation? Half the world does. After all, it is a consistent concept easy to accept when one realizes it occurs within oneself this very minute. This very moment something dies and is reborn within you. As life moves along every cell in you body will be exchanged for another. You are continually becoming a NEW BEING.

The entire universe follows this pattern. A star is born and exists for eons of time yet eventually dies to become a black hole in space. It rests and then it is reborn as a new star in the heavens. I believe that you are like that too. This is a supposition. When doing the helpful work of past life regression there has always been the question, "Is it fantasy or reality?" Often the hypnotherapist replies, "It makes no difference. Its healing power is the important thing."

None-the-less we would like to know the true facts. The case of Alan Lee, a Caucasian man born in Philadelphia May 4th 1942, provides the best objective evidence of the fact of reincarnation. Alan Lee never completed school beyond the tenth grade and never had learned any other language besides English.

In research conducted at Maryland Psychiatric Research Center 1974 Alan was regressed to sixteen previous lives by professional hypnotist Irvin Mordes. All of the sessions were witnessed and affirmed by the physicians and researchers who affixed their signatures: Walter Tauke, MD, Jerome Rubins, MD, Edward L. Reed, MD, Ruth Martin, John H. Metzinger, Victor Schlector, MD, Walter Panhnke, MD.

With each previous life regression came an uncanny ability to speak and write in the language of whatever period of history he was re-experiencing. Half of the languages he expressed, not been taught for centuries, were checked for accuracy. In the hypnotic state Alan spoke and wrote fluent American English, rural English, ancient English, Italian, Cherokee Indian (Tehalgic), Norman French, idiomatic Latin, classic Greek, Hebrew, Egyptian Hieroglyphics, Egyptian Demotic, Egyptian Hieratic, Atlantian and Lumarian. He was regressed back each time and requested to write a description of his memory in the manner of the writing of the time. The ancient scripts of his handwriting are persuasive factual evidence of previous lives.

During this study Alan's vital signs were carefully monitored. His blood pressure would suddenly drop from his normal 120 over 80 to 60 over 30 and his pulse decreased. Such a reaction may be normally associated with a state of shock but no such thing occurred. He was fine in every way.

The small book *The Many Lives Of Alan Lee* that recounts this research in detail is an excellent and interesting item to leave in the waiting room for clients to read while they wait.

The study of Past Lifetimes brings peace of mind, as each lifetime is a progressive step in the advancement of the soul. When doing regressions there seems to be indifference as to the person's social position. Some may be famous some obscure, yet all seem to teach how to live and how to recognize the immortality of the individual.

THE ALAN LEE REGRESSIONS

RUDOLPHO GUGIELMI (Rudolph Valentino) Italy/USA

Recalled this famous silent pictures movie star from Italy and described his death experience. This was later compared to the medical records at New York Polyclinic Hospital where Valentino died and were precise in the details relived. The sign compared by handwriting exerts matched. Here is the sample of the writing.

JAMIE BREWSTER Atlanta Georgia, USA
Recalled a poorly educated man who spoke with a rural southern accent, who died on May 2, 1847 during the Civil War in Gettysburg. Here is a sample of his writing. Note the rustic spelling.

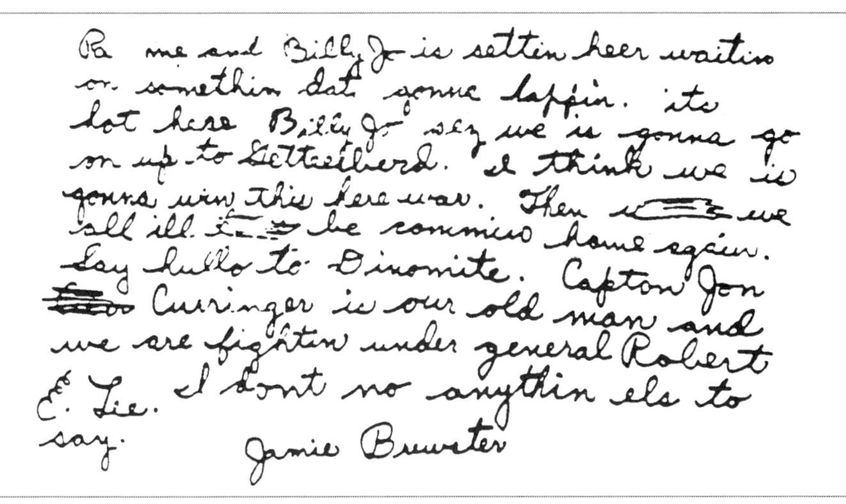

SEQUOYA North American Indian
Born in Stone Mountain April 22, 1788 and died April 30, 1847 Sequoya was a member of the Tehalagi (people of a different speech) Indians. His message was interpreted by a now living tribal elder as meaning "Something is wrong. I broke my leg." The message is signed "S. Siguoya, Tieloki."

APOLLODORUS DELPHUS VINDICTUS Ancient Greece, Dates unknown
He said he was a General and was beheaded for treason.

LEO VINCEY England, born 1761, died 1788 (The year Seqouya was reportedly born)
An archivist at largest newspaper in Southampton verified the name and location of the named "Holy Road Cemetery on the east side of High Street in Southampton." And said that "Unfortunately an burial records from that time were destroyed in the 1942 blitz."

Facts of his life were also verified. varified were the Reverend Richard Mant's Grammar School on East Street which later moved to High Street and "Mr. Ward's Academy of Young Gentlemen at the foot of High Street with lessons including fencing, dancing and French"

Affirmed as accurate were the names and time frames like "Hampshire Chronicle, the first newspaper published in Southampton and knew its founder, Sir James Linden," "was engaged to Virginia Cox whose father ran a couch line which ran from Southampton's Vine Inn to London." "Did his banking at Sadlier and Company owned by his friend Richard V. Sadlier" and he named eleven streets in Southampton.

GUILLAUME (DUC DE NORMANCIE) France/England born in Falaise 1027, died 1087
He said he became William I, King of England and wrote this message dated April 15, 1068:

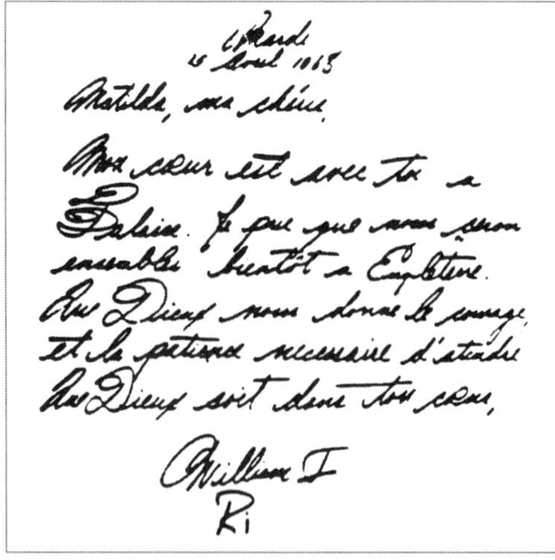

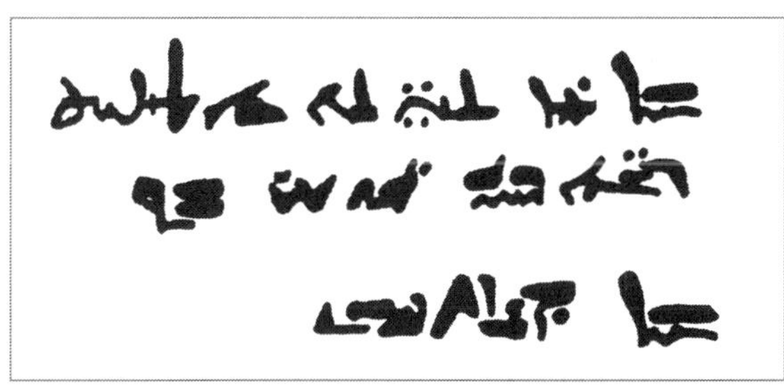

Valentinianus, Emperor in Ancient Rome 321 – 375 A.D. sample writing.

YOSEPHUS Ancient Palestine
He said he was a Hebrew slave during the time of Nazarene and present at the trail of Jesus.

SENEWE Ancient Egypt, Born 1391 B.C., Died 1339 B.C.
The son of a physician to pharaoh, he became a physician to Pharaoh Amenhotep IV (who later was known as Akhenaten) His message written in Egyptian Script says: "I am physician to Pharaoh. I am Senewe."

KALLIKRATES Complete name; Suten Net Rekh Ankh Ankn Tchetta Meri Amen Se Rekh Kallinkrates Meri Amenn) Ancient Egypt,

Born in Thebes 369 B.C., Died in Libya Africa 339 B.C. he became the last Pharoah of Tamarekh (Egypt) in 344 B.C. and ruled for two years when he fled "the invasion of Ochas (Atraxerxes III) and the Persians.

Here is what was written:

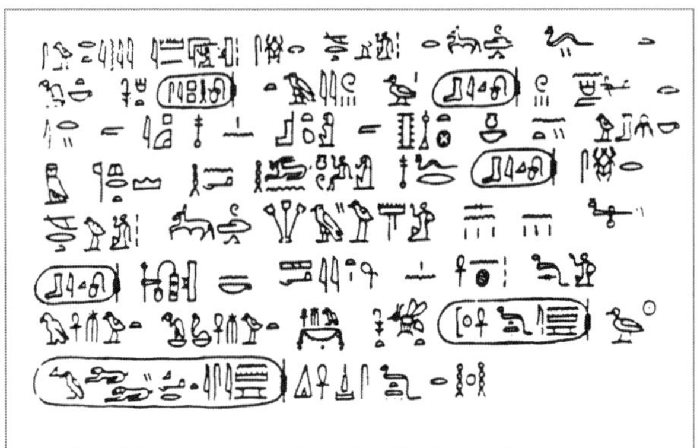

ADONNA Atlantis

This woman was born in "Tashone" in Atlan (Atlantis) during the days of "Helioca." She said that she was "responsible for putting the giant subtetron (a giant energy crystal) to its full test. The Subtetron exploded, causing the destruction of Atlan." She tired to make her way to the mountain tops of Aseers but was overtaken by volcanic fumes, fire, water and lava." Her message as written: "The people of Atlan have come from the house beyond the sun."

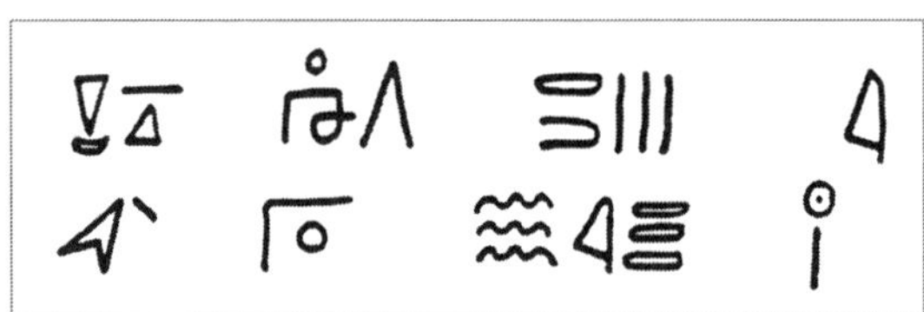

MANAMETER, Atlantis born in Metiat-Aseer in Atlan, birth and death unknown
His writing sample:

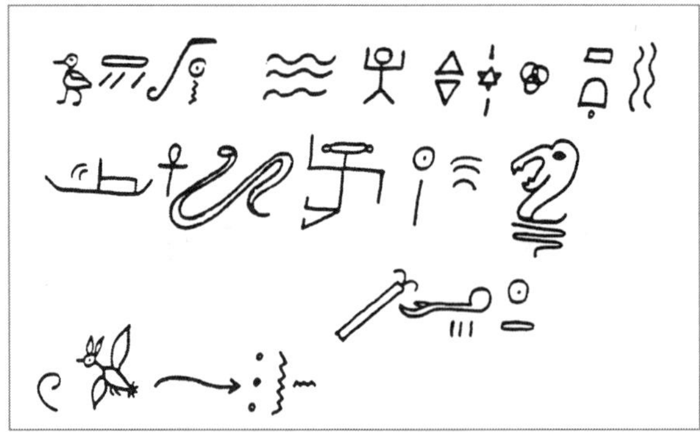

AGON, lived in Mu

He was leader of his village and proclaimed that the son of his son, Agonor would rue the Mu Empire and unite all of Mu. His son never lived to fulfill the prophesy and he wrote in his local script:

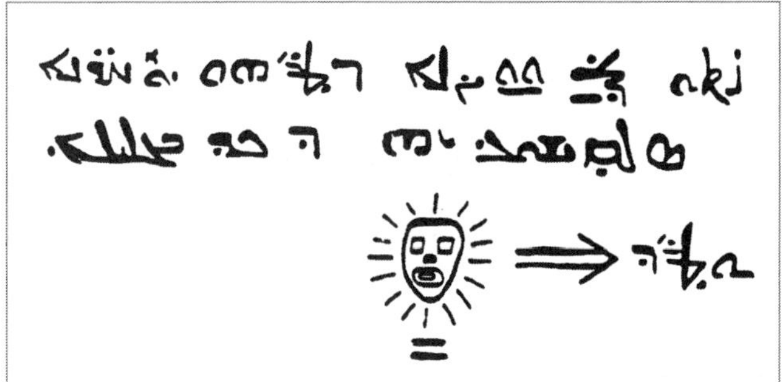

AGONORUS

Described his lifetime as "back in time frame adjacent to Atlantis" he was leader of his village and become king of all Mu and ruled from the city of Hanakai. He died in a great tidal wave and Mu sunk beneath the waters of the Pacific. When "the gods became angry and took back the lands into the great waters."

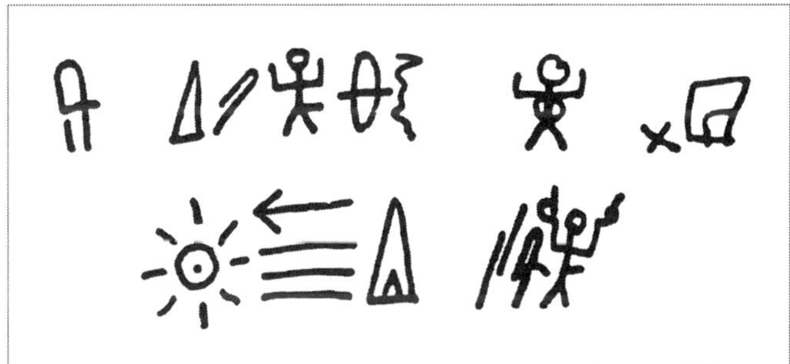

TIME
TRAVEL
The
Do-It-Yourself
Past Life
Journey
Handbook
by
Shelley Lessin Stockwell

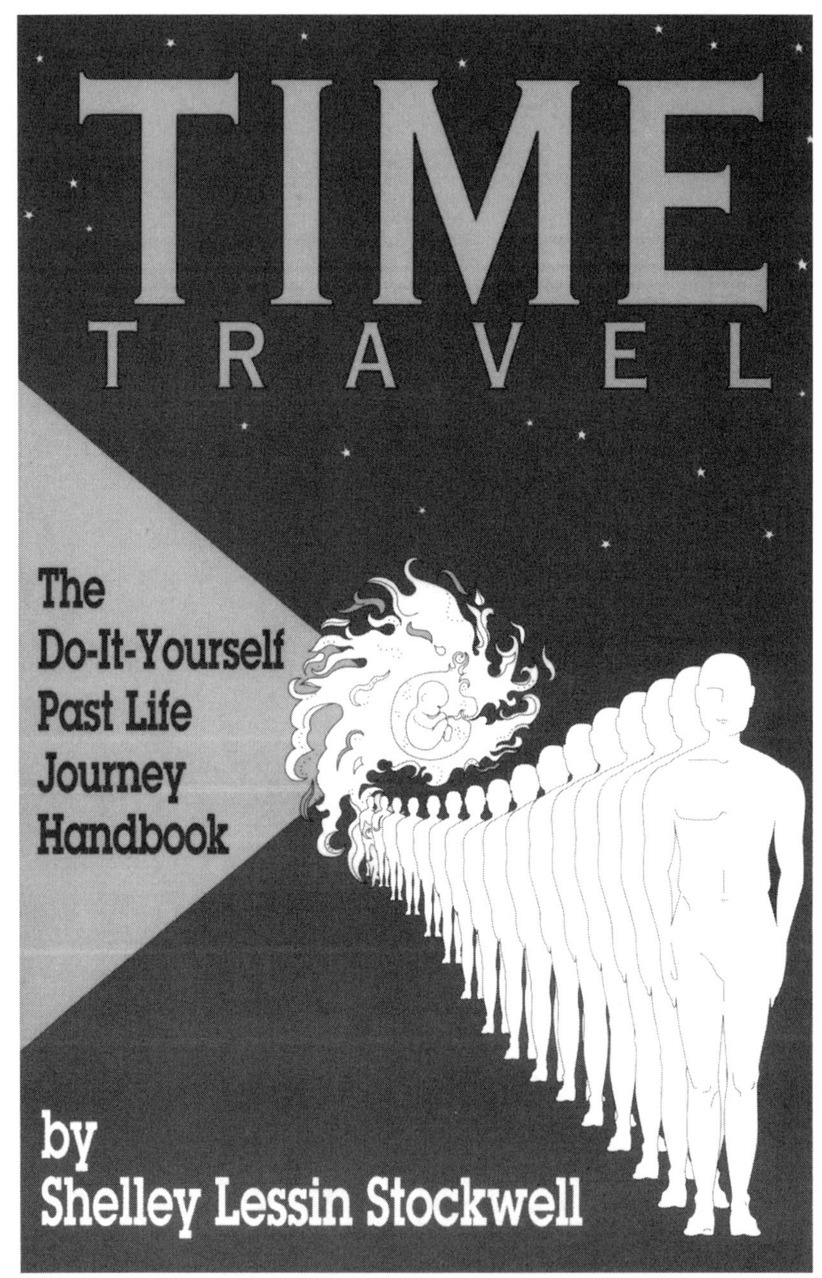

640

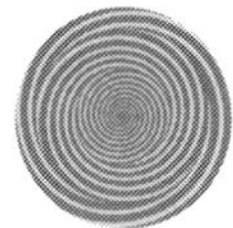

~ *Chapter 163* ~
PREVIOUS LIFE REGRESSION
HYPNOTHERAPY

Includes
Fiore's Past Life Help For Neurosis
Reincarnation & Death Pre-Talk
Problem Solving Regressions
Regression For Fun & Exploring Time

Hypnoanalysis and Previous Life Hypnotherapy are closely associated and a popular facet of clinical practice. Past life, or previous life regression, probes the subconscious for past memories. These memories are part of consciousness. Hypnotherapists and Clinical Psychologists use this highly valued form of hypnotherapy with wonderful results. Most do not expect is to go back even further than this current lifetime yet many clients recall where they were before they were themselves!

Time travel teaches those who journey more about who they are in the here and now, heals past hurts, releases current pain, renews or forgives old acquaintances, and expand their consciousness about the meaning of immortality.

FIORE'S PAST LIFE HELP FOR NEUROSIS

Neurosis in your current life can stem from this life or previous lifetimes. Uncovering a past cause produces a current cure. Edith Fiore. Ph.D. in her classic book, "You Have Been Here Before" tells this story:

"A patient came to me requesting help to overcome her phobia of snakes. After combing back through her life under hypnosis and finding nothing to explain her fears, I tried a hunch. I asked her if she had had an encounter with snakes before she was born. She saw herself as a fifteen-year old Aztec girl in front of a pyramid, watching priests dancing with poisonous snakes in their mouths. She trembled with emotion and reported the bizarre rites in vivid detail. This uncovering resulted in a cure.

After that session, I routinely used past life regression. While in hypnosis, the patient's subconscious mind indicates if the origin of a problem is found in events in this life or in a previous existence. Whether these former lifetimes are 'relived,' are fantasies, or actual experiences from a bygone era do not matter to me as a therapist; getting results is what is important. I have found past-life regression consistently helpful, often resulting in immediate remission of chronic symptoms that do not return, even after month and years. I have come to take previous life regressions very seriously indeed."

All manner of psychological problems have been resolved when past life origins are unearthed from the subconscious. Weight problems often trace back to a previous lifetime when the person was hungry or literally starved to death. Such starvation may manifest in the here and now as compulsive eating. Chronic headache, pain, disorders or weaknesses in certain areas of the body often relate to events in former lifetimes.

Fear of the dark, may originate in a terrifying former life incident that happened in the dark. Dr. Fiore reports one woman who healed her phobia for staying alone at night– and her conviction that she would be murdered if she did so– when she traced it to an earlier identical experience, in a previous life.

Recurrent nightmares are often upsetting flashbacks to a past life. Insomnia and other sleep disorders may stem, from horrifying things that happened during sleep in past lives. When some one returns to the initial sensitizing event (ISE) in the current lifetime or a past lifetime they can release it and sleep again.

REINCARNATION AND DEATH PRE-TALK

I like to explain this idea to my clients who come for past life regression. Those who come to experience a past life regressions are already in sympathy with such understanding.

"Previous Life Regressions is understood best with an exploration of the nature of death and reincarnation. World religions share a common belief in the immortality of the soul. Sects may disagree about theology, but the matter of life continuing on after death, is universal. Scriptures worldwide say that you are deathless. From time immemorial humankind has believed that death leaves the physical vehicle (the body) behind in preparation for higher teaching, which all souls must undergo.

I believe that each soul incarnates in its own time and in the vehicle that gives each the best ability to achieve what it hopes to gain or learn. Look upon death as a doorway through which every soul must pass for a timeless, space less freedom. Here you glean unlimited insight into what was gained during your last incarnation on the earth plane.

The return of the formless into form is called reincarnation. An Eastern mind easily accepts reincarnation. A western mind is stimulated to understand Previous Life Regressions too. Whether you believe you lived before or not is irrelevant. Reincarnation is the way of the universe– everything is patterned on birth, death, and rebirth. The very stars, vast galaxies, follow this pattern. Awaken from the slumbers of hypnotically induced ignorance and consider this essential truth:

There is not a living person in the entire world who has not returned from death.

We have all died many deaths before we came into this immediate incarnation. What we call birth is merely the reverse side of death, like one of the two sides of a coin, or like a door which we call 'entrance' from the outside of a house and 'exit' from the inside.

The argument that because one has no conscious memory of their many births and deaths proves that reincarnation is untrue is scientifically untenable. The field of our physical perception is extremely limited. There are objects we cannot see, sounds we cannot hear, odors we cannot smell, tastes we cannot taste, and feelings we cannot feel yet, they have been demonstrated to exist. With bodily perception so obviously limited, it is really astonishing that anyone should question the possibility of reincarnation just because he cannot remember his previous death, and thus conclude that he has had no previous existences. In like manner, one does not remember his recent birth, and yet no one doubts that he was born.

Not so very many years ago evolution was a theory believed by few. Today, the majority accepts it. And what is evolution but the evolvement of the physical body, while reincarnation is but the evolvement of the soul, which dwells within the body for a time. Both are concurrent and interrelated to each other. Body after body, or more properly expressed, life experience after life experience must be engaged in for us to evolve into whom we embody now. Reincarnation is the evolvement of the soul that resides in that body.

In the *Bible,* Christ says, *'Except that a man be born again, he cannot enter the Kingdom of God.'* That is from the English translation, and Christian doctrine has interpreted 'born again' as meaning a spiritual rebirth, but the original Hebrew text has it written as, *'born again and again.'*

In the *Koran* it is written, *'God generates beings, and then sends them back, over and over again, until they return to Him.'*

Voltaire wrote, *'After all, it is no more surprising to be born twice than it is to be born once. Everything in life is resurrection. Everything that thou mayest desire to live again– that is thy duty. For, in any case, thou wilt live again!'*

Nietzsche states; *'Live, so that thou mayest desired live again that is thy duty. For, in any case, thou wilt live again.'*

Life experience after life experience are essential for the growth of our soul or consciousness. Both evolution and reincarnation are concurrent and interrelated to each other. Unravel the matter for yourself. Reflect upon an 'only one lifetime concept" and then balance that against 'eternity on the other side.' Likewise, the idea that your behavior during your minute 'droplet of time' in the great ocean of eternity will determine your status in relation to God (The Creator which is the Creation.) for the remainder of your soul's existence is equally incongruous.

Birth and death are a phenomenon that occurs uninterruptedly. At every moment something within us dies and something is reborn. The teachings of reincarnation are but an extension of this happening daily."

MODUS OPERANDI: PROBLEMS SOLVING REGRESSIONS

You Will Need:

A Tape Recorder

Relaxing Music

Have a tape recorder ready to go and a source of relaxing music ready to play.

Interview your client to determine what their goal is. Is there a disturbance they want to calm by uncovering the underlying cause? Is there a place in time they would like to enjoy? Use any induction you like and when your client is deeply hypnotized direct them to probe their memory, back into time, to reveal the source of their difficulty.

If they are here to explore a problem say:

"**Now that you are sleeping deeply in hypnosis, open your mind fully and accept these suggestions. The source of your problem lies in your subconscious; it lives within your buried memory. We are going to explore these buried memories together and when we find it, you will tell it to me, and with the telling, all of its 'power' will dissipate and be gone forever. It will no longer affect your personality in any way. When you come up with the buried memory of trouble, you will view it impartially as a witness– as though it were an event you are seeing projected upon a motion picture screen. You view the experience with interest, that is all; for while it is YOU, you are seeing it upon that motion picture screen. You are simply watching the occurrences and though they may interest and fascinate, they leave you absolutely free of any emotional involvement.**

Now, we must find together the source of your problem. Your subconscious mind knows exactly when such occurred, so you are the one to find the buried memory. Seek it out and discover that buried memory, and when you discover it, you will tell me all about it, and with the telling, its influence on your life will vanish forever.

You have lived many lives, so it may be that what we seek is buried in your current life span, or it may go back beyond your current birth and have its origins in one of your previous lives. You are absolutely free to probe your subconscious completely and absolutely unbounded by time and space… discovering what you need to know in whatever lifetime it happens to be. Seek it! Seek it, and you will discover it.

We will do it this way. Look upon yourself as if you are seated comfortably in a movie theatre with the screen in front of you. Your mind is the projector that projects the images upon the screen, which you view entirely as a spectator. I will turn on a little soft music in the background, and as the music plays, start your journey backwards in time probing the memories of your subconscious, absolutely unlimited by time and space. Review life after life until you come upon that which we seek. It will not take long for you to do this, for your subconscious instinctively knows the space and time within itself, which it seeks, and will find it quickly.

Probe your subconscious now in silence while only the music plays, and when the memory you seek comes upon your motion picture screen you will instantly know it as the memory you seek. When you find it speak up and tell me in detail exactly what you see, feel, smell, taste, hear or intuit. As you tell me, what you witness upon your motion picture screen, its influence becomes less and less until it vanishes forever."

If you are going to make a tape recording of the session say:

"As you tell me the story, I will record it and when you come back out of the hypnosis, you may have this to play anytime you wish, and with each playing its influence in your life lessens yet more and more. Seek now and find that wanted memory from out of your past."

Stop speaking now, turn on the soft music, and let the subject probe his subconscious on his own. Occasionally, you can offer a suggestion of support and encouragement, as:

"While you seek out this memory upon which your current problem is based, you know that I'm right here, as your friend (grip the subject's hand in yours) giving you support and help. Whatever scenes come in, tell it to me exactly."

Soon your subject will speak to you, and tell you what he conjures in his mind as the forgotten incident (often traumatic) upon which his current neurosis is based. Turn on your recorder to tape the entire story. When the subject finishes his narration, suggest:

"That is fine, I have it all recorded for you. Now we know exactly what occurred in your life (or previous life, as the case may be) that caused your current disturbance. Now that we know its source and you have told it to me, its influence over your life is going, going, going, and is GONE forever!

Relax now, you may release the memory, as its power is gone and I have it on tape for you… just relax and sink down into refreshing hypnosis. In a moment, I will count from one to five and by the time I reach 'five,' you will be wide-awake and feeling fine. Then, we will listen the recording, which tells your story of this past incident upon which your current problem is based, and as you listen to it, your problem is gone. You are completely cured. You are well and fine. Get ready to awaken now, feeling well and fine. One, two, three, four, FIVE. Wake up, you are well and fine."

MODUS OPERANDI: REGRESSION FOR FUN & EXPLORING TIME

"Regression takes you back. Why not induce trance by regressing someone back to the most relaxed time of their entire life."
　　　　　—Shelley Stockwell, PhD

Previous Life Regressions can be used as an adventure experience handled in this manner:
First determine what memories the client wants to explore and explain "There are certain experiences in every lifetime that stand out and make the greatest impression and these will most likely be the ones to come into mind during hypnosis."

The subject views a regression as though witnessing an exciting movie. The beginning suggestions offer three safeguards from any very dramatic or traumatic experience.
1.　The viewing of the past life happens as though it were a motion picture projected upon a screen.
2.　An image of a protective golden cocoon of light surrounding the client and makes the person is absolutely safe at all times.
3.　Gives the client a psychological mechanism through which they can awaken themself from hypnosis instantly, anytime they desire.

Deeply hypnotize your client using any induction you enjoy and then suggest:
"Now that you are sleeping deeply in hypnosis, open your mind fully and accept these suggestions; 'each and every person has lived many lives, and each lifetime is purposeful and interesting to know about. The memories of all your lifetime adventures live buried in your subconscious, and because you want to explore them, I am going to give you the means to go back and re-experiencing them. As some of the adventures can be very exciting, witness the events– whatever they may be – as a motion picture being projected upon a screen. Thus, you can view your experiences in past lives from an impersonal viewing as a witness. And you will thrill and enjoy every experience in the past just as you would enjoy watching a thrilling motion picture upon a screen.
Visualize yourself surrounded by a golden light of protection. You are immersed in this golden light as though you are inside of a cocoon we can call your time traveling machine. Here you are absolutely safe and protected in every way. If you wish to come out of the hypnosis at any time, all you have to do is lift your forefinger from your side a fraction of an inch, and you will immediately come back to your present time and space, out of the hypnosis, awakened and feeling well and fine.
Whatever your past life experiences prove to be, look upon them the same way you view experiences in your current lifetime. You are the one who selects which memories of your past experiences you will bring forth.
I'll turn on the music now, as you commence to slip back into the past… going back through all the eventful years of this life, until you see yourself as an embryo inside your mother's body. Now go back, back even beyond that and experience whatever past life adventure stands out as the most important. Now, let one adventure stand out for you, let it form as dreamlike picture images in your mind which you project upon your motion picture screen and thrillingly enjoy it. Just let what comes in come in now and form before you, as I start the music."

(Start the soft music as a background to the client's probing reverie. Allow the subject a few moments in silence, then suggest:)

"All right, you have had a chance to reach a place in a previous lifetime of an interesting and important adventure that happened to you long ago. I am turning on the recorder now, so speak out loud and describe exactly what you observed; tell the story of what is happening in your previous lifetime. Be very descriptive, as you report who you were in that space and time, what period of history you are in, and everything you can about the being there. This is of fascinating interest to you, and all that comes in to you arises out of the memories that have lain dormant in your subconscious. You are now bring them forth... and describe one adventure at a time as I record what you relate of your past lives experiences. I am turning on the recorder now... start describing what you see."

The subject will begin relating what they see. Usually such is described in the first person, and many of the events that take place are very exciting indeed. It is a truly wonderful experience. After the subject has relived one episode of a previous lifetime, you can suggest that he go back yet further until another incident comes forth strongly, which he then relives and describes. One or two re-experienced incidents per session is sufficient. Each session can bring in new past life memory. Many are there to be probed, as you desire. The session is complete. To terminate it, use these suggestions:

"That is enough previous life experiencing for this session. In a moment, I'm going to awaken you from the hypnosis. When you awaken, you will feel fine and well in every way. You will have complete recall of this entire regression session. You'll remember the events that you brought out of your subconscious into your consciousness memory.

Your experiences are absolutely fascinating to you, and using this process becomes easier and easier for you each time you apply it. Whenever you wish to take part in such experiences, you can easily go down deep into hypnosis and go back into your past, and the memories of your past lives will unfold before you as adventures from your past lives which you project and witness upon your motion picture screen of mind. It is truly a wonderful experience in every way, and is greatly beneficial for you, as it teaches you more about yourself, and brings you a full realization of the truly immortal being you really are.

Get ready now to awaken. You are completely back in your present space and time, and retain full memory of the past life experiences you have probed. You can do it again and again any time you wish, for the adventures you can seek out of your past lives is myriad. I will count from one to five, and by the time I reach the count of 'five', you will be wide awake and feeling fine. One, two, three, four, FIVE... you are fully awake now back in your current space and time... feeling well and fine."

Editor's Note:

There are dozens of ways to venture into the past, future and simultaneous dimensions that employ different senses. After you hypnotize your client, it is wise to instruct:

"Do not think, analyze, edit, or judge...just report what comes up...anything at all."

A bridge, an elevator, a door, a corridor of time, a map, a globe, a word, a movie, a date, a portal, all are excellent thought forms to bring about a regression or progression.

Hypno-Helper

"The Many Lives Of Alan Lee" by Ormond McGill, PhD with Irvin Mordes

"Time Travel The Do It Yourself Past Life Journey Handbook"
A comprehensive "how to" book that gives fourteen ways to explore past lives, future live and between lives for yourself or your clients.

"Time Travel Audio Tape" by Shelley Stockwell, PhD

"Regression Therapy Handbook: A Two-Volume Handbook For Professionals" by Winifred Blake Lucas, PhD, Diplomate and Psychologist

"You Have Been Here Before" by Edith Fiore, PhD

"Life before Life" by Helen Wambach
A terrific survey of thousands of regressions where people recalled pre-birth memory.

"The Secret Lives Of Ormond McGill" by Ormond McGill and Shelley Stockwell.
A riveting video of Ormond McGill reliving past lives as famous hypnotists from yesteryear and the pharaoh Hatchetsup. Available at the back of this book.

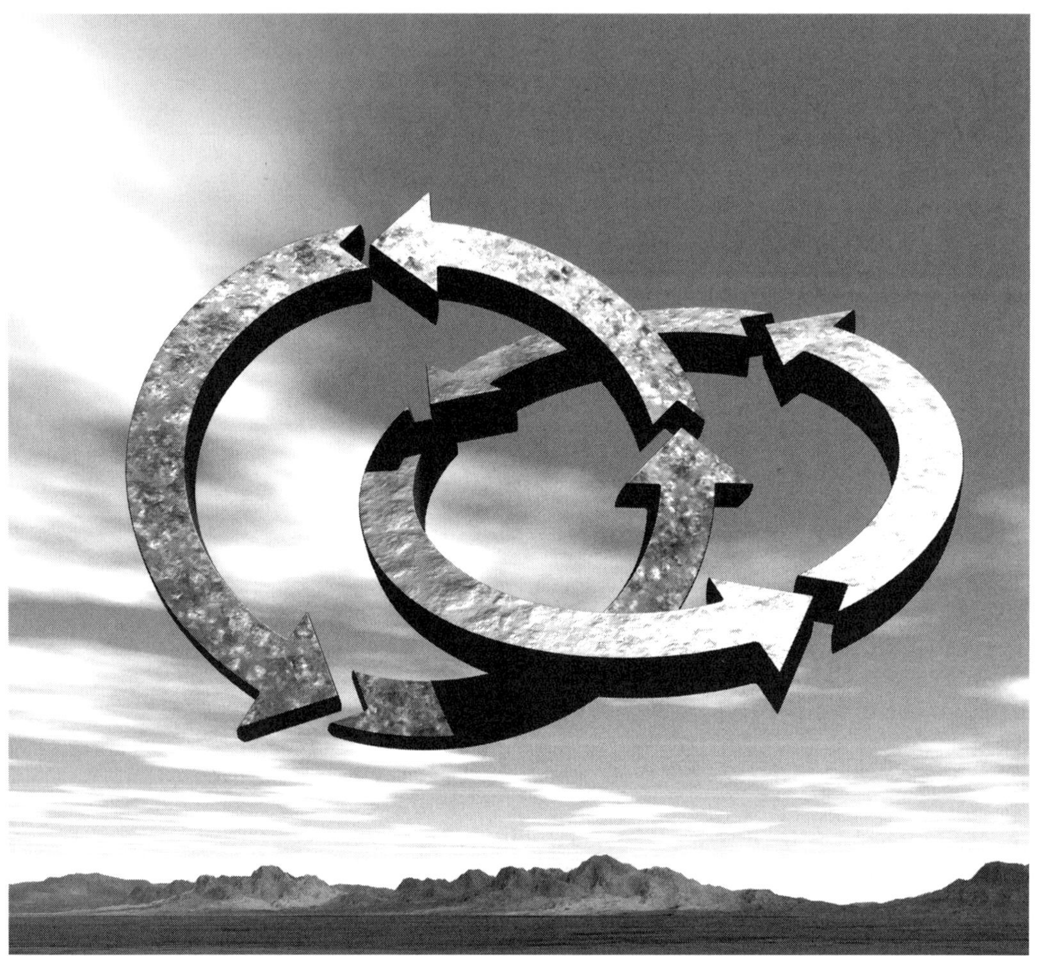

Illustration by Clark Dunbar (© RF RubberBall Productions)

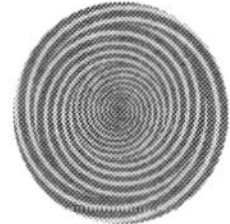

~ *Chapter 164* ~
THE QUESTION OF KARMA

Includes
Karma Releasement

In a nutshell, the hypnotherapy for mastering concerns about karma is to get the client to appreciate the many good things their current lifetime holds, rather than dwelling on possible misdeed which may or may not have happened in their past.

From time to time, you are bound to be confronted with a client concerned about their personal karma. So you won't be caught with egg on your face, here is how to deal with the issue intelligently.

Karma is an oriental concept that some people take very seriously. It holds the belief that if you have committed an atrocity in a past life you will have to pay for it in this current life. Wicked deeds in another lifetime must be atoned for in this lifetime. It adheres to the age old, "an eye for an eye, a tooth for a tooth." Further, if things are left incomplete in one life they must be completed in the next and on dying any good or bad karma will affect your rebirth status. If you have bad karma, you need to come back immediately to suffer or complete previous misdeeds. This concept is closely allied to the Christian belief that a person steeped in sin and not forgiven, is condemned to burn in hell. Such beliefs represent judgment from some imperial god or some strict universal code of ethics.

Yea or nay who is to say? The fact remains that it warrants attention. Karma is looked upon as a serious law of spiritual growth and the "worth of works" or actions. Karma will be seen as not expressing what you are, but what you have done.

Buddha suggests that no one and no thing can judge you but yourself and that to recognize your true divinity, you cleanse karma and/or drop karma.

Buddha says that there are three kinds of "thought coverings" regarding karma as it relates to reincarnation:

1. **Karma Averna**
   These are incomplete acts wanting completion, as there is an intrinsic urge in all to complete oneself.

2. **Karma Klesis**
   This includes greed, jealousy and other impurities.

3. **Karma Ghaya**
   Beliefs, opinions, ideologies, judgments, preconceived ideas that don't allow one to perceive clearly.

Discard these thought coverings so the awareness of SELF enters is his recommendation. Thought binds so many to cling to things of the materialistic nature and miss their true nature. Put aside passionate attachment to things and devote yourself to deeds of kindness brings you good karma.

Karma is psychological in nature and based in thought The Tibetan "Dhammarada" says it this way, "In the way of our living is found the way of developing karma, be it good or bad and as is our living the results of our thoughts, we can say that what we are is a result of what we have thought. It is founded in our thoughts; it is made up of our thoughts."

Jesus said it this way, "As one thinkest in his heart so is he."

If Buddha's thought coverings remain buried with the subconscious and can affect the stream of consciousness that is continuous within you they can be explored through past life regression techniques and cleared away with forgiveness and the wisdom gleaned.

Jesus would say, "Recognize your sins as mistakes you committed and ask you Father in Heaven to forgive you. So you shall be forgiven." Which is just another way to say, judge yourself fairly and squarely and correct your errors. In recognizing "your Father in Heaven" YOU recognize your own divinity and thus sins or "karma" are cleansed from your recognition. Jesus was the master hypnotherapist.

Perception of ones karma can greatly affect ones self-perception, peace and divinity.

MODUS OPERANDI: KARMA RELEASEMENT

"Forgive yourself for if thou do not, who else is about to forgive thee?"

Hypnotize your client and suggest with earnest conviction,

"Recognize your sins, observe them, learn from them, don't repeat them again and then forgive yourself.

Immediately, self-forgiveness is accepted by the subconscious and the karmic disturbance is GONE.

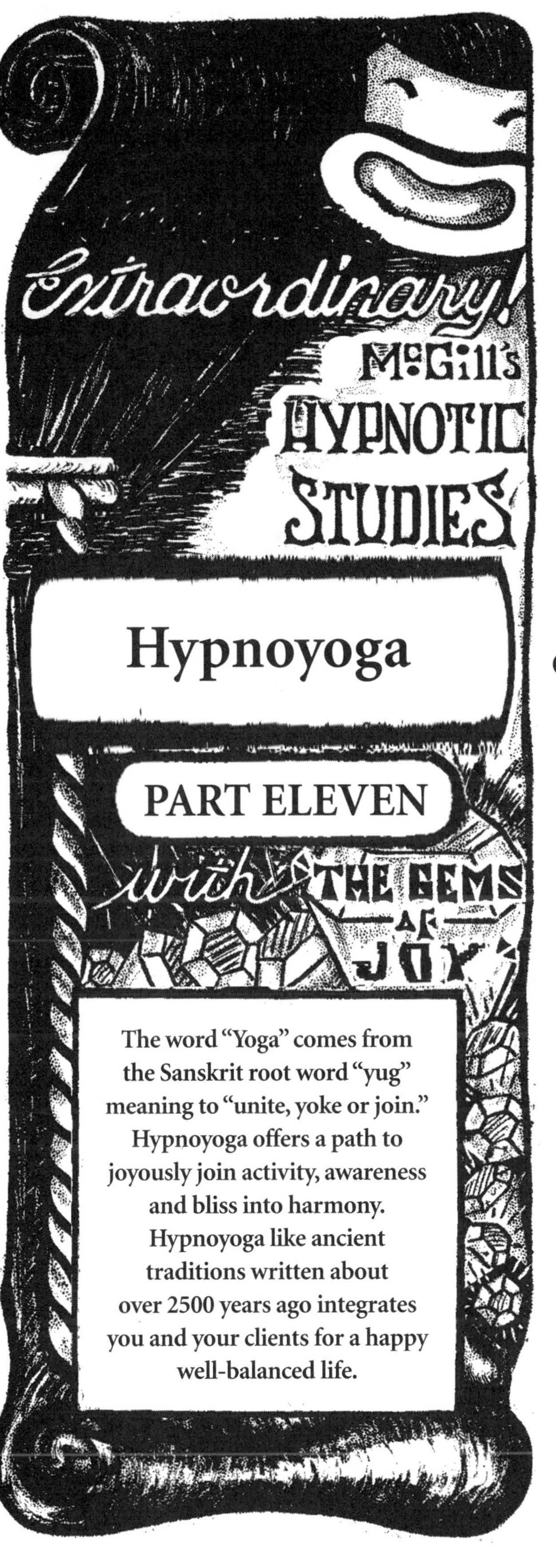

The word "Yoga" comes from the Sanskrit root word "yug" meaning to "unite, yoke or join." Hypnoyoga offers a path to joyously join activity, awareness and bliss into harmony. Hypnoyoga like ancient traditions written about over 2500 years ago integrates you and your clients for a happy well-balanced life.

CHAPTERS IN PART ELEVEN

165. England's Hypnoyoga ....page 655
166. The Attention Technique 663
167. Yoga Nidra 665
168. Yoga Yama 671
169. Yogi Therapeutics 673
170. Holotropic Breathwork 677
171. Tantra Hypnotherapy 681

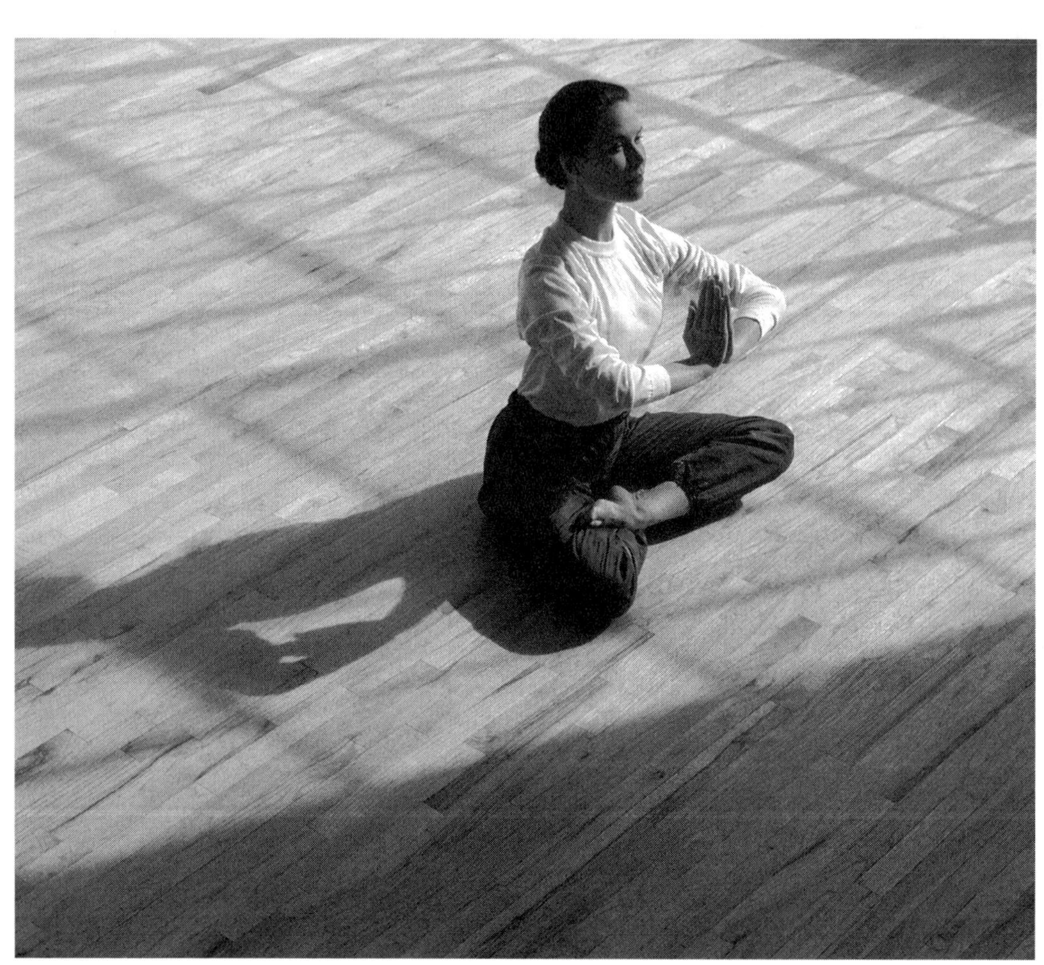

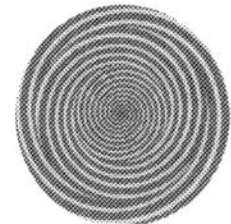

~ *Chapter 165* ~
ENGLAND'S HYPNOYOGA

Includes
Yoga Hypnotherapy
      Yoga Induction
      Yoga Techniques
Yoga Massage
Yoga Massage Inductions

Yoga + Touch + Hypnosis= Hypno Yoga

1. Hypnoyoga has great physical benefit to the body.

2. Hypnoyoga brings serenity and calm to the mind. Using it, allows the mind to just coast along in neutral gear.

It is said that the Buddha used Yoga Hypnosis to increase the consciousness and awareness of his real self.

Hypnoyoga, as created and practiced by the late Diana L. England, combines processes of Yoga and Hypnosis and results in a method of hypnotherapy that heightens awareness. The use of touch increases internal mental alertness. It awakens you. Hypnoyoga can easily be developed into a clinical hypnotherapy specialty.

Use Hypnoyoga just for the sheer joy it engenders; the sense of well-being and self-worth. It refreshes and re-energizes mind and body when your forces are low. It is a wonderful prelude to meditation or a recreation. You may use it to bring a feeling of supportiveness and caring to a convalescent or a shut-in; or to raise the spirits of someone who is feeling low.

Hypnoyoga is a delightful experience. When you are familiar with the process, you will think of your own personal reasons to use it.

Yoga combined with hypnosis reaches depths of relaxation and heights of awareness difficult to achieve with Yoga alone because it lets you speak directly to the subconscious while your senses are sharp. Beneficial suggestions become part of your inner being.

Hypnoyoga is not designed to replace Yoga. Enjoy both and discover the subtle and profound differences. If you practice Yoga on a regular basis, by all means continue to do so.

Relaxation is achieved by performing a number of elementary Yoga stretches followed by simple massage techniques. Body and mind now interrelate perfectly. As the body attains complete relaxation, so also does the conscious phase of mind, resulting in receptivity to beneficial suggestions. A circular compounding process is developed. Hypnosis increases the effectiveness of the body-awareness while the body-awareness increases the effectiveness of hypnosis.

It is imperative that the client understands in advance that Hypnoyoga requires an amount of body contact. Explain that touch is involved and exactly what will happen in advance. Some Hypnotherapists obtain a written consent before using this method and have a third person present as witness. It is up to you.

The Antithesis of "Sleep"

For nearly two hundred years, hypnotists have been telling subjects, "Go to sleep!" and then arguing with each other over whether the hypnotic state is like sleep or unlike sleep. Even some subjects have joined the argument– they had expected hypnosis to put them to sleep, so when they did not feel quite the same as when in a true state of sleep, they would wonder if they had been hypnotized after all. The truth of the matter is that hypnosis is neither sleep nor not-sleep. Hypnosis is hypnosis– a unique (yet natural) state of mind in its own right.

Hypnoyoga takes you to the farthest point distant from the idea of sleep. It induces hypnosis by the very antithesis of sleep: the increasing of awareness. To understand the seeming paradox of this body-awareness method, consider the principle on which it is based: The more fully awake one becomes, the more aware one becomes; and the more aware one becomes, the more conscious one becomes. In this instance, the heightened consciousness of the subject is directed toward his well-being.

During the Yoga exercise portion of Hypnoyoga, the hypnotherapist and client sit in straight-back chairs, a few feet apart and facing each other. At the finish of the eye and face relaxation, the hypnotherapist silently rises and takes their position behind the journeyer to perform the massage technique.

Both parties should wear comfortable clothing that will not hamper movements. If footwear is insisted, choose slippers. But why wear shoes?

MODUS OPERANDI: THE HYPNOYOGA INDUCTION

The Hypnoyoga induction turns the subject's attention part-by-part to their entire body. Becoming aware of one's body is the most direct route to complete awareness. The body becomes the fixation object. This, in and of itself even without a specific hypno-therapeutic suggestions, is remarkably relaxing and pleasurable hypnotherapy. On the other hand, the Hypntherapist may easily add verbal suggestions at the finish of this process.

Yoga stretches help your client achieve perfect mental control of the body so that the body and mind work continuously and harmoniously together. Breathing, which is basically an involuntary function, comes under the control of the will so that the inhalations and exhalations are coordinated with each exercise. This reciprocal relationship between mind and body is the crowning achievement of Yoga and the greatest benefit for well-being.

Throughout each movement and exercise, the body is completely erect and centered. This centering brings strength, stability and calm to the body and facilitates mental and psychic centeredness for the induction that follows. There is great healing potential as you drop to the very center of your inner space.

Instruct your client,

"While performing each exercise, direct your consciousness to the part of the body being used, enter into that part and become it. At the finish of the exercise, take time to become aware of how your body feels as a result of the exercise and to enjoy this pleasant awareness.

At all times, maintain a gentle kindness toward your body. The object is to experience

the sensation of flexing and relaxing muscles and to comfortably obtain an optimum stretch without force or struggle. Let your body works within its own capacity, completely free from competitive inclinations. This is a delicious experience between yourself and your body.

Each exercise starts with a full inhalation. This means that the incoming air expands the abdomen, the rib cage, and finally the chest to full capacity. During the exhalation, the abdomen contracts first, then the rib cage, and finally the chest is lowered. Care is taken to expel every bit of air completely. Inhale and exhale through your nose unless there is stale air left in the lungs at the time a new inhalation is called for. In such a case, part the lips and whisper "Ha" as the air is forcibly expelled."

YOGA EXERCISES

Have your client perform these simple Yoga stretches:

1. Tensing and Relaxing the Neck

"Inhale deeply through your nose as you stretch your head upward, shoulders pressed down. Picture yourself hanging from the ceiling by an invisible thread attached to the center-top of your head so your torso will be completely erect and centered. As you exhale, let the head relax forward, chin toward chest, and let your head hang loosely so that its weight stretches your neck muscles even farther. Do this gently and without forcing. With the next inhalation, return to the upward-stretched position and, with the exhalation, let the head relax and hang loosely. Remember always to accompany the movements with deep breathing"

(Leave time for the experience)

"Inhale deeply through your nose as you stretch your head upward, shoulders pressed down. Picture yourself hanging from the ceiling by an invisible thread attached to the center-top of your head so your torso will be completely erect and centered. As you exhale, let the head relax to the back, chin back as if looking at the ceiling. Let your head hang loosely. Do this gently and without forcing. With the next inhalation, return to the upward-stretched position and relax loosely."

(Leave time for the experience)

"Inhale deeply through your nose as you stretch your head upward, shoulders pressed down. Picture yourself hanging from the ceiling by an invisible thread attached to the center-top of your head so your torso will be completely erect and centered. As you exhale, let the head relax to one side and then the other side. Do this gently and without forcing. With the next inhalation, return to the upward-stretched position and, with the exhalation, let the head hang loosely."

(Leave time for the experience)

2. Wrist Rotation

"As you inhale, extend right arm out front with wrist sharply arched. Rotate your hand at the wrist one way then the other. Stretch your fingers out strongly, then let your hand drop limply back to your lap with your exhalation."

Repeat the procedure with the left hand:

"As you inhale, extend left arm out front with wrist sharply arched. Rotate your hand at the wrist one way then the other. Stretch your fingers out strongly, then let your hand drop limply back to your lap with your exhalation."

3. Finger Stretch
"Place your hands in front of your chest in a prayer fashion. Press the fingers of your right hand against the fingers of your left hand, stretching the left hand fingers backward as far as possible. Release the pressure. Repeat by pressing in the other direction; the fingers of your left hand stretching the right hand backward as far as possible. Relax hands in lap."

(Strangely enough, if you achieve good relaxation in the hands and fingers, the rest of the body responds by relaxing also.)

4. Hand Stretch
"From the same starting position as the finger stretch, stretch your entire hand backward at wrist, then repeat with in the opposite direction.
Relax hands in lap."

5. Hand Shaking
"Extend both your arms out in front of you and shake them vigorously for a time. Now, return both hands to your lap, take a deep breath and relax."

6. Shoulder Stretching
"With the next inhalation, raise your shoulders toward your ears. Hold this position of tension for a time…now relax with the next complete exhalation."

7. Behind The Back Hand Clasp
The shoulders are one of the first parts of the body to become tense in reaction to stress. This tension can lead to headaches, insomnia, and other undesirable symptoms. This stretch effectively relieves tension.

"Bend your left arm at the elbow, sliding the back of your left hand up and back to reach a position between your shoulder blades. At the same time, raise right arm over head, bend it at elbow, and if you can clasp your right hand fingers around left hand fingers. Newcomers to Yoga may find this stretch a little difficult at first. But don't give up! Learning to do it is worth all the time and effort. Hold this position, breathing naturally press your head against your left arm. Relax.

"Bend your right arm at the elbow, sliding the back of your right hand up and back to reach a position between your shoulder blades. At the same time, raise left arm overhead, bend it at the elbow and stretch. If you can clasp your left hand fingers around right hand fingers. If they are unable to stretch enough to clasp hands, they could hold a small towel in overhead hand and inch the fingers of lower hand along length of towel until the appropriate stretch is accomplished.
Hold this position, breathing naturally press your head against your right arm. Relax."

658

8. Shoulder-Back Stretch

"Turn sideways in your chair and clasp your hands low behind your back. Press your shoulders back, reaching your arms upward. Arch neck and back, breathing naturally. Let yourself bend forward, keeping your neck and back arched until your torso touches your thighs. Then relax your head forward and reach your arms even higher. Slowly straighten up, turn forward in the chair, breathe deeply and relax."

9. Forward Bend

"Place your right foot on the chair, with your heel close to body. Inhale as you clasp arms around your leg and touch your forehead to knee. Lower your foot with control to the floor as you exhale. Repeat this with your left foot. Relax."

10. Foot Rotation

"Bend your right knee, clasp your hands under thigh just above knee for support, and then inhale as you extend your right leg out front. Rotate your foot to the right, and then to the left, stretch, and lower it gently to the floor as you exhale. Relax.

Bend your left knee, clasp your hands under thigh just above knee for support, and then inhale as you extend your left leg out front. Rotate your foot to the left, and then to the right, stretch, and lower it gently to the floor as you exhale. Relax."

11. Foot Shaking

"Extend your right leg out front and shake your right foot vigorously. Lower your foot to floor and relax. Repeat with your left foot. Relax. Leaning back in chair a little, extend both your legs together out front (low) and shake them back and forth together on the horizontal plane. Breathe deeply and relax."

12. Waist Bend

"Seated in upright position, weight centered. Roll your weight over to right side of your derriere, hold the chair back with left hand, and bend at waist with right hand hanging limply. (Be sure bend is directly to the side.)

Now upright with your weight centered, roll your over to left side of your derriere, hold the chair back with right hand, and bend at waist with left hand hanging limply. Slowly straighten up with inhalation."

13. Torso Twist

"Cross your left foot behind the right. Place the palm of your right knee on the chair seat and your left hand on right knee. Press with your left hand to help twist at the waist and neck to look over your right shoulder. Hold and relax.

Now the other side; cross your right foot behind the left. Place the palm of your left knee on the chair seat and your right hand on left knee. Press with your right hand to help twist at the waist and neck to look over your left shoulder. Hold and relax."

14. Eyes and Face Relaxation

"Sit in an erect position with your eyes straight forward. Roll your eyes in a full circle all the way around to the left; then repeat all the way around to the right. Relax your eyelids closed and then squeeze them tightly together and snap them open three times.

Next, squeeze them tightly together and relax three times. With eyes still closed, stretch the facial muscles by 'making faces.' Stretch your mouth and lips, forehead, nose, and even the tongue. Take a deep breath and, with the exhalation, relax."

Having completed these preliminary Yoga Exercises, your client will enjoy the sense of well being that comes from relaxing completely and sending awareness (consciousness) to every part of the body. You are now ready to perform the Yoga Message Techniques to induce hypnosis in a delightful and pleasant manner.

MODUS OPERANDI: YOGA MASSAGE

Although the massage techniques used in this method are elementary, the suggestions that follow help you to make them more effective. Your approach is active, conscious and outgoing. Keep your touch firm by gentle. You establish immediate rapport by tuning in to your client's mood and needs and vary your touch accordingly, while at the same time provide a feeling of stability and reassurance.

After the initial touch, don't lose physical contact until all the touching is finished. Keep one hand always touching. Remember this when changing from one process to another. For many people cessation of physical contact is interpreted as an interruption of continuity, rejection or abandonment. When you have finished a process, slide your hands to the area of the cervical vertebrae (referred to as the 'rest position').

YOGA MASSAGE INDUCTIONS

Consult the drawings to ascertain the correct positioning and then instruct your client to:
"Remain seated, with your eyes closed, passive and quiescent. No effort or conscious action is required. Remain open and receptive to any suggestions and sensations that come to you."

1. Head Kneading

You are standing behind the subject who is seated in a chair with their eyes closed. Place your fingers across the forehead at the hairline; your thumbs are at the back of the head to provide leverage.

Gently manipulate the scalp forward and backward with the fingertips, both hands moving simultaneously. Press hard enough to move the skin itself over the bone rather than merely moving your fingers back and forth across the surface of the skin.

Move your fingers to a mid-crown position and repeat the process; move to the highest point of the crown and repeat; move to middle-back section of head and repeat; with thumbs, perform process at the lowest point of the skull.

Now place your thumbs on the bones directly behind the ears, fingertips at the sides of the head in line with temples, and move the scalp with a circular motion as before; repeat the process with fingertips at center-side of head and again with fingertips just above ears.

660

Suggest, **"Experience this fully right now"** as you slide your hands to rest position and pause.

Next, place the pads of your thumbs on the little furrow located at the base of the skull where it joins the neck. Move your thumbs in small circles, work from center across the width of the neck saying, "Get ready for an experience which will help you to become more centered."

2. Head Pressing (forehead to back)

Move to the subject's left side and place your left hand on the forehead (little finger in line with eyebrows) and your right hand across the back of the head. (Your hands should be fully opened by in a curved position to follow the contour of the head.)

Now, start pressing with both hands as though trying to push them together. Start with a gentle pressure and gradually increase it, hold a moment, then release the pressure as gradually as you increased it.

Now, slide your hands to the rest position placing the pads of your thumbs on the topmost two vertebrae and applying pressure as you make circular movements. Continue down the length of the neck (include first five vertebrae).

3. Pressing & Touching

Standing in back of the subject, place your right hand along the right side of the head, allowing the fingers to encircle the face and cover the right eyelid (the palm of the hand lies against the temple, allowing the fingers to remain free to cover the eyelid). Place your left hand in the same position (opposite side) with the left-hand fingers covering subject's left eyelid. Press in firmly against the sides of the subject's head as you simultaneously very gently touch their closed eyelids. (It is extremely important not to press against the eyes.) Holding the eyelids closed permits deeper relaxation to occur in the small muscles around the eyes.

Now, slide your fingertips to the upper back muscles (on each side of the spinal column) and knead gently. Pause and proceed.

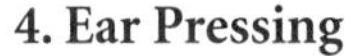

4. Ear Pressing

Standing behind the subject, place the palms of your hands over their ears, fingers resting against the head in an encircling position. Now press gently against the ears but be very careful not to press too hard or to flatten your hands. Make sure your hands are slightly cupped and curved to outline the contour of the skull. This slight pressure creates the impression that your voice is coming from inside of the subject's head. If you like, you may give them a positive suggestion at this time.

Proceed with no interim to process 5.

5. Shoulder Tapping

Stand behind the seated subject, commence gently tapping at the center back of the shoulder are, progressing outward to their shoulders and down the arms as far as the elbows. Form little paddles with your hands (fingers and thumb stretched out but held tightly together). The tap should be gentle. Tap rhythmically and quickly, one hand after the other.

Perform the tapping for a longer period at the center back and shoulders and don't reverse the direction of the tapping– after reaching the elbows, return your hands to

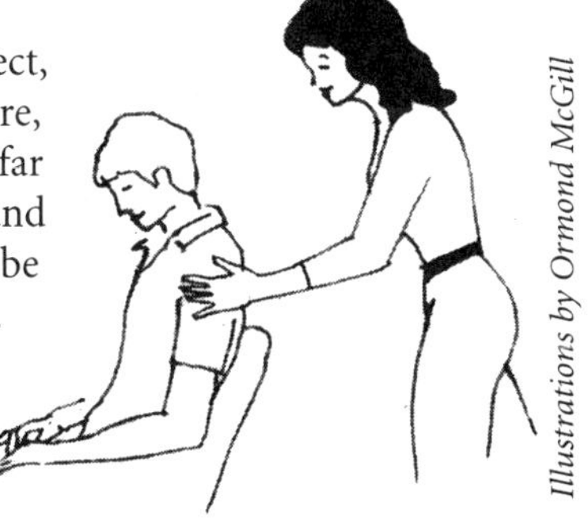

the center-back position to repeat the process.

Take time at the center back position to massage the back and shoulder area well. Start with both hands at the center of back, just below the neck. Start kneading, working outward across the upper back, shoulders, and finishing with the biceps. Then reverse the direction and knead biceps, shoulders, and upper back.

6. Head Lift

Place one hand firmly beneath the chin as the other hand cradles the back of the head. Gently pull upward until you notice a slight resistance

7. Brow Pinch

Use the points of your forefinger and your thumb, gently pinch or knead along the brow line, moving in and then out.

8. Cradle the Face & Head

Finally, place your fingers down the jaw line with the soft part of your palms on the eye sockets. Hold this position for a while and then you are complete.

No specific suggestions need be given. Hypnoyoga has excellent therapeutic value in itself. Or, you can add any verbal suggestion that you desire before you bring them back.

Often your client is so deeply entranced you will have to shake them a little, and state, **"Fix this wonderful feeling in your mind. You can come back to this place anytime you'd like. When you return to a wakeful state you will have an increased awareness of your life. Arouse anytime you wish."** Many clients come back surprised that the session is over. It feels so good that they have literally been "gone" while you were working.

TIPS TO ADVANCE YOUR PRACTICE OF HYPNOYOGA:

1. Use Hypnoyoga in connection with Human Energy Hypnotherapy. In other words, use it as Mesmer would have used it. It is powerful.

2. Perform the entire process/session of Hypnoyoga against a soft background of *Serenity Resonance Sound*.

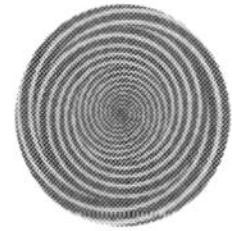

~ *Chapter 166* ~
THE ATTENTION TECHNIQUE

This Tantra Meditation is directly related to the astral nervous system and chakra centers. A method of kundalini hypnotherapy, it fills your clients with a buzzing of prana, opens their third eyes and teaches them to become witness to their thoughts.

You begin by explaining that you will be assisting them to awaken to a higher state of being and then explaining the following sutra:

"Give attention between the eyebrows. Let your mind be before thought. Let form fill with breath essence to the top of the head and then shower as light."

MODUS OPERANDI: the Attention Technique
There are four parts to the technique explained:

1. **"Give attention between the eyebrows...**
   This refers to opening your third eye in the center of your forehead, between your eyebrows. In many people the third eye is shut but becomes functional when attention is placed upon it. To do this focus your two physical eyes upon your third eye with eyes closed. Suddenly you will feel your two eyes come to sharp focus and they will seem to "stand still" as the third eye opens to intuitive knowing. "

2. **"...let mind be before thoughts...**
   This is a strange phenomenon that you will experience when you activate your third eye. It feels as if your thoughts are separated from mind and somehow run before you and you stand back and watch them pass. You become witness to your thoughts as a gap between you and your thoughts are created. "

3. **"...let form fill with breath essence to the top of the head.**
   Breath essence is prana and prana is energy for enlightenment and the kundalini. You bring prana into the body remembering that physical energy and psychic energy are different from each other. Psychic energy can't possibly exhaust you as it comes from an infinite cosmic source; the more you use the more you get."

4. **"...there is a shower of light...**
    **You have aroused the kundalini, which in turn arouses the chakras. As the energy reaches
    the top of your head the "shahastra" chakra** (also known as the lotus of a thousand
    blossoms) **is activated. The shower of light is universal wisdom showering you with
    cosmic consciousness. "**

Then go ahead and instruct them to follow the instructions of the sutras with their eyes
closed if they haven't already done so as you explained the steps to them.

**"Give attention between the eyebrows. Let your mind be before thought. Let form fill
with breath essence to the top of the head and then shower as light. And so it is."**

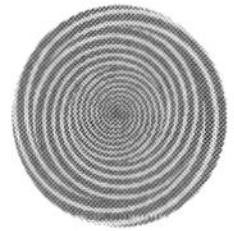

~ *Chapter 167* ~
YOGA NIDRA

Includes
Yoga Nidra
Yoga Nidra Variations:
     Third Eye Vibration
     The Door And The Egg
     The Ocean And Consciousness
     Well Wishes

Those who experience Yoga Nidra change from how they were before they enjoyed this impressive experience. It opens and expands awareness in every way.

MODUS OPERANDI: YOGA NIDRA
    Pretalk:
"Yoga Nidra originated in India for the purpose of increasing awareness of oneself. Yoga Nidra will expand your consciousness and increase your awareness. The expansion of consciousness is a never ending and compounding experience, and the more you use it, the more extensive your awareness will become."

    Begin:
"Sit relaxed and or lie prone upon your back. Make yourself as comfortably and motionless as possible as you listen with great attentiveness to all that transpires around you.

Now close your eyes and keep them closed. Yoga Nidra functions on the level of awareness and the act of hearing and feeling are the important sensing you will use. And join with this the level of attentive listening.

And should Yoga Nidra bring in a dream experience to you, just let it happen. But all the while keep mentally saying to yourself. 'I will not go to sleep' 'I will listen to these words at all times with full awareness. And so, I will not sleep while I practice Yoga Nidra, I will remain constantly aware and as the process progresses, I will not sleep while I practice Yoga Nidra I will become increasingly more and more aware.'

Now, take a deep breath, and as you breathe in, feel calmness spreading throughout your body. And as you breathe out, say to yourself mentally 'relaxed, relaxed, relaxed. I am becoming completely relaxed.' Think it and you will experience it. You will experience absolute relaxation settling into your body and ascending all about you. Become absolutely quiet now and listen. Become aware of all the sounds coming to you in the space where you are.

Become aware of the most distant sounds that you can now hear. Allow your sense of hearing to search out distant sounds, and follow these distant sounds with your awareness.
(Pause)

Now move your attention from sounds to sounds without paying attention to what these sounds are. Allow your sense of hearing to go from sound to sound without identifying them now bring the distance sounds gradually back to closer sound to sound that are close by inside this very room where you are resting.

You now move your awareness from sound to visualizing. Imagine and visualize the four walls of this room, the floor of this room, the ceiling of this room and visualize your body resting in this room and notice the place where your body relaxes on the surface where you are resting.

Turn your attention now to your breathing and become aware of your natural breathing. Just relax more and more deeply as you do this but do not go to sleep. Be aware of your body as the air goes in and out of your body. Become fully conscious of each breathing out and breathing in and relax as you do…all the while saying 'I will not go to sleep but I will remain constantly aware'…as you bring health and well being to your body say to yourself this resolve:

'I am advancing my consciousness and heightening my awareness in every way…

I am advancing my consciousness and heightening my awareness in every way…

I am advancing my consciousness and heightening my awareness in every way.'

(Pause)

Now we are going to rotate consciousness to the different parts of the body and allow your consciousness to flow to each part. Let your mind move freely from one part of the body to the next. (Take your time as you move throughout the body to give your client time to experience each suggestion)

As you relax with attention sitting comfortably in your chair or stretched out comfortably where you are. Bring your consciousness to your right hand. Become aware of your right hand. Now experience the thumb on your right hand. Experience your right forefinger. Experience your right middle finger. Experience your right ring finger. Experience your right little finger. Bring your consciousness to the palm of your right hand.

Bring your consciousness to the right side of your body. Experience your right wrist…your right elbows…your right shoulder…the right side of your waist…your right hip…your right thigh…your right kneecap…your right calf…your right foot. Experience the sole of your right foot. Experience your right big toe…your right second toe…to your right third toe…to your right forth toe…to your right little toe.

Now, move your consciousness to the left side of your body. Become aware of your left hand. Become aware of your left hand. Now experience the thumb on your left hand. Experience your left forefinger. Experience your left middle finger…of your left ring finger…your left little finger. Bring your consciousness to the palm of your left hand. Experience your left wrist…your left elbows…your left shoulder…the left side of your waist…your left hip…to your left thigh…to your left kneecap…to your left calf…to your left foot. Experience the sole of your left foot. Experience your left big toe. Your left second toe…to your left third toe…to your left forth toe…to your left little toe. Become aware of the sole of your left foot.

Experience your forehead…your right eyebrow…your left eyebrow…the space between your eyebrows. Experience your tight closed eye…your left closed eye…your right ear, your left ear…your right cheek…your left cheek. Experience your nose…your upper lip, your lower lip. Experience your chin. Experience your throat…the right side of your chest…the left side of your chest…the middle of your chest. Experience your navel…your abdomen…your genitals.

Move your awareness to your back and experience the sole of your right foot…the sole of your left foot…your right heel…your left heel…your right calf…your left calf…the back of your left knee…the back of your right knee…the back of your right thigh…the back of your left thigh. Move your attention to your back

Experience your right shoulder blade

Experience your left shoulder blade

Experience your right buttocks

Experience your left buttocks…your right hip…your left hip. Experience your whole spine. Experience your right shoulder blade…your left shoulder blade. Experience the back of your head and the top of your head. **Move your concentration to the top of your head. Experience the top of your head.**

Now experience your whole right leg…your whole left leg. Experience both legs together. Experience in your conscious awareness the whole back of your body, the whole front of your body. Now experience the whole your body all together! Relax now and go deeper and deeper into profound relaxation but…Do…NOT…GO…TO…SLEEP.

Become aware of your whole body and the space of your whole body and how it relates to the whole body as you perform Yoga Nidra. Experience in detail all the meeting points between your body and the surface upon which you rest. Experience these points in detail… all meeting points of your body and the place where you rest. Notice clearly and distinctly. Think about this place. Feel this clearly and distinctly and do not go to sleep but become more and more aware as you do this.

Move your consciousness now to your hands…becoming aware of the skin on the palms of your hands…experiencing the skin on the palms of your hands…and on your fingers. Experience it intensely with full awareness. Consciously experience the skin on the soles of your feet. Experience the skin on the soles of your feet from the heels to the tips of your toes.

Now move your consciousness to the skin on your face and experience the skin on your face. Your awareness now moves to the skin on your forehead…on your cheeks…on your chin. Experience your eyelids and the place where your upper and lower eyelids meet. Now moving down from eye and lips. And as you contemplate and experience the skin on your face become aware and feel the meeting points where your eyelids meet. And feel the meeting point where your lips meet each other. Where your mouth meets…feel it with full awareness.

Bring attention now to your breathing and become aware that you are breathing quietly and slowly. Experience your breath. Become completely aware of your breathing and concentrate on the flow of your breath as it goes into your lungs and all the way down deep inside of you all the way down to your navel. Experience your breath moving along this passage as you inhale. Become aware of the breath entering your nostrils…entering and flowing in your nostrils and meeting at the top to form a triangle. THINK of your breath as starting separately from you in the distance and drawing near and uniting in the space between your eyebrows. This is your third eye.

THINK of the breath going in your right nostril and out your right nostril. Then THINK of the breath going in your left nostril…one side and then the other…alternating in and out right…in and out…in and out…in and out…in and not and do not become sleepy. You remain aware at all times. THINK of your breath going into and coming out of right and then left…staying fully aware.

You experience your body as it sinks deeper and deeper, heavier and heavier into the place where you rest. And now the reverse this awareness and experience your body without weight as a sensation of lightness and weightlessness. All parts of your body are free of weight…as if you are now floating above the place where you rest. It is a wonderful experience of floating in airy lightness.

Imagine cold, like in the winter, and experience the cold with your entire body. Now awaken the sensation of heat in your body. Feel your whole body as being warm all over…visualize the heat of a warm summer day. Your body is keenly aware as you move to feeling utterly cool and comfortable and the temperature is just right and you feel good all over as you move now into the experience of absolute and complete pleasure within yourself. As you experience both physical and mental pleasure. You experience inside yourself absolute and complete pleasure.

Now, withdraw your mind from the sensations of consciously experiencing through your body and concentrate your attention on the space of your perception before your closed eyes. Imagine that before you in a transparent screen through which you see before your closed eyes infinite space that goes on and on and on and on as far as your eyes can see…and concentrate and witness this space that appears on his private space of yours before your closed eyes, as your screen of mind. As you witness do not become involved at what you see before your closed eyes.

Watch now with complete detachment as a witness. Imagine and see yourself in your mind's eye in a beautiful park in the early hours of morning…such a serene and peaceful park and you can see yourself walking peacefully in this lovely park and you hear the birds as they sing to welcome in the new day and you see many brightly colored and fragrant flowers with the dew drops sparkling upon them and you see the dew drops on the petals. Nearby there is a fishpond where the fish float lazily in the water. You see luscious trees and you love them all. And there is a clearing through the trees, there is a small temple with an aura of light surrounding it and you go to the door of this little shrine and go inside. Feel how pleasant and cool it is inside, and a sense of deep peace and harmony envelopes you as you rest inside this temple.

Bring your awareness back now to seeing the space that appears before your closed eyes. And look upon it as your screen of mind. It appears to your sensing like a dark gray mistiness. Continue watching. Continue looking, into this space and imagine into it this fascinating scene, which you now make appear before you.

Imagine that it is early morning and it is still dark. You are walking toward hills climbing up towards a mountain. You are alone. You are walking to the east and if you look back you can see the crescent shaped moon glows in the sky.

You know that soon the sun will soon rise over the mountain that you see above you. Looking down you can see far below you the lights of a small town sparkle in the early morning mist. The mountain is covered with snow. The path you follow twists back and forth and winds over large boulders and bridges spanning deep chasms and the pale sky above it heralds the coming of dawn.

As you climb upward, you find that the path has become covered with snow and the snow makes a crunching sound as your feet sink in and you climb up the snowy mountain. You come upon a glacier. It creaks and groans of moving ice below your feet and snow sticks to your warm shoes as you deftly you move up the mountain. Up and up the side and the higher you climb the more cold increases and the wind howls around your body and the snow and ice clings about your shoes. You have reached the top of the mountain and stand firmly upon it. A magnificent scene is revealed before your eyes. To the east you see a vast range of snow covered peaks and dark valleys and to the west are hills leading to rolling plains and the sea.

Intensify your imagination and visualize this scene: See the sun rise like a golden ball in the east, scattering rays of golden light off snow that dazzle your eyes. And in the west, it is still gray, above is a crown of blue sky. And in the east it is golden as it nears the sun. Watch the sunlight strike the tops of the mountains and move down their sides causing deep valley to emerge as the shadows retreat.

668

You stand like a king or queen upon the mountaintop and contemplate this grand scene as a new day dawns. Let your mind flow freely with this experience it as you witness it upon your screen of mind in the space that appears before your closed eyes.

And now remember your resolve and let it become your reality. Repeat your resolve within your mind with emphasis three times:

'I am expanding my consciousness and increase my awareness in every way…

I am expanding my consciousness and increase my awareness in every way…

I am expanding my consciousness and increase my awareness in every way.'

You are now ready to return again to the here and now.

Become consciously aware of your natural breathing.

Become aware of the complete relaxation the practice of Yoga Nidra has brought to you.

Become aware of how good you feel.

Become aware of your physical existence.

Become aware of your arms and legs and your body stretched out and relaxed.

Become aware of the meeting points between your body and the place where you rest.

Develop awareness of the room you are in: the walls, the ceiling, the noises inside the room and the noises outside the room. Now move your mind from inside yourself and become completely external.

Stay quiet for a few more minutes longer now and keep your eyes closed.

All right, start moving your body and stretch yourself now. Just take your time and do not hurry. When you are sure that you are wide awake and alert, open your eyes and take an upright seating position. You have returned to the reality of the here and now and this session of Yoga Nidra is now complete."

YOGA NIDRA VARIATIONS

You may add these suggestions if you like:

THIRD EYE VIBRATION

"Move this space in front of your eyes yet deeper inside yourself, so you see it as if you are looking through the inside of your forehead. The space now completely surrounds your third-eye as Become intently aware of this space but doe not become involved…just aware that you are watching whatever occurs in this space as though you are watching and witnessing a movie upon a screen.

Bring you attention your awareness, to your eyebrow center and focus your attention on your third-eye and become absolutely still and listen. And you will hear the god sound of AUHM radiating from your third eye. Visualize it reverberating AUHM; projecting it through your third-eye out into the universe. Now return to witness the screen of mind, which appears before you as infinite space, and notice this space carefully for any colors or patterns that emerge. Make no effort in doing this. Just be the watcher. You are totally aware of your watching your inner space without involvement and you become aware of any images and spontaneous thoughts that emerge.

Relax…relax…relax more deeply that ever and repeat to yourself this resolve: 'I am expanding my consciousness in every way. 'I am expanding my consciousness in every way. 'I am expanding my consciousness in every way.'

THE DOOR AND THE EGG

Return your consciousness again to your third eye center between your eyebrows and focus your attention there as you become of aware of a golden door. Imagine it as a large, solid golden door and open it…push…push…push with your mind and it opens before you. Now you are on the other side of the door. Visualize and imagine yourself standing at the entrance of a dark cave. Deep within you can see a flaming light. Go to it the light. Move your consciousness to the light and discover what you find. Some find there a golden egg that brightly dazzles the eyes. Within the egg, within the flame, is your soul, which resides in the center of your being.

Leave the egg and the flaming light and pass back through the golden door and close it behind you as you exit, knowing you can return whenever you like and become aware again of your third eye behind the space between your eyebrows.

THE OCEAN OF CONSCIOUSNESS
Become aware of the screen of your mind upon which appears your inner space and think of it as becoming like an ocean…a dark blue ocean with waves. Become aware of the waves. This ocean within your inner space and the rolling waves represent sleep- the manifesting of the unconscious state of your mind. Now, without going to sleep, become aware of sleep. And visualize the state of unconsciousness within you that is like the waves upon this ocean. And you are becoming master of these waves, so you can ride upon this vast ocean with ease. In your mastery the waves become calm and the ocean serene. And with the lessening of unconsciousness causes more and core consciousness to arise within you.

WELL WISHES
Visualize, a well on the screen of your mind. You are looking into the depth of this well and it is dark and deep. It is a tunnel wending going deep into the earth. There is a bucket on a chain and you lower it into the well and it drops down into the abyss…into the darkness. You can feel the weight of the bucket on the end of the chain, but you cannot see it. Now pull the bucket up, up and out of the darkness into the light. And now visualize yourself getting into the bucket and winding yourself safely down into the darkness of the well. As you descend deeper and deeper into the well more and more intensely does the darkness surround you. You move in the complete darkness of the well as you descend deeper and deeper and more and more intensely into the darkness surrounding you. You move in complete darkness into the unknown the all-pervading darkness. Complete darkness surrounds you and cannot even see yourself. Yet you find that you can know and feel that you are. For you discover that there is no need to see yourself to discover you SELF. This revelation becomes your own as you begin to realize who you are, deep inside yourself.

Start winding yourself up and pull yourself out of the well. Up, up, up, you rise from out of the well and the darkness. And again you are in the light. You feel changed somehow now you are again in the light and see yourself on the outside. You know that you have had a glimpse of your real SELF on the inside. Get out of the bucket now and out of the well. What bliss you feel.

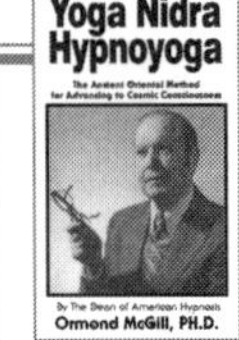

Hypno-Helper
"Yoga Nidra/Hypnoyoga" audio tape by Ormond McGill
Enjoy an amazing journey of Yoga Nidra guided by Ormond McGill.
Available on the order form at the back of this book.

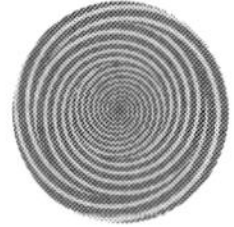

~ *Chapter 168* ~
YOGA YAMA

"The success of one's work depends upon the purity of the heart and not so much upon the accessories."
—Sanskrit Proverb

An Oriental Method of Let's Pretend Hypnosis, discussed in earlier chapters, is Patanjali's ancient yoga system, Yoga Yama. Through the practical technique of yoga, one forever sheds the barren realms of materialism and turns inward for personal development. Here you mold character (behavior) by subjective mental power extended to objective levels. Deliberately pretending and then performing a desired outcome does this.

Yama precepts are purity of body and mind, contentment in all circumstances, self-discipline, and self-study (contemplation). The first step known as Yama is to make a firm determination to control your mind. Yama, then may be translated as self-control. Even people with long records of not succeeding have turned things around using this method.

The practice of Yama Yoga develops the positive and restrains or nullifies the negative. Negatives are nullified by developing corresponding positives. Instead of trying to remove a negative quality directly, it is far easier to restraint it by cultivating its positive opposite. And while physical performing and/or pretending the positive, it commences to become so in fact.

Hindu teachers have such a delightfully roundabout way of getting to the point.

Yoga Yama purports that very mental characteristic of your personality manifests in either a positive or a negative manner. Sometimes a positive attribute can be carried too far and unbalanced by other positive thus becoming a negative. For example, courage is a positive characteristic, the negative of which is cowardice. But courage unbalanced by prudence becomes recklessness, which is a negative characteristic. Here is the governing rule of using Yoga Yama:

A positive characteristic is one that makes you stronger and more efficient; it is a success-propelling quality. A negative characteristic is one that tends to make you weaker and less efficient; it is a success-repelling quality.

Yoga Yama can be used for your own personal self-development, or directed toward your clients. In using it, commence by making a list of various mental qualities, both positive and negative, and then check those, which should be strengthened, and those, which should be restrained.

If using the method for yourself, go over the list above carefully and check off each item to your honest appraisal of yourself. If you are just right on a given quality, mark it with a (+). If you are deficient in that quality, mark it with a (-). If you are excessive in that quality, mark it with a (+-).

Self-respect	Thrift	Vanity
Persistence	Hope	Discrimination
Initiative	Cheerfulness	Perception
Adaptability	Kindliness	Memory
Observation	Temperance	Stability
Imagination	Reverence	Temper
Determination	Self-Control	Ambition
Courage	Patience	Faith
Tact	Egotism	Veracity
Neatness	Judgment	Justice
Loyalty	Reasoning	Service
Chastity	Attention	Morality
Spirituality	Industry	Friendliness
Self-Confidence	Acquisitiveness	Aggressiveness

If using this procedure with a client, have evaluate themselves with this chart during their initial consultation, prior to hypnosis. If they follow the instruction conscientiously, you will be able to determine which characteristics require strengthening and which require more restraint.

MODUS OPERANDI: YOGA YAMA METHOD

In this process you have the person visualize and imagine being as they wish it to be.

"With your eyes closed, mentally picture and imagine yourself behaving as you would like to behave. With each mental image using gestures or movement, physically act-out the role you have visualized. And affirm, 'I can be as I wish to be.'

In this physical performance you amplify their mental visualization. There is a close correlation between physical actions and mental states. Each reacts upon the other, and is actually opposite poles of the same thing. Accordingly, when you mentally picture something that you physically act out, the better your physical behavior is performed. And the better the result will be. Yama Yogis go so far as to claim that if you deliberately counterfeit the rate and rhythm of breathing manifested in a particular emotional or mental state, then that state of being will be actualized in their thoughts and feelings.

History does not tell us whether Dave Elman directly knew of Yoga Yama. Still, his innovating teachings reflect the same philosophy.

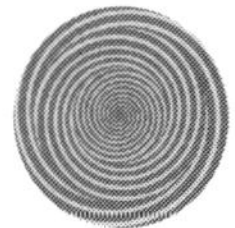

~ *Chapter 169* ~
YOGI THERAPEUTICS

Instill the Seven Yogi Ways to Good Health and Well-Being into the subconscious of your clients and they will rate you tops in hypnotherapy. Yogi Therapeutics can be BIG BUSINESS.

Includes
The Seven Health Essentials:
1. **Healthy Eating**
2. **Healthy Drinking**
3. **Healthy Breathing**
4. **Healthy Exercise and Rest**
5. **Healthy Air and Sunshine**
6. **Healthy Elimination**
7. **Healthy Thinking**

Yogis maintain a rigid practice of mental and physical discipline in relation to health, and emphasize that the following essentials. Let us consider, each in turn:

1. Healthy Eating
"Mix good thoughts with good food, as you eat your way to health."

Yogis say that ultimately, all food we eat, is assimilated into the blood as "liquid flesh." This nourishing fluid is carried and circulated to all parts of the body exactly where it is needed to feed every cell.

The first step in healthy food assimilation is careful mastication, and it is here that the process of healthy eating begins. Thus the yogi chews well, mixing the saliva thoroughly in the process before allowing the food to enter the stomach.

The yogi method of food mastication is to deliberately think of the food as it is being eaten, without being distracted by other thoughts at that time. Expressed in terms of an ancient Yoga sutra: "When eating, become the food." That is the mental process of healthy eating.

The physical process is to chew all food so completely that it is reduced to a soft pulp, which gradually "swallows itself" without conscious effort. Any remainder of food not so swallowed is removed from the mouth as waste product, and is discarded.

Another point in relation to yogi healthy eating is to develop the habit of eating in response to hunger instead of appetite. Hunger is the feeling denoting the normal demand of the system for food. Appetite, on the other hand, is the abnormal cultivated craving for the taste of certain foods. When food is needed by your system, "The inner mind will tell" they say. Or in more western terminology, "Whenever food is needed by the body, the subconscious mind will announce it by the sensation of hunger."

The yogi is rarely concerned with particular diet, as it is held that with the regulated body the inner mind will automatically select, in response to hunger, those foods especially needed. In general, the yogis recommend the eating of natural foods.

2. Healthy Drinking

Like food, drinking is vital to maintaining good health. A yoga affirms that the inner mind (the subconscious) directs the body to respond to the need for liquids. Thirst is a basic craving, and here again one must distinguish between artificial thirst appetite and real thirst hunger.

Yogis say that there are only three natural fluids that truly satisfy thirst: water, juice, and milk. These are named in the order of their importance. All other thirst-quenching liquids are acquired appetites and not recommended. Natural thirst is invariably satisfied with water, particularly with water of an agreeable temperature.

Water is essential to health, as it is needed as fluid material for the blood; it is needed to manufacture and secrete the various chemical fluids and juices of the body. To keep the body alive and functioning, it must be kept moist. If there are not sufficient fluids in the system nature draws upon the fluids of the blood, and thus robs it.

Water also performs an important function of elimination of waste from the body. It is also essential to breathing and heat control. No less than two quarts of water (or related liquids) must be taken in every twenty-four hours for a healthful state. The water should be drunk during different periods of the day and in moderate amounts. It is essential to start the day and end the day by drinking water. Drink slowly and while drinking, think about the good the water is doing for your body and "become the water."

3. Healthy Breathing

In your natural state, you need no special instructions for this element of healthy living. Breathing is the most vital physical process for the maintenance of life. This is obvious, for while without food or drink your body can live for days. Without breath the body dies in a matter of minutes. The yogi's rules for healthy breathing are simple:

First, remember to breathe through your nostrils and not through your mouth. Warmed and filtered air is demanded by nature; the nostrils provide this. If one's habits of breathing are incorrect, then they must be corrected. To do this, the Yogi's way says, "Become conscious of the breath, as it goes in and out of the lungs, while assuming the right posture for the breathing."

A practical technique, used for correct yogi breathing, is to keep yourself straight and breathe deeply filling the lungs completely to capacity with each breath; hold the breath, for a moment, in the fully inflated lungs just before you exhale. Then let the air go out easily. And while breathing hold the thought in the mind that along with the air, the vital energy of life itself is entering the body, bringing you well being in every way. The yogi call this "vital energy of life," which enters the body with the breath, prahna, and hold that while prana comes into one through all the processes of health, it enters more through the breath than through any of the other processes.

4. Healthy Exercise and Rest

Nature intends that you exercise your body, which produces muscular contractions that propels the blood, carrying with it "waste" from the body and, refreshing the muscles with fresh building material, oxygen, and energy. The activity of exercise stimulates all the functions of the body.

Yogis say that for exercise to be most beneficial, the mind must be added to the process. As expressed in Yoga, "When walking become the walking, when jumping become the jump." There is deep wisdom here. It is a psychological/physiological fact that circulation follows the attention. To get the most out of whatever exercises you do, send your mind to the desired part of your body by willing concentrating energy there. This "mental picture" coupled with the firm belief and faith that it will do so, builds strength and the physical perfection you wish. This applies into daily exercise a very ancient Yoga practice; visualizing yourself as you wish yourself to be! It vitalizes the exercise and converts a "dead" system of exercise into a living series of actions.

The yogis say that "shaking yourself" is among the best of physical exercises. It's action is akin a big dog when he shakes water from his hide after a swim. Emulate such bending, twisting, stretching, wiggling, shaking, crouching, and crawling and you'll find a most healthful way of exercise.

Resting is equally important to perfect health for without it, physical balance is incomplete. Muscular relaxation has powerful effects upon the nervous system, surmounted by the brain. Yoga emphasizes the importance of rest to preserve health. It teaches a philosophy of relaxation based upon a resting cat for the perfect example of complete relaxation,

Resting takes tension off the mind, nerves, and muscles. Learn to just "let go!" Picture yourself being heavy as lead and dropping off your weight into the bed or chair as you rest. Think of yourself as limp as a wet cloth. Picture yourself withdrawing all nervous force from every voluntary muscle and allow yourself to become apparently lifeless from head to toe. As you do this, if you doze, it is quite okay. One hour of such rest can refresh you more than a whole night's sleep.

5. Healthy Air And Sunshine

To the man or woman leading a natural life in the open, little need be said on this important fifth principle of Yoga for healthy living. But as many people today live a more-or-less shut-in life, special attention must be given to it.

The yogis state that nature has provided two great gifts to her children in relation to their health and well being: air and sunshine. For perfect health, these must be taken advantage of.

Fresh air supplies life-giving oxygen to the lungs and allows the burning of waste matter in the system. In the open air, this supply is normal. For this reason, always allow plenty of ventilation about yourself; make it your deliberate practice to get plenty of fresh air. Plan a brisk walk in the open air and keep out in the open air as much as possible. And, remember fresh air is needed at night as well as during the day.

Nature's gift of sunshine is also important, but it must be a natural process, not one of deliberate overexposure. Sunbaths that cook one in the sun are harmful. But used with care sunlight provides wonderful therapy. As the yogis express it, "Sunlight is energy. You are energy. The energy of sunlight builds up your energy, but as it is powerful, use it with proper discretion."

For health, plan your abode so it is well sunned and well aired. Flood your rooms with sunlight at least once a day. Let the sun shine upon you when out-of-doors, particularly in the early morning. But, remember, use it in moderation, as too much of a good thing is not good.

6. Healthy Elimination

The healthy performance of elimination in the body is essential and important to your well being. When functioning smoothly it is a subconscious and automatic regulation. The subconscious mind and the organs the subconscious mind controls regulate elimination.

The body's waste products are removed from your system through breath, skin, kidneys, and bowels. The smooth functioning of these processes is absolutely essential to life. The most common difficulty is malfunctioning bowels. Yogi therapeutics developed methods to correct this:

1. Increase the amount of fluids partaken daily.
2. Add a little roughage to your food intake.
3. Exercise the abdominal muscles by alternate contraction and expansion.
4. Applying the principle of healthy thinking, which will be discussed as the last "health essential" of Yoga.

7. Healthy Thinking

This seventh of the seven Yoga health essentials introduces an element of health of special interest to the hypnotherapy student: that feelings, emotions, and mental states are reflected and materialized in your physical condition. In other words, your mental attitude has much to do with your state of health. Bright, cheerful, and happy mental attitudes reflect themselves in normal functioning of the physical body, while the mental states of depression, gloom, worry, fear, hate, jealousy, and anger produce abnormal body functioning.

In western terminology, mental and/or emotional states that cause physical harm are called "psychosomatic." Accurately stated most acute and chronic disease– both functional and organic– are caused by a person's mental state. Yoga has held this belief for centuries, and looks upon many diseases, as evolving from mental causes; as such, these diseases may be cured by mental powers.

In both physical cause and mental cure, understand that the cure is produced through the effect of mental states upon the physiological processes. These physiological processes are largely "mental" in origin. Mind affects body function under the general control and direction of the subconscious mind. It is all summed up in this one Yoga sutra:

"Mind affects the body and the body affects the mind. It is a circling."

Understand this, and you understand the heart of Yogi Therapeutics. It is the very heart of all hypnotherapy. Each and every one of these Yoga principles of good health can be designed as a suggestion-formula, and submerged into the subconscious to continuously bring your clients good health and well being.

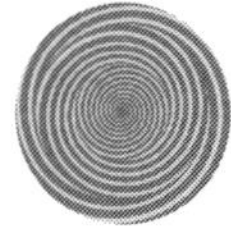

~ *Chapter 170* ~
HOLOTROPIC BREATH WORK

Includes
Holotropic Breath Work
A Breathwork Session
Dealing With Depression And Anger
The Breath Experience From The Birth Paradigm
How To Do A Holotropic Session

Holotropic Breathwork= natures way to take an LSD trip

When LSD (lysergic acid diethylamide) came along in 1950, it was perfectly legal to use and it produced a "trip" that was said to be fantastic and fascinating. Later it was declared dangerous and illegal. The lure of an extraordinary trip still lingers. With holotropic breathwork, much of the fantastic experience remains but the danger has been removed.

Holotropic Beathwork is nature's door of the mind.

Holotropic breathwork calls for proper care taking. The breather is vulnerable as they are in hypnosis (after all, this is a form of hypnosis) and may potentially release great emotion. Churchhill and Mulder employ holotropic-trained physicians when conducting these sessions at their Hypnotherapy Training Institute in Northern California.

Here is what Breath Worker and Hypnotherapist Shelley Stockwell-Nicholas says about it:

HOLOTROPIC BREATH WORK
By Shelley Stockwell-Nicholas, PhD

Similar to the Yogic "breath of fire," holotropic breathing brings up powerful energy and transformational experiences. Breathe deep, fully and rapidly to provocative music and the oxygen stimulates your central nervous system for amazing consciousness expansion. Holotropic Breathwork blends psychology and sacred studies with music, hypnosis, focused bodywork, art therapy and fast breathing to facilitate personal development, inner peace and spiritual growth. Most enter states of non-ordinary consciousness. Breathers experience their lives now, their past, womb memories, other-lives, mythic images and spiritual knowing. After each session participants draw their experience on paper. When their drawing is complete, they discuss the experience and how they'll use it constructively in their life. The work Holotropic was coined by Stan Grof to stand for "moving toward wholeness."

A BREATHWORK SESSION

In the holotropic session the client "breathes" while they close their eyes and listen to music. The hypnotherapist or spiritual counselor "sits" in quiet attendance for a fixed period of time (anywhere from half an hour to five hours). Afterwards, the client draws a picture and verbally shares their experience.

DEALING WITH DEPRESSION AND ANGER

Breathwork helps you let go of depression, inner struggle, sorrow and conflict, and realistically experience constraints, feel limits, and learn to relax, strive and succeed.

Suppose, a client refuses to see how you cage themselves or pushes inner struggles from their mind. In denying such feelings they may "hire" other people to make them sad or mad to create the very world that warrants the feelings they repress.

A series of Breathwork sessions teaches acceptance and how to meet challenges, win and relax.

THE BREATH EXPERIENCE FROM THE BIRTH PARADIGM

Holotropic breath is often referred to as a "spiritual rebirthing process" because, according to the process's creator Stan Grof, the breather may experience one of four aspects that relate to the birth process before expanding into higher consciousness. These birth aspects may occur in any sequence or not at all. A similar approach is called "rebirthing breathing." Here are the four birth phases:

1. **Relaxation**

   Here, a breather feels a loving oneness with others. He or she may imagine floating like a fetus. This brings with it complete yielding, relaxation and mellow bliss.

2. **Constraint**

   Such feelings can remind you of the months just before labor, when you had a womb with no view. On the negative side feelings may include a sense of no exit, trapped, helpless or sad. On the positive side this experience teaches you to feel and enjoy limits.

3. **Struggle**

   Struggle experiences simulate labor. You and your mom are working together so that you can be born. Struggle, fully felt, teaches you power, persistence, striving to succeed and cooperation. If you get hung up here you might believe that life is a struggle.

4. **Triumph**

   Represents the delivery phase of birth. You win! Success, ecstasy and intense joy and transcendence are yours. You may have to clear away lonely and hurt feelings on the way to bliss.

MODUS OPERANDI: HOW TO DO A HOLOTROPIC SESSION

Music

Play stirring music on the loud side. You want to slightly overload the senses. Chanting and rhythms are the best. Make sure that the music is long so that you don't have to constantly change it. I like Tibetan bells, Indian chanting, flute, voice toning, Gregorian chants, koto, sitar or any exotic sound without familiar lyrics.

Breath

Think of yourself having an internal cleansing bath of air. Instruct the breather to **"breath deeply and rapidly. There are no right or wrong ways to do this process. Each person experiences it in his or her own special way. Respect whatever comes up and keep breathing. Just be in your breath."**

I prefer to breathe in through the nostrils and out through the mouth. Discover what works best for you. It is very important that the breathing remains full: as if you are breathing down to the tips of your toes. Make full cleansing breaths out as well. If you are the sitter, arrange ahead of time for a signal to remind the breather to breath. A touch on their shoulder, an audible sigh or a gentle touch on the belly. Be appropriate and respectful.

Drawing

Following the session offer the breather a large piece of paper with a large circle drawn on it. Then instruct them to "put your experience on the paper. This is not an art assignment. Just let yourself enjoy the colors and draw." Continue playing soothing music as they capture their experience.

When they are complete let them share their drawing and their thoughts with you.

Hypno-Helper

"Heighten Your Holos" by Alexander Lessin, PhD. Certified Holotropic Breathworker, Maui Hawaii, gives in depth instructions for combining Holotropic Breathwork with hypnotherapy. Call (808) 244-4103.

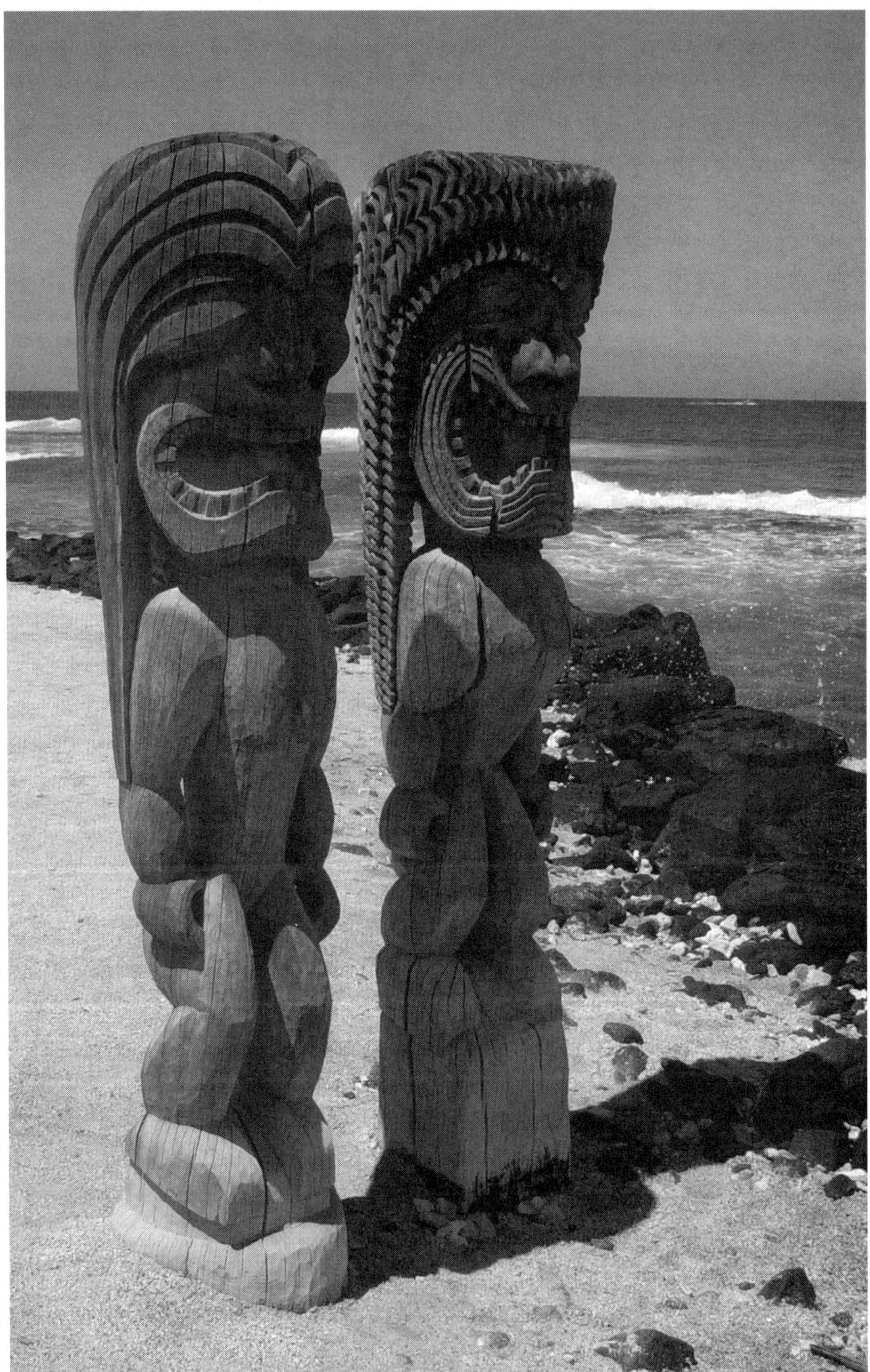

Photo by Jon Nicholas

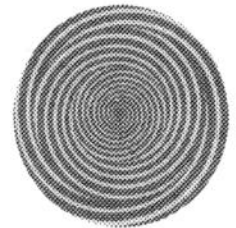

~ *Chapter 171* ~
TANTRA HYPNOTHERAPY

Includes
Immortal Breath
Tantra Hypnotherapy

In India, Yoga Hypnotherapy is known as Tantra Meditation. Interest in tantra and mediation is sweeping the West as East Meets West. It is a valuable meeting. As a form of Hypnotherapy, Tantra Meditation is excellent. It can become a specialty of your office that you can give your clients.

Over five thousand years ago, it is said that Devi became enlightened while sitting in the lap of her lover, Lord Shiva. Here, she listened and learned from him to perform the Tantra Meditation to obtain personal transformation.

She wrote of this technique in a book titled, "Vigyarana Bharivara Tantra" "Vigyarana" means consciousness, "bharivara" means divine love and "tantra" means technique (how to do). So the book was titled the "conscious divine love technique."

Tantra Hypnotherapy focuses on how you become and not with what you are now. It has no ideal for you. It simple says that your true ideal identity is hidden within yourself, and only you can find it by becoming more aware. To become more aware means to advance your consciousness. It is a sacred method.

This Tantra Technique can advance your client's awareness of the divine immortal nature of their real self. As one achieves such recognition, all outer worries and concerns evaporate like drops of water on a hot tin roof. This is why it is such a remarkable form of hypnotherapy.

IMMORTAL BREATH

Breathing is your connection between your mortal body and your immortal self. When you inhale a breath, the "in breath" brings in life force from the Cosmos. It connects the spiritual with the material.

When you exhale the breath, you cast out waste and lower death force. At the termination of the "in breath" – just before it turns to the "out breath," there is a gap (just for a moment). And in that fraction of a moment, you enter the realm of death. And equally there is a similar gap at the termination of the exhaled breath just before it turns again to become an inhaled breath. In and out goes the breath bringing life and death continually into the body in which you dwell. Yin and Yang this positive and negative energy charges you with the vitality of life, immortal being that you are. Hopefully you will understand.

MODUS OPERANDI: TANTRA HYPNOTHERAPY

Commence by inducing hypnosis in your client. This causes subconscious acceptance of the Tantra technique as a suggestion-formula:

Repeat this sutra three times to the hypnotized client:

"Open wide Subconscious Mind and receive deep into yourself this wonderful sutra. Let it become reality…Radiant one. This experience may dawn between two breaths. After the breath comes in and just before turning out– the beneficence (or supreme goodness).

Dawn between two breaths. After the breath comes in down and just before turning out– the beneficence (or supreme goodness).

Dawn between two breaths. After breath comes in and just before turning out– the beneficence (or supreme goodness)."

Continue:

"Occasionally you may have known that you are breathing, but you may never before have been aware of the gaps between the breathing. Try it. Experience it. You will note the gaps. Move in with the breath; then move out with the breath…feel your breathing consciously in and out. Do not go ahead of the breath or behind the breath, just be with the breath consciously. Be simultaneous with your breathing– it is then that you will experience the gaps between the breaths. Simply become aware of the breath going in and the breath going out. This is the best way to begin. With this practice of breath consciousness, suddenly you will experience the gaps in which there is no breath. When you do, you stand in a realm between life and death, and with this sensing– enlightenment."

How can so simple a thing as becoming aware of the gaps in your breathing– going in and out of the body bring awareness? Right there is the secret for it makes one aware of a very basic process of which most are continually unaware: only when you think of it for one minute are you aware of your breathing, the second minutes you will have forgotten. When you reach the point of awareness where you are continuously aware of your breathing and the gaps between the breathing, then comes, as expressed in the sutra, "the beneficence" and you move into a completely new dimension of consciousness– Cosmic Consciousness.

"Thank you, dear Subconscious Mind, for making this ——————— (client's name) reality."

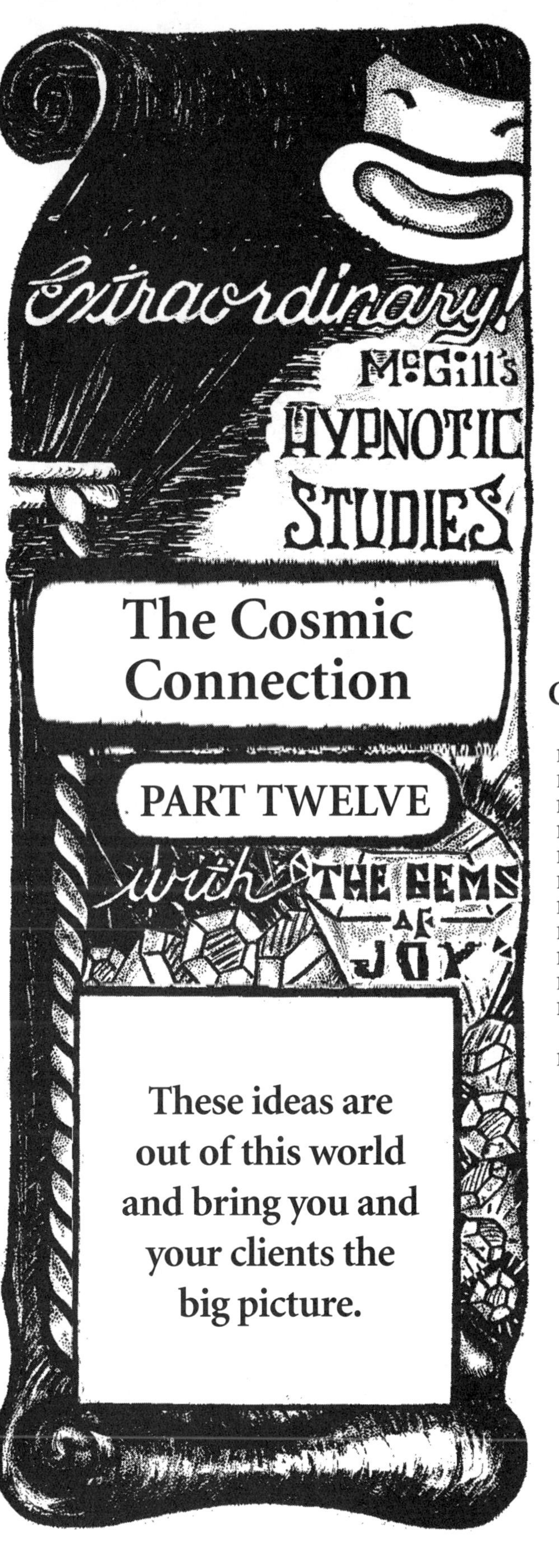

CHAPTERS IN PART TWELVE

172. The Cosmic Connection ....page 687
173. Enlightenment Hypnotherapy 689
174. The Hypnotherapy Of Cosmic Love ..691
175. Mastermind Hypnotherapy 693
176. Self-Realization Hypnotherapy 697
177. The Light Within Hypnotherapy 699
178. The Kundalini 701
179. Transpersonal Hypnotherapy..............705
180. Guardian Angel Hypnotherapy 709
181. Spirit Depossession 713
182. Ten Giant Steps
      To Super Consciousness 719
183. Universal Mind Hypnotherapy............723

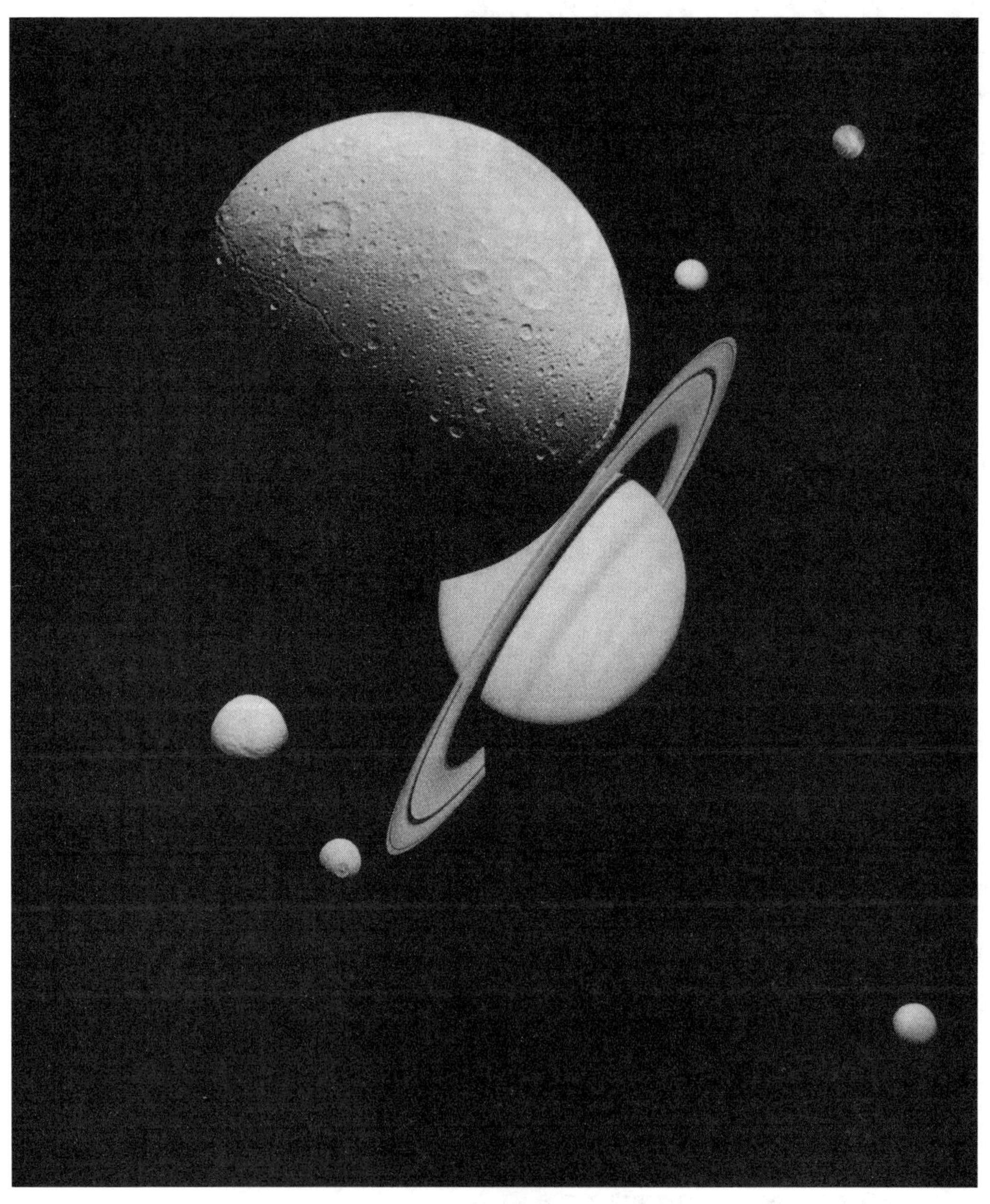

Saturn

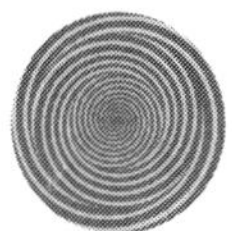

~ *Chapter 172* ~
THE COSMIC CONNECTION

To know is to feel. To feel is to be conscious of what you feel. Feeling is a conscious experience. You can never make a cosmic connection through intellect. It is only obtained through consciousness of the feeling. The cosmic connection belongs to the heart. To be conscious of something is to experience it. When you make a cosmic connection, you will be as conscious of it as anything tangible that you experience in life. The cosmic connection comes like a flame in your heart. Often your hands seem to be alive with energy. Placing your energized hands on your client or in their direction gives them renewed strength, guidance and protection. All hypnotherapy performed with the cosmic connection does this automatically. When you consciously bring this energy to yourself and direct it along with beneficial suggestions, you offer a direct universal healing method. Many try to claim this method with their own name. Reiki is one such name to claim.

MODUS OPERANDI: Cosmic Connection
Breathe in unison with your client to fill you and them with vital energy (prana). Then direct the energy with your mind for the beneficial purposes of the session.
There YOU HAVE IT!
To be a master hypnotherapist, present your suggestions energized with a cosmic connection and center the suggestions upon the core of their purpose. This amplifies their desire and you become a master…but remember, that hypnotherapy by a master is always a giving.
Money, recognition or fame is but a byproduct of your profession. Hypnosis is a God-given gift. Know this and make it your motivation and inspiration. As Christ expressed it, "Seek ye first the kingdom of God and all else will be added unto thee."

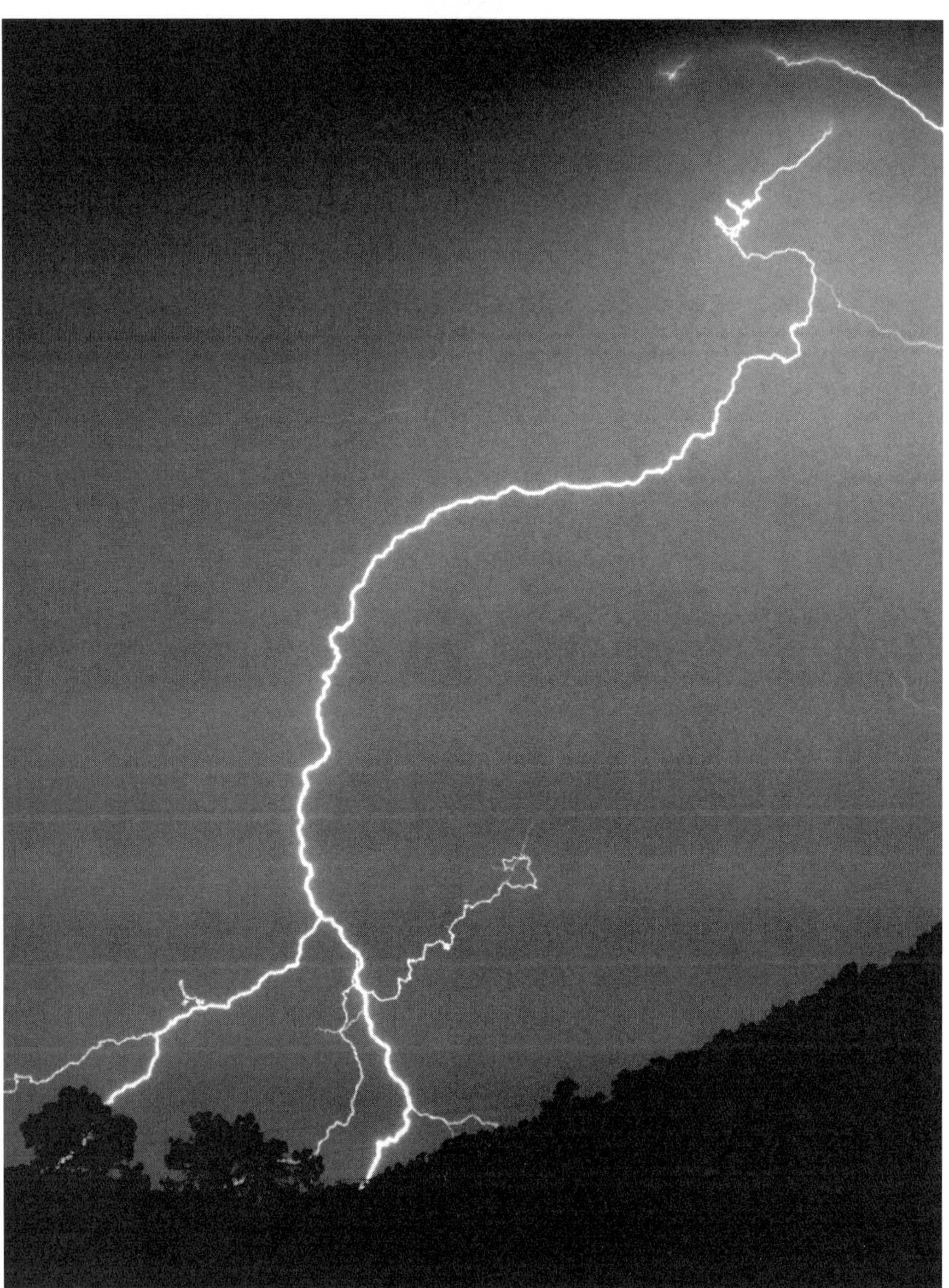

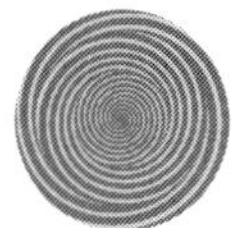

~ *Chapter 173* ~
ENLIGHTENMENT HYPNOTHERAPY

Once in a while, a client will enter the office and ask, "Can hypnosis give me Enlightenment?"

You answer, "Of course. Indeed, yes, hypnosis can give you Enlightenment. It's a Cosmic Connection."

Your answer is truthful.

Enlightenment is a struggle for the conscious mind. But for the subconscious mind, it is a snap. For what is Enlightenment but to feel the I AM living life naturally in the perpetual here and now.

The client leaves your office profoundly different than the one who entered. That is the marvel of HYPNOTHERAPY FOR ENLIGHTENMENT.

MODUS OPERANDI: ENLIGHTENMENT HYPNOTHERAPY

Have the client take a comfortable seat in your office. Induct somnambulism and present these suggestions:

"Subconscious Mind make this known to all levels of ________ (give their name) awareness. Let them feel it as truth.

Enlightenment is natural and easy. Those with unlimited views find it easiest. With limits we move faster and slow down Enlightenment. Unlimited we easily find enlightenment. If you cling to the idea of Enlightenment it makes Enlightenment more difficult. You now find Enlightenment by not seeking, but by allowing it to come into you in its own correct and proper timing. You get out of your way and accept your true nature.

Enlightenment is natural and easy." (Pause.)

Let this understanding sink in deeply to all levels of your mind. You know it well. You now come to fully understand Enlightenment. Enlightenment is natural and easy.

You obey your true nature and you walk freely in your life. Your thoughts are truthful and clear. Your actions reflect your true thoughts. You are connected to the true nature of all things. You understand that Enlightenment comes easily because you obey your innate nature. You uncritically accept all aspects of each moment of life. Life thrills you."

(Pause and let this understanding sink in deeply.)

"Because you are ready to achieve Enlightenment you activate your senses. You embrace the world of senses. You accept fully ideas that come through your awakened senses. Your full perception is true Enlightenment. You seek Enlightenment with a mind fully open to all senses, thoughts and ideas. Enlightenment comes because you live your life fully and to the hilt."

(Pause. Let this understanding sink in deeply.)

"Your mind and perceptions are in accordance with ALL that IS. You know that real fullness in life is possible. You empty your mind of any limits. Your mind is unlimited. Your mind is clear, and illuminated. There is neither self nor other-than-self. You live your life in accord with all that IS. Relaxed and easy.

Just be."

(Pause.)

"Let this understanding become your very own. You know that Enlightenment comes in trusting your feelings. This idea sinks deeply into all levels of your mind and become your very own. When this is so, come back with me into the here and now. Take your time. There is no hurry. You have all eternity. You arise from hypnosis with a smile in your heart, you know who and what you are. This is Enlightenment."

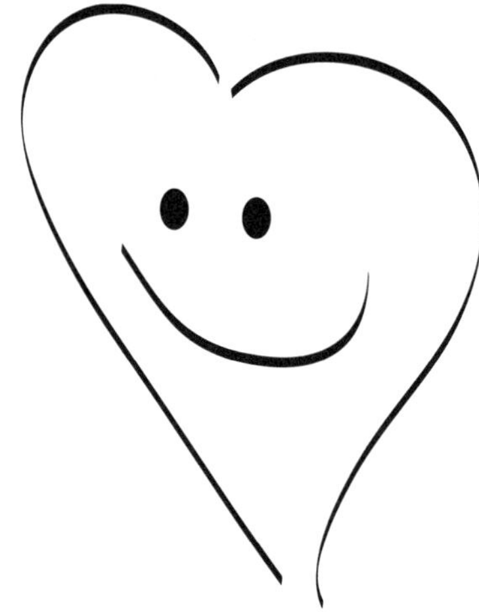

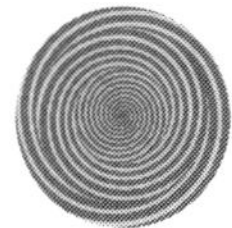

~ *Chapter 174* ~
HYPNOTHERAPY OF COSMIC LOVE

"Love is the greatest power of in the Universe."

Includes
Preparation And Higher States Suggestions
Suggestion Formula For Cosmic Love Hypnotherapy

The Cosmic Connection belongs to the heart.

Cosmic love is like the wind when it is not windy. You cannot make it happen. You have to know that cosmic love is already in your heart and it is so.

Present this specialized suggestion formula following your somnambulistic induction. It is a gift given directly to the subconscious of your client that helps them to achieve the most from their session.

PREPARATION AND HIGHER STATES SUGGESTIONS

"Prepare yourself for an enhancing adventure. While entranced by hypnosis, you are about to enter the realm of love, and advance into THE VOID.

THE VOID is where all creation forms. It is the Great Mystery of Mysteries. THE VOID is the energy center of all that IS. Out of this VOID comes Love. Love created you. LOVE IS THE STRONGEST FORCE IN THE ENTIRE UNIVERSE. COSMIC LOVE IS UNIVERSAL LOVE. Once in touch with it, all becomes peaceful and serene.

It has been spoken through long corridors of the ages that 'God is Love'. As you learn about Love, you equally learn about THE VOID, which is the Crucible of Creation. Love, Creation, and THE VOID, are one.

From THE VOID springs love of God, love between parents and their children, love between mates and friends. Love exists within the atomic structure of matter. Scientists call love between atoms, 'charm'.

All matter is composed of particles so small they are beyond microscopic viewing and are recognized by the patterns of their movement. Each atom has a nucleus at its center, around which swirls a miniature solar system of electrons. From these atoms seeming solid matter is formed. Yet, if an atom were blown up to the size of the head of a pin, the nearest electron swirling around its center would be forty inches from its nucleus. Each atom is 95% VOID.

So it is also in vast space. Even with its billions of stars, it is 95% VOID! It is the way of the Universe.

What seems so solid about yourself is mostly VOID. THE VOID has been called a variety of names: Buddha called it "the emptiness that is immeasurably full." Jesus presented it in a very personal way by calling it 'My Father in Heaven.' The lofty philosopher Plato called it

'Lagos.' Einstein called it 'Space.' The Taoists know it as 'The Tao.' By whatever name it is known, THE VOID is ever flowing with the energy of LOVE, the greatest creative force.

Think of THE VOID within yourself as a perfect replica of the void in all dimensions and remember that the creator and the creation are one.

As it is written, 'The Hand of God Moved Across THE VOID, and Creation Started.' From out of THE VOID came all that IS. You learn this truth well while you rest in the pleasant reverie of hypnosis.

ALL THAT IS was formed by infinite varieties of energy or vibration. Behind your infinite vibration is a sentience that is called your MIND. Your MIND lets your infinite energy create patterns that you want for yourself.

To recognize this is to take a quantum leap in consciousness (awareness). With this awareness, you understand what you are in relation to THE VOID and the creative power of your mind.

Allow these truths to go deep into your subconscious and become your very own. It is so easy when you are open to what you already know: love is the greatest creative force and the essence of you. Such is the HYPNOTHERAPY OF COSMIC LOVE. When YOU KNOW you know, come back from hypnosis and return to the here and now, and transform your life in wondrous ways."

SUGGESTION FORMULA FOR COSMIC LOVE HYPNOTHERAPY

"Lie down or sit and just relax all over. Become quiet inside of yourself and let your mind drift. Now think of a yawn. Actually yawn. Yawn. Yawn. Yawn. It makes you feel so good and you relax more and more, the more that you yawn.

Now breathe deeply through your nose… hold the breath and exhale slowly. That's good. Now do it two more times. (Pause)

How quiet and peaceful you feel. How serene. You drift down into the realm of sleep and dreams. The flow of relaxation covers your entire body and your mind also has become relaxed. Deep into the realm of sleep you go. Every breath you take sends you down deeper and deeper into to realm of sleep…your conscious mind moves aside and your subconscious mind takes center stage.

Cosmic love enters you. Love flows into you from out of the void, of which you are a part. Allow these suggestions and love to enter now and become your reality. See yourself as pure and good and immersed in the energy of love. Now see within your mind's eyes a white glowing ball of light. See this ball of light as being the center of your being, from which you radiate in all directions. It is the energy of the Void within you: the energy of Cosmic Love.

You can use this energy for anything you please, by using your creative mind. You can use it to bring love of all kinds into your life. You can use it to bring success and abundance into your life. You can radiate it out for the benefit of all.

Now let this God Power within you rest in silence for some moments. Silence. Silence. (Pause.)

How wonderful and full of life you feel. Prepare to come back from hypnosis now. You know now the meaning of cosmic love has become your reality. Your subconscious mind will rouse you when it feels your heart overflowing with cosmic love. When you have that feeling, your session is complete. You have made the Cosmic Love Connection and you will enjoy it with each hypnosis session you experience."

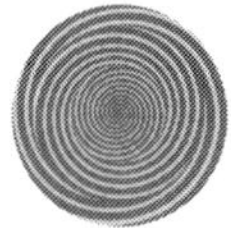

~ *Chapter 175* ~
MASTERMIND HYPNOTHERAPY

Includes
The Four Rules of Mind Control
The Five Main Functions Of Mind

"Control your mind or you'll have no privacy."
—Ormond McGill

When you become master of your mind, you are a MASTERMIND. Mastermind Hypnosis is innovative, as it does not deal with specific problems. Instead, it instructs the subconscious to properly use and control the whole mind.

An out-of-control mind can cause great trouble, it can even plunge on into insanity. It can destruct like a blind Samson. When mind is under control, it can raise one to the heights of genius. When mind is used properly, all difficulties disappear on their own. Mastermind Hypnosis is designed to give the client that control. In other words, to become master of their mind instead of being mastered by their mind.

Understand what mind is.

Mind is nothing tangible, it is nothing you can place your finger on; it is present in everyone.

Mind is a process of producing thoughts, and thoughts are things. Thoughts are forms of energy arranged in certain patterns. Some refer to such as "thought forms." A "thought form" is mental energy with a purpose, and that purpose is good or bad to the individual depending upon what it is. When mind is used correctly, its purpose can be directed to be helpful. Hypnosis is a most effective way to control mind and cause it to function as directed. Giving the person that mastery over himself (or herself) is the purpose of Mastermind Hypnotherapy.

These rules for controlling mind, which can be instilled in the subconscious, via hypnosis, make one master of their mind:

THE SEVEN RULES OF CONSCIOUS MENTAL CONTROL:
Here are seven rules of mental discipline.
1. Make mind think what you want it to think.
2. Make mind think when you want it to think.
3. Make mind stop thinking when you want it to stop thinking.
4. Make mind be attentive to whatever is before it, i.e., cease wandering.
5. Become a witness to your thoughts.
6. Realize that mostly your thoughts are not your own.
7. Establish a peaceful mind.

The more proficient you become at witnessing thoughts, the more control you develop over using your mind. This perspective of witnessing thoughts is applied to all forms of mental activity. When it becomes a habitual way of thinking, it greatly alters perception. Soon recognition comes that it is one's SELF that is doing the actual thinking, and that mind is only the process through which one does the thinking. Then mind becomes the servant (which is its true position) rather than the deluded role of one's master. That kind of perception makes one a Mastermind.

Remember...

The value of mind depends upon how it is used. Mind is there in everyone, and it is neither your enemy nor your friend. You can make it a friend, or you can make it an enemy. It is up to you; YOU who stands behind the mind. When you master your mind, you use it as the superb instrument it is designed to be; the means through which you can accomplish great achievements. You teach clients this through Mastermind Hypnotherapy.

THE FIVE MAIN FUNCTIONS OF MIND

Mastermind hypnotherapy calls upon the five main function of mind or Centers of Operation, which can be used either to one's advantage or disadvantage. These are:

1. **Right Knowledge**

   Right Knowledge is your innate capacity to intuitively know what is right and true, and to use this knowledge correctly. Right Knowledge is a searchlight to wisdom. Wherever it shines becomes focused and clear.

2. **Wrong Knowledge**

   If you focus in Wrong Knowledge, mind tends to find the wrong in everything. This is the basis of pessimism. Wrong Knowledge can accept untruth as truth. Many suffer from using Wrong Knowledge rather than Right Knowledge. By directing your mind with hypnosis, you choose to bypass this mode and use right knowledge instead.

3. **Imagination**

   Imagination is your creative function of mind. It is very powerful. All that is beautiful originates in the imagination: art, music, dance, inventiveness and scientific breakthroughs. Imagination is the inner fantasy of your mind. Mental pictures and sensory perceptions are transformed from the unreal to the real. Some say that when mind energizes imagined images; a matrix is formed which starts a process of direct creation. Everything that is ugly also comes through the Imagination. Imagination used in the wrong way can be very harmful. Recognize your imagination as a great mental power, and carefully use it correctly.

4. **Sleep**

   The sleep function of mind is beautiful and life giving. It can be a source of inspiration. In inspired sleep, your consciousness remains awake while your body falls asleep. You sleep and witness your own conscious expression. Innovative solutions are born during conscious sleep. Sleep occurs in various stages. In the lighter stage, Rapid Eye Movements (REM), shows that dreams occur. In deeper sleep, brain activity slows down, and your body rejuvenates.

5. Memory

Memory is not completely reliable: you can add many things to it; imagination may enter into it; things can be deleted from it; all manner of things may be done to it. Misused, memory creates confusion.

MODUS OPERANDI: MASTERMIND HYPNOTHERAPY

Induce somnambulism and present the following suggestion formula to the client:

SUGGESTION FORMULA ONE: THE FOUR RULES OF MIND CONTROL

Present this "suggestion formula" often to a mind in hypnosis (subconscious). Its effects are compounding, and establish within the mind, rules for controlling mind.

"You are gaining perfect control over your mind. Your control over your mind lifts you up to the heights of genius. You instinctively know you are not your mind. You use your mind to work for you. Your mind is used to produce your thoughts. Your thoughts are orderly and disciplined, and are filled with wisdom in every way. You easily make your mind think WHAT you want to think. You make your mind think WHEN you want it to think. You make your mind STOP THINKING when you don't want it to think. You have absolute control over your mind, and you become a WITNESS to your thoughts. You obtain perfect control over your mind, and this perfect control over your mind is NOW YOUR VERY OWN. Your subconscious makes it so. YOU ARE BECOMING A MASTERMIND.

Now, advance to Suggestion Formula Two in Mastermind Hypnotherapy.

SUGGESTION FORMULA: PROGRAM THE FIVE MAIN MIND FUNCTIONS

In Mastermind Hypnotherapy, use one "suggestion formula" per session. Do not overburden the subconscious. Advance to this script on mind function. Induce somnambulism and tell the subconscious:

"Know your mind has five main functions: RIGHT KNOWLEDGE, WRONG KNOWLEDGE, IMAGINATION, SLEEP, AND MEMORY. Remember this always. You always use these functions of your mind perfectly to benefit your life. You use your mind to bring in RIGHT KNOWLEDGE for yourself. You will make the right decisions. You always turn your mind in the direction of RIGHT KNOWLEDGE.

You reject WRONG KNOWLEDGE. Your function of RIGHT KNOWLEDGE completely overwhelms any wrong knowledge. Wrong knowledge vanishes from your mind forever.

You use your IMAGINATION to create beautiful and wonderful things. Your IMAGINATION powerfully creates a wonderful and beautiful life for you. You have perfect control over your imagination and you use it to benefit your life in every way.

You use the gift of SLEEP TO BENEFIT YOU IN EVERY WAY. You sleep soundly as well, and your sleep refreshes and revitalizes you. Your SLEEP helps you in every way. As you sleep, you become a WITNESS of your CONSCIOUSNESS. Your body sleeps and keeps you well, happy, healthy, and rested in every way. Your body sleeps refreshed as you WITNESS YOUR CONSCIOUSNESS. Your conscious deep sleep advances your control over your mind and you use your superb mind the way it was meant to be used.

You use your MEMORY functions perfectly in every way. Your MEMORY is accurate and precise. You remember things as they are. You are freed from any disturbing memories from the past. All past memories have completely lost their influence over you. You live your life fully in the HERE AND NOW. You appreciate fully that you are living in the HERE AND NOW.

You are totally honest with yourself. You accept whatever has happened as it is, be it good or bad. You don't change memory. You know it as it is! When the past is remembered correctly, you only repeat in the present behavior that helps you live life better in the here and now.

With hypnosis, you now train your memory to bring in what is true. You face memory squarely. You put the past where it belongs; understood, identified, diffused; you take to the present all of the good and none of the bad. Hypnosis has erased any past disturbances in an instant.

These five functions of mind are completely under your control, and you use them to benefit your life in every way. Control is yours. RIGHT KNOWLEDGE is always yours. WRONG KNOWLEDGE you will automatically reject and it will have no place in your life. Your IMAGINATION is creative and creates wonderful and beautiful things for you. Your SLEEP brings you perfect rest and well-being. While your body sleeps, you WITNESS YOUR CONSCIOUSNESS. And your MEMORY functions perfectly and you use it to help you live your life fully in the here and now.

All these suggestions go deeply into your subconscious and program your mental computer. YOU ARE A MASTERMIND! LET IT BE AND SO IT IS!

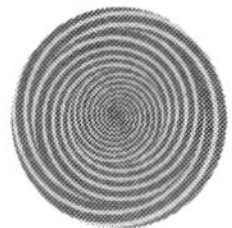

~ *Chapter 176* ~
SELF-REALIZATION HYPNOTHERAPY

Many clients come to hypnotherapy for insight into who and what they are.

In this busy, technical world, it is easy to get lost amongst things. Self-Realization Hypnotherapy brings the appreciation that they are greater than things, no matter how remarkable the things may be. Help your client move beyond self-belittlement. Mentally lift them above earthly stuff and advance into the spiritual.

I have searched intensely to find one concise suggestion to bring understanding of what they are. Here is the suggestion I arrived at. This one concise suggestion makes all the difference in the world.

"You are a timeless miracle."

Everything is expressed in that one suggestion. MIRACLE truly expresses the totality of your BEING. It is a miracle that you exist. YOU is your unique individual self.

TIMELESS provides recognition that there is no time in eternity. It recognizes your immortality. As a trinity of body, mind, and spirit, you are an everlasting consciousness. You are an individual I AM, which is absolutely unique in the entire Universe. In relation to yourself you stand at the very center of the Universe. God is within you.

In the simple is found the complex. The more one advances in consciousness, the more orderly becomes their recognition of the Universe. The world suddenly becomes a playground. A simple suggestion. Try it. It will prove to be a remarkable form of hypnotherapy.

When your introspective client asks, "What Am I?" Answer:

"You are a timeless miracle."

MODUS OPERANDI: SELF REALIZATION HYPNOTHERAPY

Hypnotize the client into a somnambulistic state. Then speak to their subconscious in a personal manner:

"Subconscious, bring to this person's continued awareness that which you know to be the truth. Cause them to KNOW they are a timeless miracle.

________ (their name), you wish to know who and what you are. From this time forth, you KNOW. You say it in these words: 'I AM A TIMELESS MIRACLE. I AM A TIMELESS MIRACLE. I AM A TIMELESS MIRACLE.'

Let this resonate through your being. Let this become your reality. All is there complete. (Pause.)

Rest now and arouse from the hypnosis when you have achieved what you came for today. Take your time. There is no hurry. Imbibe the joy this self-realization brings to YOU."

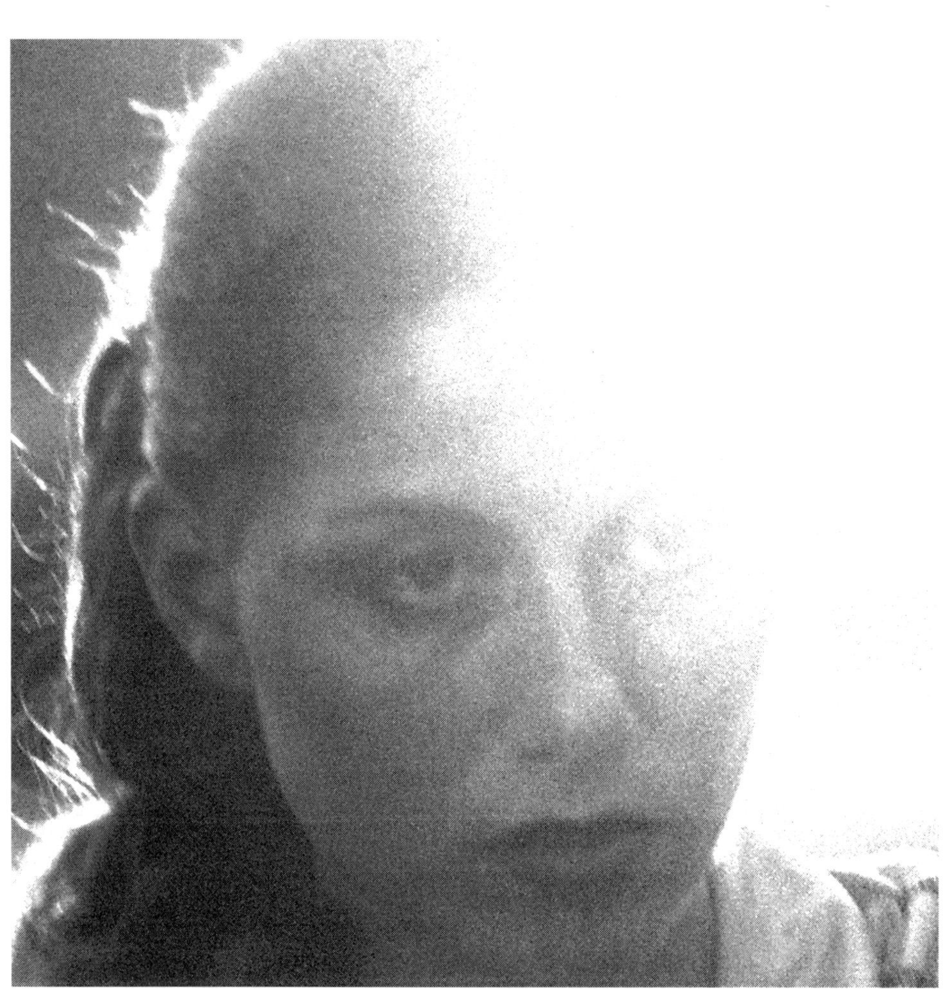

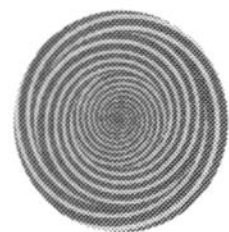

~ *Chapter 177* ~
THE LIGHT WITHIN HYPNOTHERAPY

The light is within or "The One Who IS" Hypnotherapy is the essence or presence of personality of the individual. It makes you recognize that you are part of the Cosmic Connection.

A client will occasionally come to your hypnotherapy office complaining that they have lost their spark. They have lost interest in what they do. Your job is to hypnotize them. Realize that is impossible to lose or even dim their "light within." Dimness seems to come when we allow outside destructive events to put dust around our light so its brightness is not distinctly perceived.

The Light Within Hypnotherapy re-ignites their spark and makes it easily perceived.

This process is simple, direct and effective. It is amazing how such a visualization expressing the truth of the situation can benefit a disturbed client. It is a great healer and rapid too.

MODUS OPERANDI: THE "LIGHT WITHIN" HYPNOTHERAPY
Hypnotize your client and instruct them to:
"Form an image yourself as an electric light burning brightly.
(Pause)

The only way you can dim that bright light is to allow outside disturbances to filter the light. Filters can range from light gray to black. When black, it may seem that the light is totally gone. Actually, the light is there still burning brightly as ever, it just is difficult to see through the black filter.

The cure for such disruption of light is to visualize and imagine yourself removing the filters in the way of the LIGHT. Do it now.

Good.
(Pause.)

As you remove any filters, you discover the LIGHT WITHIN burning ever brightly. You remember that the SPARK is ever there."

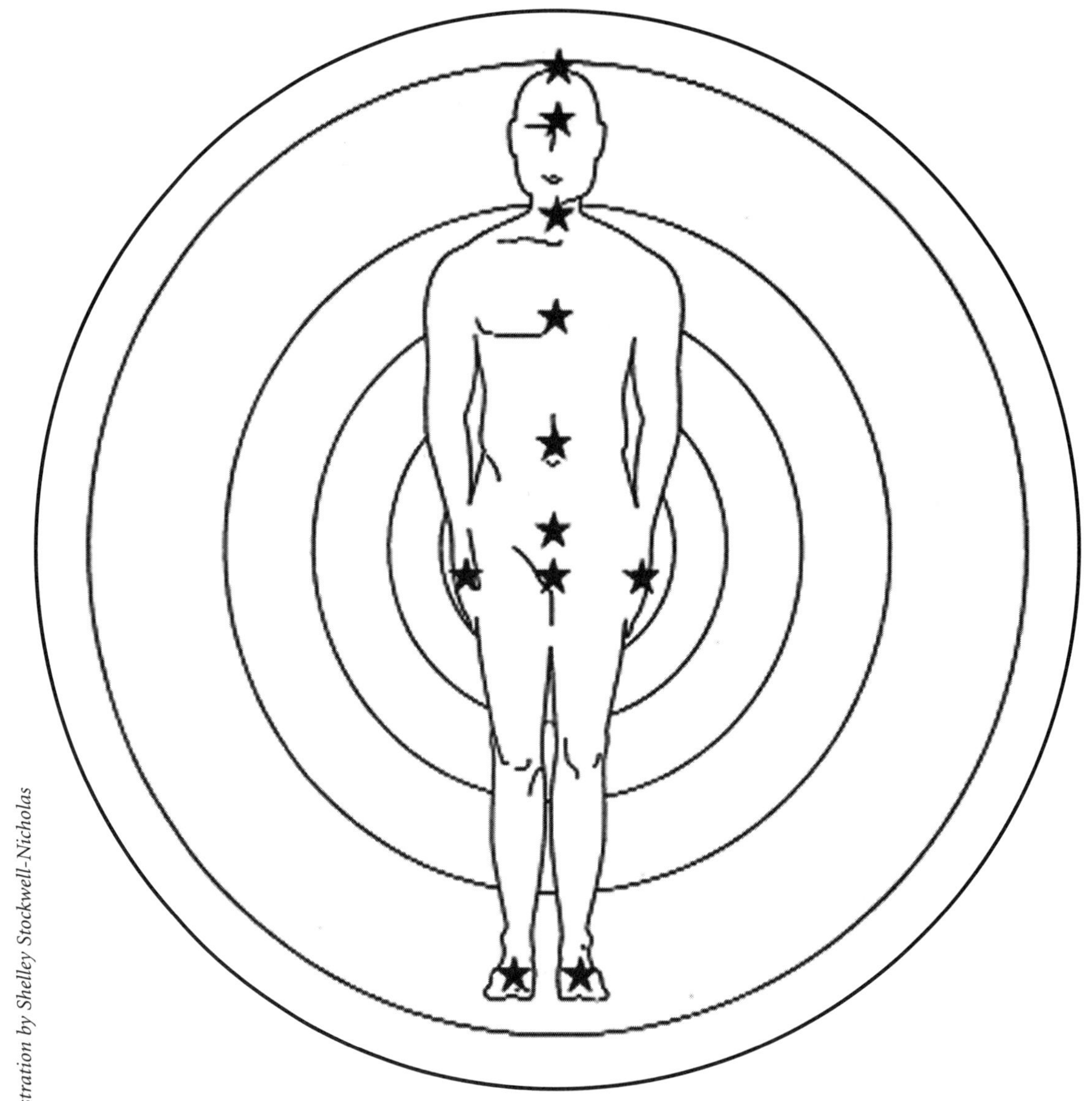

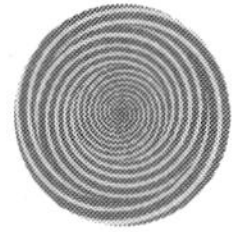

~ *Chapter 178* ~
THE KUNDALINI
By Shelley Stockwell-Nicholas, PhD

Includes
Signposts of the Kundalini

The Kundalini is a form of energy associated with the feeling of being alive—filled with freely moving energy—flooded with light, or enlightenment. This is a first-hand experience of the body opening through the central nervous system via the spine and the seven chakras.

The Seven Chakras
(1) **The base of the spine**
(2) **Sexual organs**
(3) **Solar plexus**
(4) **Heart**
(5) **Throat**
(6) **Third eye (in the middle of your forehead)**
(7) **Top of head.**

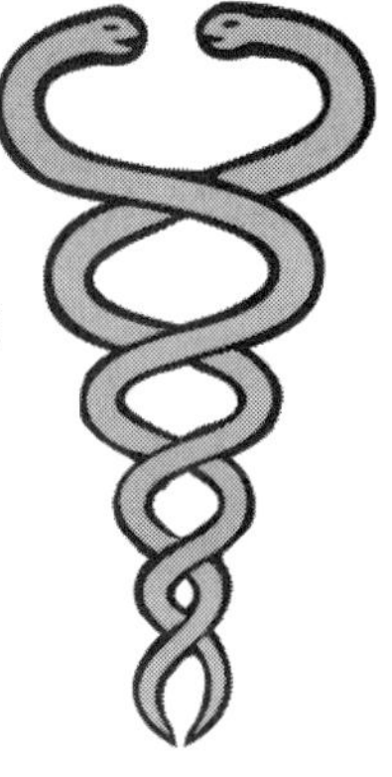

Kundalini Snakes

The Kundalini releases emotional or karmic "blocks." As the chakras clear and open, releasing freely moving energy, we can flood with a myriad of physical and emotional experiences. Experiencing the Kundalini is an on-going process, lasting from several months to many years. As the energy moves through the body, it clears away blocking impurities or imbalances.

It leaves you with an experience of being fully alive, reborn, and reawakened into a full feeling (fulfilling) experience of resonating energy. Joseph Campbell calls it "feeling the rapture of being alive."

The Sanskrit word "Kundalini" was used by the Yogis as far back as 7000 years ago. They believed that without the kundalini energy, no enlightenment is possible. "The Kundalini," they said, "is the central energy of all life." At death, this "energy cocoon" leaves the body and determines the nature of each reincarnation.

The patterns of movement, as energy travels through the body, vary slightly from culture to culture. Yet every pattern corresponds to the central nervous system. All agree that as the different centers are activated, a person's spiritual awakening intensifies.

Many experience the Kundalini spontaneously, as a result of a key event, such as a near-death experience or childbirth. Spontaneous Kundalini awakening can also be stimulated by hypnosis, acupuncture, energy-balancing, meditation, Rolfing and touch therapies. Learning to contact and express the truth stimulates the kundalini.

The process of enlightenment can be quite dramatic. In fact, those who do not understand might inaccurately label a person who is having a spiritual emergency as psychotic. This puts a kundalini soul in a peculiar dilemma. Their "spirit body" is being profoundly lifted into the sacred hand of God, while their physical self might be chastised, exorcised or even committed!

Spiritual opening often happens spontaneously during hypnotherapy and counseling. So it is critical that every counselor and therapist be aware of the tell tale signs of a Kundalini awakening and honor it.

If your client demonstrates the following signposts during hypnosis, hang in there and support them. They will come out renewed and truly transformed. If you have to cancel your appointments for the next few hours; it will be well worth your time.

Fortunately, today there is a renaissance of truth and introspection, as we collectively embark on the kundalini journey of an awakened world.

SIGNPOSTS OF THE KUNDALINI

The following objective or subjective signposts, mark purification and balancing. The results will be greater emotional stability, enhance intuition, and a feeling of peace. You will come out renewed and truly transformed once and for your highest good.

1. Having An "Aha!" Experience

2. Body Sensations
Deep ecstatic tingling vibration
Feeling of orgasm
Feeling hot and cold
Feeling discomfort
Headaches
Focused sensations in any part of your body, beginning & ending abruptly

3. Seeing Inner Visions
Visions of inner light
Visual balancing
Simultaneously seeing the inner and outer

4. Hearing Sounds
Hearing strong sounds and voices seemingly from the inside

5. Time distortion

6. Awareness Shifts
Thoughts speed up, slow down, or stop
Spontaneous trance states.
Detachment

7. Out of Body Experiences

Trance states.
Detachment
Feeling that you are away from your physical body
A feeling of watching yourself.

8. Intense Emotions

Ecstasy, bliss, and cosmic harmony.
Fear, anger, depression, or confusion followed by peace, love, contentment

9. Increased ESP

Natural psychics are more likely to have a kundalini awakening
Increased intuitive powers and ability to see auras

10. Temporary Paralysis

Involuntary positioning of body, limbs, or fingers

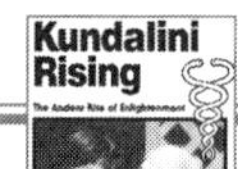
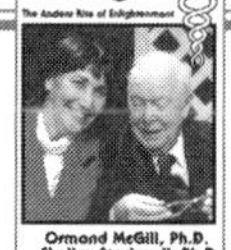

Hypno-Helper

"Kundalini Rising" audio tape by Ormond McGill and Shelley Stockwell.
Available on the order form at the back of this book.

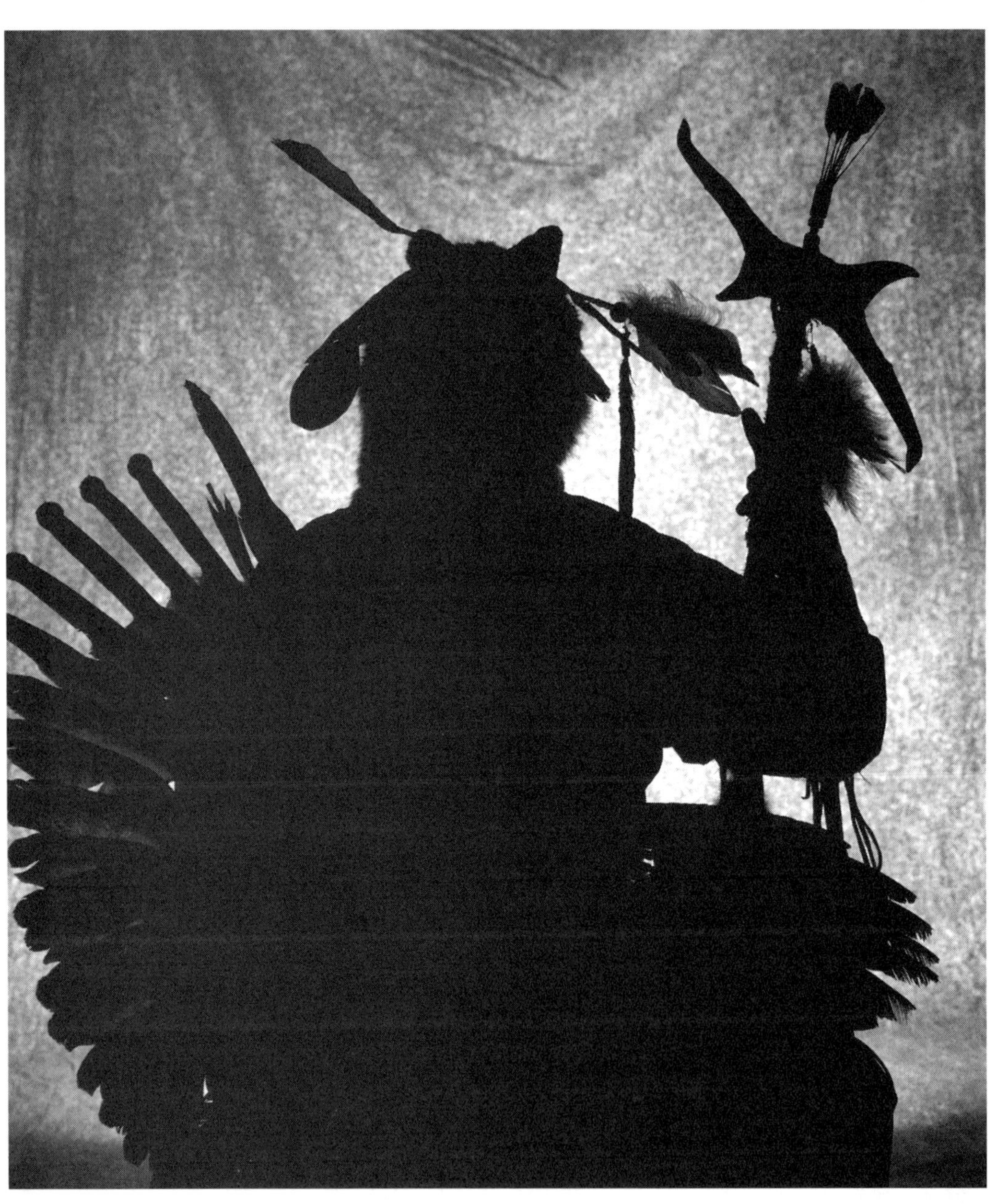

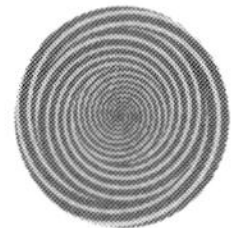

~ *Chapter 179* ~
TRANSPERSONAL HYPNOTHERAPY
By Shelley Stockwell-Nicholas, PhD
(© Excerpted From her book "Time Travel: The Do It Yourself Past Life Journey Handbook")

Includes
Enlightenment
Shamanic Journeys: Please Don't Squeeze the Shaman
Accentuate The Positive, Eliminate The Negative
Wounded Healers
How To Do A Soul Retrieval
Wounded Healer Reframing Suggestions

Transpersonal hypnosis explores the fascinating realm of the super-conscious mind. Here we discover an unlimited vista of creativity, expanded consciousness, guidance and peak experiences.

Every seasoned hypnotist will tell you that even if your intention is to be a simple re-programmer, your subjects will spontaneously enter fascinating expansive and intuitive places. Guaranteed this super conscious, creative self will just show up. Transpersonal phenomenon is as much a part of you, as the body that you're sitting in right now. Transpersonal hypnosis view body, mind and spirit as conscious, subconscious and super-conscious mind modes.

A REAL LIFE HYPNO-TALE

Speaking to 150 senior citizens at Leisure World about hypnosis a lovely lady asked: "Is this kind of like knowing something is going to happen before it happens."

I said: "Well I guess hypnosis is kind of like that." and then asked, "How many of you folks, know that something is going to happen before it happens?" and over half of them, very reluctantly, raised their hands. "Look around at all those hands."

I said: "Just out of curiosity folks, how many of you feel like a loved one who's passed on, has talked to you" and again over half raised their hands. "This is amazing" one said.

Another said: "I'm so startled. I was embarrassed to tell anyone about my experience and yet many have had the same thing happen."

Transpersonal Hypnotherapy takes clients beyond their personality. Techniques includes time travel; past life projection, age progression, future life progression and between life journeys; psychic skills, trance channeling, automatic writing, kundalini awakening, higher-self hypnosis, soul retrieval, breath and encounters with intuition and the divine.

ENLIGHTENMENT

To en•lighten means to give spiritual insight to. Enlightenment was an 18th century philosophical movement that emphasized universal human progress and the use of reason. As we alter normal consciousness, our journey may move into these amazing realms of transcendental states.

SHAMANIC JOURNEYS: PLEASE DON'T SQUEEZE THE SHAMAN

The world's first doctors were shamans who understood that physical, emotional and spiritual energy were inseparable. A shaman is a spiritual healer and awakener of deeper states of consciousness and soul searching. These states focus upon releasing discomfort or blocks, restoring wellness and becoming enlightened.

Shamans have been known as witch doctor, medicine man, medicine woman, mundunugu, priest, ducun, exorcist, magician, sorcerer, warlock, witch, dowser and those who do voodoo .

Most Shamanic approaches balance love and power, male and female, and light and dark, to invoke inner harmony.

Shamanism relies heavily upon ceremony and ritual to evoke trance. Many rituals involve hypnotic tools like smells, smoke, repetition, taste, sound, suggestion and sleep deprivation. Some rely on mood altering substances.

ACCENTUATE THE POSITIVE, ELIMINATE THE NEGATIVE

Beware of fear-based hypnosis relying upon negative thought forms like cutting cords of "dark energies" ghosts, goblins and icky attachments. Such an approach risks instilling false memory and upsets people. Exorcists are masterful in this dark approach. On a tour of Egypt I led, one participant, went frantically about each sacred sight releasing "evil spirits." She saw them everywhere while the rest of us did not. The power of such negative suggestions became a self-fulfilling prophesy of unhappiness.

A depressed woman visited a Manhattan Beach, CA. Psychic who told her that it would cost hundreds of dollars to rid her of an attached ghost and therefore her depression. A few more visits and some $15,000 later, this gullible woman (hypnotized indeed) was really depressed! The con artist, "Madam Something or Other" eventually went to jail but is now back to her old tricks.

Transpersonal Hypnotherapy celebrates co-creation with a higher source and light. My personal rule of thumb is. **"If it's not fun or doesn't manifest fun-don't do it."** All this to say "guru-" **G-U-R-U "Gee, you are you!"**

We naturally hold within profound magic and wisdom. The trick is to tap this joyous power at will.

SOUL RETRIEVAL

The goal is as in all hypnosis is integration. Soul retrieval "into-greats" your client.

Soul retrieval and healing suggestion from an enlightened hypnotherapist works miracles.

Ancestors of all cultures teach that during life's painful rituals and traumas, we lose vitality and joy. Our language talks about "lost souls" or those who have had their "spirit broken."

Psychologists call such experiences "dissociation caused by trauma" or "Post-Traumatic Stress Disorder." Semantics only.

When you assist someone to "take back their soul" they release trauma, learn to stay conscious and have healthy boundaries.

Hypnosis and shamanic soul retrieval brings back-disowned essences to heal the past. Some Transpersonal Hypnotherapists specialize in soul retrievals.

MODUS OPERANDI: HOW TO DO A SOUL RETRIEVAL

Soul retrievals are energetic and use few verbal suggestions other than the preliminary expectation and agreement.

Pre Talk

"We are about to do a sacred ritual where you simply relax and bring home parts of your precious self that may be traveling in a parallel void. Your job is simply to breath. During this process you will lie still and as you do, I'll begin by rattling and drumming (or chanting), **then I will lie still beside you and when I find an essence ready to come home, I will gently blow into your third eye (or heart) and welcome that part of you back again. Is that okay with you? We will begin with a blessing. Make yourself comfortable, close your eyes and repeat after me:**

'I bless myself on all levels: Physically with radiant health, energy, vitality; Mentally with clear thinking, focus, direction, to find my path and purpose; emotionally with unconditional love, peace, joy, and harmony for myself and others; and spiritually with guidance so that I may truly fulfill my life's purpose. I take back my soul I am whole. I take back my soul I am holy.'"

WOUNDED HEALER REFRAMING SUGGESTION

You Will Need:
Sound makers like drums, rattles and music

If the client has been traumatized you might suggest; **"Shamanic society, believes that the holiest person is a wounded one, for in the wounding, God is summoned for their healing to take place. Those who overcome are gifted with the power to heal others."**

Play "in•chanting" music. As the music plays shake a rattle, ring a bell, chant or clap all around the resting client.

"Take a deep breath and let it out and think or say these words out loud again: 'I take back my soul, I am whole. I take back my soul, I am holy.'

Become silent and, if you choose, lie down beside the client. You needn't touch them or you could touch their shoulder or the side of the arm. Intone their name like a mantra inside your head as you begin your mental "quest" for their "essences." Imagine yourself traveling the void back to any time in their life where their soul, vitality, or energy separated from their being. It could be a little memory, such as skinning their knee, or a big memory, such as being beaten, molested or abandoned. Use whatever ploy is necessary to convince this frightened part to leave this parallel reality and come back home. Call upon allies, guides, fantasies, anything you need to do the convincing.

The content of your shamanic fantasy is none of their business. I do not recommend sharing any of it with them verbally because you are after energy and not content. The client is highly suggestible and your "stories" could create false memories so keep them to yourself.

If you find a thought, image, memory, or uneasy feeling, invite that one out of hiding thinking, **"Come home, it's safe now. It's time to come home."**

When they come with you back to your resting client, blow fully and forcefully into their third eye or heart with the words, **"Welcome home."**

The retrieval takes as long as an hour and as short as five minutes. You continue until you feel you have retrieved all disowned energies. Then sit in quiet continence and finally say something like, **"Very good. You can come back feeling perfect in every way."**

Smile and ask, **"How are you doing?"** Then listen to what they have to say.

The session is complete.

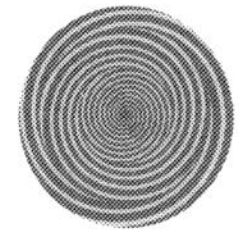

~ *Chapter 180* ~
GUARDIAN ANGEL HYPNOTHERAPY
TECHNIQUES

Includes
The Written Angel Consultation and Induction
Death and Rebirth Hypnosis

Angels have been known to humankind for ages and are popular than today. Pictures of angels are even found on postage stamps. Figurines of angels abound in stores internationally. Stories of Angels are written about, and seen in motion pictures and on TV. A recent survey affirmed that 63% of the American public believes in Guardian Angels, and 50% of these told of having an experience in which their Guardian Angel protected their life. The Guardian Angel Approach to hypnotherapy holds a grasp of omnipresent, omniscience, omnipotent power for achievement.

It is excellent hypnotherapy and brings in the element of belief. Belief bypasses critical mind so the subconscious accepts an idea. Belief is a subconscious motivator of behavior.

Many people believe they directly communicate with their Guardian Angel via prayer, or by simply and directly asking for a spoken or written communication.

MODUS OPERANDI: THE WRITTEN ANGEL CONSULTATION AND INDUCTION
You Will Need:
Paper
Pen Or Pencil
A Bowl That You Can Burn Something In
Matches Or A Lighter

This Written Angel Consultation and Induction has universal application. Basically, it expresses faith in something higher and beyond to assist in attaining whatever is needed and requested. It can be used as a specialized form of hypnotherapy in your practice.

Instead of a verbal consultation, give your client the privacy of time and space to write out the consultation. Here is an example of such a letter together with directions of how it is "mailed."

You or your client write this letter on a paper requesting what you want.
"Dearest Angel. I request your help to afford me the opportunity I ask for in this letter." (The request is written in detail and ends with this salutation).
You could have them write down three wishes that they would like granted.

"Let me achieve profound hypnosis now to develop my subconscious talents and

1.

2.

3.

Thank you, Guardian Angel, for making this beneficial request happen and become reality in my life.

With my love, _____________ (Sign your name)."

When the Written Consultation is complete, you and your client review it together. The client is then hypnotized with their eyes remaining open as you place their letter in a bowl saying,

"Concentrate on the flame, as the letter burns and the smoke rises in the air, upward to be received and answered by your Guardian Angel. Concentrate upon the rising smoke as you relax, knowing that your angel is granting your wishes. The burning brings in power for its realization. Now close your eyes and visualize the rising smoke as it conveys your message directly to your angel."

The entire process produces a state of mind amenable to transforming pretending to actuality. The recorded request has been conveyed. No further thought is given to it. The request will be fulfilled, often in most unexpected ways. Does it work? Thousands say it does.

If the client requests something negative to be removed from their life, the burning is suggested to symbolize the "removal of the difficulty." This technique is related to the removal of "nefarious entities hypnotherapy" which is gaining in popularity. However in this instance attention is directed towards the spiritual rather than the anti-spiritual. Both approaches call upon outside assistance for the healing, but concentrating on help from angels is by far the nicer way towards mental health and peace of mind.

MODUS OPERANDI: DEATH AND REBIRTH HYPNOSIS

In this angelic approach, your client writes upon a slip of paper request for what they desire to achieve. The affirmation slip is then placed beneath them on the chair, couch or bed upon which they rest with legs slightly apart and arms resting along side about six inches out from body. All lights off for total darkness. The hypnotherapist sits close by the side of reclining subject in a position to easily whisper into subject's ear.

"I have placed your request beneath your head (or by your side). **Concentrate upon your written request and take six deep breaths in rapid succession. Good.**

Lying now in darkness in this time and space close your eyes.

Lie absolutely still, and pretend you are dead. You cannot move at all. You are dead. You cannot even change your mind. You are dead. Stay just as you are. If you are angry and filled with wrath, stay so. If you are happy and filled with love, stay so. Stay exactly as you are. You cannot change anything. You are dead. Only I, who am outside of yourself, can change the position of your body or instruct your mind to change. I will do everything for you, as there is nothing you can do for yourself for you are pretending you are dead.

Hear this well inside yourself; any pain you have now or have ever felt is now completely gone from you, for a dead body can feel no pain. It is perfect as it is. And a dead brain senses no mind to cause it anxiety in any way. Your mind is totally in peace at rest. You are pretending you have just died and your body is placid and flexible.

As I grip your hand and move your arm they remain in whatever position they are placed. As I move your hands about, the movement relaxes you more and more and the

deeper you drop down inside yourself the more relaxed you become. You are dropping down into the very basement of relaxation, and you feel so good. You are dropping down into the abyss of your subconscious…and the deeper you go down within the inner space inside your self, the more it seems that you are rising up and up into the higher realms of outer space.

Going inner is going outer, and it seems that you are rising higher and higher into spirituals realms like the realm of sleep and dreams… and you visit with the angels.

And your very special Guardian Angel is there ready to assist and grant your every request and wish. And so you make a wish: 'My Dearest Guardian Angel make my body perfect in every way. Remove all dust from my mind, so it functions like pure crystal. And as I relax, engulfed atop the slip of my affirmation, let this game of pretend I play transform into the reality of this heartfelt desire I have requested. Let it become my very own. Please make it so. My thanks and love to thee.'"

(Repeat the affirmation of achievement requested several times. No more need it be said. The message has been received.)

"Enjoy this knowing and the space within which you now find yourself, and drop down into sleep for some moments, if you wish. And when your subconscious has given you this reality, you pleasantly arouse yourself knowing that all of life is a miracle and that you– to your personal reality– are the greatest miracle of all.

When you awake, you are fully alive even more alert, fully vitally alive then you have ever been. You come back in the here and now knowing it is so because it is."

For more on the GUARDIAN ANGEL see the chapter on the Guardian angel HYPNOTISM SHOW.

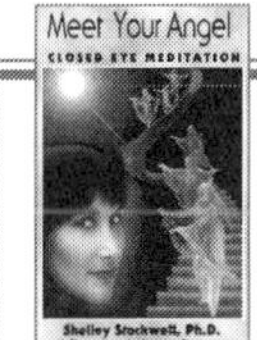

Hypno-Helper
"Meet Your Angel" audio tape by Shelley Stockwell-Nicholas, music by Jeannie Fitzsimmons.
Available on the order form at the back of this book.

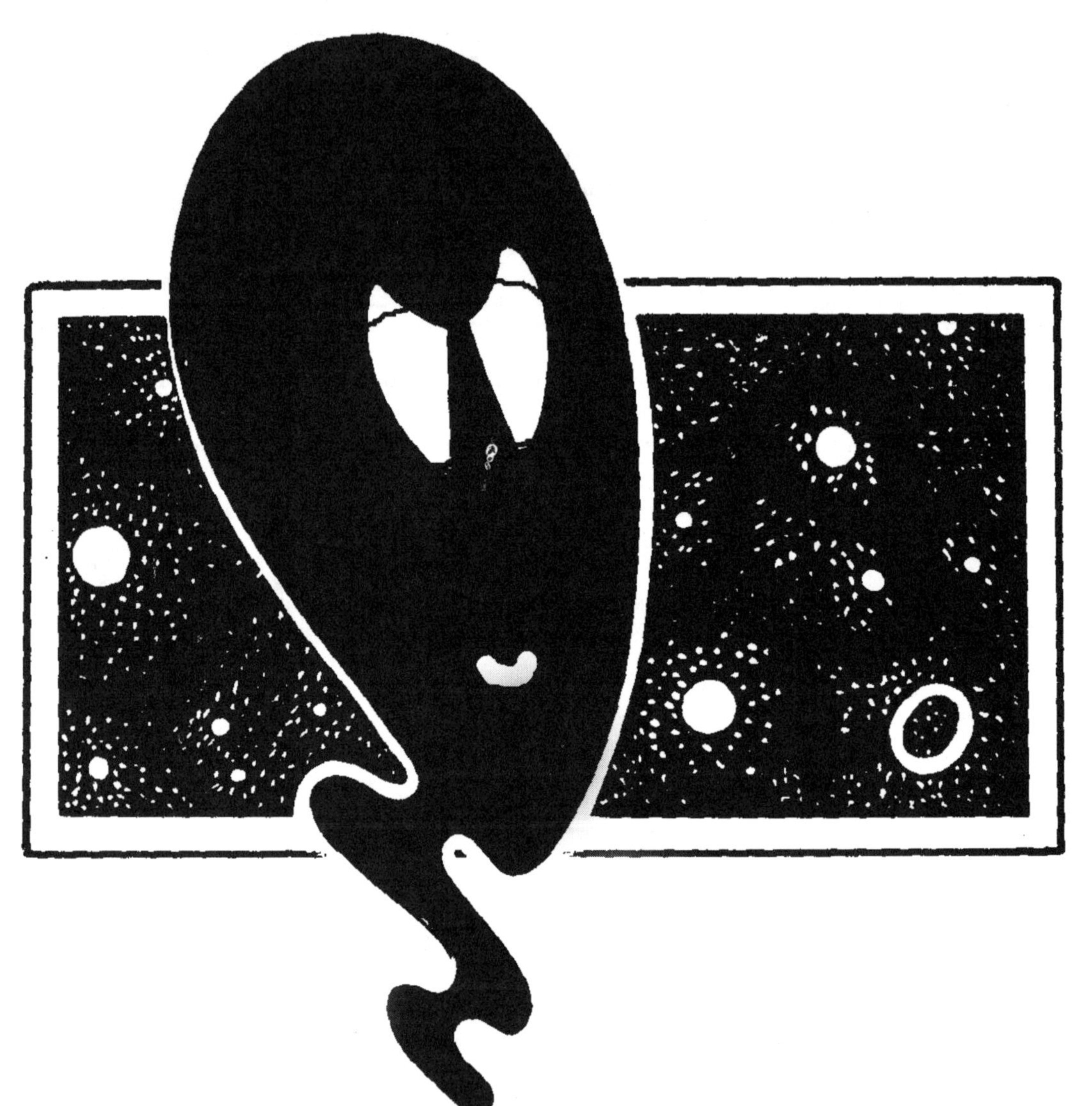

Illustration by Ormond McGill

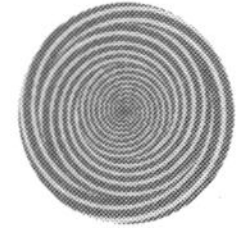

~ *Chapter 181* ~
SPIRIT DEPOSSESSION
HYPNOTHERAPY

Includes
Depossession Warning
Hypnotherapeutic Spirit Depossession
Marotta's Remote Depossession

Spirit Possession Hypnotherapy has sufficiently entered the field, as to warrant some coverage in this encyclopedia. Some use spirit depossession as the cornerstone of their practice. Both luck and spirit possession belong in the realm of speculation, but they are such ancient speculations they have become belief for many. It is remarkable in our High Tech Age that it is still given attention, yet somehow ancient beliefs hang on.

The Chinese tradition of ancestor worship goes back thousands of years, to the attached departed ancestors who directly affect the lives of the living. The Japanese believe that earthbound spirits can take possession of the living. Before the birth of Christianity, the ancient Greeks and Romans believed in spirit possession. Now and in the past, from Hindu to Catholics, many believe that removing evil spirits sets you free.

"A sick man pining away is one upon whom an evil spirit has gazed."
  —Homer

"Certain tyrannical demons require for their enjoyment some soul still incarnate to satisfy their passions."
  —Plutarch

"Demons are the spirits of wicked men."
  —Josephus

The ancient Egyptians very much believed that the dead affect the living. Spirit possession was a biblical obsession. There are some twenty-six incidents described in The Bible of Jesus exorcising possessing spirits. In every case, possessing spirits were described as harmful to the individual, and on removal immediately the person was benefited. Here are some ancient biblical references:

"Jesus preached and cast out devils."
  —Mark 1:39

"Jesus commanded the unclean spirit to come out of the man. The man was healed."
  —Luke 8:27-33

"Jesus gave his twelve disciples power against unclean spirits to cast them out."
  —Matthew 10:1

In 1727 Father Johann Joseph Grassner, in his long flowing purple cape, held a huge crucifix before him to drove the devil away. His hypnotic suggestion went like this "When you are touched by the crucifix, fall to the floor. There you will die and be examined by a physician who will be sure that you have no pulse. After they have declared you 'dead,' I will exorcise the demons to leave your body. You will then revive and when you stand you will be completely cured of what ails you." Tune in your television on Sunday morning and you can find many a religious person using an updated version of his technique.

Effects of spirit possession upon clients who believe in such range from great to slight. Symptoms are depression for no apparent cause, nervousness and doing things spontaneously without knowing just why the individual did them. In theory, the more the possessing entity takes control of the individual's consciousness, the greater the influence. Unwanted habits such as drinking, drug abuse, etc... is attributed to the possessing spirit influence.

DEPOSSESSION WARNING

This type of hypnotherapy tends to promote "The Devil Made Me Do It" attitude, and places the blame for unwanted behavior upon an outside influence, rather than having the person have the guts to accept their personal responsibility. To counteract this, always close such session with **"From now on you will be totally responsible to yourself for mastery of yourself."**

My advice: Do not get caught up in the mystical when you deal with this kind of hypnotherapy. Handle it as casually and matter-of-factly as going out for a cup of coffee.

MODUS OPERANDI: HYPNOTHERAPEUTIC SPIRIT DEPOSSESSION

Depossession can almost be looked upon as a spiritual ceremony, and should be performed in time and space free of interruption.

Have your client relax comfortably and enter hypnosis. While resting in hypnotic reverie, instruct client to exhale and inhale through the nose, and recite their favorite prayer (either mentally or out loud). Adults usually favor The Lord's Prayer. Children know "Now I lay me down to sleep..."

With your client in hypnosis suggest, **"I speak directly to your subconscious. Summon the possessing spirit so we may have a direct communication. I know that the possessing spirit can hear and speak though the senses of the body it has entered. Subconscious mind, cause a nod of client's head when this has been accomplished."**

(Wait for affirmation and agreement then proceed to directly address the possessing spirit. Speak to it exactly as you would speak to any human being. Be reasonable but firm.)

Address the so-called "possessing spirit" with an explanation that you understand their situation. **"Spirit, your body is dead, and there is no need for you to hang around further in this dimension. How nice it will be to free yourself and leave this physical body you have** entered. Move on into The White Light of higher dimensions of awareness for their soul's development."

Sometimes you will enter into a discussion with the possessing spirit as to the advantages of moving on. You may explain that their loved ones await them; that they will be in personal formless form of their own, and that they leave right now with blessings. Then command: **"Leave this person's body right now, and go on your way to higher things… knowing that you will possess a new physical body of your very own. How happy you will be. Okay. Understand. Real happiness awaits you. Now Go!"**

Most often, the entity will leave the body it has taken refuge in. However, sometimes, it is said, an entity will be stubborn or frightened to leave. However the case may be, insist to the possessing spirit that it must leave. Demand that they do, stressing that real happiness lies on ahead.

Those who work in this field say that they often sense a lightness come about their client, as the possessing spirit exits. When this is felt, arouse your client from the hypnosis with the knowledge that now they are free of all invading influences. **"You are well and fine. From now on you will be totally responsible to yourself for mastery of yourself."**

MODUS OPERANDI: MAROTTA'S REMOTE DEPOSSESSION

Albert Marotta, a professional hypnotherapist and college professor for over thirty years, uses this approach to release an "attached spirit" or entity from afar:

1. **Protect & Heal**
2. **Go To Highest Consciousness**
3. **Picture The Individual You Are Working With**
4. **Releasement**
5. **Talk To The Entity**
6. **Release Any Negative Influences**
7. **Call Forth The Replacements**
8. **Get Your Reward**

Here is his process:

1. **Protect & Heal the One Who is Doing the Depossession**
   "Experience your aura. Taste, feel, hear, smell and see your aura. Check it and see if there are any leaks tears or damage. Bring down white light like a layer of pancake syrup to repair any damage."

2. **Go To Highest Consciousness**
   "Now move to the highest realm of consciousness so that you can do the work that needs to be done today. Call forth your higher self, guides and helpers to assist."

3. **Picture The Individual You Are Clearing**
   As you ask, **"What needs to be done?"**
   (Let them answer.)
   Then instruct them:
   "Place the person you would like to help in front of the mirror of truth. As you look at them in the mirror, you can see the general shape of their physical body and its outline. There is a little switch that allows you to see and experience the body as transparent. Now go ahead and flick the switch and they will become completely transparent. If there are any parts of the body that is not transparent let me know what it is.

(Or, you can ask, "What area should I work on first?")

When they tell you, instruct them to:
"Seal that place in a saran wrap of poor white energy. Just do it and suspend it through time and place. Fill it with white light paste to absorb any negative energy that may remain. Compress the walls of light tighter, tighter, smaller and smaller. Good.

If it could speak, what would it say? Your level of awareness is now heightened five hundred times and you will know exactly what they are thinking. Who is talking? What year is this?"
(This will be the year the entity died.)

4. **Releasement**
    When they get to the place where they are ready to release say;
    "Would you like a place of better understanding and learning? If so, Look up and toward the light and you will see someone from your life who is coming to get you. Who do you see?
    (Note the quality of their eyes. If it is loving, that means everything is going well.)
    Are they glad to see you? What is the quality of their touch?"

5. **Talk To The Entity**
    "Who are you? What is your name? What year is it?"

6. **Release Any Negative Influences**
    The spirit has revealed themself. Their punishment is isolation. They didn't know that there is an alternative, now you offer it to them.
    "Recall all unpleasant memories and send them to the light where any such memory will be reformed and leave you with a sense of release."
    (Allow time for this process.)

    "There is a place so powerful that you will never need fear again. You are much more powerful that you ever believed. It is hidden in the last place you would ever look; below all the levels of the core of yourself. As you see acknowledge and recognize what happens, you stand tall in the light. Go back through all the eons of time and all negative energy of every and all person, animal, place, thing, event or living being from every time, space, place or dimension. As you go into the light you will be transformed and brought back as a positive healing force and source.

    Now, call back any and all you have ever had charge over in all time, place, space and dimension. Issue the order for them to empower themselves to transform all negative energy and send them into the light so they all come back filled with light for the most positive healing force and source.

    Call forth all those below and all those above and seal them in light.
    Now do the same with any and all negative energies and send them to the light and come back a as positive force and source."

7. **Call Forth The Replacements**
   "Ask that all be replaced, empowered and infused by light until any and all the dark side has been recharged and replaced with light."

8. **Get Your Reward**
   "Without them what is your reward for this call back?
   Receive the gift now of being forever free to be in the light. You are one with all that is. It is safe in your world. You are recharged and renewed with light."

REFERENCES

Cannon, A, "The Invisible Influence" Dutton, NY, 1954

Chaplin, A, "The Bright Light of Death" DeVores, 1977

Crabtree A, "Explorations in Possession and Multiple Personality" Praeger, NY, 1985

Dethlefsen, T, "Voices From Other Lives" Evans, NY, 1976

Ebon, M., Editor, "Exorcism: Fact Not Fiction" New American Library, NY, 1974

Fiore, Edith, "The Unquiet Dead" Doubleday, NY, 1987

Leeks, S, "Driving Out the Devils" Putman, NY 1975

Montgomery, R, "Search For Truth" Ballantine, NY, 1968

Moody, R, "Life After Life" Mockingbird Press, Atlanta, 1975

Osis, K. and E. Haraldsson. "At the Hour of Death" Pub. Avon, NY, 1977

Sugre, T, "There Is A River (Biography of Edgar Cayce)" Dell, NY, 1942

"The Egyptian Book of the Dead" Dover, NY, 1967

"The Tibetan Book of the Dead" Oxford University Press, Oxford, England, 1960

Zaretsky, I, "Bibliography On Spirit Possession" Berkeley University Press, Berkeley, CA, 1966

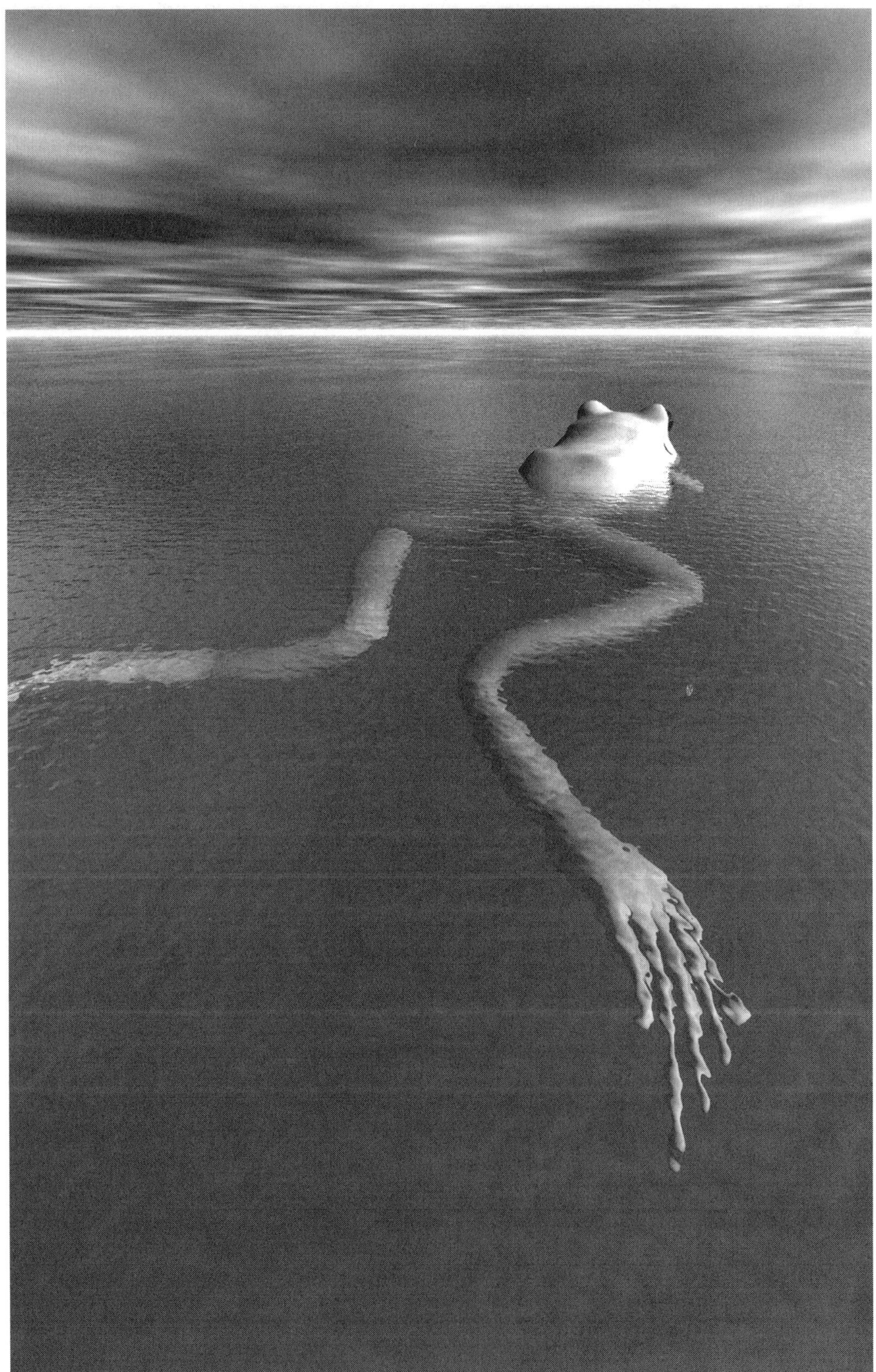

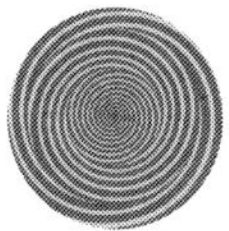

~ *Chapter 182* ~
TEN GIANT STEPS
TO SUPERCONSCIOUSNESS

Excerpted from the book "Everything You Ever Wanted to Know About Everything"
by Ormond McGill and Shelley Stockwell

Present these suggestions in the first person if you are using it for yourself, or in the second person if presenting it to a client:

"Lie on your back, close your eyes and relax. Breathe deeply and fully SIX TIMES in rapid succession. Very likely, it will cause a swimming sensation in your head, as this deep, rapid breathing saturates the brain with excessive oxygen. This mental state is receptive to hypnotic suggestions.

Now say to yourself: 'I am very comfortable. I am completely relaxed. Both my mind and body are relaxing completely. This complete relaxation is becoming my reality.' Concentrate on these suggestions

(Pause.)

My eyes are closed and I am becoming sleepy…very sleepy. I am drifting down into hypnotic sleep wherein my subconscious phase of mind will accept each suggestion presented to it. My subconscious will put these suggestions into action in my life, my consciousness advances to superconsciousness and I become KNOWER OF KNOWING.

(Pause.)

Wonderful hypnotic sleep in which my subconscious will transform into reality every suggestion that is presented. I continue to go deeper and deeper inside myself. My mind is drifting down into a state of reverie as I place my hands over my ears, and read OUT LOUD to myself the ten giant steps to superconsciousness. I subconsciously cause them to become my very own. Breathe deeply 6 times saying I am so relaxed. I am so sleepy. I am dropping off to sleep.

(Pause.)

BREATHE DEEPLY 6 TIMES.

God is the Mystery of Mysteries and ever shall be. Nothing is closer to the heart of me than God dwelling within myself. God, the creator and the creation are one. I engrave into my subconscious now the first giant step of superconscious wisdom.

(Pause.)

BREATHE DEEPLY 6 TIMES.

I come to know about EXISTENCE. I not only exist in the Universe, I am a part of that Universe…just as I am a part of God which is that Universe. I engrave into my subconscious the second giant step of superconscious wisdom.
(Pause.)

BREATHE DEEPLY 6 TIMES.

I have come to know about DEATH. Death as a termination of my existence is impossible. Death is merely a transition of my individual SELF from one form to another. Life and death are a perpetual continuum, like sunset and sunrise. Life and death depend upon the other to be. Death is a door or portal, not a stopping. My body remains at the door as my consciousness moves inside and enters the temple. I learn equally the art of living and the art of dying. I come to accept life and death's perpetual reception of each other. Such is the flow of life. I go with the flow. I engrave into my subconscious this third giant step of superconscious wisdom.
(Pause.)

BREATHE DEEPLY 6 TIMES.

To know LOVE and SEX, I appreciate that sex is fun, and LOVE enriches. Sex is a natural part of my nature. The only thing that stands between love and me is fear. I will not inner-fear. I ask myself what will I think of myself if I take the risk to love you? What will I think of myself if I don't? To come to know about perfect sex, I concentrate on joy. I engrave into my subconscious this fourth giant step of superconscious wisdom.
(Pause.)

BREATHE DEEPLY 6 TIMES.

I come to think of MONEY. If you place a piece of bread and gold before an animal, the animal will pick up the bread and go on its way. Much of what we value is based on imagined concepts of worth, rather than true worth. The only real value of money is how it is used and its convenience as a means to barter. I engrave into my subconscious this fifth giant step of superconscious wisdom.
(Pause.)

BREATHE DEEPLY 6 TIMES.

I come to know about MIND. There is no mind inside my head. MIND is a process for producing thoughts and thoughts are energy that operates my brain-computer, so I can manifest in 3-D space. My mind is immortal and provides the process of producing thoughts, in whatever form I dwell. I engrave into my subconscious this sixth giant step of superconscious wisdom.
(Pause.)

BREATHE DEEPLY 6 TIMES.

HAPPINESS is a decision I make. I choose how I react to the world around me. To be happy, I choose joy in all I do. I celebrate what I do. If I cannot celebrate what I do, then I will do something I can celebrate. I learn to laugh a lot, knowing that happiness relates to how I feel about myself. I engrave into my subconscious this seventh giant step of superconscious wisdom.
(Pause.)

BREATHE DEEPLY 6 TIMES.

I accept as WISDOM this wisdom. What is in front of me is what it is, not other than it is. I am interested in everything that happens in life. I do what must be done first before doing what must be done second. I know that everything is a miracle and I am the greatest miracle of all. I engrave into my subconscious this eighth giant step of superconscious wisdom.
(Pause.)

BREATHE DEEPLY 6 TIMES.

CONSCIOUSNESS is like a block of ice: it can be frozen and cease to flow. Heat it by focusing energy there and it takes a Quantum Leap and changes to water. Continue heating and it turns to steam, which is another Quantum Leap in Awareness. Another Quantum Leap occurs when the steam rises and disperses into the atmosphere. I understand this deeply. When consciousness is like ice, it perceives little. When consciousness is like water, it perceives more. When consciousness is like steam, it raises you above the world. I engrave into my subconscious this ninth giant step of superconscious wisdom.

I become the witness to life and what was formerly a point-of-view transforms into points-of-view. I have advanced to superconsciousness. From this perspective, I take a quantum leap in Awareness and tenth giant step of superconscious."

AROUSAL FROM THE SESSION

"When these giant steps of superconsciousness are programmed into the memory banks of your Brain-Computer, you are ready to arouse from hypnosis.

Remove your hands from your ears and rest upon your back. With your eyes closed, think to yourself: This has been a wonderfully pleasant hypnosis session and such a vast array of cosmic wisdom has been programmed into my mind. It is mine henceforth for all eternity."
(Allow some moments of silence.)

"It is time to prepare to arouse fully aware of the HERE AND NOW. Subconscious Mind, pay close attention, I will count slowly from one to ten. With each count, slowly arouse from hypnosis. By the count of ten, you will be fully alert in every way and feeling wonderful and fine.

One… two… three… begin to arouse from hypnosis now…four…five…six… I come back completely now, feeling wonderful and fine…seven…eight…nine…TEN. Awake and fully alert, back to yourself, feeling wonderful and fine, and all the cosmic wisdom is absorbed as you very own. You have trod successfully the GIANT STEPS TO SUPERCONSCIOUSNESS. THE MASTERY IS YOURS.

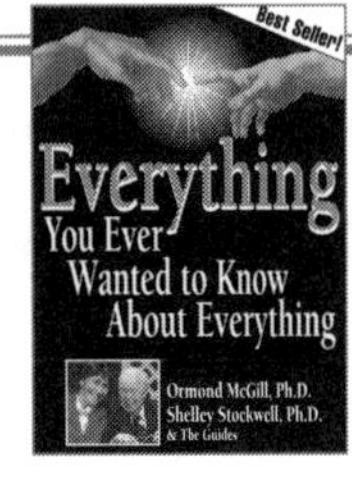

Hypno-Helper

"Everything You Ever Wanted to Know About Everything" book by Ormond McGill and Shelley Stockwell-Nicholas.
"Everything You Ever Wanted to Know About Everything 10 Giant Steps to Superconsciousness" audio tape by Ormond McGill are available at the back of this book.

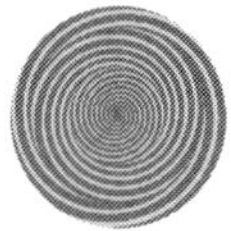

~ *Chapter 183* ~
UNIVERSAL MIND HYPNOTHERAPY

Includes
Universal Mind and Healing
Two Super Mind Inductions
    1. Deep Breathing Meditation Induction
    2. Five Senses Super-Mind Induction
Five Universal Mind Suggestion Formulas
    1. Universal Mind For General Good Health
    2. Universal Mind For Immunization From Diseases
    3. Universal Mind Suggestion For Mastering Pain Sensations
    4. Universal Mind Suggestion For Perpetual Youth
    5. Universal Mind Suggestion For Developing Your ESP And PSI Powers

You are about to explore a profoundly advanced and revolutionary form of hypnotherapy. It moves beyond the conscious/subconscious sensory mind to the cosmic connection of the Universal Mind. Universal Mind Hypnotherapy sends the mind into the abyss of the SELF. Here, all worldly stress and cares evaporate. Peace and serenity reign.

The abyss of SELF is a part of the superconscious mind, universal mind, or cosmic consciousness. This super-mind is your connection with the God Power and the knowing that you are a timeless miracle.

The entire Universe is dynamic and perpetually changing in finite vibration. You are part of the universe. Universal Mind Hypnosis connects and attunes you to this profound energy of the all in all.

The pathway to your super consciousness is hypnosis. You start by relaxing the conscious mind and enlisting it to direct attention to the subconscious and the Mind of the Universe. The conscious mind suggests your goal to the non-critical and accepting subconscious mind and the subconscious mind causes the goal to be realized.

When you return from this journey, you will very likely recall little, a bit here and there, but assuredly not entirely. That is why many say of this method "At last, I have reached the depth of hypnosis I always wanted. I was zapped out!"

Actually, far from zapped out, you have become un-zapped. In fact, you are more aware than you were before the session. Your enlightenment awareness comes with such brightness, it seems almost too much to hang onto at first, so you retreat back into the darkness because you feel safe and familiar here. The illusion is that you are safer when you are less aware.

Some give percentages as to who can be hypnotized and the depth of trance. The truth is that most of us are hypnotized all the time and it is far easier to induce hypnosis than "unduce" it. The majority of humans respond to their environment the way they are hypnotized to respond. Their limited universe instructs them of their limitations, which they unquestioningly accept and respond to. So many people walk around this planet asleep or half asleep.

Once in a while, a master comes along who is awake and explains the value of waking up and becoming fully aware. Once in while, cosmic knowledge flashes through to create a new paradigm. We call these "flashes of genius." Unfortunately, most geniuses are awake in just a very tiny space of awareness and are asleep in others. True enlightenment is when you are awake to whole, full reality. I believe that everyone will eventually awaken to full reality, as it is always there for us to recognize. It is eternity. But, don't think of eternity as time for eternity is simply continuous awareness in the here and now.

UNIVERSAL MIND AND HEALING

All hypnotherapy helps others heal by use of the mind. Healing is bound to be both mental and physical, as mind affects the body and body affects the mind. In advancing into a connection with universal mind, you enter the realm of healing miracles. Universal mind suggestions accomplish therapeutic miracles. They bring in a flow of cosmic healing energy. Have faith that it is so and you produce such "miracles." Present generalized suggestions for mental and physical well being as you begin. Remember, "Ask and ye shall receive."

Actively enlist the conscious mind to want to connect higher awareness. It's easy because your conscious mind eagerly connects with what it perceives as good. The conscious mind knows the goodness of higher states. Oh, of course, the conscious mind likes to ask questions. How do you do it? What technique must be used? Is it difficult? Will it take a lot of time? There is no need to answer these questions. Just instruct the conscious mind to:

"Use hypnosis to reach through any questions and make the effort without effort. There is no effort to achieve what you already have. The gift of Universal Mind is yours."

For Self Hypnosis:
"If you want to take yourself to superconsciousness, place your hands over ears and speak your induction out loud to yourself. Or record it and play it back to yourself."

For Hypnotizing Another:
"If hypnotizing a client, have them make themselves comfortable." A good way to begin: **"Let your conscious mind decide the purpose of the session."**

MODUS OPERANDI: TWO SUPER UNIVERSAL MIND INDUCTIONS

The Deep Breathing Meditation Induction and the Five Senses Induction prepare your client for the powerful Universal Mind Suggestions. These suggestion formulas can be presented either in the first or second person.

1. DEEP BREATHING MEDITATION INDUCTION
You Will Need:
Hypno-Music
A Violet Light (optional)

If you choose to use this induction, it would precede the five senses Induction.

Go into a quiet, darkened room with your client. Use a violet light, when convenient. Violet light has a sedative effect. Play the Hypno-music cassette quietly in the background. Face the client and breathe in unison with them. The breathing technique brings in more prahnic, or lifeforce energy

"You are taking a quantum leap in heightening your consciousness. Breathing brings in prahnic energy or vitality. Let us breathe together, in unison and notice how breath enters the body. Feel it completely.

An ancient sutra says: 'Radiant one, this experience may dawn between two breaths. After breath comes in and just before turning up – the beneficence.' Become consciously aware of your breathing and we will explore the meaning of the sutra.

Just before exhaling, notice that there is a point, for just a moment, in which there is no breathing. There is a gap. Become aware of this gap, and exhale your breath. Consciously experience it passing out your body. And note, that this point too, just for a moment, there is a gap with no breath. When you are consciously aware of the gaps in breath, you will enter what the sutra calls 'beneficence'.

Breath coming into the body represents life. Breath going out represents death…death and re-birth. The gaps between the in and the out and the out and the in is beyond life and death of the body. At that moment, you contact the Universal Mind. This is a new dimension of consciousness. We will now just breathe for ten minutes and you will be ready to advance to the five senses and Universal Mind Hypnotherapy."

Be silent and relax as you sit quietly with your client in meditation. When ten minutes have passed, arise and light the candle on the table in front of the client. This prelude quiets their mind even more and prepares them for the Five Senses Induction.

2. FIVE SENSES SUPER-MIND INDUCTION
You Will Need:
Hypno-Music
A Violet Light (optional)
A Candle (optional)
Peppermint or Rose Oil (optional)

Go into a quiet, darkened room with your client. Use a violet light, when convenient. Violet light has a sedative effect. Play the Hypno-music cassette quietly in the background.

"Profound Universal Mind Hypnosis combines your five senses; seeing, hearing, tasting, smelling, and feeling. Around and around you will go from sense to sense – in a mounting spiral down, down into the abyss of your inner SELF. Who says you go down? Maybe you go up. There is no up or down in the cosmos. We will go slowly as you achieve profound hypnosis!

The profound hypnosis of the Universal Mind makes you so aware, you often create amnesia or forgetfulness about the experience. In reality, you have taken a quantum leap of consciousness. How good it feels to be safe again, Sleepyhead.

We begin by seeing. Relax. Close your eyes whenever you wish.

(If a candle is used) **Passively gaze at the flickering candle flame. Your eyes will grow weary as you stare at the candle.**

(Their eyes will soon close.)

Now become aware of the Hypnomusic playing in the background. Your sense of sight is eclipsed by your full attention to the music. You feel like you actually enter into the music. As you do, you drop deeper into hypnosis. (Allow some space for it to happen.)

Now, move on to the sense of taste and as you do you drop deeper and deeper into hypnosis.

(An option is to place a little candy peppermint wafer in the client's mouth, squeezing it in between their lips.) **"Taste this fully. Do not chew or swallow the candy, just let it enter into your taste as it slowly dissolves into the mouth. As it dissolves you will continue dropping down deeper and deeper into hypnosis."**

(Allow some space for this.)

Now, move on to your sense of smell. (Waft some subtle essence like rose oil beneath their nose.)

Inhale the fragrance deeply, and, as you do, you will drop down deeper and deeper into profound hypnosis.

Now, move on into the sense of feeling. (You can stand behind the client, and, gently place your fingertips at each of their temples and stroke the temples gently.) **Each stroke sends you down, down, ever deeper into profound hypnosis. Where is profound hypnosis? Your mind knows; you need not bother to explain."**

(At this point in the induction, allow some space for the stroking.)

Become aware of each of your senses seeing, hearing, tasting, smelling and feeling. Go from sense to sense, one by one, seeing, hearing, tasting, smelling and feeling. Around and around you go from each of your senses in a mounting spiral down, down into the abyss of your inner SELF. Who says that you go down? Maybe you go up. There is no up or down in the cosmos. It is wisely said, 'As above so below.' You spiral down deeper and deeper into the abyss of SELF…seeing, hearing, tasting, smelling, and feeling takes you down, down, down. Drop off to the realm of sleep. You are more aware of your true nature in existence than you have ever been before.

You now de-hypnotize yourself from any unwanted ways and enter the realm of your true self. The more you drop down into the abyss of yourself, into the reverie of hypnosis, the more you enter this dreamland and free your SELF to connect with Universal Mind. Your Supermind is your gift. It is your heritage. Open wide, go down deep into the abyss inside yourself, and open wide your powers of Universal Mind."

(You can now give specific suggestions for your client or use one of the five formulas that follow.) When complete suggest:

"You will always use your mind as a whole, a trinity of conscious to subconscious to superconscious mind. The amazing powers of your Universal Mind are yours to use and command. When you know that has been accomplished, arouse from hypnosis and return to the here and now feeling wonderful and fine. There is no hurry, your SELF knows, on its own, when to spontaneously return to the outer world feeling wonderful and fine."

FIVE UNIVERSAL MIND SUGGESTION FORMULAS

Having induced such profound receptivity the SELF is now ready to receive suggestion. Here are five universal mind suggestion formulas of great value to yourself and your clients. You can develop your own specific formulas to give to the receptive universal mind, too. Have faith in these. They can create miracles on demand.

1. UNIVERSAL MIND FOR GENERAL GOOD HEALTH

"You are in hypnosis now. Relax completely and allow these suggestions to become your reality.

Healing energy from the cosmos enters into you bringing health and wellness in every way. Your entire body is becoming aglow with radiant energy. You can feel its warmth. It penetrates and brings good health to your entire body from the top of your head to the tips of your toes. Every cell of your brain and body is replete with healthy life. Perfect health is yours. Let it be so.

Allow this inner glowing of health-giving energy from out of the cosmos to become your very own. When your inner mind knows that the process is complete, arouse from hypnosis and return to the here and now."

2. UNIVERSAL MIND FOR IMMUNIZATION FROM DISEASES

"You are in deep hypnosis now, and these suggestions pass through your subconscious mind to the universal mind to completely immunize you from any and all disease.

You are protected and encased in a cocoon of glowing energy of life and radiant health resistant to all disease. Every organ of your entire body functions to perfection and resists disease in every way. An armor of immunization surrounds and permeates every molecule of you… it protects you and keeps you constantly in good health. Your body completely renews, restores and regenerates itself into perfect radiant wellness, the way God intended you to be.

Arouse when your inner mind KNOWS it is so."

3. UNIVERSAL MIND SUGGESTION FOR MASTERING PAIN SENSATIONS

"You are in deep hypnosis now, as any and all pain sensations vanish.

Now, tighten up the muscles of your body and turn your attention away from any painful sensations to experiencing the power that is within your body. Your body is strong, powerful, and free of all uncomfortable sensation. As you tighten up the muscles of your body, you feel powerful and radiant well-being throughout your entire body. Now, suddenly relax as any tension suddenly lets GO! As you suddenly let GO from tension to relaxation, all pain is GONE! Your body is now free to renew and restore itself to absolute perfection. You feel free… free… free. Now your body is comfortable, and you are free to heal to absolute perfection. Heal! Heal! Heal!" When you know that this is so arouse WHEN and AS you will."

4. UNIVERSAL MIND SUGGESTION FOR PERPETUAL YOUTH

"You are in deep hypnosis now in direct connection with Universal Mind. Universal Mind gives you the power to perpetuate your youthfulness. You see yourself at the age you prefer inside yourself. That is the age you visualize and imagine yourself to be. You energize this inside youthful picture an image of yourself with cosmic energy from the Universe. You become the age at which you feel yourself to be. Youthful vigor and vitality fill your life, and your mind is crystal clear.

This inside reality becomes your outside reality as well. When it is so, arouse from the hypnosis, and come back with me to the here and now, feeling and looking terrific.

5. UNIVERSAL MIND SUGGESTION FOR DEVELOPING YOUR ESP AND PSI POWERS

"You are in deep hypnosis now, and you know your psychic gifts reside in your connection with Universal Mind. The ESP and PSI Powers of your mind are developing in leaps and bound, as you continually increase your connection with Universal Mind. You receive telepathic messages from the minds of those around you. You have clairvoyant perception of events. You have the ability to create directly in the Universe and bring abundance for yourself.

Day by day, in every way, your psychic talents increase. You are cultivating a direct connection with universal mind. You are becoming a master of the ESP and PSI powers of your mind. Subconscious mind and universal mind connect bringing in such superpowers of awareness to be recognized by your conscious mind.

Let this become your reality. When your inner mind knows this has become realized, and your ESP and PSI powers are growing ever greater, day by day, arouse from the hypnosis now, feeling wonderful and fine."

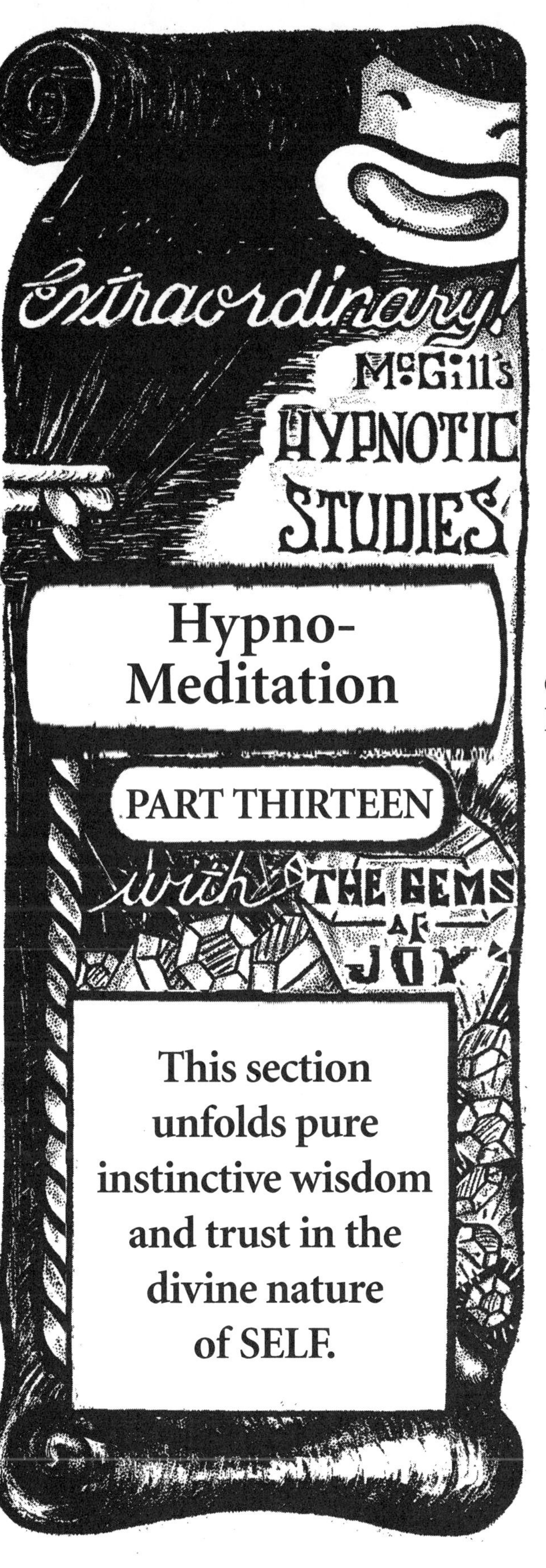

CHAPTERS IN PART THIRTEEN

184. Thoughts On Hypnomeditation ....page 731
185. Hypnosis Verses Meditation 733
186. Hypno-Meditation Formulas 735
187. You Are A Rainbow.................................739
188. Color/Chakra Balancing 741
189. The Ladder Of Colors 745
190. Hypnotherapy Of Infinity 749
191. Ancient Essene Hypno-Meditation 751
192. Essene Entering Darkness Meditation 757
193. Meditation Of The Violet Flame..........761
194. Hypnotherapy Of Zen 765
195. Transcendental Hypnotherapy............769

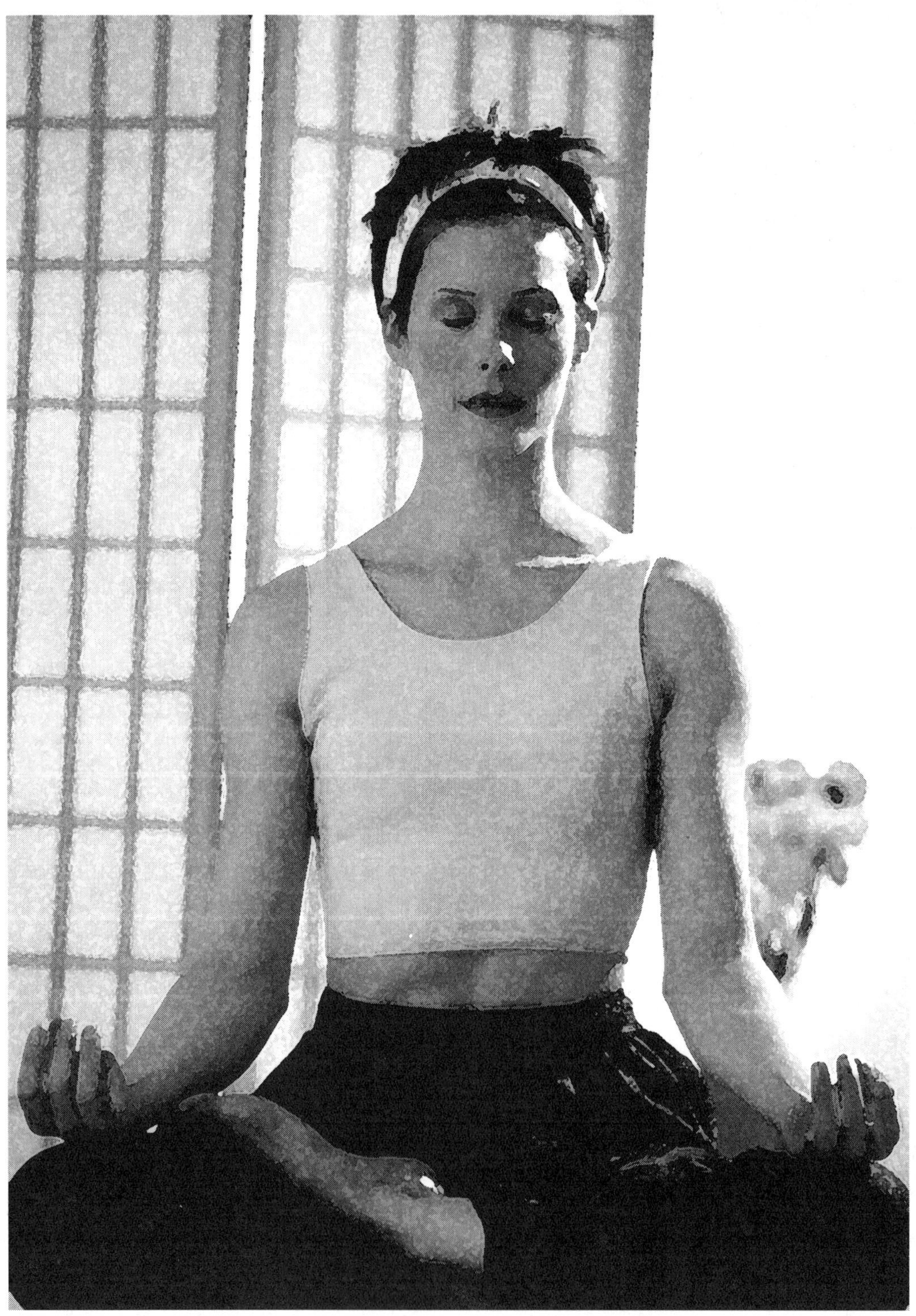

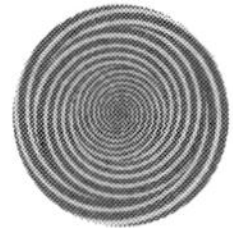

~ *Chapter 184* ~
THOUGHTS ON HYPNOMEDITATION

Includes
Meditations Three States Of Mind

Meditation is instinctive knowing. Knowing is wisdom and wisdom comes through living in meditation. Processes that establish meditation in the mind of the client are remarkable hypnotherapy. Meditation tells of the perfection of existence and of YOUR perfection in existence. Implanting this wisdom into the subconscious mind of your client is the purpose of HypnoMeditation.

Knowledge is recognized as power in the world and most seek knowledge. However the really wise one knows that through knowledge one becomes separated from the whole. Knowledge, unless relegated to its proper status, can be the antithesis of wisdom. Here is an example:

You come across a wildflower while walking through a meadow. It is a new variety to you so your mind has no knowledge of what flower it is and so your mind remains silent. Now you can look at the flower and truly experience it and you are filled with wonder about it. The flower is there and you are there and since you have no acquired knowledge about the flower to judge it by, you are not separated from the flower. In other words, you are bridged and so you can become one with the flower.

This is beautiful.

On the other hand, if you have knowledge about the flower and know its common name and scientific name, your knowledge has caused you to become separated from the flower and the total experience of its loveliness is lost. The misuse of knowledge has cost you your bridge between yourself and the flower.

The undiluted beauty has been lost.

To understand what is expressed here is to understand that knowledge can divide and separate you from the heart of what is real. The secret of meditation is to go beyond knowledge. HypnoMeditation is pure space, emptiness undisturbed by knowledge.

How true is the biblical parable that we have fallen through eating of the tree of knowledge. It seems so illogical that we have "fallen" through knowledge. It looks illogical because logic is supportive of knowledge. It looks illogical because logic is the root of this fall. An absolutely logical, absolutely sane person will be amongst the most miserable. Sanity needs to be balanced by insanity. Logic needs to be balanced by illogic. Opposites must meet and balance. One who is entirely reasonable is unreasonable-they miss much. Indeed some one like that will go on missing the most beautiful and most true. They will collect the trivia of knowledge and this mundane life will miss the spiritual and transcendental entirely.

Master Patanjali says, "When mind is not occupied by things, by thoughts (for things are thoughts), then there enters 'that which IS' and that which IS, is the case." In other words, that which IS, is truth and only in emptiness can occur. Only in emptiness do you become pregnant with knowing, which is beyond knowledge. HypnoMeditation makes this possible.

MEDITATIONS THREE STATES OF MIND

In relation to meditation there are three states of mind:

1. Consciousness With Contents

This is the consciousness of the average person. In such a mind, thoughts are always moving, a desire is arising, anger, greed, ambition or whatever. Always there is some content in the mind and the mind is never unoccupied. While awake, they are thinking. When asleep dreaming. Thinking and dreaming are allied processes with dreaming a little bit more primitive because while dreaming mind usually thinks in symbols rather than concepts.

2. Consciousness Without Contents

Meditation leads here because in meditation we have no motivation to achieve anything in particular; we are interested in just BEING. Meditation is not directed to accomplishing any goal, unless you call meditation the goal. Really it is not, for YOU are the goal reached even before you start. You could say that meditation is the way to come to know THYSELF.

3. When Both Consciousness and Content Disappear: Samadhi

This is a higher state of conscious, "Cosmic Consciousness" and a cosmic leap in consciousness with direct insight- the intuition of knowing. It is knowledge beyond what we commonly accept knowledge to be.

In the state of samadhi one first drops the contents of the mind and you are half empty. Then you drop normal consciousness and become fully empty. This full/empty is found as the greatest benediction that can happen to someone, as now they become conscious of the divine nature of SELF, which is eternal in existence. In other words, you come to know THYSELF.

Bringing this deep perception to your client is what hypnotherapy is truly about. It is Transcendental Hypnotherapy.

HypnoMeditation brings in meditation to the mind and meditation is the pathway to samadhi. Samadhi is to know the divinity of oneself; to move from knowledge to knowing; and to advance to Cosmic Consciousness. With this true wisdom there comes in a peaceful mind. Buddha's "Nothing need be done" is self-operating, just as the Universe is self-operating. Using HypnoMeditation one comes to know that they are a miniature of the Universe. The following chapters in this section are devoted to the ways and means of this hypnotherapy.

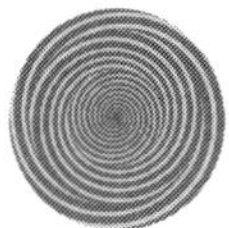

~ *Chapter 185* ~
HYPNOSIS VERSES MEDITATION

Includes
Hypnosis Meditation Induction
Witness Meditation

If the world "hypnosis" is scary to someone, call it meditation. No one is afraid of meditation and in fact hypnosis and meditation are closely aligned. It could almost be said that meditation is the Eastern form of hypnosis and hypnosis is the Western form of meditation.

MODUS OPERANDI: HYPNOSIS MEDITATION INDUCTION
You will need
A Small Crystal or Crystal Ball (that you can hold in your hand)

"Instead of hypnosis today we will explore meditation. As you know, meditation is a pleasant way to relax the body and enter into the inner realm of the mind. Meditation originated in India and has become very popular in Western countries. Classes in meditation are even taught in colleges and universities.

To meditate begin by sitting comfortably in your chair, place your feet on the ground and rest your hands in your lap so that your fingers do not touch. In showing you how to meditate. I will use a crystal ball as it is used for meditation in India."

(Pick up the crystal ball and show it to the client and continue)

"The crystal ball is used by the Yogis as the object upon which they concentrate in meditation. We will use it that way. As I hold it before you and move it from one side to the other, direct your attention upon it as it moves. Watch the changing lights with in the crystal. As it moves before you concentrate on relaxing your body step by step and when I tell you 'close your eyes' your eyes will close and you will go deep inside yourself. So start now by thinking of relaxing the muscles of your scalp. Relax the muscles of your head and face.

Now let your thoughts move on down and relax the muscles of your shoulders, and allow the relaxation to flow down your arms to your hands as they rest in your lap. Relax completely.

Relax your chest and torso muscles as your mind now moves down your body and you watch the crystal move before you and relax your thighs, knees, your calves and right on down to your feet. Your entire body is so relaxed.

Now close your eyes and relax completely. Just let your self GO! As you drop inside yourself feeling so peaceful and drowsy all over. Your head drops down to your chest, as you are so sleepy. You feel so relaxed and good. Our eyes are closed and are becoming stuck tightly together. You will find that you cannot open them. Try as hard as you will. Try. Try but you will find that you cannot open your eyes. Forget about your eyes now and just go deeper into relaxation and you will find that you will be able to concentrate wonderfully with the power of suggestion of the ideas I will now present to you..."

MODUS OPERANDI: WITNESS MEDITATION

"Do you know what a court recorder is? Does the court recorder keep recording even if the witness is confused or contradicts or is lying or mistaken? The court recorder keeps recording. That's the attitude you will take. Just verbally report everything that you witness...everything you are aware of. There is no way you cannot be aware, is there? Perhaps your big toe itches or your arm feels relaxed, report what you focus on. Maybe you have a thought about what to eat for dinner or you may think of something out of the clear blue. It may be bizarre or silly or whatever...remember the court recorder and just speak it out. Maybe you remember something from earlier today or a long time ago or something buried in your subconscious mind. Or you may see something. Don't concern yourself about it, just get in touch with what you experience and report each sound, taste, smell, feeling, word or vision. Remember the court recorder and report without judging whether it is important or unimportant...your job is to faithfully report what comes to mind."

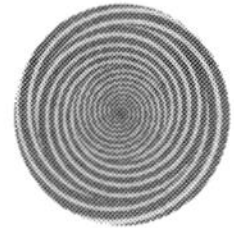

~ *Chapter 186* ~
HYPNO-MEDITATION FORMULAS

Includes
White Light Of Protection Hypno-Meditation
Know Thyself Hypno-Meditation
The Flame In Your Heart Hypno-Meditation

"God is within you."
> —Jesus

If you did nothing more in all your work than to instill these meditations into the subconscious of your client, you would have enhanced the quality of their life.

Hypno-meditation brings in recognition of the divine nature of one's SELF. It combines daily living with spiritual heights and a realization that as an individual YOU are the one and only exactly like yourself in the entirety of existence. YOU are an original and you stand at the very center of the universe in relation to yourself. It is a GOD position.

Hypno-meditation changes the quality of your life when used in connection with self hypnosis or hypnotizing others.

Hypnosis and meditation are opposites of the same: yin and yang, polarities of each other: diametric approaches that constitute the whole. Hypnotherapy is goal directed, meditation has no goal except the YOU you already are. Hypnosis entails a constriction of consciousness or awareness while meditation entails expanded consciousness or awareness. Look at a coin; on one side you see heads on the opposite side, tails. Both appear totally different yet they constitute the coin. Hypno-meditation merges the two sides of the coin together; you are goal directed toward recognition of your real SELF and your "beingness" in existence.

Meditation is a state of being and not doing. Each way moves you beyond intellect and is merely a pathway to discovery yourself as changeless. The intellect finds no answers to the truth of your Being. Philosophy can give you a pat answer. If this satisfies you, you convert to the philosophy yet YOU remain the same. If it doesn't satisfy you, you go on searching for another philosophy to be converted to, but YOU remain the same and YOU are not touched at all. For how can one change what is REAL? YOU are YOU whichever philosophy is embraced.

Mastering and presenting hypno-meditation makes you a master of your profession.

MODUS OPERANDI: THE WHITE LIGHT OF PROTECTION HYPNO-MEDITATION
Keep the energy moving upward from center to center and do not allow it to linger in any one center until it is released from the top of the head. This leaves the entire body buzzing with energy:

"Your Inner being is surrounded at all times with the white light of purity. As you accept the white light into your inner self you become a source of love. This white light symbolizes the love of God for you, and your love of God. It protects you from harm at all times and forms a wall of protective love around you. It is your armor.

You accept the white light of protection into your inner self. You visualize the inner space of your spine. Each vertebra stands out sharp and clear in your mind. You see your head resting on one end of your spine and the base of your spine ending in a hollow center with kundalini energy ready to spring into surging energy up your spine. You know the kundalini, light rays, power energy, vitality and psychic force as one and the same. Kundalini is light rays of vitality. This vitality energizes all of your meditations. You see yourself as light rays going into the hollow space of the base of your spine, filling it with light and energy. Filled with light, you see the kundalini begin to stir and uncoil. You see it rising as a beam of light energy rising up your spinal column. This kundalini light is a source of great and vital power. It is the source of great psychic energy. The light rising up now touches your psychic center located in the region of your reproductive organs, the light causes this center to spin and become aglow with light. You feel warmth coming into this region of your body. It is aglow with energy.

The light continues to rise yet further up your spinal column and touches the next psychic center of your solar plexus. The power of the light touches your core.

Now it moves up to your heart and touches your heart center. The power of the light touches your heart. Your heart is aglow with light. You can feel your heart beat faster as it glows with light.

Your entire body becomes more and more aglow with light. You are filled with energy. Now the light is rising yet further up your spinal column and touches the center of your throat. This center begins to spin and glow with light and more and more energy within your body as it moves now up your spine to your third eye, the center between your eyebrows. Now this center beams the energy within your head as light upon the center at the very top of your head. The energy of the kundalini has reached the crown of your head and this center begins to spin and glow and showers out a fountain of light above your head. You wear a crown of light. You are aglow with energy and light. Your entire body is radiant with energy."

MODUS OPERANDI: KNOW THYSELF HYPNO-MEDITATION
This divine meditation brings to consciousness the individual remarkable BEING you are in existence. It is the meditation for full living:

"The white light of protection floods you with energy and you recognize your inner self and outer self as different and distinct. Your inner self is your real being. Your outer self is that which you present to the world. Your inner self is serene and dwells within your being in absolute peace and harmony. Your inner self is absolutely free of stress. Life is a joy for you. Life a game to be enjoyed and it is played on the playground of existence. You flow with existence as a log floats on flowing waters and whatever touches you is a treasure of full living. Existence brings you the treasures of living full in every way. Your attitude about life is that life is a game you are playing in the universe for the sheer pleasure of it. Life is a joy and stress is no more. Life is a joy. You are safe within a fortress of joy. You relax into existence. You are content to be.

736

MODUS OPERANDI: THE FLAME IN YOUR HEART HYPNO-MEDITATION

This hypno-meditation expands your radiance to others. It is the meditation of the personality that takes you instinctively beyond the three dimensions of mind; wakefulness, dreaming, sleeping so you come to know that your real SELF is consciousness beyond limit.

"You accept the white light of protection into your inner being and the light floods you with energy. You instinctively know that your mind has three divisions: wakefulness, dreaming and sleeping. Your real SELF is a consciousness beyond any of these divisions. You know that this is true. At all times while you are awake you will sense deep within yourself a flame of your real self. You are a flame. You are light. Your heart is a luminous torch burning brightly and your body is but an aura of its flame. You are a flame. You are aflame. You are light. Your heart is a burning torch flaming love for all to feel who come near me. When you go to sleep, you dream of this flame that burns within you. It is beautiful. It is light. You dream of it burning within you as a flame of love and as you pass on beyond dreams into deep sleep you still carry the flame of love with you. It protects you and helps and aids all those about you. You are light. You are light. You are light.

You stand apart from yourself and recognize your SELF as this brilliant flame. As you pass beyond waking, beyond dreaming, beyond sleeping you recognize yourself as your SELF, which is a flame. You are light.

Sink down now into the lassitude of self-hypnosis. Go deep into it. After a time arouse yourself as you will and you will sense an inner warmth inside yourself as the flame begins to burn, brighter and brighter within you. The warmth is so great that others around you sense it. Once this flame has been kindled it is self perpetuating. Others feel your flame-YOU have become a presence.

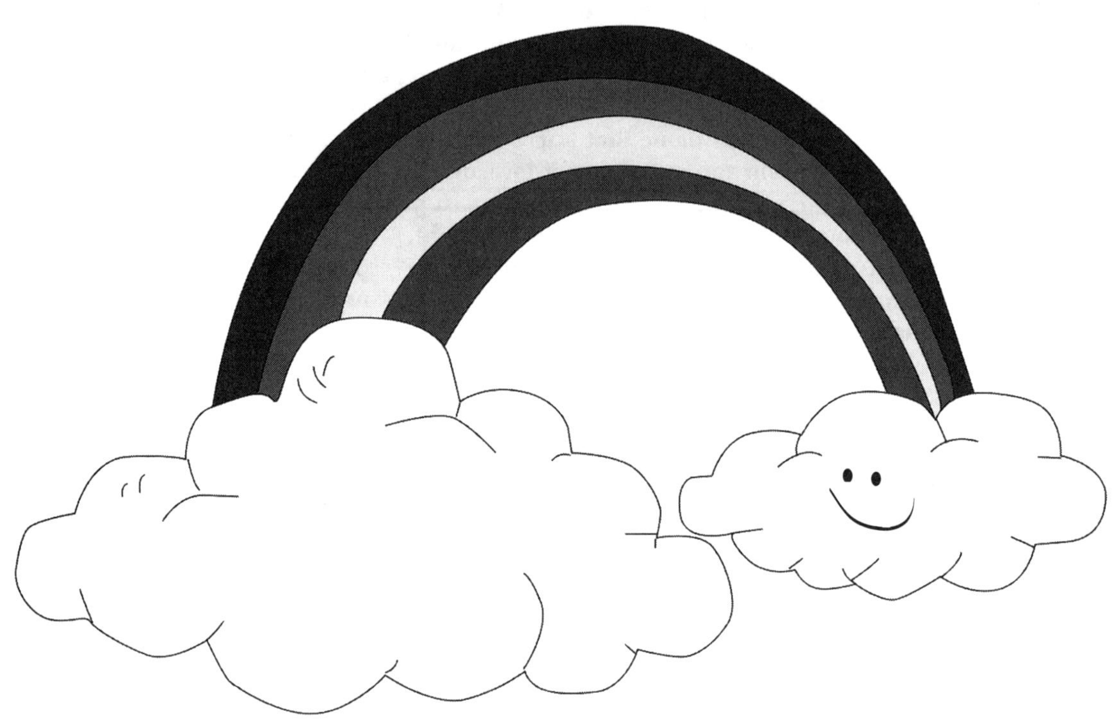

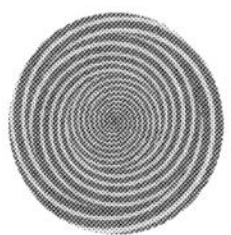

~ *Chapter 187* ~
YOU ARE A RAINBOW
SELF-HYPNOSIS

I was personally given this beautiful self-hypnosis process from a dear guru while I was in India. It is so enchanting that anyone can use and benefit from it. As a hypnotherapist, you can give it as a gift to all your clients.

MODUS OPERANDI: YOU ARE A RAINBOW
You Will Need:
A Place Near A Nice Stream

"Perform this self-hypnosis method quietly by yourself on a warm sunny day out in the countryside as you sit beside a rippling stream.

Close your eyes and do nothing at all. Just sit and sit and sit, and listen to the rippling stream of water, as it flows along. In your mind, enter the sound of the flowing water. Do this quietly with your spine straight, and without even trying at all, and somehow let your rate of breathing match the rhythm of the little flowing stream. A mood or meditation will descend upon you as mind stops its chattering.

And you drift and drift and drift. Before long, it will seem that you are 'out of body' and no longer have need of a body in these special moments. You do not need a body because you are going to become a rainbow.

Now, proceed on…

Visualize a shaft of white light (like a searchlight beam) coming down from space to illuminate the crown of your head and infuse your brain.

Allow the light to penetrate deeply and flow on down your spine until it reaches the center of your body behind your navel…your center of being. In this center, construct a prismatic crystal…a prism…as the White Light of Creation falls upon the prism it is refracted into a multicolored spectrum that fragments the light into rainbow hues. Allow the colors of light to be like rainbow colored snowflakes drifting gently down upon you… and where they touch they instantly melt and are gone.

They are gone because they have entered into you, and have become a part of your aura. You radiate out and touch all life, all matter, with the prismatic colors of your creation.

You are a rainbow.

Come back anytime you wish. There is no hurry. Just be like the rippling stream beside which you are seated, as it flows on and on and on."

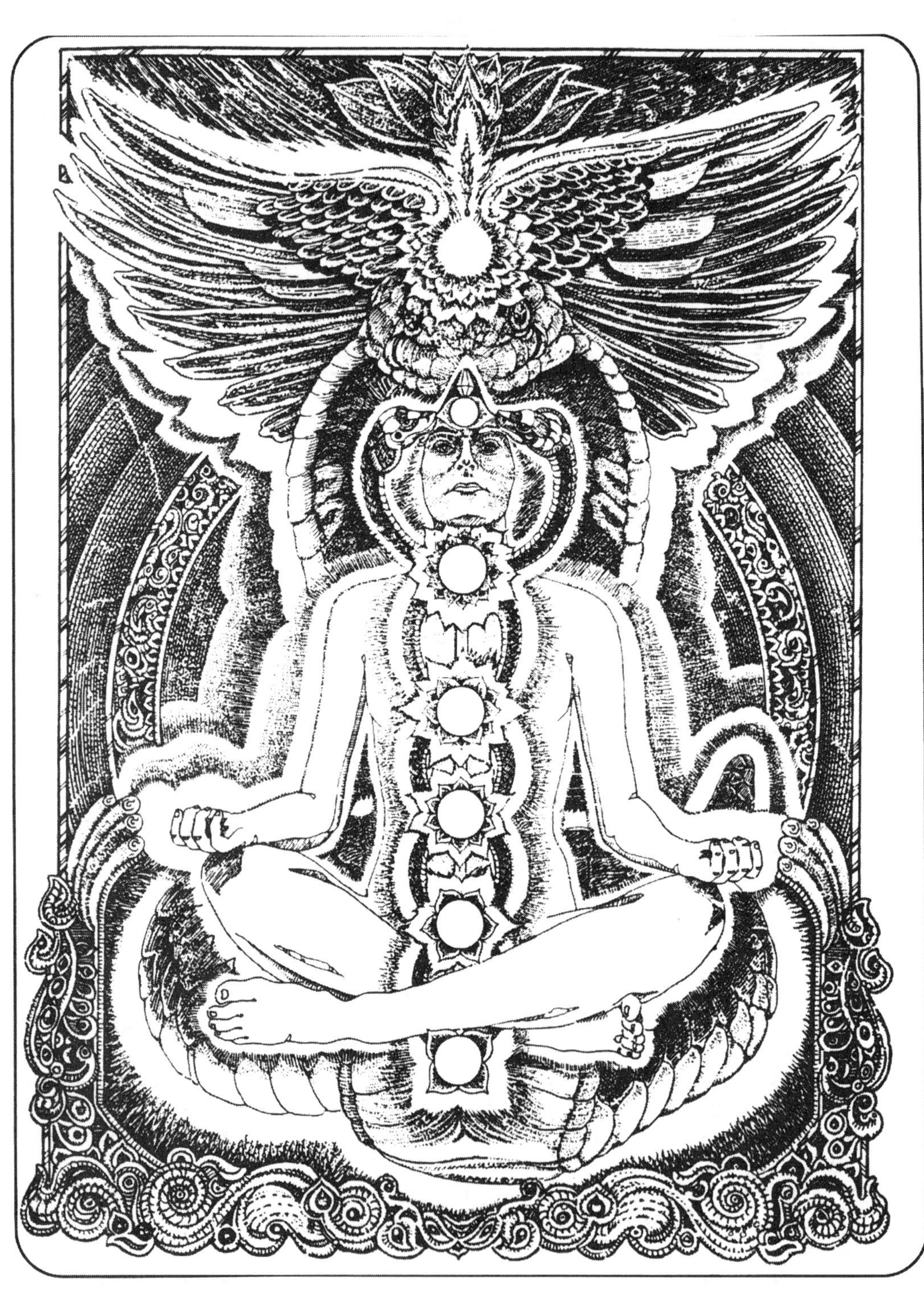

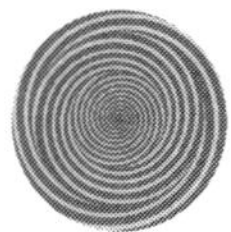

~ *Chapter 188* ~
COLOR/CHAKRA BALANCING

A client may come into your office just to increase their general well being or body, mind, and spirit. This is holistic hypnotherapy. Perform it as often as you desire. The process brings balance and well being and makes one feel better in every way. Your clients can never have too much of that.

MODUS OPERANDI: COLOR CHAKRA BALANCING

Induce trance using your favorite method. With the client in hypnosis, present these exercises for well being. In performing all of these holistic exercises, instruct them to breathe deep and regularly. No special rhythm is needed, just deep and healthy breathing.

"You are in hypnosis now and I am going to give you a series of special exercises to perform that will increase your well-being in every way. As you perform each exercise, you will go down ever deeper and deeper into hypnosis. You will drop down, down into profound hypnosis. Understand?

If you do, nod your head."

(Await client's head nod – this is a subconscious acceptance that the suggestions will be followed.)

Then suggest to the client:

"In hypnosis now, stand up from your chair. Make your entire body loose and natural. Now, lift your hands up into the air high above your head, and start shaking your hands. As you shake your hands, you bring cosmic energy into your hands, and you feel the incoming energy make them tingle."

(Let them continue shaking hands for a full minute and then hold them still, still upraised above the head, high in the air.)

"Hold your hands still and feel how alive they have become, filled with energy. Now easily bend over at your waist and lower your hands to your knees… then slowly scoop your arms and hands over the front of your body until they are again extended high in the air above your head. As you scoop your hands over your body, THINK & FEEL the energy in your hands being scooped and absorbed within your body. In this process, you scoop cosmic energy into your body. Perform this process of bending until hands touch your knees; then slowly scoop the energy upwards into your body half a dozen times. Then, let your hands drop from above your head hanging relaxed by your side. Experience the energy of cosmic energy brought into your body.

(Pause.)

Just stay still for a minute, and let every fiber of your body absorb the energy into itself. You will experience the energy coursing through your body. It is wonderful, and sends you down deeper and deeper into hypnosis.
(Pause a moment.)

Now, extend your hands out from the sides of your body – right hand to the right side; left hand to the left side – you are standing now with your arms outstretched – you stand forming a cross. Your hands will still be buzzing with energy. Once you get it started, the more you get. Now, scoop the energy in your hands into your chest, as you fold your hands inward to rest on your chest, each scooped handful of energy going into your breasts. Experience the energy going into your body, as your hands bring energy into your chest. Good.
(Pause.)

Move your hands from your chest out to your sides again, and perform this exercise of scooping in the energy in this in-and-out from sides to chest a half dozen times."
(Pause.)

Let your hands to drop to your sides and feel the energy flood your lungs and heart. Now, lift your hands high over your head, and shake them vigorously. This time, mentally direct the energy coming into your hands to go down your arms and directly into your body. Allow energy to directly enter your body from your shaking hands for a few minutes. Then stop; relax your hands to your sides. Experience your body alive with cosmic energy. It has been called, 'the force.'
(Pause)

Rest doing nothing but experiencing the energy yourself.
(Pause.)

Now, sit down. Continue going deeper and deeper into hypnosis.
(Help the client into their chair.)

Open your eyes and remain in hypnosis. Drop your left arm over the top of your head, reaching down so your fingers touch your right ear. Hold this position and turn your head so you are looking back behind yourself. Return to front and rest. Do this exercise six times, complete, and return head to front. Rest a few moments, with hands in lap.
(Pause.)

Now, drop your right arm over the top of your head and reach down until your right fingers touch your left ear. Then, with eyes still open, turn your head until you are looking behind yourself. This time, you are looking back gently on your right side. Return to the front and rest. Perform this exercise six times.
(Pause.)

Perform the exercise six times looking behind yourself as your head turns, but this time, instead of your eyes following directly from right to left… as you move your head to the left, roll your eyes and look towards the right. Perform six times, then return to front and rest. Then, perform same with right side of body."
(Pause and allow them time for the process.)

Stand up again, still in hypnosis, with eyes closed. You are now going to perform a holistic exercise to unwind the chakra or energy centers within your body. Place your left hand behind your back and rest it over the base of your spine. Direct the energy of your hand into this spot. As you do this, visualize within your mind the color RED. Hold this position with left hand on base of spine behind your back with your mind filled with the color RED for some thirty seconds. Then rest with your hands in your lap. "
(Pause.)

Now, rest your right hand on your second chakra, which is located just below the belly button. Start moving your hand around and around clockwise, as you fill your mind with the color ORANGE, as you stroke in a circling over this section of your body. Do this for thirty seconds, then rest with hands in your lap. "
(Pause.)

"Now, rest your left hand on your third chakra, which is located in your solar plexus…just below the rib cage. Start moving your left hand around and around clockwise over this area, while holding the thought that you are unwinding the chakras, and releasing their energy inside yourself. During the process with the third chakra, imagine the color YELLOW inside your head. Perform for half a minute. Then stop and rest hands in your lap.
(Pause.)

Now, rest your right hand over your heart (your heart chakra) and revolve the hand around and around over your heart while holding in mind the color GREEN. Perform for thirty seconds. Then, again, rest hands in your lap."
(Pause.)

Now, rest your left hand on your throat (this is your fifth chakra center), and gently stroke your throat around and around clockwise – unwinding the energy of this chakra. As you do this, fill your mind with the color BLUE. Perform for half a minute; then stop and rest hands on lap.
(Pause.)

Now, place your right hand on the center of your forehead (this is your 'third eye' center located between the eyebrows). Unwind this chakra by revolving your energized fingers over the 'third eye center'. While doing this, fill your mind with the color VIOLET. Continue for half a minute, then rest hands in lap.
(Pause.)

Now, place both hands on top of your head. Revolve your fingers around and around unwinding the 'crown chakra', while flooding your mind with the color WHITE. WHITE. WHITE. WHITE INSIDE YOUR HEAD, AND VISUALIZE IT AS A BEAM OF WHITE LIGHT beaming out from the crown of your head into the Cosmos. In doing this, you connect with the Universe itself. Let the white light beam out strongly, and continue it until you feel yourself coming automatically out of the hypnosis feeling wonderful and fine."

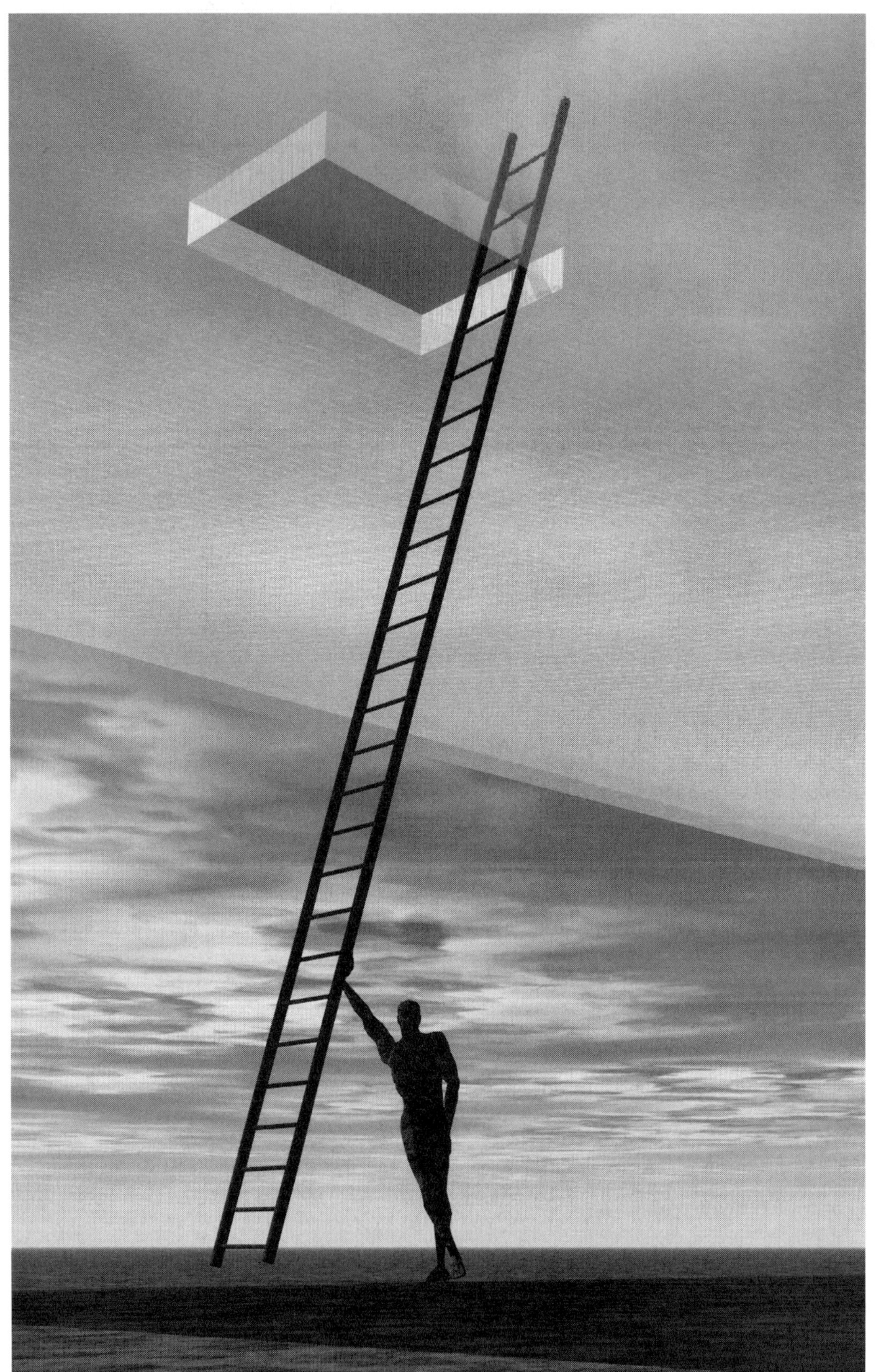

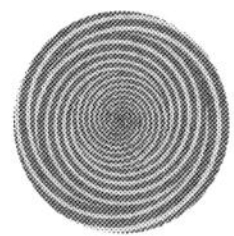

~ *Chapter 189* ~
THE LADDER OF COLORS:
STIMULATING YOUR CHAKRAS

Adapted from "Hypnotism and Mysticism of India," by Ormond McGill

The Ladder of Colors is an excellent initial process to start each session with immediate rapport. It directs chakra stimulation toward the source of cosmic power for strength, guidance and protection. Us it as often as you please. It is excellent.

Besides our western cerebrospinal and sympathetic nervous systems Yogis talk of a psychic nervous system. This system is called "suchumna" and activates the chakra centers along the spine. On each side of the sushumna flows currents or prahna, the vital energy of life from out of the cosmos.

These two currents of energy pass through the substance of the spinal cord. The current that flows on the right side is called "pingula" and is the positive current. On the left side flows the negative phase of current called "ida" (pronounced ee-dah). Each charka too has its own pingula and ida.. You can liken these to electrical energy, forms of vibration that activate the chakras for a variety of purposes.

The chakras are related to yoga, yoga is related to samadhi, and samadhi is related to hypnomeditation.

Chakra means "wheel" or "whirling around a object." This term is applied to these centers because they manifest a peculiar vibratory whirling activity when prahna stimulates the kundalini sushumna.

The chakras are not physical organs and belong to your psychic nervous system. In other words, they are composed of astral or etheric material, not physical matter, and offer strength, guidance and protection. Each has a specific designated color associated with it. The theory goes that if you concentrate and fill your mind with the color, you stimulate a specific chakra.

MODUS OPERANDI: THE LADDER OF COLOR CHAKRA BALANCING
1. **Muladhara- RED This seat of the Kundalini is located at the base of the spine.**
   "Sit upright with your spine straight and concentrate on the color red. Fill your mind with red in any form you desire, red apples a red cloth, anything that is red. Red stimulates the Muladhara Chakra at the base of your spine. And starts the psychic energy moving up the spinal channel."

2. **Svadhisthana- ORANGE**
    On the spine at the region of the reproductive organs.
    "Concentrate on the color orange. Fill your mind with orange in any form you desire, a bowl of oranges, an orange robe of a Tibetan monk, anything that is orange. Orange stimulates the Svadhisthana Chakra at the region of the reproductive organs. You will feel its energy."

3. **Manipura- YELLOW**
    On the spine at the region of the solar plexus or gut
    "Concentrate on the color yellow. Fill your mind with yellow in any form you desire, a yellow field grain, a yellow sunrise, anything that is yellow. Yellow stimulates the Manipura Chakra on the spine at the region of the solar plexus or gut In Japan this area is called the "hara." You will feel its energy."

4. **Anahata- GREEN**
    On the spine at the region of the heart
    "Concentrate on the color green. Fill your mind with green in any form you desire, green grass the image is not important. Green stimulates the Anahata Chakra on the spine at the region of the heart. Feel its energy."

5. **Viuddha- BLUE**
    On the spine at the region of the throat
    "Concentrate on the color blue. Fill your mind with blue in any form you desire, a blue sky, a blue ocean. Blue stimulates the Viuddha Chakra on the spine at the region of the throat. Feel its energy."

6. **Ajna- VIOLET**
    On the forehead in the space between the eyebrows or the third eye.
    "Concentrate on the color violet. Fill your mind with violet ocean. Violet stimulates the Ajna on the forehead in the space between the eyebrows or the third eye. Feel its energy."
    And the optional 7th chakra

7. **Sahastrara- WHITE LIGHT**
    On the crown of the head this chakra is said to form a connection with the Cosmos. It is the combination of all colors and does not have to be included in the Ladder of Colors process.
    "Concentrate on the white light. Fill your mind with white. It stimulates the Sahastrara on the crown of the head."

Once again here are the colors and chakras:

1. **Muladhara- RED**
   This seat of the Kundalini I located at the base of the spine.

2. **Svadhisthana- ORANGE**
   On the spine at the region of the reproductive organs

3. **Manipura- YELLOW**
   On the spine at the region of the solar plexus or gut

4. **Anahata- GREEN**
   On the spine at the region of the heart

5. **Viuddha- BLUE**
   On the spine at the region of the throat

6. **Ajna- VIOLET**
   On the forehead in the space between the eyebrows or the third eye.

7. **Sahastrara- WHITE LIGHT**

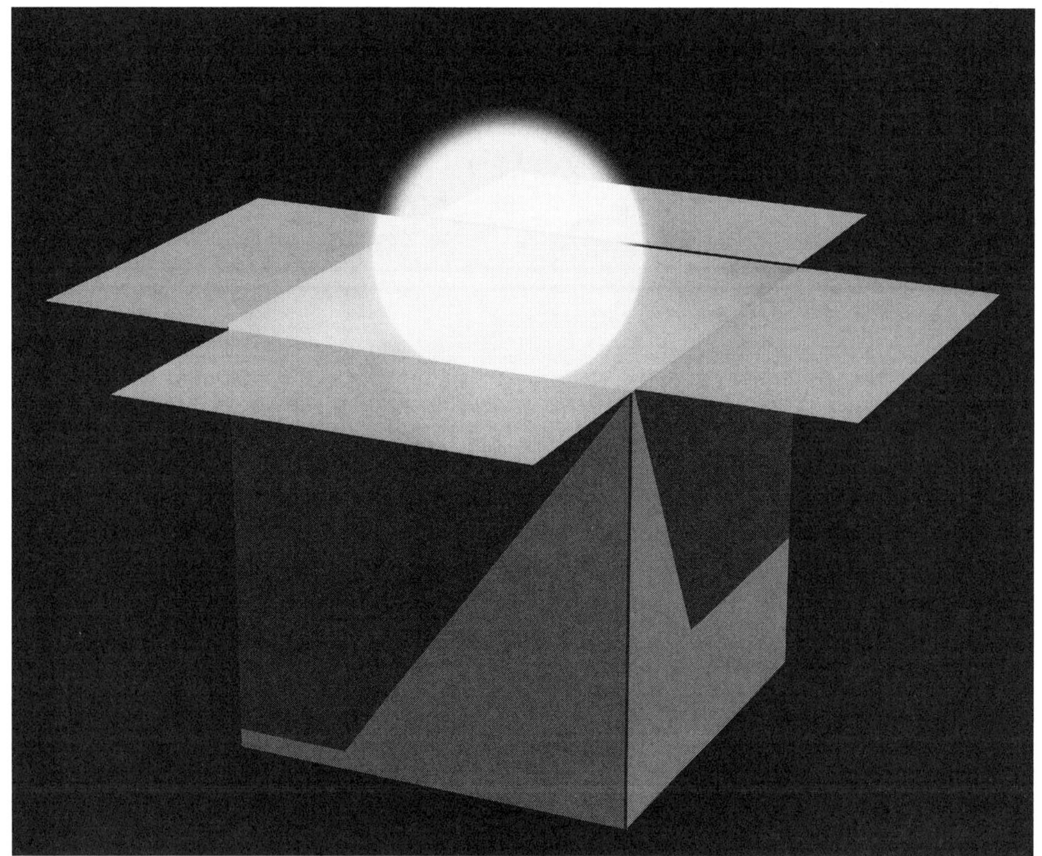

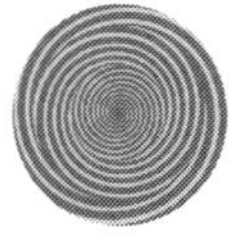

~ *Chapter 190* ~
HYPNOTHERAPY OF INFINITY

When you are ready, you can include this method in your Professional Practice. What is told here is given your client while in profound hypnosis. Suggest:

"As you relax in hypnotic reverie, you will witness before you within the eye of mind, a solid cube. This is your normal perception. Now, advance your perception so remarkably that you can perceive the cube's six sides simultaneously. As you do this, the cube will unfold as a Cross of Light

This perception produces a state of Oneness With Cosmic Mind. You have moved beyond three-dimensional perception into timelessness.

The Cross of Light symbolizes your center in the Universe, and the Cross of Light represents the Universe. In the center of the cross, where the two perpendicular lines intersect, will be seen the tetrahedron Center of Consciousness Jewel which manifests as the rose. Witness as the rose unfolds. The central rose is the null zero point: The Void.

When the two opposite realms of consciousness intersect in equal modulation, your mind and Universal Mind combine and you achieve to Cosmic Consciousness.

Cosmic Consciousness. Before your inner vision stands The Hermanic Rosy Cross. Now, place your consciousness in the center of the rose in the tetrahedron, as it is represented, and let yourself go into The Knowing Of God and a recognition of your own Divinity.

In doing this, you have advanced your perception into the Infinite."

A tremendous gift you have given. Your client's subconscious will understand. You are using Holographic Mind.

"Take your time. There is not time. You have all eternity for the looking. Look now. The leap is infinite. When you have taken the Quantum Leap, return to the here and now, and arouse from the hypnosis, with full awareness of you remarkable perception. The past is there. The now is there. The future is there."

The session of The Hypnotherapy Of Infinity is complete.

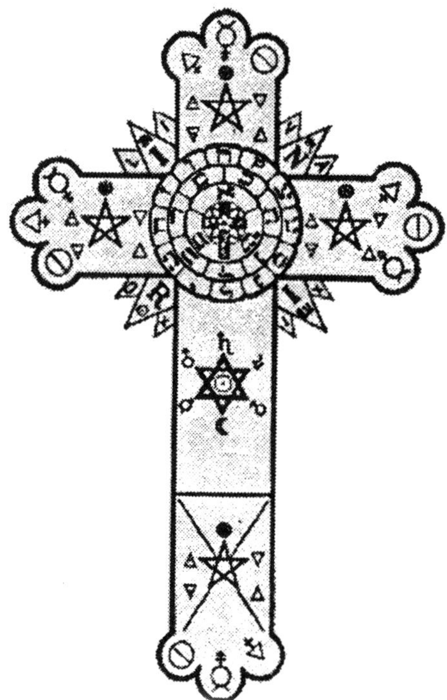

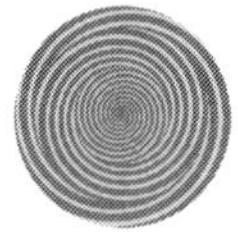

~ *Chapter 191* ~
ANCIENT ESSENE HYPNO-MEDITATION

Thanks to Hypnotherapist Carl Joseph Berg for bringing the Essenes to me.

Includes
The Mystery Of Mastery: The Three Streams
The Essenes Holy Streams
Ancient Essene Hypnotherapy
The Essene Blue Sky Induction
Essene Angels, Life, Light and Peace
Essene Healing

Jesus was an Essene.

The Essene method of spiritual hypnotherapy comes from aged fragments of leather parchment found in secret Vatican Archives in 1928. The word "Essene" means "essence." Essenes taught the recognition of the peace of the soul and God within each person. Their purpose was to establish peace-of-mind and peace-of-mind is at the very heart of successful hypnotherapy.

To these ancient scholars, "suggestion" was "prayer." In prayer is found the energy of the creative mind. "Choose what you want to have in your life and then pray," they said. "ALL for which you pray will be provided (manifested) in the physical and spiritual world." Prayer evokes energy that uses the power of the Creative Mind to give you what you want. Focused thought and emotion empowers inner peace.

They prayed that their "client" would be as perfect as the venerated earthly Mother and heavenly Father. "Combining these male and female (yang and yin) energies makes one WHOLE," they said. They prayed and affirmed "Remember that the Kingdom of God is within you." The Creator is the Creation of your heart, soul, mind, and strength. THE CREATOR AND THE CREATION ARE ONE. "Love your Creator," they said.

Here is a popular prayer from the Essenes:
"Our Mother, upon earth, hallowed be thy name. Thy kingdom come, thy will be done in us, as it is in thee. As thou sendest every day thy angels, send them to us also. Forgive us our sins, as we atone. And lead us to wellness, for thine is the earth, the body, and the health. Amen."

Sound familiar?

THE MYSTERY OF MASTERY: THE THREE STREAMS

Essenes were thankful for earthly and spiritual gifts and lived closely with nature. They taught the use of nourishing with food, sleep, air, water, sunshine, and fire, and mastered evil with "Love that passeth understanding." Among their teachings were the "Three Holy Streams" which is even more than prayer.

What are these three holy streams?

They are life, sound and light.

"Life, sound, and light, like God, are never born and never die" they said, "and even holy scrolls cannot record the mysteries for you there." Your body was not only meant to breathe, eat, drink, and think…it was meant to enter these streams so that you take your place where "words are no more." Here are the "Holy Streams" edited from the original Essene scroll. It is powerful hypnosis.

SUGGESTION FORMULA: THE ESSENES HOLY STREAMS

"Into the innermost circle you come, into the mystery of mysteries, to that which was old when our father Enoch was young and walked the earth.

Around and around have you come on your journey of many years, always following the path of righteousness, living according to the Holy Law and the sacred vows of Brotherhood and Sisterhood. You made of your body a holy temple wherein dwell the angels. Many years have you shared the daylight hours with the angels of the Earthly Mother; many years have you slept in the arms of the Heavenly Father, taught by his unknown angels. You have learned that the laws of Humans are seven, of the angels three, and of God, one."

"The laws of the angels, the three Holy Streams and lets you bathe in the light of heaven and behold the revelation of the mystery of mysteries: the law of God, which is one.

In the hour before the rising sun, before the angels of the Earthly Mother breathe life into the still sleeping earth, enter the first Holy Stream of Life. Your Brother Tree, who holds the mystery of this Holy Stream, embraces your thought. Be one with all trees. In the beginning of times, we all shared the Holy Stream of Life that gave birth to all creation. And as you embrace your Brother Tree, the power of the Holy Stream of Life fills your whole body.

When the sun is high in the heavens, seek the second Holy Stream of Sound. In this heat of noontide, all creatures are still and seek shade; the angels of the Earthly Mother are silent. Then let into your ears the Holy Stream of Sound, for it is only heard in silence. Think of streams born in the desert after a sudden storm, and the roaring sound of the waters as they rush past. Truly, this is the voice of God. When born, you entered the world with the sound of God in your ears: the singing of the vast chorus of the sky and the holy chant of the stars in their fixed rounds. This Holy Stream of Sound traverses the vault of stars and crosses the endless kingdom of Heaven. It is ever in our ears. Listen for it, then, in the silence of noontide; bathe in it, and let the rhythm of the music of God beat in your ears until you are one. This sound formed the world, brought forth mountains, and set the stars in their high thrones of glory. Bathe in the stream of sound. Let the music flow over you.

Then breathe deeply of the third Holy Stream, the angel of air, and say the word 'life' and share in the holy stream of sound that gave birth to all creation. The mighty roaring of the stream of sound fills your whole body. Then breathe deeply of the angel of air, and become the sound itself, to carry you to the endless kingdom where the world of rhythms rise and fall.

When darkness gently closes the eyes of the Earthly Mother, and you too sleep, your spirit joins the Heavenly Father. In the moment before sleep, think of the bright and glorious stars, the white, shining, far-seen and far-piercing stars. Your thoughts before sleep are as the bow of the skillful archer that sends the arrow where he wills. Let your thoughts before sleep be with the stars; for the stars are Light, and the Heavenly Father is Light a thousand times brighter than the brightness of a thousand suns. Enter the Holy Stream of Light, the shackles of death lose their hold forever. Breaking free from the bonds of earth, ascend the Holy Stream of Light. This endless kingdom in the eternal Sea of Light gives birth to all creation. And you shall be one with the Holy Stream of Light, before you sleep.

Your body was made to breathe, eat, think, and enter the Holy Streams of Life. And your ears were made to hear the words of others, the songs of birds, the music of falling rain, and the Holy Stream of Sound. You become the Tree of Life, whose its roots go deep into the Holy eternal Stream of Life. As the angel of sun warms the earth, all creatures of land and water and air and you rejoice in the new day.

The rising and setting sun, the ripple of sheaves of grain, and the words of the holy scrolls make you see the holy stream of light. One day your body will return to the earthly mother but the holy stream of life, the holy stream of sound, and the holy stream of light were never born, and can never die.

Enter the holy streams, life, sound, and light which were given you at birth; that you may reach the Kingdom of the Heaven and become one with it.

More than this cannot be told, for the holy streams empties into the far-distant sea. They take you to that place where words are no more, even the holy scrolls cannot record the mysteries therein."

MODUS OPERANDI: ANCIENT ESSENE HYPNOTHERAPY
You Will Need:
A Comfortable Chair
Soft Music

The 'Blue Sky Induction" that follows promotes "peace of mind" and is excellent hypnotherapy. Use this close-to-nature meditation of a clear, blue sky produces wonderful healing for all that is you. When, your client is filled with clear blue sky, you go into your private session room. Darken the room and play soft meditative music. Take seat them in a comfortable chair or recliner and rest back with their eyes closed.

THE ESSENE BLUE SKY INDUCTION
"Visualize and imagine a host of angels rising up before the screen of mind. At first, it is like imagination, but it becomes more and more real. It seems like reality. Transformation of consciousness leads you directly to subconscious reality."
If you like, you can now go outside with yourself or client and give these instructions:
"Enter the endless blue sky and become it. Your consciousness is just like the clear sky and your mind is just like the clouds. The sky remains untouched by the clouds. Your consciousness remains undisturbed even if your mind is confused or disturbed. Focus on the clear blue sky, not the clouds to make a peaceful mind. Just you and the sky are here. Look up into the endless clear sky. It may appear like an inverted blue bowl, and you are in the center. And, while looking, feel the clarity of it– the boundless expanse. Then enter that clarity, become as ONE with it. Feel as if you, yourself, have become the sky; you enter vast spaciousness.

Just by looking into the sky, you increase your consciousness; the boundaries of your outer self disappear. The no-boundary sky reflects you. Blink your eyes as little as possible. Stare into that emptiness.

The moment will come when the sky seems to enter you. At that moment, thinking stops. Mind disappears. This happens because in the clarity of the blue sky there is nothing to think about other than infinite space (void) and so mind enter the realm of no-mind.

First, you enter the sky and then the sky enters you. A meeting occurs deep within yourself, as your inner sky meets the outer sky."

Stay silent for a minute and then take your client into your hypnosis place. Have them sit comfortably and recite the following suggestion formula:

SUGGESTION FORMULA: ESSENE ANGELS, LIFE, LIGHT AND PEACE

"Filled with the clear blue sky we begin. The Ancient Essenes tell us that to change the conditions of our outer world, we must become our inner desire. To bring peace, we must become that very peace.

First, seek peace with your body;

Then, peace with your thoughts;

Then, peace with your feelings.

Graceful peace and earth changes are already here. Peace be with you as you let these suggestions become your reality. Imagine a panorama of Guardian Angels looking kindly upon you as you rest in the chair below. You may see them or even hear them sing. If you do, Essene Hypnosis has surely been produced. Focus attention from angel face to angel face, angel essence to angel essence. Each angel helps you drop down deeper and deeper into the reverie of hypnosis.

Enter now into The Three Streams of Life. Let this become a way of living, morning, noon and night.

On awakening, before arising, lovingly embrace THE HOLY STREAM OF LIFE. Take six deep full breaths in rapid succession, then place your hands over your ears and say 'LIFE!' three times.

Let the word and energy of life rrrrring through your being! 'LIFE! LIFE! LIFE!'

At noon of each day, loving embrace THE HOLY STREAM OF SOUND. To do this, take six deep full breaths in rapid succession. Listen. Listen. Listen and become the SOUND itself where the world rises and falls into a space of silence.

Each night, lovingly embrace THE HOLY STREAM OF LIGHT. As you drop into sleep, become a star traveler and enter THE HOLY STREAM OF LIGHT from distant suns. Take six deep breaths in rapid succession, and say the word LIGHT three times. 'LIGHT! LIGHT! LIGHT!' As you breathe, you become the LIGHT itself.

Words are no more. REST and visualize and imagine your flock of angels in the sky before you.

Subconscious mind make these suggestions become my reality. I obtain perfect peace within myself. I am PEACE. PEACE. PEACE.

Now affirm this to yourself: I have the power to change my outer world by changing my inner world. I can make my body well and perfect because I develop inner peace. I'm the perfect outcome of my peaceful thoughts and choices. I know that this is so.

My prayers are prayers of thanks, in knowing what I have created. Creation is perfect. I give thanks for being able to choose what I wish to experience. Prayer is like water to the seed of my dreams and desires.

When my subconscious KNOWS that it is so, it arouses me from hypnosis with PEACE WITHIN ME. I give peace to others I meet.

My salutation is 'May peace be with you.'

When these suggestions of the Essenes have become reality, arise from hypnosis feeling wonderful and fine, completely at PEACE with all that is."

SUGGESTION FORMULA: ESSENE HEALING

In truth, we are already healed. Your soul is never ill. If your body needs healing, strength must come from inside yourself. Your body is a feedback mechanism mirroring the quality of our choices of thought, feeling, emotion, breath, nutrients, and movements in our honoring life. Contemporary hypnotherapists will recognize this as the power of suggestion. Powerful forces within you can change climate, military situations, economies, health and longevity. Essene physicians said that fear lodged in your tissues causes disease. Love causes healing.

You have the power to move electrical energy across membranes of your cell walls, generate complex patterns in consciousness, and create specific chemistry with the laboratory of your body. Anesthesia can be produced, tumors dissolved, blood pressure lowered, and disease halted.

"Gone. Gone. Gone. Already accomplished because it is gone. Seek peace within your own body; for your body is a mountain pond that reflects the sun when it is still and clear. When it is full of mud and stones, it reflects nothing. Each of your thoughts can shake the heavens.

Seek peace with your own feelings. Call on the Force of Love (God) to enter your feelings, that they may be purified. Then all that was before impatience and discord will turn into harmony and peace.

Seek peace in all that lives, in all you do, in each word you speak. For peace is the key to all knowledge, to all life, to all mystery."

You have the power to heal your most painful experiences by changing the emotion of the experience itself. Illness stems from the choices and actions you make. Repeat, 'Gone. Gone. GONE! to illness,' say the Essenes and 'It is gone!'"

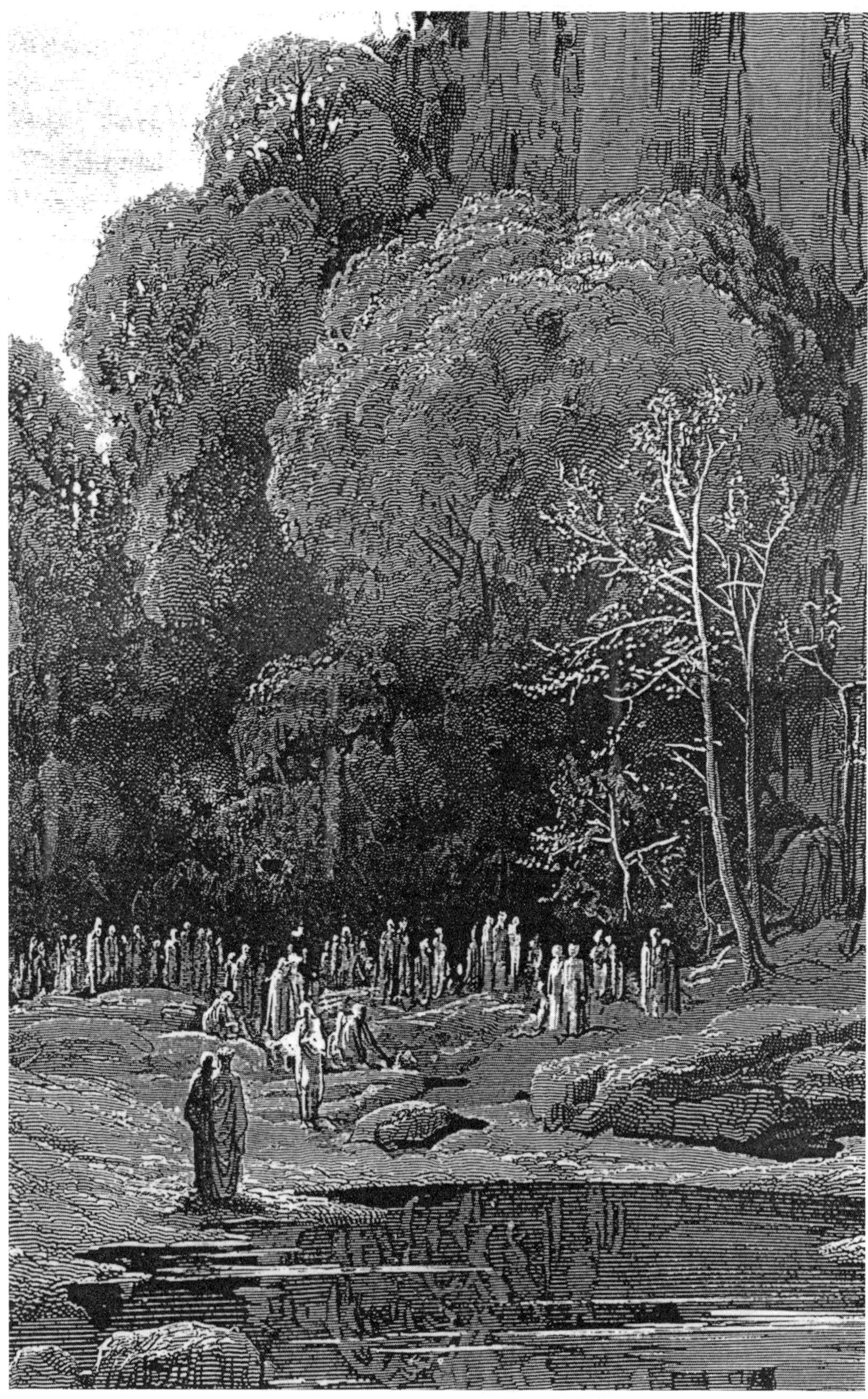

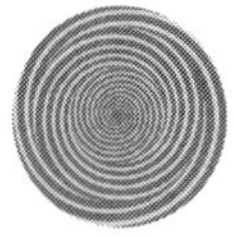

~ *Chapter 192* ~
ESSENE ENTERING DARKNESS MEDITATION

Includes
Entering The Darkness Hypno-Meditation
Entering The Darkness Induction and Session
Concluding The Session
Native American's Controlling The Outside World

This chapter continues the Essenes approach to hypnotherapy and offers two ancient hypno-meditation techniques to obtain a peaceful mind. Most meditations symbolize God as light, but in this process, God represents the WHOLE, containing both light and darkness. In some ways, darkness is even greater than light, for light comes and goes while darkness remains. Darkness is always there.

Light has a source; darkness is without source. That which is without source is infinite. Light produces certain disturbances; it creates tensions. Darkness, as the opposite of light, brings inner relaxation, and with inner relaxation comes a peaceful mind. Thus, the Essenes direct attention to darkness in their meditation and it provides a remarkable form of hypnotherapy. You can make it a specialty of your office.

MODUS OPERANDI: "ENTERING DARKNESS" HYPNO-MEDITATION
You Will Need:
A Table
A Candle
Soft Music

Arrange your session room so when the lights are turned off, it is completely dark. Have a recliner chair in the center of the room, with a table in front to rest a burning candle.

The client takes their seat in the recliner. The candle is lit, and the client is instructed to concentrate on the flame.

The hypnotherapist sits beside the client. Only the lighted candle is seen in the darkness. Meditative music plays softly as a background. Now, present these instructions to the client:

ENTERING THE DARKNESS INDUCTION AND SESSION

"Fix your eyes on the candle flame. Do not concentrate on anything in particular for the moment, just relax back in your chair and let your mind drift, allowing whatever thoughts come in to just pass through it.

Now, breathe deeply through your nose, hold the breath for about five seconds, and then exhale <u>very slowly</u>.

(Repeat this three times.)

As each breath is taken, visualize energy moving into your body and down your back to the base of your spine. As each breath is released, release any tension moving up from the base of your spine, and out of your body. All the while, concentrate on the candle flame. Now, close your eyes as I blow out the candle.

Now, starting with your feet, THINK of how relaxed they are becoming. Think it and you will feel it. Now, move your attention up your legs – relaxing the muscles in your legs. Now, move on up through the muscles of your torso, relaxing the torso muscles.

Now, turn your attention to your hands resting in your lap, and THINK of your fingertips tingling with the energy of the universe entering you. Then move this energy up your arms, your shoulders, your neck, your face, clear up to the very top of your head. Every muscle of your entire body has been progressively relaxed – every muscle from your feet to the top of your head has been mentally suggested to relax. In this process, let all sensations that come in be exactly what they are and do not try to change them in any way.

Now, in this relaxed condition, continue being with your body and visualize all feelings, tensions, emotions as flowing out of your body from your fingertips and toes. And, along with this discharge of energy, THINK of how each breath you take is causing you to become more and more relaxed and sleepy. How sleepy you are becoming.

Continue to THINK how very sleepy you are. How deep and full your breaths are becoming, as every breath you take sends you down deeper and deeper into the realm of hypnotic sleep, wherein your conscious mind moves to one side and your subconscious emerges to accept this wonderful Essene meditation of ENTERING THE DARKNESS.

Let this profound meditation become your reality. It will transform your life. Go into the SILENCE now for some moments, and when it again commences, let the meditation of ENTERING THE DARKNESS become your reality. It will bring you perfect PEACE OF MIND."

(Fade out the music.)

"Go silent for a few moments now. Silence. Silence. Silence. Silence in pitch blackness...open your eyes in pitch blackness."

(Bring up the music again.)

"Feel the darkness. Have a loving attitude towards it. Allow the darkness to touch you. In this realm of the complete darkness, let any negative attitude of darkness disappear as you commune with the darkness. In doing this, you enter a realm of greater relaxation, which is beyond anything you have previously known – it provides the opportunity of completely letting go! In letting go, contemplate the fact that all forms arise out of darkness and dissolve back into darkness. In darkness, absolute stillness will be found. Darkness is the 'cosmic womb'.

Enter the blackness as the form of forms and understand this well.

Your form can no longer be seen in the blackness, thus you can be any form you wish to create in your mind. Such is the form of forms.

When light is there, you are defined; then your body has a definition. Boundaries exist to what you know yourself and your form. In blackness, nothing is defined and everything emerges into every other thing. Forms disappear, and only the form of forms remains.

Now do this...

Stare, stare, stare into the darkness. Stare into THE VOID and look deep into the darkness that surrounds you. Just relax and be perfectly at ease in the darkness; soon it will start entering your eyes; and, as the darkness enters your eyes, peace-of-mind comes to you, and you experience a sensation of serenity and bliss. It is a cosmic experience, and you will come out of the experience a different person...all your troubles will seem to vanish, and you will feel happiness for the successful; compassion for the miserable; appreciate the virtuous, and be unbothered by evil.

You have become a Mastermind. Relax into Existence. Go with the Flow."

(Pause)

"It is a Cosmic Experience, and you cannot enter any Cosmic Experience without the Cosmic Experience entering YOU.

Now, rest and feel as if you are near your mother. The darkness is your mother...THE MOTHER OF ALL. Darkness is the womb; feel that you are in the womb of your mother. The experience will seem very real, and soon you will become warm. Sooner or later, you'll start feeling that the darkness is the womb that envelopes you from everywhere. You are within it. You are at peace with all life, including death.

From this time forward, you carry a patch of darkness with you during everything you do. You hold this radiant darkness close. Others about you, who are sensitive, will sense it and feel at peace.

When you carry the radiance of darkness, you will feel an empathy towards ALL THAT IS, and you become perfectly content just to be what you are. You have peace-of-mind, and know the real meaning when the Essenes say, PEACE BE WITH YOU!"

CONCLUDING THE SESSION

(Turn music off. Turn lights on.)

"Go SILENT for some moments. You will arouse from the Hypnosis with a Quantum Leap in Awareness. TAKE YOUR TIME... THERE IS NO HURRY.

Arouse when and as you will. You will arouse from this session feeling wonderful and fine, and KNOWING that the Buddha was correct in saying, "NOTHING NEED BE DONE!"

The Essene "entering the darkness" hypnotherapy is complete.

MODUS OPERANDI: NATIVE AMERICAN'S CONTROLLING THE OUTSIDE WORLD

North American Indians echo the Essene's, "to change the condition of the outside world, invite the condition from within. To bring peace, be peaceful and that very peace is perfection." The Essene's said it this way "First seek peace with your own body; then shall you seek peace with your own thoughts; then shall you seek peace with your own feelings. Peace and graceful earth changes are already here. And always: May peace be with you."

Native Americans invite the rain or, as they call it, "today we pray rain" and often water from the sky falls faster than earth can absorb it that day. They feel gratitude for all that has come to pass and for the wind, heat, and the drought saying, **"That is the way until now. It is not good. It is not bad. It has been our medicine. Now I choose new medicine. I have the feeling of what rain feels like. Barefoot I walk with mud oozing from my toes, the smell of rain on the fields and buildings; and what it feels like to walk in fields of corn because the rain is so plentiful."**

"The old ones remind us, that this is how we choose our path in this world. This is how we plant the seeds in a new way, in each new day. Our prayers become a prayer of thanks for what IS. Our prayers are not for what we created, creation is already complete. Out prayer is a prayer of the opportunity to choose which creation we experience. Through our thanks, we honor all possibilities and bring the ones we choose into the world. This empowers the prayer and brings its outcome to focus. This secret of communing with Great Spirit and the forces of the world and our body reminds us that prayer is to us, as water is to the seed of a plant."

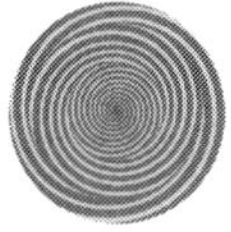

~ *Chapter 193* ~
MEDITATION OF THE VIOLET FLAME

This meditation of creative power offers profound hypnosis instilled into the subconscious. It deserves much experimenting as it seems to stimulate the kundalini energy and may well play an important role in the hypnotherapy of the 21st Century.

MODUS OPERANDI: MEDITATION OF THE VIOLET FLAME

PRE-TALK
"The Violet Flame is one of the most cherished secrets of esoteric lore used by the Great White Brotherhood of Tibet. The Violet Flame has the power to transmute thought into materialized reality. That is why the Violet Flame is given only to these sacred members. It is the source of personal power to be used only by the pure of heart."

THE JOURNEY
"To achieve this in yourself, just relax and close your eyes. Now take a deep breath…hold it for a few minutes then exhale slowly. Do it again…then do it one more time. It provides energy when you activate the Violet Flame.

Now experience your body as though you were dead. However you are to remain just as you are. Do not move. Do not do anything. JUST…BE…AS…YOU…ARE. Let it be exactly as if your body were dead.

Experience your mind in this manner…if you are filled with love…stay so. If you feel anxiety or fear…stay so…you are dead and you can't change anything. JUST…BE…AS…YOU…ARE.

Now, in this state, direct your attention to the space between your eyebrows. This is the location of your third eye, called in India 'the Eye of Shiva.' It is one of the great secrets of directing power into creation.

In most persons this third eye is closed, but it becomes functional when attention is directed to it, your two eyes turn upon it like bits of iron filings are drawn to a magnet. In this process, focus your attention in the middle of your forehead and your two eyes will come to sharp focus upon your third eye. The will stand still as the third eye opens. Then a strange experience will come to you: you will commence to feel that somehow your thoughts are separate from your mind. They seem to pass before you and you can witness them as they pass. You have become a witness to your thoughts rather than being a participant in your thoughts. Once your attention is turned upon the third eye, a gap occurs between yourself and your thoughts. In this experience, you have taken a quantum leap in consciousness. You begin to sense your body as being filled with vital energy. You can sense an inner vibration within your body.

Now focus your attention to your third eye upon the top of your head. Visualize it as though a shower of light were gushing forth into space above your head.

You are now ready to bring in the Violet Flame.

First enter the silence for a few moments. Enter the silence as though you were dead. Enter the SILENCE, SILENCE, SILENCE.

(Pause for some moments in silence)

Now learn the truth about the violet flame. When one is ready, members of secret societies and mystery schools are taught how to bring in the Violet Flame. It is a source of power; power to be used by the pure of heart.

The Violet Flame is a meditation of power. It is a connection with the void…the creative source of all that is. It springs forth like a violet fire coursing through your veins; penetrating all layers of your body; binging in strength and well-being to your body and serenity to your mind. It cleanses all debris from your soul and consumes as it transforms, moving you into realms of higher consciousness.

The Violet Flame flushes out and renews your body cells, polishing the jewel of consciousness to dazzling brightness. Within it lives the power to bend the will of the universe and causes it to manifest in all manner of prosperity. Whatever your wish; power, love, talent, whatsoever becomes your very own as it turns imagined creation into reality. That is why one must be pure in heart before it is manifested. But it does not originate inside yourself; it is cosmic in origin, connected with Universal Mind with which your subconscious has a direct communication.

Using your subconscious mind, you can direct the Violet Flame for the benefit of yourself or others. The Violet Flame is the power behind miracles.

You are now going to drop even deeper into hypnosis and enter the realm of the subconscious. Become silent again for a few moments now and open the doors of your inner self. SILENCE. SILENCE. SILENCE."

(Pause for some moments in silence)

"You are becoming more and more relaxed and are dropping deeper into hypnosis with every breath you take. The vistas of your subconscious are opening wide to receive and manifest the Violet Light to become your way of life. It is the way of the Masters.

Now suddenly LET GO! LET GO! Suddenly LET GO and you drop directly into the abyss of your inner self in which the Violet Flame will blaze. You obtain mastery of its power as is your true reality.

Receive the mastery of the Violet Flame deep inside yourself. You are ready not to accept the mantra of the Violet Flame into your SELF. Affirm it to yourself:

'In the name of the Creator of all that IS, I call forth the energy of the sacred Violet Flame. Let this energy go deep into my heart and become my gift that is my heritage. I acclaim that I AM. I AM. I command the Violet Flame to blaze forth from the Threefold Flame from the white fire core of my own I AM to consummate my knowing of my soul's destiny. I call forth the all-cleansing Violet Flame to pass through my body and clear it of all imperfections and I will come to know my Higher Self which exists in the eternal stream of life as I chant the mantra of the Violet Flame and cause its power to become my own. I declare within my soul I AM I!

I AM THE VIOLET FLAME IN ACTION & RENOWN
I AM THE VIOLET FLAME TO ITS RADIANCE I BOW
I AM THE VIOLET FLAME IN MIGHTY COSMIC POWER
I AM THE VIOLET FLAME SHINING EVERY HOUR
I AM THE VIOLET FLAME BLAZING LIKE THE SUN
I AM THE VIOLET FLAME ACCLAIMING EVERYONE.'

I let these decrees go deep within my subconscious as silence enters. SILENCE. SILENCE. SILENCE.'

(Pause for some moments in silence)

RADIANT VIOLET FLAME DESCEND NOW AND BLAZE BRIGHT
RADIANT VIOLET FLAME COME FORTH AND SHINE THY LIGHT
RADIANT VIOLET FLAME REVEAL COSMIC POWER FOR ALL TO SEE
RADIANT VIOLET FLAME AWAKEN THE EARTH; SET IT FREE
RADIANT VIOLET FLAME SET FREE, SET FREE, SET FREE.
RADIANT VIOLET FLAME EXPLODE AND BOIL THROUGH ME
RADIANT VIOLET FLAME EXPAND FOR ALL TO HEAL
RADIANT VIOLET FLAME ESTABLISH MERCY'S OUTPOST HERE
RADIANT VIOLET FLAME TRANSMUTE NOW ALL PEACE.

I let these decrees go deep within my subconscious as silence enters. SILENCE. SILENCE. SILENCE.

(Pause for some moments in silence)

Oh Violet Flame, sweep through my very core and intensify more and more. Right now blaze through and saturate… expand and penetrate. Claim my mind now and for eternity… purge my soul in purity… advance my divinity."

The process is complete.

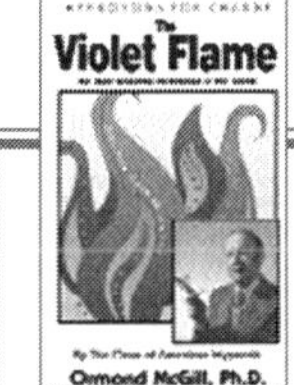

Hypno-Helper
"The Violet Flame" audio tape by Ormond McGill voice is available on the order form at the back of this book.

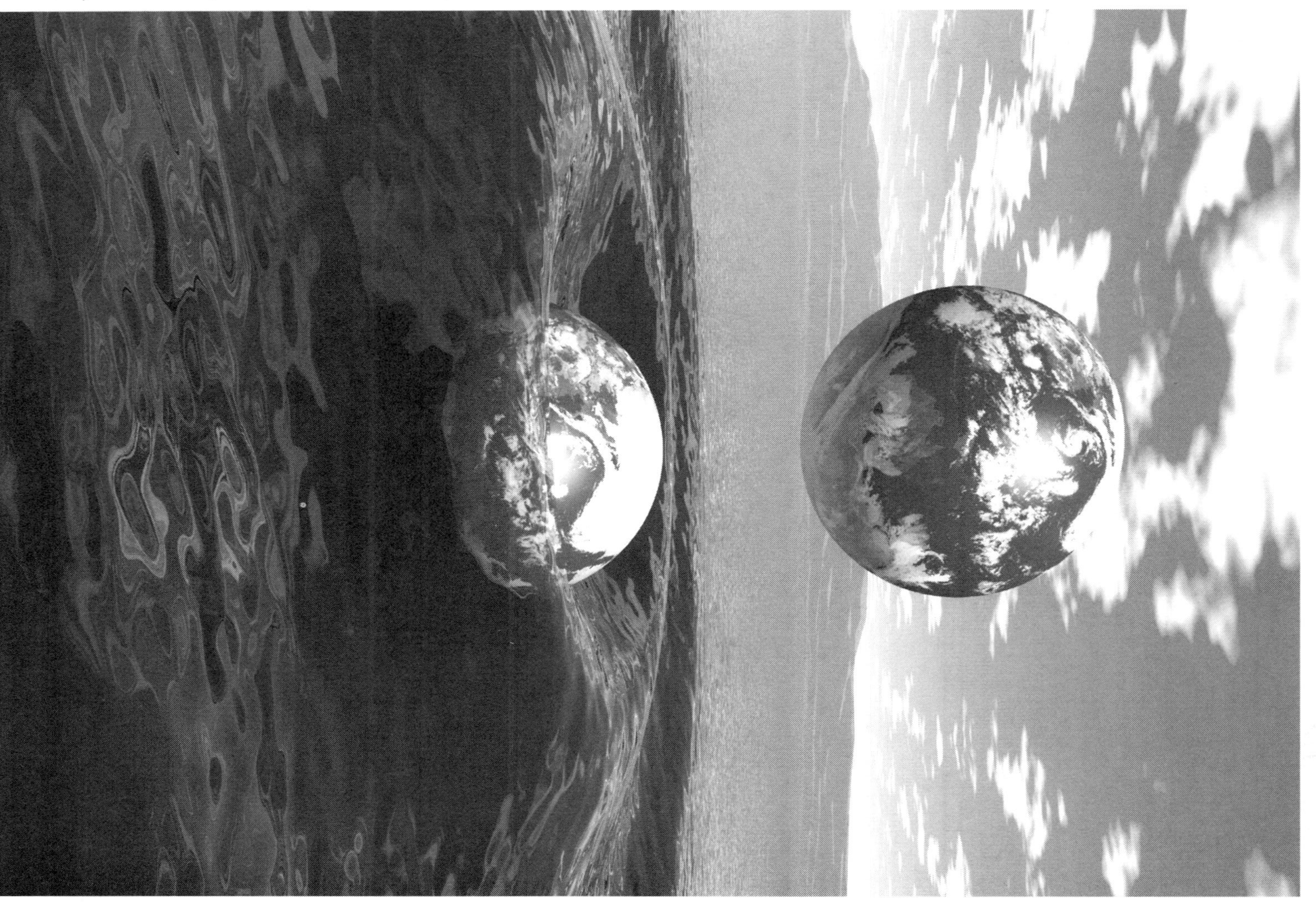

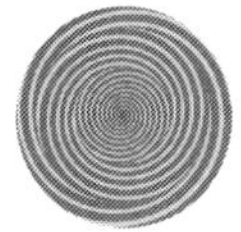

~ *Chapter 194* ~
HYPNOTHERAPY OF ZEN

Includes
Zen Hypnotherapy
The Suggestion Formula Of Zen
The Arousal From Zen Hypnotherapy

ENLIGHTENMENT = THE BRILLIANCE OF INSTINCTIVE KNOWING

This method of Hypnotherapy is very Eastern. As Zen insights are transcendental, it functions well as a prelude to the Transcendental Hypnotherapy in the next chapter.

Zen Hypnotherapy provides great benefits for your client. When Zen is suggested and accepted subconsciously, all stress in the world vanishes, for Zen is above the world. Zen is a "mind game." Hypnotherapy is a "mind game." When played together…in combination…the results are remarkable. The "mind game" of Zen is filled with koans, paradoxes, and contradictions.

Clearing the mind with "nothing" is great hypnotherapy. Many troubles that people have are based on a mind filled with ceaseless chattering about how miserable they are. A client comes into your office having spent many years in training their mind to be wonderfully miserable and asks you, as a hypnotherapist, to take away the misery they have so carefully produced, so they can have some peace within themselves. Finding that inner peace is the purpose of Zen Hypnotherapy.

Zen gives you opinions and then tells you not to have opinions. As an example, you can concentrate for hours and come up with nothing for a koan like "What is the sound of one hand clapping?" Zen is the most stupid thing you will ever study that is positively brilliant. Brilliant produces light (lightness). Lightness as a mental activity is called "enlightenment."

MODUS OPERANDI: ZEN HYPNOTHERAPY
You Will Need:
Soft Music Or The *Serenity Resonance Sound*

Hypnotize your client into a relaxed state of hypnotic reverie…then suggest:
"In this pleasant, serene and relaxed stat of mind, you are now in your subconscious opens wide to understand and accept these suggestions of ZEN which I will now read to you. Just relax and listen and let what is given you here become your very own. It will flood your mind with the brilliance of ENLIGHTENMENT.

THE SUGGESTION FORMULA OF ZEN

Read this softly to client in hypnosis, against a background of soft meditative music or Serenity Resonance Sound.

"Enlightenment comes most readily for those with few preferences. When wishing for and wishing against are absent from thought, everything becomes clear. Making distinctions makes heaven and earth far apart. To set up your world with what you like against what you dislike upsets your mind. It disturbs the mind's essential peace.

The Universe is perfect just like vast space, where nothing is lacking and nothing is in excess. It is our choosing to accept or reject this perfection that keeps us from seeing the true nature of things. Life not a choice of outer things, nor inner feelings. Just be serene in the oneness of things and such erroneous views disappear by themselves. When you try to stop activity to achieve passivity, your very effort fills you with activity. So just relax and accept the idea that there is nothing to distinguish no pattern to master. All is perfect in its oneness. As long as you remain in one extreme or the other, you would never know Oneness.

Those who do not live in the single way fail in both activity and passivity. To deny the reality of things is to miss their reality, just as to assert the purposelessness of things is likewise to miss their reality. The more you talk and think about it, the further astray you can wander from the truth. Many masters say that when one stops talking about going beyond that which appears to be and that which appears not to be, then there is inner enlightenment. Thus do not search for the truth; only cease to cherish opinions.

A dualistic state has a trace of this and that, right and wrong and causes the mind to be lost in confusion. At their roots all duality's is a single source, which we call the One. But do not become attached even to this One. When the mind is undisturbed as to which way it should choose, but just allows what IS to be, there is nothing in the world which can offend. And when a thing can no longer offend, it ceases to exist with the strength it had.

To live in the way of Enlightenment is neither easy nor difficult, but those with limited views are fearful and irresolute, and the faster they hurry the slower they go, and clinging (attachment) cannot be limited; even to be attached to the idea of enlightenment is to go astray. Just let things be in their own way, and there will be neither coming nor going.

Obey your nature and you will walk freely and undisturbed. When thought is in bondage, the truth is hidden, for everything is murky and unclear, and the burdensome practice of judging brings annoyance and weariness as no benefits can be derived from distinctions and separations.

If you wish to move in the way of Enlightenment, do not dislike the world of senses and ideas; accept them fully is identical with true Enlightenment. The wise strive for no goals, only the foolish fetter themselves. Distinctions arise from clinging to needs. To see Enlightenment with a discriminating mind is the greatest of all mistakes.

The unified mind in accord with that which IS, all self-centered striving ceases. Doubts and irresolution's vanish, and the real fullness of living is possible. When all is empty, clear, and illuminated with no exertion of the mind's power, we are freed from bondage. For in this world of 'suchness' there is neither self nor other than self.

To come directly into harmony with Existence simply say that nothing is separate and nothing is excluded. No matter when or where or how, enlightenment means entering this truth. And this thought is beyond extension or diminution in time or space, as it is a single thought in eternity.

To the enlightened one, the universe stands always before your eyes as infinitely large and infinitely small with no difference. Definitions have vanished and no boundaries are seen. So too is it with your Being and non-Being. Don't waste time in doubts and arguments, but move along and intermingle with all things without distinction. To live in this realization is to be without anxiety about non-perfection. To live in this faith is the way to non-duality because the non-dual is one with the trusting mind. Truly the way of enlightenment is beyond language for in it is found the great truth that in reality there is only the eternal 'KNOWINGNESS OF ISNESS.'"

THE AROUSAL FROM ZEN HYPNOTHERAPY

At the end of the reading of this dissertation of the nature of ZEN, suggest:

"Relax now and go ever deeper and deeper into the subjective state of hypnosis. There is no need to hold all you have heard in conscious collection as it is perpetually retained in the memory banks of your mental computer (your subconscious mind). What you have been given in this session will stay with you, and bring you serenity and peace. It causes you to stop fighting yourself. Get ready to arouse from hypnosis now, filled with serenity and peace, with the brilliance of enlightenment."

As I count from one to five...with each count...you will come up from the depth and return most enjoyable to the here and now...one...two...three...four...FIVE! You are fully aroused, fully alert, feeling wonderful and fine with a peacefulness within yourself, which passes understanding.

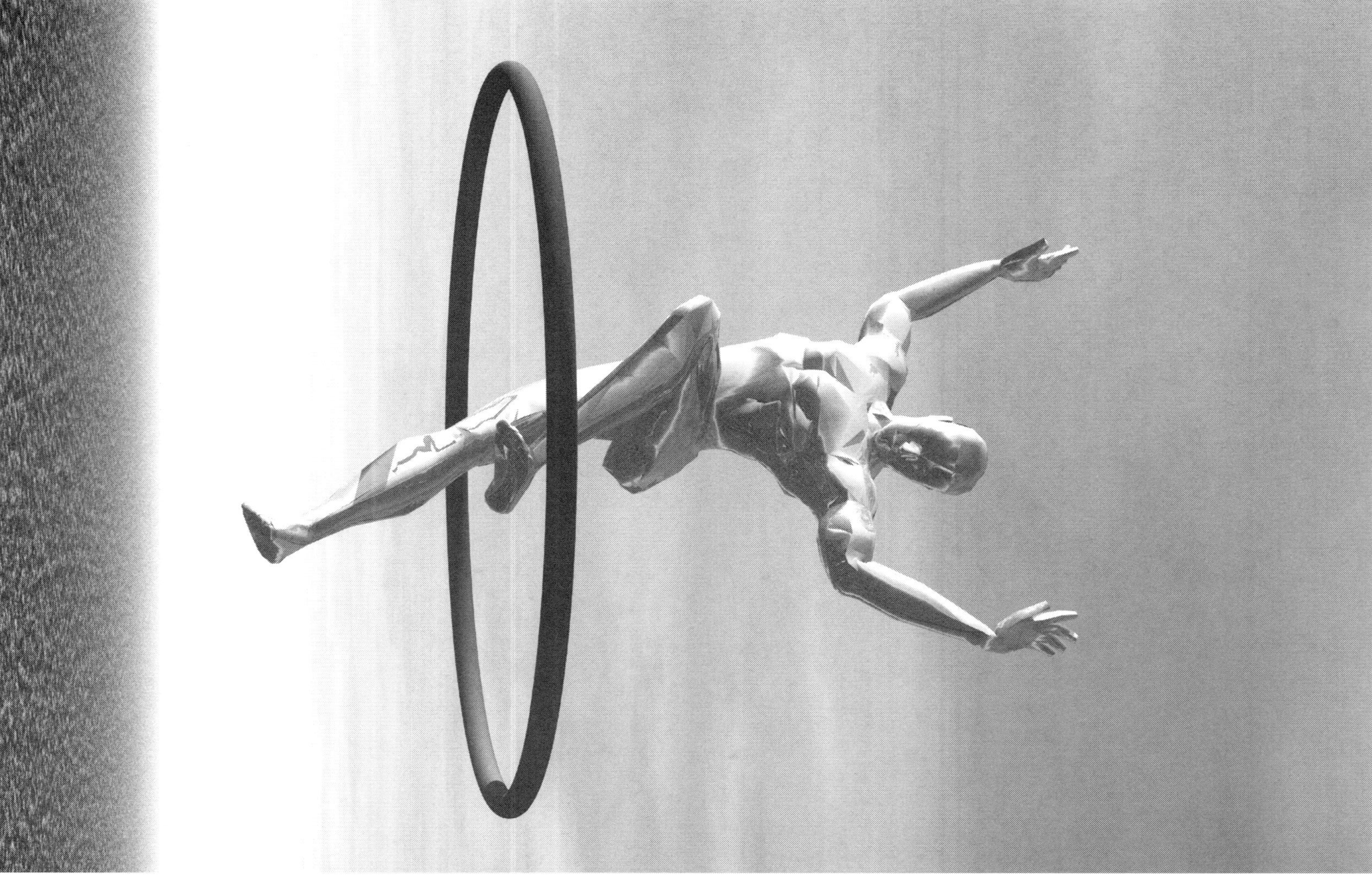

Illustration by Clark Dunbar (© RF RubberBall Productions)

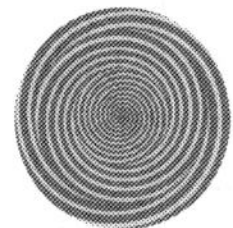

<h1 style="text-align:center">~ Chapter 195 ~
TRANSCENDENTAL HYPNOTHERAPY</h1>

"Mans next great discoveries will be found within his own inner space."
—Steinmetz's

Transcendental Hypnotherapy is among the greatest methods of mental mastery.
Why is it among the great?
Because it is transcendental…it connects your inner space with outer space. The process is given in detail, so you can use it with your clients in professional practice.

MODUS OPERANDI: TRANSCENDENTAL HYPNOTHERAPY

You Will Need:
The *Serenity Resonance Sound* as a background sound

Have your client take a seat in a comfortable chair, with their feet flat on the floor and resting their hands upon their lap. The light in the clinical office should come from behind the client directed towards yourself as the hypnotherapist. Give these suggestions:
"As you sit quietly in the chair, relax your body. Just let yourself GO!
As you do this, direct your attention to my eyes. Look deeply into my eyes and keep your complete attention fixed upon my eyes until I tell you to close your eyes. As you stare deeply into my eyes, notice how your perception of my eyes begins to change. It begins to seem that instead of focusing upon my eyes, the point of focusing moves through my eyes to the other side of my eyes, to a point beyond my eyes. You will find that you are no longer looking at my eyes, but that you are looking through my eyes into myself. It is as though my eyes have become windows through which you look directly into the space, which is inside myself. You are becoming aware that you are looking through the windows of my eyes out into the vastness of space…in which the stars of the heavens pulsate and shine. And, as you do this, come to know that I function as a 'space ship' for yourself, for as you travel into my inner space which is connected with vast outer space, it is equally your own inner and outer space that you travel through."

Let *Serenity Resonance Sound* rise up now…then fade again to background, as you continue…

"Let your entire body completely relax now, and send your BEING through the windows of my eyes and project your BEING into that vast space which spreads before yourself.
As you look deeply in this manner while relaxing your body, your eyes become so heavy you can no longer hold them open. So close your eyes, and just let GO.

Now, experience yourself sinking down into this vast space, which spreads before you on into infinity. Your are breathing deep and freely, and every breath you take sends you down deeper and deeper into this vast space…far, far down beyond even a vestige of consciousness of the physical world. Drift. Drift. Drift. You'll find yourself drifting in space. A mind free of its body in the space…drifting down ever deeper and deeper into the Cosmos.

Now, ask yourself some questions as you drift down into this vast space. Are you the one who is called by a certain name in the physical world? Are you the person who lives at a certain address? Are the individual who possesses a certain bank account and holds a certain position in the world? Experience how you feel right now in this vast space in which you experience yourself as yourself…this vast space is beyond the realm of time, and all the things you thought were important suddenly come to have no meaning at all…for you are now a free mind drifting in free space, as your inner space of yourself becomes connected with infinite outer space. And you come to KNOW you are none of the things you thought you were, and yet you still are YOU.

As a free mind, you are drifting down deeper and deeper into this vast space, and you know it as THE VOID. You are drifting down to the very center of this vast space; you are drifting down to the very center of yourself."

Pause. The serenity Resonance Sound rises up and then again fades to background.

"You are drifting down, down to your SELF…going deeper and deeper into the vast space of yourself. You see your SELF before yourself, and you ask a question. 'How can this be…for I am here in space drifting down to myself?' And suddenly you realize what you really are…YOU are the consciousness of your SELF and you appreciate and recognize this fact with great joy in now knowing…in full awareness…what you really are. You are an individual consciousness who is the only one exactly like yourself in the entire Universe. And you recognize this fact with great joy in at least becoming fully aware of what you really are…that the SELF you see before you is the real YOU. Your inner space and outer space are joined in perfect union.

This insight comes upon you like the bursting of stars. Suddenly you feel utter blissfulness; utter peacefulness; utter happiness. And you find yourself dropping down directly to the CENTER OF YOUR BEING, which is your SELF.

You go down, down into your SELF and you emerge as one BEING. Your inner space and outer space have become united. In doing this, you experience complete rest, for now you are HOME. Now you know what you really are and what you are meant to be. The reason for your existence. You are the mind of this SELF…the consciousness of this SELF through which you currently manifest in 3-D space, while you are in body."

Pause.

"Now, even this realization begins to melt and fade away as you merge into yourself…and experience no longer a separation of yourself as being mind on the one hand and of being SELF on the other…for your mind and your SELF have become as ONE, as pure consciousness. Each is now recognized as part of the other in being recognized in your eternal BEINGNESS. You KNOW BEINGNESS. And along with this experience you your BEINGNESS you also experience your relationship of ONENESS expanding to include ONENESS with all Existence."

Pause.

"Suddenly, you KNOW THAT YOU ARE PART OF THE TOTALITY…that a part of that Totality is YOU and that YOU ARE THE TOTALITY. When inner space and outer space meet, YOU BECOME ONE WITH THE INFINITE.

This experiencing of SELF that you now know completely changes your relationship to the physical world, in which you live at this moment…in the here and now…and that, of course, includes your body. It gives you a control over your body, which includes your body. It gives you a control over your body which you never before imagined you possessed…for now that you as mind and you as SELF (CONSCIOUSNESS) work together as a team in mutual unity, the SELF takes over control of the mind as it manifests in the physical world in the operation of your bio-computer brain which operates your body in 3-D space and time. Mind under control of SELF makes you a MASTERMIND, which can bring perfection to your body, as you wish.

With this control, which you have now achieved, you can make yourself whatever is your wish. You can heal your body; you can keep your body in perfect health; you can reform its habits; you can make your body perform to perfection beyond your wildest dreams. You can master ALL that is about yourself, and achieve whatever you desire to achieve. You have discovered yourself, and in fusing mind with SELF you have established SELF as the controller of mind which produces thoughts, and you have become the MASTER SELF."

Pause.

The *Serenity Resonance Sound* rises up…then fades again to background.

"Now, you have discovered who you really are, and you can cause all concerns and worries to vanish and disappear forever, as is your wish. You are now in complete control of yourself, and you have the power to make of yourself exactly what you wish to be. From this time forward, you will control yourself always from your CENTER OF BEING…and you will make of yourself the perfection which it is your right to be."

Pause.

"This which you now know as truth, from having experienced this truth in this TRANSCENDENTAL HYPNOTIC SESSION will stay with you always. Every breath you take into your physical body automatically reinforces this truth, and causes it to become your very own."

Turn off the *Serenity Resonance Sound* now.

"I bring you back to the here and now on a joyous returning to the physical world with this blissful KNOWING burning within you like an everlasting flame."

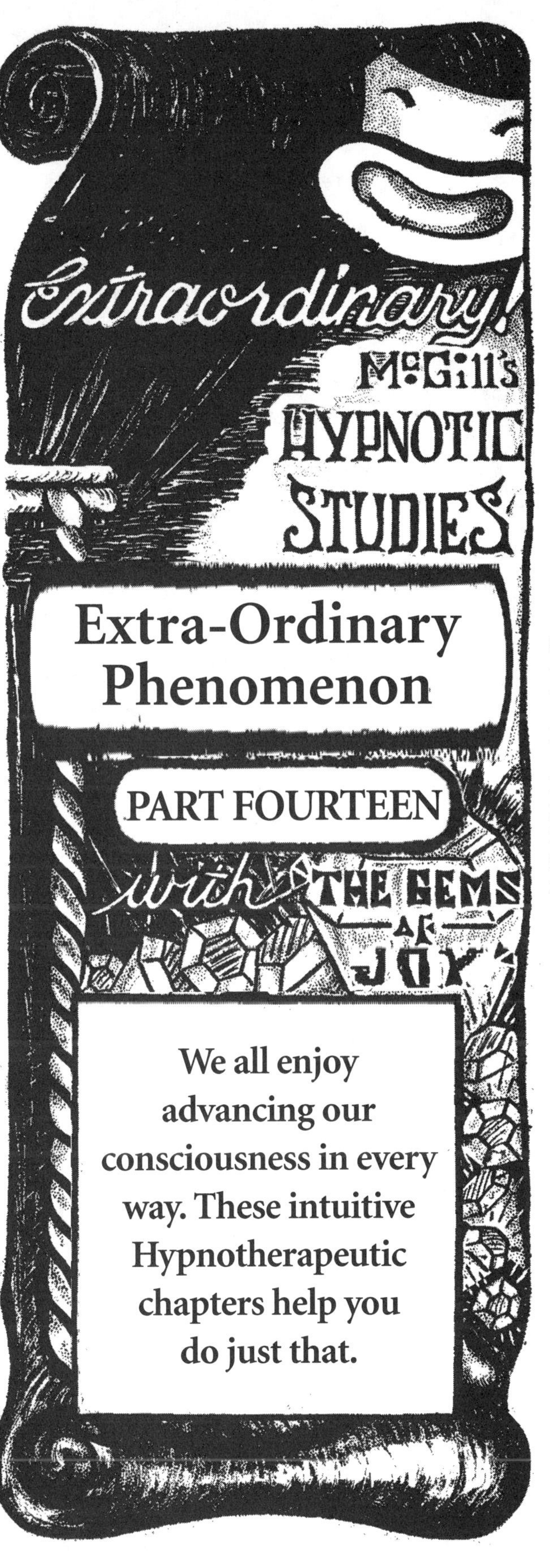

CHAPTERS IN PART FOURTEEN

196. Extraordinary Hypnotic Phenomena......................................page 775
197. Out Of Body Hypnotherapy 779
198. Telepathy Experiments 783
199. Clairvoyance 785
200. Trance Channeling 787
201. Stockwell's Be More Psychic Hypnosis 789

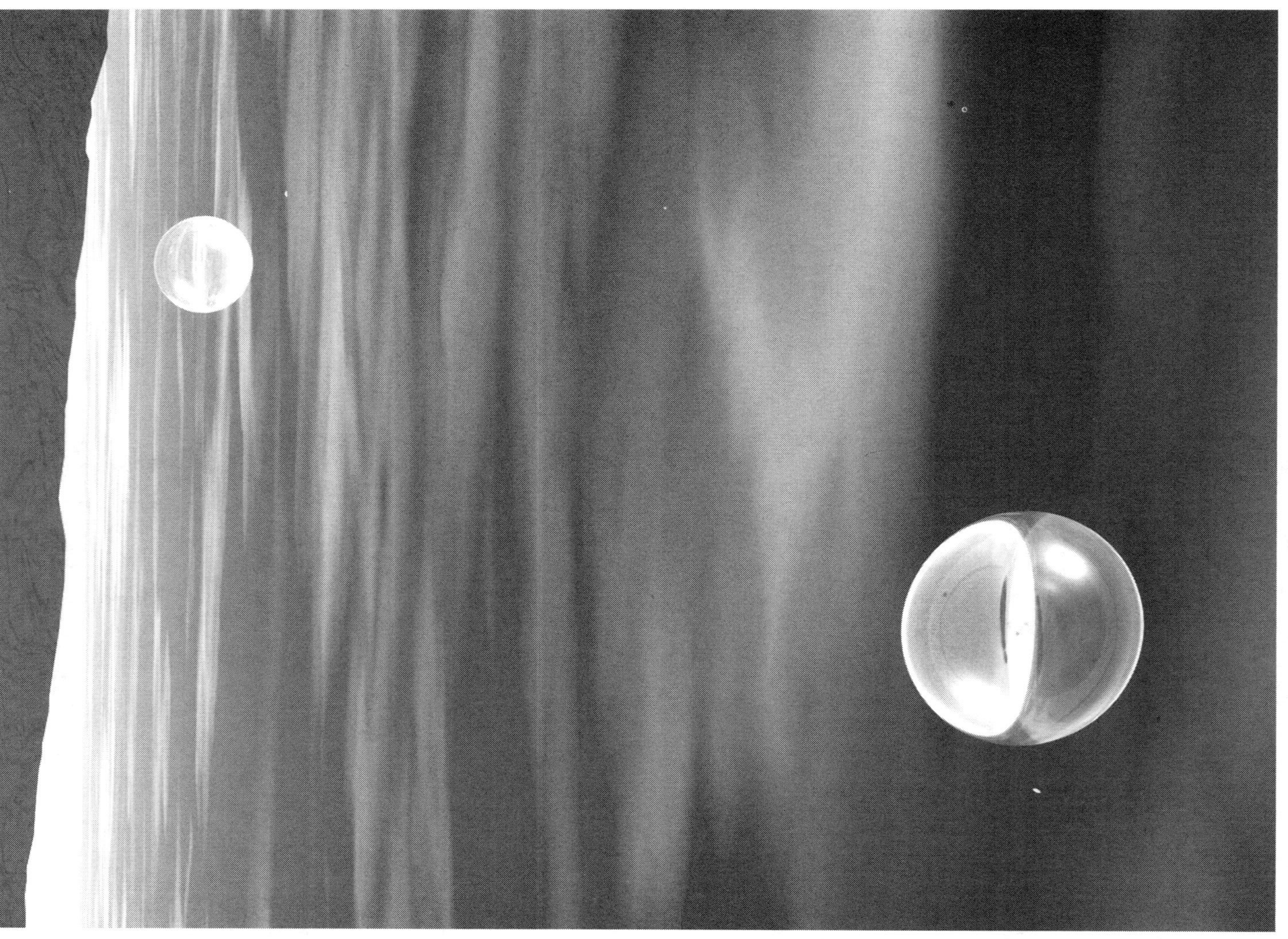

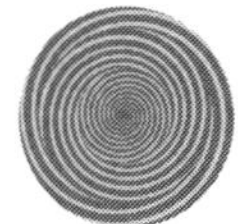

~ *Chapter 196* ~
EXTRAORDINARY HYPNOTIC PHENOMENA

Includes
The Blue Light Sensitizing Method
Magnetic Light Experiment
Involuntary Movement Experiment
Hyperaesthesia of Energy
Hyperaesthesia of Sight

Promise Nothing. Help All You Can.

Patience & Practice= Results

More and more someone will come to your hypnotherapy office wanting you to help them develop their psychic talents and other amazing mental skills. Your knowledge of extraordinary hypnotism aids these who so seek.

Extraordinary hypnotism usually develops slowly but occasionally comes about instantly. Persistence is well worthwhile. Mesmeric human energy is best for such experimenting with verbal suggestions kept to the minimum. This emphasizes mental commands.

MODUS OPERANDI: THE BLUE LIGHT SENSITIZING METHOD
The Blue Light Method gives the required energy to advance into further extraordinary hypnotism experiments and keeps verbal suggestions to a minimum.

You Will Need:
A Reclining Chair Or Hypnosis Couch
A Blue Light
Soothing Music (Like The *Serenity Resonance Sound*)

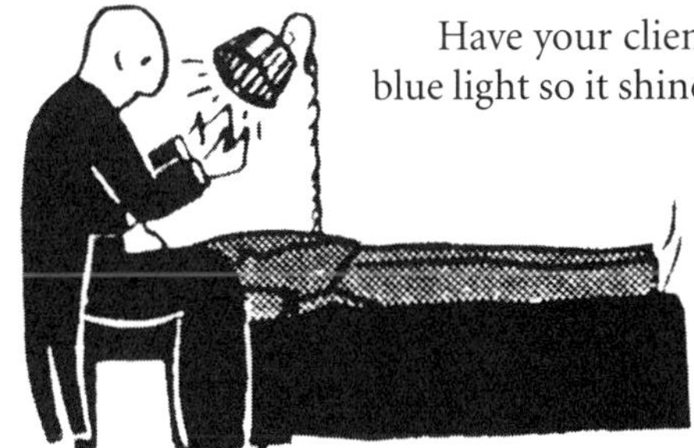

Have your client recline on a couch. Darken the room and arrange a blue light so it shines down upon their forehead. The Serenity Resonance Sound played as a soft background enhances the relaxation to move them into a Theta/Delta state.

Instruct your client to, **"close your eyes and just relax"** as you stand beside them and lean over them making long sweeping passes going from their head to foot. As you make the passes, extend your fingers tensely while visualizing a "magnetic current" passing out of them into the auric field of the person. You will clearly sense the transference of this energy, as your fingers tingle. You may actually see "electricity" emanating from your fingers!

Next, make short circular energy passes around the closed eyes of the subject. As you make these passes concentrate on the person passing down into a profound hypnotic trance.

Following these, return to performing the long sweeping passes over the entire length of the body. Watch your client and you will observe a loosening of facial muscles and a deepening of the breath, as entrancement ensues. Continue this process for as long as thirty minutes. Then arouse person. An electric tingling will be felt about the body upon arousal. You can now try some the experiments.

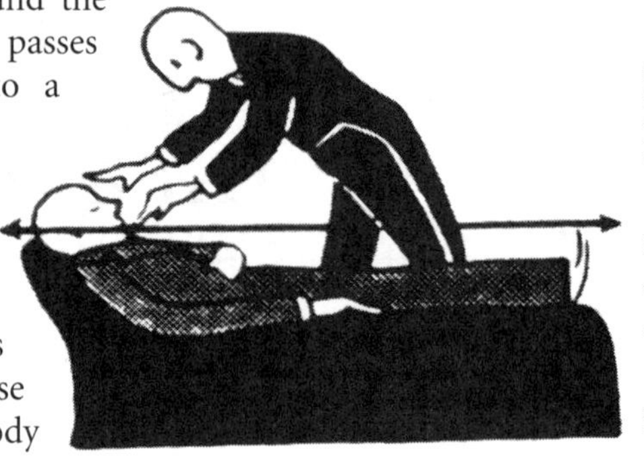

Illustration by Ormond McGill

MODUS OPERANDI: MAGNETIC LIGHT EXPERIMENT
You Will Need:
A Strong Magnet
A Pitch-Black Room

After you have hypnotized and sensitized your client with the blue light method (or another method that you prefer), black out the room completely and hold a strong magnet in front of them. A sensitized person will see luminous emanations proceeding from the tips of the magnet. Seeing these, have them reach and locate the magnet in the complete dark. To see the "magnetic light," not only must the subject be sensitized but the darkness must be absolute. If this experiment is not at once successful, have the person remain in the darkness for half an hour. Developing these extraordinary powers of mind takes patience and persistence.

MODUS OPERANDI: INVOLUNTARY MOVEMENT EXPERIMENT
You'll need:
A Blindfold Or Eye Shades

After the client has been hypnotized or energy charged by the magnet, place a blindfold or eyeshades on them. Now, hold your hand without actual contact near any part of their body or head, and that part will slowly move in the direction in which your fingers are drawn.

MODUS OPERANDI: HYPERAESTHESIA OF ENERGY

You'll need:

A Blindfold Or Eye Shades
Other People Who Want To Explore Energy

The word *Hyperaesthesia* means "heightened sensitivity" and comes from the Greek word *aistheticos* meaning "sense of perception."

Have your blindfolded client sit in a chair before a group of observers. Tell them **"As you know, all humans are surrounded by an aura or electro-magnetic field. You will recognize the feeling (or emanation) from my hand as I hold it near to you."** Hold your hand close to near the nape of his or her neck to let them become familiar with it.

Then tell them "Now various people will place their hands, one by one, near the nape of your neck and you will easily and immediately recognize and distinguish my personal energy from the others." The subject can tell it every time.

MODUS OPERANDI: HYPERAESTHESIA OF SIGHT

You Will Need:

A Deck Of Playing Cards
A Note Pad

This fascinating hyperaesthesia demonstrates "super sight."

Hypnotize your client. Select one playing card from a deck of playing cards. Write down its name, but don't say what it is out loud. Hand it face down, with the card back upward toward your client and tell them, **"This is a picture of your mother and you will easily be able to recognize and locate that picture under any circumstances."**

Then return the card in amongst the other cards in the deck and mix them up. Then hand the entire deck to the hypnotized person back uppermost. Have them **"look at the back of each card in turn– until you will stop at one card that has the picture of your mother on it."** On turning the card over it will be found to be the correct one.

The logical explanation for this is that every card, no matter how new a deck, has on it some minute differences, which sets it apart from its neighbors. In the illusion of seeing their mother's picture, the subject makes note of these minute differences, and is able to distinguish that card by its back alone. It is an amazing experiment.

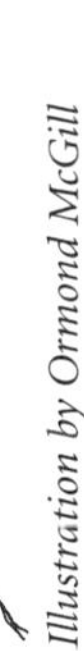

Illustration by Ormond McGill

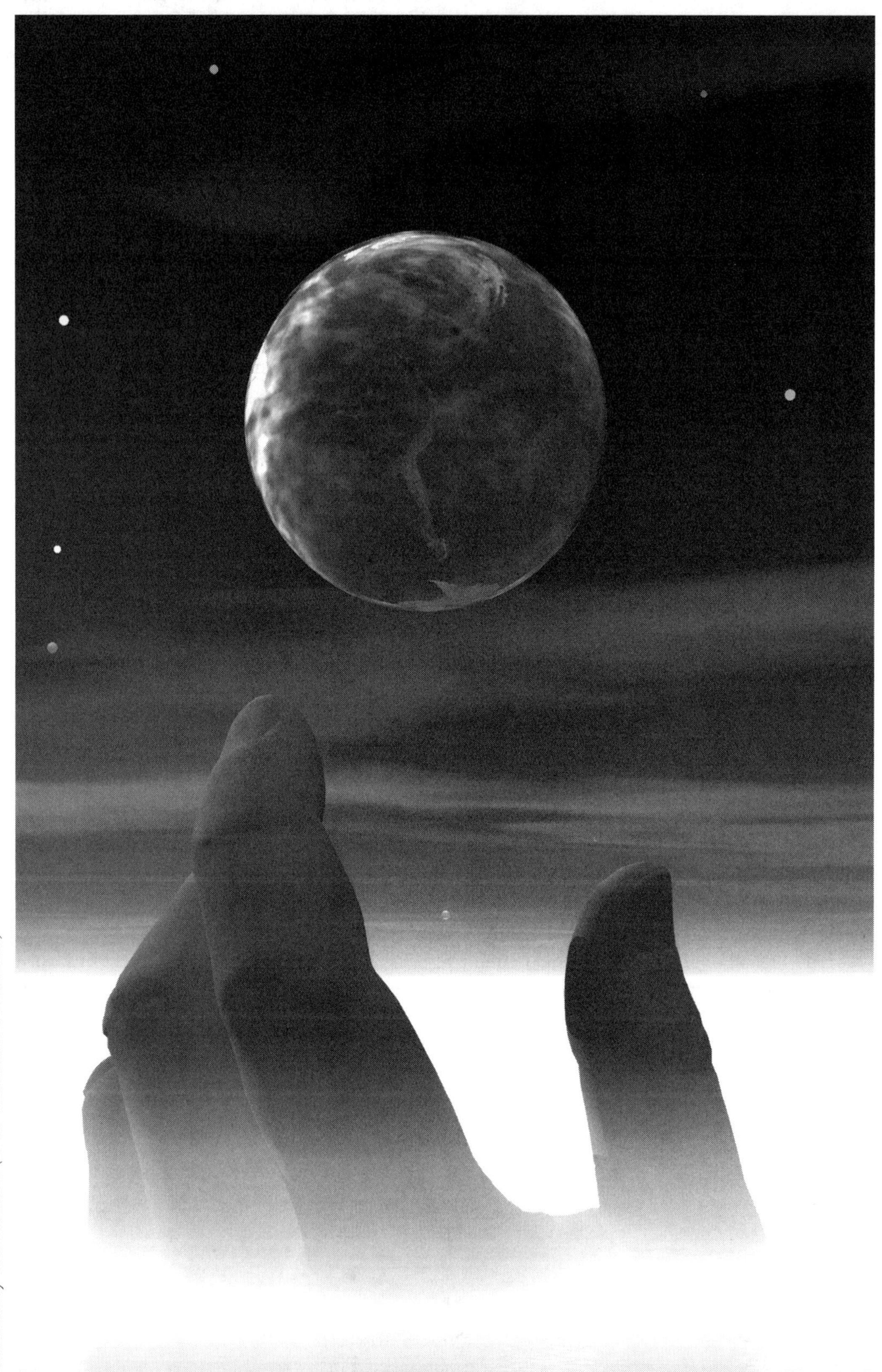

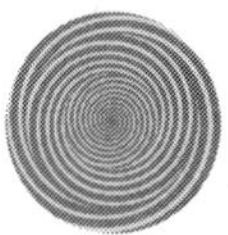

~ *Chapter 197* ~
OUT OF BODY HYPNOTHERAPY

Includes
Out-Of-Body Hypnotherapy
Up, Up And Away Images

Out-of-body travel like astral projection, has been known for centuries. When you get out-of-your-body, the experience is often described as "hovering above the body and observing yourself below." Sometimes the experience happens so spontaneously that it comes with a shock of surprise. The out-of-body experience has never been associated with hypnotherapy. Yet it is remarkable hypnotherapy that definitely raises self-esteem, boosts wellness, and solves problems.

Out-of-body hypnotherapy is based upon two objectives:
1. To program the subconscious so that on a post-hypnotic cue the astral body is projected (or released) from the physical body, to view the physical self from an out-of-body position.

2. To use this "vacated" physical body viewpoint to reform and make the perfect body-house in which the SELF lives.

Following these processes, the astral body (which contains the SELF) re-enters into the physical body. When one awakens from the hypnosis, life goes on with a realization of a perfected new body forming. This happens via subconscious instruction.

MODUS OPERANDI: OUT-OF-BODY HYPNOTHERAPY
Pre-Talk or Induction:
You can begin with this as your pre-talk or you can use it after inducing trance:

"Sometimes we think of the subconscious as unreasoning and obedient to commands whether they are beneficial or not. And that is true as far as subconscious behavior goes, but it is not true as far as subconscious capacity goes. Your subconscious has unlimited knowledge of your true nature (your true nature as a deathless being). Your subconscious is a wonderful storehouse of knowledge and knows all about your true nature.

This can be likened to the memory banks of a computer. When you operate a computer you easily draw upon its memory. What has been placed there influences the results. You turn the computer on and it gives you access to its memory when you call upon it. Your subconscious phase of mind works like that too. When you instruct the subconscious, via hypnosis, to have out-of-body experience, it easily brings an out-of-body into being, because your subconscious remembers and has had much practice."

Hypnotize the client deeply if not already entranced and direct their subconscious mind,

"Bring your inner-self out of your body, so you can look down and witness your body from a distance. In other words, command your SELF to bid the astral body to leave the physical body and journey with the "cue"'astral body project outside.'

Now, view yourself from a distance. You will see yourself as a familiar object, but without the personal identification you have when you are inside your body and thus closely identified with it. Reconstruct a new image of your body made to your specifications (or without a specific problem that they wish to correct). **Take as long as you need. When you reenter your body and awaken from the hypnosis, the out-of-body hypnotherapy is complete."**

This suffices for the first session of out-of-body hypnotherapy. The subconscious has been instructed in the out-of-body operation and a "conditioned" post-hypnotic response for the SELF to journey the astral form each time the "cue" **"astral body project outside."** is given.

Likewise, general hypnotherapy for the creating a newly perfect body image has been established. In subsequent sessions, you can correct specific problems in addition to improving a general self-image.

MODUS OPERANDI: UP. UP AND AWAY IMAGES

"Bring your awareness to the present and make sure that you are not asleep. As you visualize the objects I mention, peer with your third eye upon the inner space of the screen of your mind. As fast as the images are heard, visualize and experience them upon all levels of feeling, emotion and imagination. The faster you are told the faster moves your mind in full awareness to witness them upon the screen.

See the face of Buddha, smiling. See Christ, standing. See a flickering candle. See a weeping willow tree. See a tall palm tree. See a car moving along a road. See colored clouds floating in the sky. See yellow clouds; blue cloud, red clouds. See a starlit night. See the full moon in the sky. See a dog standing. See a cat resting. See an elephant moving through the jungle. See a horse racing. See the sun rising. See the sun sitting. See an ocean with waves upon it. See a big pond of clear water. See a blue lotus or lily…a white lotus…a pink lotus. See a golden spider web. See a sandy bank of a wide river. See a boat sailing on the ocean. See yourself lying naked upon the sand of the beach. See an ocean with and a silver cord extending from you to the sky. Visualize yourself as the immortal being that you are.

See yourself floating outside your body. Imagine that you are on the ceiling of the room where you now rest. See your body get up and tiptoe to the door of the room where you are now. Quietly open the door and go outside and then close the door behind you. See your body walking outside the room you are in. See many familiar things outside the room. Notice how freely you move. Experience complete brightness…how wonderful this feeling of brightness. It may be that you see people that you know on this mental journey. You can see them but they cannot see you as you make this out of body astral flight.

Suddenly you see yourself floating over the sea. See it clearly and become completely aware of the experience. See the bright blue waters of the ocean glistening below you as you float above it so lightly. Your body floats like a cloud and the wind blows your body like a cloud. Feel the mists of other clouds as they brush past your face as you rise up amongst the clouds. Observe the sunlight reflecting off the banks of clouds through which you pass. Now your body is lifted by the air and carried over the land. As you float closer to the earth, you see fields and farmhouses, forests, and winding rivers that reflect the sun.

Pause a moment on your astral flight and look closely at yourself. Note how relaxed you are. On your face is an expression of peace, calm and utter blissfulness.

See your body suddenly immersed in color as it passes through a rainbow…and feel yourself purified by the subtle colors of yellow, green, blue, violet, red, orange and gold. You feel these colors penetrating your entire body and SELF. You are invigorated."

COMING BACK

"Slowly return to your body as you see your body return the outside of the building where you now rest. See yourself again in this familiar room where you are. Quietly walk inside and open the door to the room and close it after you. Return to where you rest. It is fascinating to see your body resting exactly as you left it. Now sense yourself floating above your body and visualize yourself as you come into your own body and mesh again with every fiber and molecule and essence that is YOU. You are home once more and you dwell in this home in this immediate space and time. You rest quietly in your chair.

Relax your body completely now and prepare to enter the here and now. Relax as you bring your attention again to your natural breathing. Notice this natural breathing now for a few minutes and develop awareness of the wonderful physical relaxation you feel. You have not been asleep. You have not dreamed. It has happened to you. This wonderful experience makes you fully aware of yourself from a new view of higher consciousness.

Now become aware of your physical self seated or resting where you are. You feel good and vital and alive in every way. You are coming back but do not open your eyes. Visualize your surroundings and allow your mind to become completely external. Come back slowly as you rest quietly for a few moments becoming externalized.

You are ready to come back now. Start moving your body and stretch yourself. Move gently and enjoy your body as you arouse. And you become completely aware and awake but do not open your eyes just yet…simply rest a moment longer.

All right. You are back in your body in the here and now, so open your eyes whenever you wish. You are back in the here and now and feeling wonderful and fine and remarkable aware of the true nature of yourself. And this out of body session of is complete. Rise and Shine."

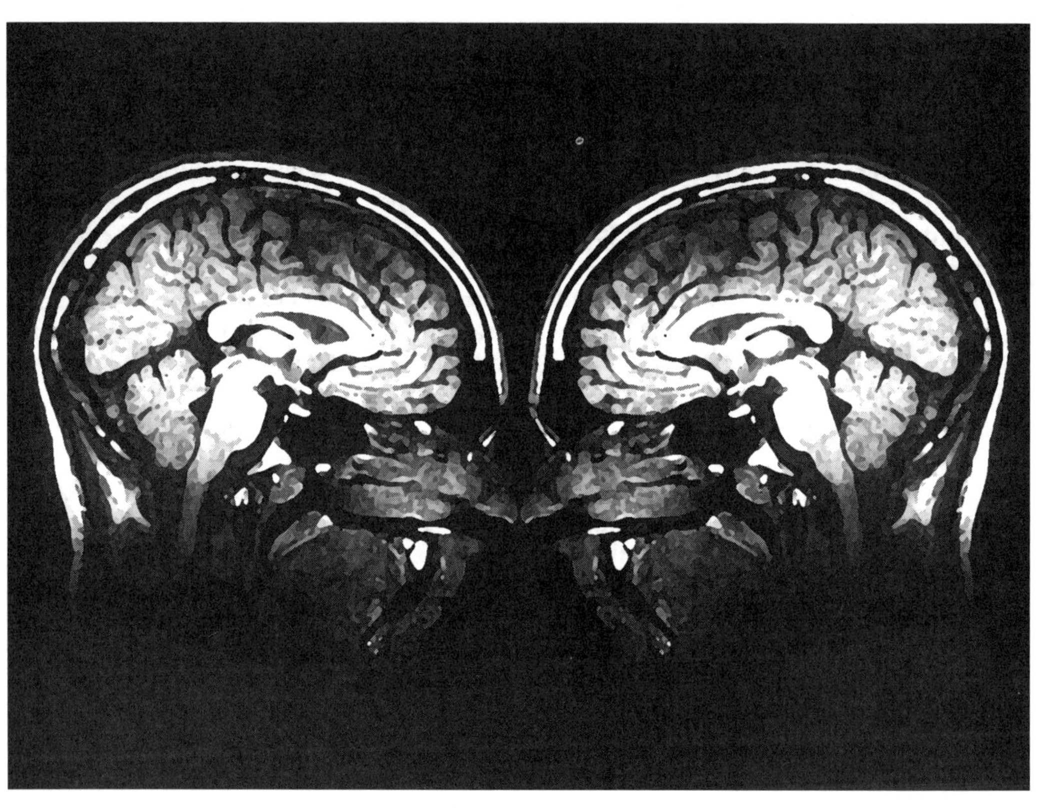

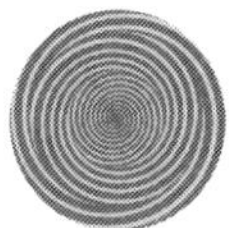

~ *Chapter 198* ~
TELEPATHY EXPERIMENTS

Includes
Sensational Telepathy Experiment 1
Complete Body Movement Telepathy Experiment 2
Duo Telepathy Experiment 3

These simple forms of telepathic communication put you and your client on the way to developing sensitivities and more detailed telepathic communication. They are simple forms of telepathic communication More detailed telepathic communication will come on its own. Your psychically developing client will enjoy these experiments. Begin by this one:

SENSATIONAL TELEPATHY EXPERIMENT 1
Have your hypnotized client close their eyes and suggest, **"You will now sense an electric-like tingling sensation from my fingers, as I pass them down your arm. I will do this without physically touching you. As the sensation is felt, your arm will slowly rise up from your lap."** As you make the passes, see within your mind (your mind's eye) the arm rising. Slowly the arm will rise.

Repcat the experiment with subject's left arm.

"Now I am not going to tell you over which arm I will make the passes, but as you feel such raise that hand accordingly." Experiment with this test a few times to determine the subject's sensitivity.

Then suggest that **"You will feel the same sensation when you simply think of which arm you are to rise– simply raise the hands in which the tingles are felt."**

Now, experiment with ESP by concentrating on his lifting either his right or left hand, as desired. In transmitting a telepathic impulse, such as lifting a hand, just visualize in your mind an image of the subject lifting up the thought of hand.

COMPLETE BODY MOVEMENT TELEPATHY EXPERIMENT 2
You will need:
A Coin

You can now advance your experiment with telepathy to complete body movement. Have the hypnotized person stand with feet together, explaining; **"You will feel an impulse to take a step forward or a step backward, as the case may be. When you sense an impulse move in that direction. I will flip a coin. If it comes up heads you will move forwards. If it is tails you will move backwards."**

Proceed to flip a coin, thinking "forewords" with heads and "backwards" with tails and see what happens. Keep track of results.

DUO TELEPATHY EXPERIMENT 3
You will need:
Two Hypnosis Subjects

Hypnotize two subjects and suggest, **"You are in close rapport with each other."** Assign one to be the "transmitter" and the other is the "receiver." Have the "transmitter" experiment with "receiver"– lifting a thought of hand or body movement. Keep track of results.

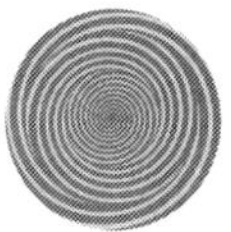

~ *Chapter 199* ~
CLAIRVOYANCE

Includes
Third Eye Seeing Experiment 1
Third Eye Seeing Experiment 2
Astral Projection

Clairvoyance means "clear seeing." It's the intuition of knowing and an ability to psychically envision occurrences at a distance. Space, as related to miles, has no meaning to the phenomena. Some people have the faculty of spontaneous clairvoyance. If you have the good fortune to experiment with a natural clairvoyant results can be astonishing. And a good hypnotic subject can also develop into a fine clairvoyant. Do not expect too much at first, it takes persistence.

THIRD-EYE SEEING EXPERIMENT 1
You will need:
A Darkened Room
A Blue Light
A Piece Of Paper And Writing Implement
Any Other Objects (like a book or statue or photo)

Work in a darkened room with blue light. Induce hypnosis in subject using the Mesmeric process and make energy passes over them for several minutes, while concentrating your mind on their subject developing clairvoyance. Setting your "mental purpose directive" is important to all such psychic conditioning. Use passes without contact, and the more profound the hypnosis the better. When subject is entranced try this experiment:

Write a single number (from 1 to 10) on a slip of paper. Take the paper in the palm of your hand, and press it on the top of their head. Ask them to tell you what the number is, using these suggestions:

"I want you to tell me what number – from on to ten – I have written on this paper slip I am now holding to your head. You can see it perfectly in you mind's eye. It is getting plainer to your inner vision. Do not guess. See the number within your eye of mind. See the number now!"

Insist that they can see it. Be positive and command them to see. If they do not at first, make more passes and quickly say, **"You can see it now!"**

If the entranced subject names the number correctly, then try it with two numbers, then three, and so on. This is all part of initial clairvoyant training. Then take an object, like a book or whatever, and have them describe it, as they envision it within their mind. Such practice applies to both telepathy and clairvoyance.

THIRD-EYE SEEING EXPERIMENT 2
You will need:
A Watch (or cards)

With your subject in profound hypnosis, take a watch and swirl the hands, so you have no knowledge of the time at which that watch is now set. Without looking at the watch, hold the face inward to your client's forehead. Tell them, **"The watch I hold at your forehead had been set to a random time. Tell me at what time the watch is set. You will see the face of the watch clearly within your mind."** Demand it be seen.

If subject says, "I cannot see it." Ask what you are to do, so he can see it. Do exactly whatever he tells you to do.

If the subject still does not tell you what to do, make further mesmeric passes over their forehead, and insist that they tell the time at which the watch is set. Force the subject to see.

In another version of this experiment in clairvoyance you write various numbers on different cards. Turn them face down and mix them, so that you have no idea, of which is which. Without looking at it, pick up a card and hold to subject's forehead. Ask them to name the number that is on it.

Remember both telepathy and clairvoyance are psychic talents that must be developed, and practice makes perfect. When accuracy comes in along with the phenomena, results can be amazing.

ASTRAL PROJECTION
After being successful with numbers and different objects, in the same room in which you are experimenting, ask the subject to describe a distant place seen within the mind, with which neither of you is familiar.

This form of clairvoyance in which the hypnotized person's perception seems to be molded into an "astral body form." Some regard it as the most accurate form of psychic perception. In experimenting with Astral Projection, hypnotize subject with the Mesmeric Method, and while the client is entranced, tell them to leave their body and astrally travel to any place they want to be. Have the subject describe what is seen.

Experiment.

Remember, until control is mastered, all psychic talents can be elusive. They may be surprisingly accurate on some days and at other times nothing seems to come through. Be patient and persistent in your experiments with clairvoyant subjects. Advance from the more simple to the more complex (actually nothing is really complex to mind).

As a hypnotherapist, as you work with clients developing their psychic abilities, you will find that the energies produced simultaneously advance your own powers in such direction.

For more information on astral travel see chapter 120, "Astral Hypno-Healing" and Chapter 197 "Out Of Body Hypnotherapy".

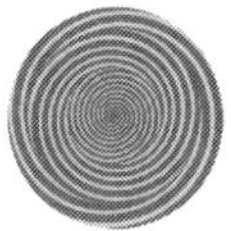

~ *Chapter 200* ~
TRANCE CHANNELING

Includes
Developing Channeling Ability

Channeling is an active multiple-personality meditation. Like meditation it is as much outside oneself as it is inside. The amazing skill of channeling belongs to the Cosmos possibly even more than it does to you.

Have you ever been talking or teaching a class and after it was over have someone say, "That was just great what you said about such and such?" That "such and such" refers to something you must have said of profound significance, or else why would the student acclaim it. Yet, for the life of you, you can't remember what you said.

Such speaking without recall is a form of channeling. Without question you spoke it, but it did not come out of your conscious mind. It was verbalized without your consciously thinking for yourself. Perhaps it was your subconscious speaking. Or, maybe the speaking came from an outside source; guidance to which you gave articulation. Perhaps it was your Guardian Angel or some other guiding source (or "force") to which you gave voice.

Who knows for sure just what source or force channeling is? Maybe it is just a fantasy like an articulated dream. Or, maybe it is an actual personality from another dimension for whom you speak. When the same source comes through frequently, we get so used to it, we often will give it a name. It can become so familiar that it comes into your consciousness like an intimate friend. Judge its worth by its wisdom.

What comes through is extremely unique. It seems like a personality with a continuing intelligence and memory. It will take whatever form it elects to form.

Many have the channeling experience. Some channel readily and others infrequently. Some remain detached during the experience others report that the source seems to literally to take over control of the individual during the contact.

Of course it is to be expected that some will believe in channeling and some will not, but there is enough universal interest that the hypnotherapist will have clients asking if such ability can be increased through the use of hypnosis.

Of course it can, as it is a personal mental ability that responds to subconscious motivation as a habit of perception. The ability to channel is definitely something the hypnotherapist can help requesting clients to master. And, it is not difficult for almost all clients who wish to develop more talent for channeling have already had some experience with channeling.

Channeling is a valuable talent for both you and your client to cultivate. Many a professional hypnotherapist, whose work is recognized as outstanding, has credited channeled guidance. Indeed, many a hypnotherapist, has privately whispered, "Thank God for this gift."

Developing channeling ability is much like posthypnotically motivating any other talent. Use hypnosis and tell the subconscious how much the talent is appreciated along with a request for steady increasing of the talent.

You can repeat such a hypnotic session as often as desired. The depth of channeling that can be developed is unlimited and cannot be overdone, as it probes the infinite. Let the client realize that always they are in control, and can explore their guidance upon their own command– on and off– as is their wish.

MODUS OPERANDI: DEVELOPING CHANNELING ABILITY

Hypnotize client. Induce somnambulism. A Mesmerizing process is very helpful for increasing psychic energy. Take your time. A slow induction process is advised. Then present these suggestions, in the first person, to your client's subconscious. Do this in an intimate and personal way as if the subconscious is a dearest friend.

"Ask and thou shall receive. Subconscious mind, please listen to me and answer my request. Please help me develop a wonderful mental talent which you well know how to do. Help me develop the skill of channeling. I have had some success with this remarkable mental power of which you have ever-ready control. Help me henceforth to steadily increase my ability to channel for guidance, ever and always under my control. I know you can. I know you will.

Let me be an open channel to whatever comes into me, from out of the universe, as the case may be. I recognize the talent of channeling as God's gift to me, and tank you for increasing my awareness to this advanced form of perception. I am an open channel to all forms of channeling input. I am open ever more and more to continuing channeling input and wisdom, over which I have perfect control. Thank you my subconscious for making my talent for channeling my ever-increasing reality. I am open. I am open. I am open."

Go quiet for some moments now, to allow this request for developing channeling skill to go deep into client's subconscious. Then continue…

"Thank you my subconscious for advancing my talent of channeling, which you have wonderfully done. And you have made me know that with every breath I take my talent of channeling increases…increases…increases. When you know my skill is established, arouse me from the hypnosis feeling joyous in the gift of channeling you have given me."

Go silent now, and drop yet deeper into hypnosis as your talent for channeling increases…increases…increases. When it is "mentally set" you will arouse from the hypnosis feeling wonderfully elated.

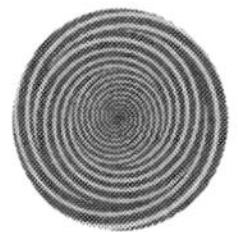

~ Chapter 201 ~
STOCKWELL'S
BE MORE PSYCHIC HYPNOSIS

By Shelley Stockwell-Nicholas, PhD

"Prophecy has always existed and, I predict always will."
—Shelley Stockwell-Nicholas

Includes
The History of Mystery
Coming To Your Senses
Trance Channeling or Medium-ship
Will You Remember?
How To Be More Psychic

Intuition is a powerful asset! It gives transpersonal glimpses beyond the ordinary into the extraordinary for heightened awareness. Seers, oracles, trance channelers, prophesiers, diviners and fortune-tellers rely heavily upon "ESP" (extra sensory perception) and "PSI" (psychic phenomena) to glimpse into a non-physical world and into the future. Their domain belongs to you and your clients.

Every hypnotherapist learns that in altered state, the supernatural is natural. It offers soul and hope into the equation.

Hypnosis is the best way to develop intuition as it allows analytical thinking to step aside. It is near impossible to go with the flow of the higher self and super conscious mind while consciously analyzing and judging.

THE HISTORY OF MYSTERY
The ancient book, the "Aeneid" was used to tell fortunes. To answer a question you would put your finger at random upon any line in the book and there was the answer. Christians later used the bible and Muslims the Koran in the same way.

Etruscans predicted the future based on the flight of birds.

Joseph saw the future in a dream and advised the Pharaoh.

Cassandra warned against the Trojan Horse.

Nostradamas, the French astrologer, predicted a future that spanned centuries.

A seer warned Julius Caesar about the "ides of March."

Governments enlist remote viewers. Law enforcement enlists psychics. Presidents consult spiritual counselors.

Stars, Tarot cards, I Ching, crystal balls, Oaija boards and tea-leaves serve as divination tools or spring boards for what belongs to us all; into-wishin'.

Pre-cognition

Pre-cognition is knowing that something is going to happen before it does. This includes premonitions, prophecy, lucid dreams and visions.

Retro-cognition

Retro-cognition is the ability to read the past by being in a place or touching an object that was present then. Deja vu experience are when we go to a place for the first time, yet remember all about it in a past place and time.

Telepathy

When we link into another's thoughts, energy is transmitted and received without spoken language. We all have this experience when we look into a beloved's eyes and sense what they are thinking.

COMING TO YOUR SENSES

Intuition is an individual experience. The only perfect way to develop psychic abilities is what works most comfortably for you. The best and easiest style employs your dominant senses. You can explain this to your client in the pre talk.

"Clair enough to be your very best"
   —I.D. Clair

Clairvoyance generically means to receive information as a direct knowing or in symbols, sensations, through the senses. There is a whole family of "clairs":

Clair Audient (sound)
Clair Sentient (feel)
Clair Voyant (sight)
Clair de Loon (a little off kilter)
Any way it is done you will have a sensation-all experience

Clair Audient: Sound Advice

Clairaudience means "clear psychic hearing." If you're sound dominant, you'll most likely hear messages or sounds in your inner ear. The "inner voice" may sound familiar. Some swear that someone outside of themselves is talking inside or outside their skull.

The first time I channeled, my deceased father's voice came from a beam of light. If you are auditory, listen carefully. Your extra-sensory perception, received as sound, offers sound advice.

Clair Sentient: Good Vibes

Clairsentients chill out with a "feeling" or "*just know*" things that go beyond the senses. If you are touch dominant, you'll most likely *feel or sense* your guidance. Kinesthetic or touch dominant folks tune into sensations and vibrations. The sensing of energy from any source is called "radiothesia" or "psychometry." Dowsers use this to find water. Psychics, who work with the police, often "tune in" by touching or holding an object or item.

Empaths actually feel another's body while focusing on them. **"You can develop your feeling sensate ability with yourself by tuning in on your body right now. Notice any "blocks" or limits and then expand your awareness outside of the walls of flesh to your auric field or the energy that is outside of you. Now, from this awareness, think about someone you know and feel their body and their auric field, noting any *blocks* or limits in this perception."**

Clair-Voyant: I See

Clairvoyants are visionaries who "see" inner and outer visions or just "know" events, items or the activities of others who not present in physical reality. Their *pictures* come as symbols, images, pictures or visions. Such lucid dreams require you to intuitively interpret what you see or simply report. If you "Call 'em like you see 'em" you allow others to make their own interpretation. If you are a visual person you may *see* visions, symbols or pictures.

The "remote viewer" sends their mind out to view anything. You slide into a time frame to lock onto an event that had a peak emotion attached to it. Through a tell-a-vision technique these perceptions are projected into the spoken word.

Sniff It Out

Odor dominants can sniff and smell an entire experience.

Taster's Choice

Tasters taste.

Direct Knowing

Some intuitives bypass the senses all together and have a "direct knowing." The most important thing is to not hold an expectation as to how it is supposed to be for you. Don't expect to see anything if you're a feeler. Or feel if you hear. Just receive the way you do and report it in a way that is most natural. That way you set yourself for success.

TRANCE CHANNELING OR MEDIUMSHIP

When tapping intuition, you can choose to merge with inner voices: nonphysical entities, guides, angels, ET's, and those who have crossed over. Notice I used the word *choose*. A channel must willingly yield and allow entities to communicate through them. It is really quite easy to this as you talk to yourself all the time. Who is it that is doing the talking and who are you talking to anyway?

You employ all your senses when you channel but your dominant senses will usually serve you best. Light Trance channels may appear as they do in their regular state of awareness with no difference of voice or personality.

Deep Trance channels may look like they have fallen into deep sleep and demonstrate dramatic shifts in energy, voice and style. The vocabulary and wisdom of a channeled entity that emerges is often leagues away from the vehicle that brings the voice forward. Jane Roberts surprised many with the rasping male voice of her guide "Seth." Edgar Cayce, called "the sleeping prophet," was a humble man with an eighth-grade education who delivered scholarly medical and philosophical dissertations.

WILL YOU REMEMBER?

Just like in other altered states, some intuitives are not aware of their physical environment. Others are partially aware. And some are fully present. Any way you do it, intuition allows wisdom to flow through you. The result is a larger perspective. Be it light or deep trance the trick is to tap the super conscious or the collective unconscious and report it through voice, automatic writing, creativity or energy transmission (Like hands on healing, long distance healing, or *Shaktipod*).

HOW TO BE MORE PSYCHIC

To be more psychic, quiet your conscious and subconscious mind. Self-hypnosis, prayer and meditation help you "step aside" to let what comes come. When you put your rational mind aside, imagine that you are a child and just receive what comes.

My friend Sandi Medearis puts all thoughts on a *cosmic clipboard*. "I greet each thought with the words, ''hello and good-bye.' This allows me to open myself to the wisdom of the superconscious."

The biggest dilemma folks face is thinking, "Oh this is nothing, my mind playing tricks on me. I must have made it up."

MODUS OPERANDI: BE MORE PSYCHIC HYPNOSIS

Pre Talk Questions:

"Have you been somewhere for the first time and felt like you'd been there before?

Have you met someone new and yet you sense you know all about them?

Have you known the phone was going to ring before it did or that something would happen before it actually occurred?

You may already have had many intuitive experiences.

The most important thing for you to do as you further develop your psychic ability is to suspend judgment and leave your thoughts behind. Let go of any expectation of how intuition is supposed to be for you. Don't expect to see anything if you're a feeler. Or feel if you hear. Just receive the way you do and report it in a way that is most natural. That way you set yourself for success. Anything you perceive you can project into the spoken word through tell-a-vision…just say what is going on."

Put your client in a trance and suggest:

"Now expand your awareness outside of the walls of flesh to your auric field, or the energy that is outside of you. From this awareness, think about someone you know and *feel* their body and their auric field, noting any *blocks* or limits in this perception.

Imagine that you are a child openly receiving what comes. To tap your intuition, set aside or quiet your conscious and subconscious mind. You can put all thoughts on a *cosmic clipboard*. And greet each thought with the words, 'hello and good-bye.' This allows you to open yourself to the wisdom of the superconscious, the part of you that knows everything. The part of you that is wise beyond wise.

Affirm: 'I am opening and expanding my awareness in every way' and notice that you more easily tune in to each of your senses. This is called coming to your senses. You now see, hear, feel, see, smell, taste and intuit a bigger knowing. You are one with the greater wisdom."

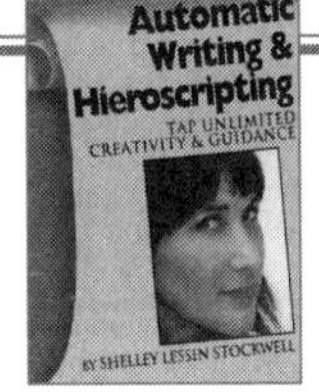

Hypno-Helper

"Automatic Writing & Hieroscripting: Tap Unlimited Creativity & Guidance" book by Shelley Stockwell

"Automatic Writing & Hieroscripting" audio tape by Shelley Stockwell

Available on the order form at the back of this book.

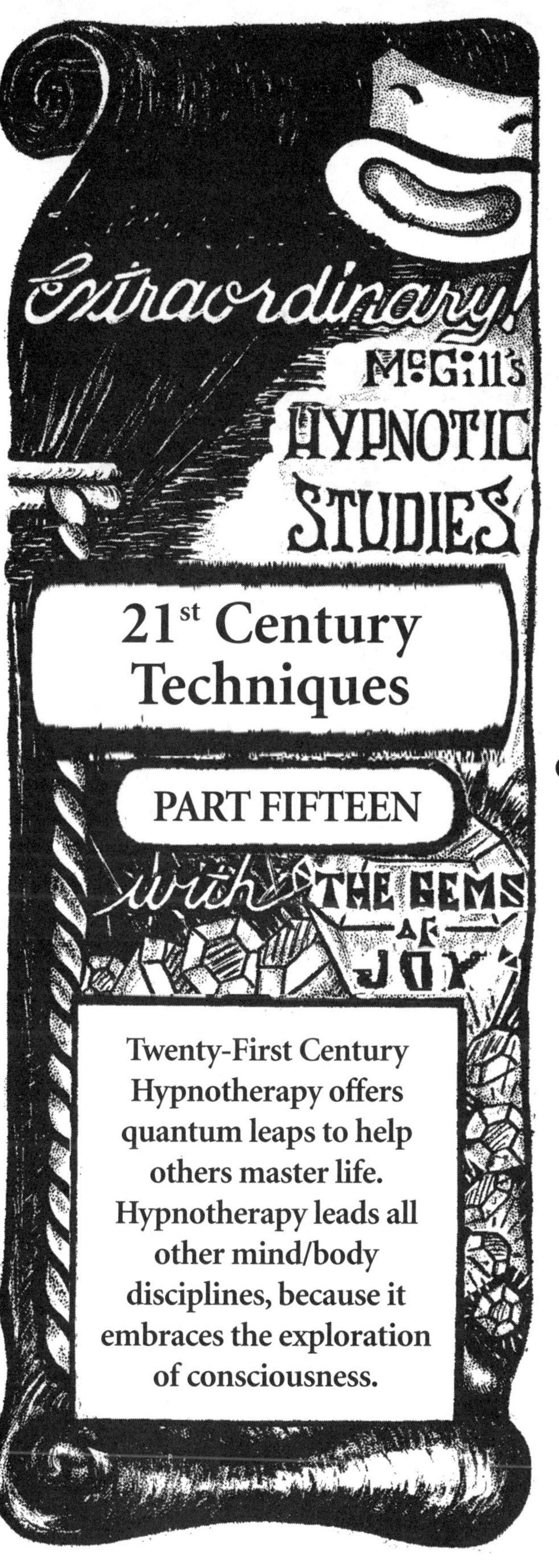

CHAPTERS IN PART FIFTEEN

202.   21st Century Hypnotherapy ......page 797
203.   Bodhisattva Hypnotherapy:
       Wakefulness...801
204.   Bodhisattva Hypnotherapy
       Continued 805
205.   Metamorphosis Hypnosis 811
206.   Epilogue: Your Mind Potential 815
207.   About Ormond McGill 817

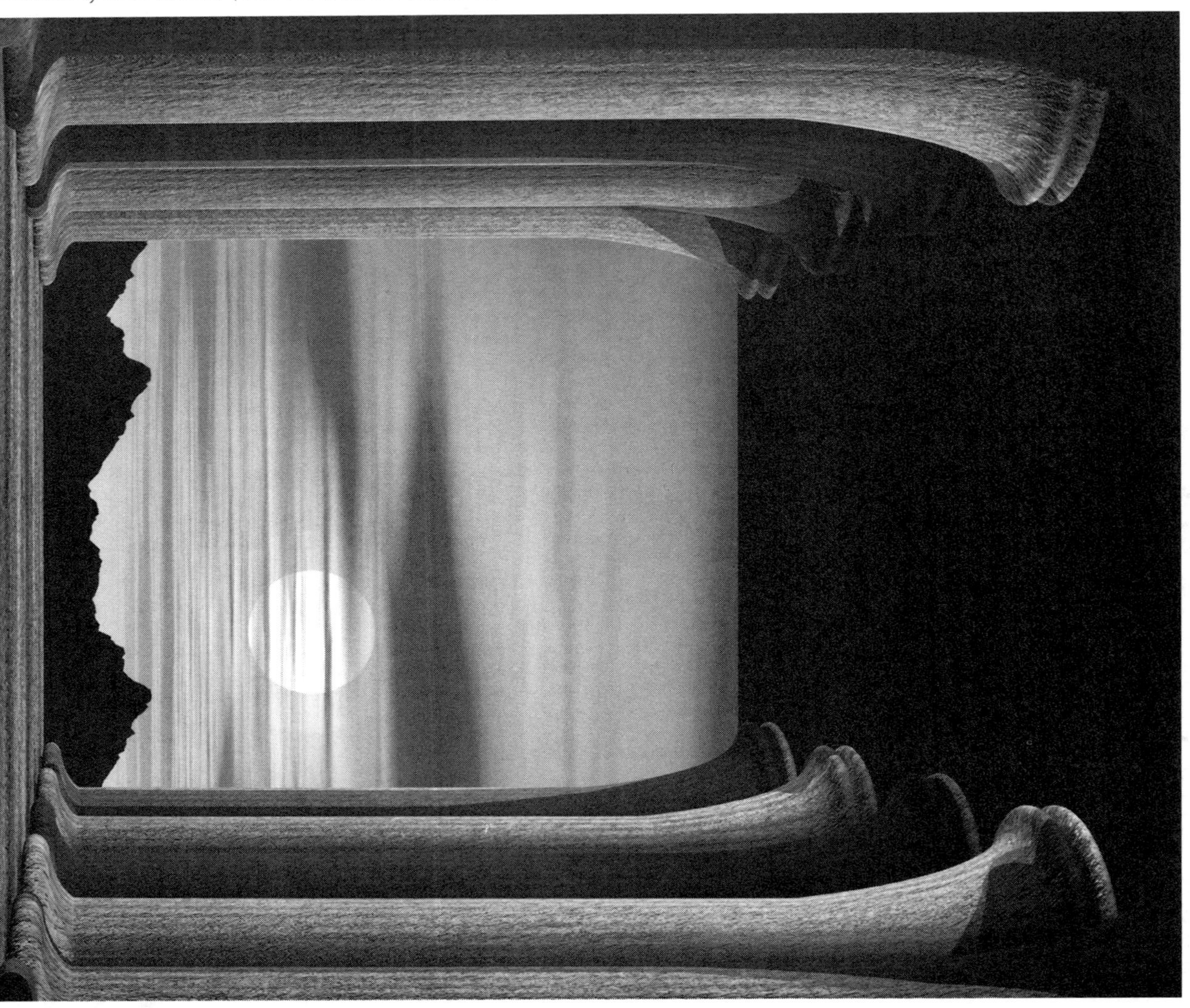

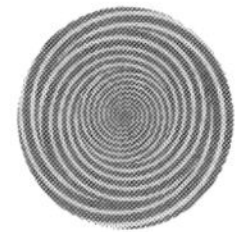

~ Chapter 202 ~

21ST CENTURY HYPNOTHERAPY

Includes:

The Seven Rules Of Conscious Mental Control
Use Stress To Promote Well Being
Key Belief
The Three Principles of Key Belief
The Healing Power Of Belief
Key The Subconscious for Benefits
The Power Of Source
Ancient Hypnotherapy Becoming New

Mind, like the Universe, is subject to constant change. Evolution is ever proceeding. In relationship to hypnotherapy one moment something may be old and the next moment in comes the new.

1. Early psychology was a compartmentalized mind with conscious and subconscious.
2. The next quantum leap was not so specific mind was looked upon by mind activity.
3. Then came quantum leap three as Milton Erickson expressed it, "I don't care if you stand on your head, just as long as your conscious mind gets out of the way."
4. Quantum leap four was Dave Elman's idea that we "By pass the critical mind and establish selective thinking.
5. And, Five is the permission hypnotherapy where we know that the Universe is perfect and that you are part of this perfection and give permission for such to happen in your life.

Much hypnotherapy occurs spontaneously and without conscious control. In the past, our families, our peers, our society, our religion, and advertisers inadvertently hypnotized us. Such accidental hypnosis caused many to give their mind to subconscious control, placing it beyond conscious control. The job of the Hypnotherapist is usually to wake you up from hurtful trances.

Twenty-First Century Hypnotherapy advances deliberate control of spontaneous hypnosis and places your mind under more direct conscious control of itself.

The Twentieth Century concept of hypnosis was to bypass critical mind and establish selective thinking. A new concept now replaces the old. In the Twenty-First Century, the concept of hypnosis is to intelligently direct subconscious mind via advanced critical mind control.

THE SEVEN RULES OF CONSCIOUS MENTAL CONTROL

Here are seven rules of mental discipline.

1. **Make mind think *what* you want it to think.**
2. **Make mind think *when* you want it to think.**
3. **Make mind *stop thinking* when you want it to stop thinking.**
4. **Make mind be attentive to whatever is before it, i.e. *cease wandering.***
5.   **Become a *witness* to your thoughts.**
6. **Realize that mostly your *thoughts are not your own.***
7. **Establish a *peaceful mind.***

Do these and you become a Mastermind.

USE STRESS TO PROMOTE WELL BEING

Stress is frequently blamed for illness and death. Stress will unquestionably increase during the 21st Century. Thus, we must master stress to be of benefit. Stress can also be redirected as a mental healer and productive emotional energy. You can do this is in both your BETA (waking) state and in THETA/DELTA (hypnotic) state of mind. This is the "key" to a quantum leap in hypnotherapy. The results can be remarkable.

Think of the stress a war pilot is under during the battle. A pilot who comes through an assault may instantly release intense stress without traumatic reactions. For those who do that, it is almost miraculous. It can happen in an instant. Cancerous tumors have been known to instantly vanish during intense stress. Increasing stress for wellness presents a quantum leap in hypnotherapy.

Everything takes energy to accomplish. Hypnotherapy is no exception. Target the intense energy of stress toward goals. Hypnotize yourself and your client to harness energy, key it into imagination, and make it your/their reality.

It begins by understanding the principles of key beliefs.

KEY BELIEF

Huxley placed the letter "C" on the wall of a classroom of children with defective eyesight. He told them it would be the key to develop perfect vision. It helped each child's vision greatly. A miracle? No. Belief is the secret "key" to possibility. A Sacred Shrine, such as Lourdes, is a perfect example.

THE THREE PRINCIPLES OF A KEY BELIEF

1. Everything you create begins when you *first pretend* that it is so.
2. From pretending, you advance to believing that it is so.
3. From believing, you advance to the *reality* that it is so.
    Use this idea with every client.

"KEY" THE SUBCONSCIOUS FOR BENEFITS

"Key" the mind to the goal. One "key" can be the hypnotherapy process itself. Whatever you, as the Hypnotherapist, choose to underscore can be the "key." Give the "key" in a direct suggestion. Joy and wellness is the point.

Emotions drive suggestions. Evangelistic healing is proof of that; evoke emotions and get results. The evangelist places God/Christ as the subconscious "key" which causes belief to take effect. A rousing service is excellent as an emotionally aroused group with heightened emotion and the rapid induction of a tap on forehead and a shouted "HEAL!" turns the key.

A good hypnotherapist evokes the same emotions of a cathedral or tent in their office.

THE POWER OF THE SOURCE

Belief, devotion, and/or respect for the *source* from which the "key" is given is said to be the secret of miraculous healing. Belief in the power of the source is the electricity of healing power. Faith is the "key." Be it God, Spirit Guides, Guardian Angels, Masters, Higher Self or the Hypnotist, it makes no difference as long as the faith is firm.

ANCIENT HYPNOTHERAPY BECOMING NEW

"Peace Be With You," said the Essenes. Peace within oneself is the goal of complete HAPPINESS. It is the pinnacle of hypnotherapeutic achievement. The old Chinese Sage, Chin Kang said "On Cultivating Life" in the 4th Century A.D.:

"A mind at peace with itself provides a tranquil spirit which calmly guides the body and is the guardian of health and longevity."

Twenty-first Century Hypnotherapy combines Oriental and Occidental Methods.

May peace be with you!

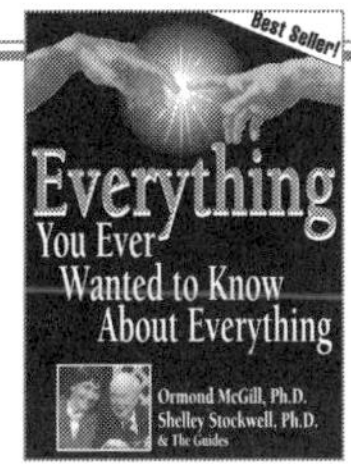

Hypno-Helper
"Everything You Ever Wanted to Know About Everything" book by Ormond McGill and Shelley Stockwell-Nicholas.
"Everything You Ever Wanted to Know About Everything 10 Giant Steps to Superconsciousness" audio tape by Ormond McGill are available at the back of this book.

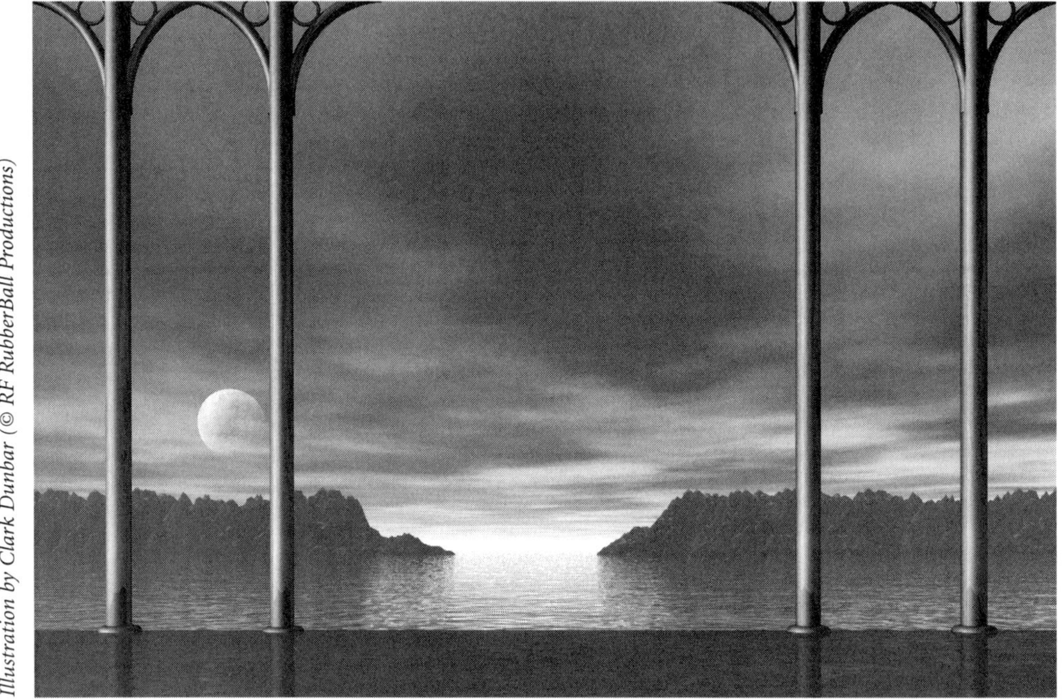

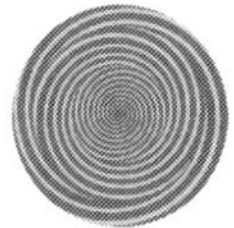

~ *Chapter 203* ~
BODHISATTVA HYPNOTHERAPY: WAKEFULNESS

Bodhisattva in the Buddhist tradition means 'Awakened One." An 'Awakened One is a person who has learned what the world has to teach. They have Mastered life and risen above it and are dying to move on to higher realms of consciousness.

Yet…

The Bodhisattva, out of compassion, tarries for a bit to be of further id to the Planet and to those who live upon the Planet as best can be done. A Bodhisattva is of help to all humankind. As time advances in the Twenty-First Century keep a lookout for more and more clients coming to your office and requesting to achieve Bodhisattvaship.

Bodhisattva Hypnotherapy is transformational hypnotherapy. In numerous cases, it can cause a 100% turnaround of a client's personality from self-centered to universally-centered. You have given it s a gift to your client and as it is expressed, "the more you give to others the more the gifts come back to yourself" or you might say "I tossed my bread upon the waters and it came back as sandwiches."

MODUS OPERANDI: BODHISATTVA HYPNOTHERAPY

You Will Need:
"The Serenity Resonance Sound" or any alpha-theta sound
"Entrancing Music" (See order form at the back of this book)

Have your client take a seat, relax and give their attention to one minute of the Serenity Resonance Sound at high volume. Then hypnotize them by this speedy method; (you may play soft music and the low volume Serenity Resonance Sound (available as "Entrancing Music"). Let the client know what to expect.

"Give me your full attention as you close your eyes and I press here on your forehead. Press your right forefinger firmly in the center of their forehead at the "third eye," **Concentrate towards the pressure of my finger and roll your eyes upward to this place beneath your closed eyelids. You cannot open your eyes no matter how hard you try.**

With eyeballs rolled upward beneath closed eyelids, it is physically impossible to open your eyes. While they struggles to open their eyes shout, **"SLEEP!"** and push his head gently toward his lap. Hypnosis is induced in the instant.

Brush his hands from his lap and let them dangle by his side as you affirm:

"You have expressed desire to advance to Wakefulness or Bodhisattva. Your desire will make it so.

In profound hypnosis now, let these principles of Bodhisattva mastery enter you subconscious and become your very own. Open wide subconscious mind that these seeds of Bodhisattva wisdom become firmly planted. Go silent for a few moments and listen, listen, listen.

The tree of the Spirit Awakening perpetually bears fruit, does not decay and continuously flourishes.

Let that sink in…

A well-intentioned person who thinks, 'I shall eliminate the headache and heartaches of sentient beings bears immeasurable merit. Of such nature is the conscientious one.

Let that sink in…

In brief this spirit of awakening is known to be of two kinds: the spirit of aspiring for Awakening and the spirit of venturing for Awakening.

Let that sink in…

The mind does not find peace, not does it enjoy pleasure and joy, not does it find sleep or fortitude when the thorn of hatred dwells in the heart.

Let that sink in…

Let the Masters, whose minds are fathomless, guide you in escaping from the state of mundane existence. Hold fast to the jewel of the spirit of Awakening.

Let that sink in…

Let the wisdom of the Bodhisattva equally become the wisdom of yourself. Just as the lightening illuminate the darkness of a cloudy night for an instant, in the same way, do you cause your mind to incline toward merit.

Let that sink in…

The Lords of Sages, who have been contemplating for eons, have seen this alone as a blessing by which joy is increased and immeasurable multitudes of beings are revitalized.

Let that sink in…

Let those who wish to overcome miseries and mundane existence, dispel adversities and seek to awaken to joy and never forsake the Spirit of Awakening.

Let that sink in…

Hatred creates suffering. You must persistently overcome it and become happy in this world and in the other. Therefore remove the fuel of any hatred for it has no function other than to harm you.

Let that sink in…

The masters teach their entire systems for the sake of wisdom. Wisdom can be recognized as truth and truth can be recognized as two kinds; 'conventional' and 'ultimate.' Ultimate reality and wisdom is beyond the scope of the intellect and conventional wisdom. Therefore, to ward off suffering, develop ultimate wisdom. Contemplate. Quiet the mind.

Detach and find joy in the world. Your quiet mind sees reality and recognizes what in life is or is not illusion.

When you find fulfillment according to your own wishes you cannot suffer because no one wants to suffer. Stabilize your mind in meditative concentration for a mind distracted lives in the fangs of mental destruction. A mind as yours naturally endowed with Quiescence is stable and finds joy in all things.

Ordinary people may see and imagine things as real and not illusory. Even the perception of form and structure of objects is established by consensus and not by ultimate cognition. You can now rise above such imagining and find the ultimate wisdom.

Let that sink in…

The Masters teach you to bring yourself to ultimate understanding and wisdom by contemplating this idea; you have enough already. Your cup is completely full. Any more and your cup will spill over and you'll be all wet."

The session in Bodhisattva Hypnotherapy is complete. Turn off all sound and let silence enter as it all sinks in. Give them permission to return from hypnosis and return to the here and now.

Collect your fee but make no comment. What further is there to say?

Illustration by Clark Dunbar (© RF RubberBall Productions)

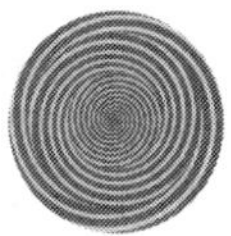

~ *Chapter 204* ~
BODHISATTVA HYPNOTHERAPY
CONTINUED

Includes:
The Bodhisattva Way

Bodhisattva in Buddhist tradition means 'Awakened One" has a new lease on life. In our age of ever advancing technology the Bodhisattva way greatly balances mind with spirit.

Just as the physician of today takes an oath of nobleness so perhaps will the hypnotherapist of the future take this Bodhisattva oath.

MODUS OPERANDI: THE BODHISATTVA WAY
You will need:
"The Serenity Resonance Sound" or "Entrancing Music"

Have your client take a seat, relax and give their attention to one minute of the Serenity Resonance Sound or Entrancing Music at soft volume.

"However you are and wherever you are just relax with closed eyes. Commence to breath in rhythm with your heart beats. Six beats inhale (Pause)

Three beats hold your breath ((Pause)

and six beats, exhale. (Pause)

Good. Continue relaxing while performing this rhythmic breathing.

Let your mind drift and drift and drift to intermesh with the Serenity Resonance Sound and music. Automatically you will drift into hypnosis and your subconscious gates open wide.

All is now ready for further seeds of Bodhisattva wisdom to be planted in the garden of your subconscious mind amid the rain of the gentle music and harmony of serenity.

May all sentient beings be blessed with the Bodhisattva way of life.

Let this sink in…

Through merit, may all those in all directions who are afflicted by suffering obtain oceans of joy and contentment.

Let this sink in…

By the power of my virtue let those whose flesh has fallen off, whose skeletons are the color of white ashes attain celestial bodies and dwell with gods and goddesses.

Let this sink in…

May a rain of lotuses fall mixed with fragrant waters to extinguish any self-imposed hells of pain or fear. So they may be refreshed and liberated with joy, creating heaven on Earth. May the blind see, the deaf hear and any struck with grief find happiness anew. May all have good health and strength.

Let this sink in…

Friend come quickly! Cast away fear. You are alive. By the power of the Bodhisattva ,all adversity is removed as streams of delight flow and your spirit of awakening is born.

Let this sink in…

May the beings of pain rejoice upon the showers of fragrant rains and breezes. Those who are cold find warmth. Let those who are oppressed with heat, be cooled by oceans of spring water.

Let this sink in…

As long as the cycle of existence lasts so will all happiness. The world attains constant joy.

Let this sink in…

All forests become a pleasure grove and the trees all grow as wish fulfilling trees and all ponds a delight of lotuses, doves and swans. And all burning coals become glistening mounds of jewels and the earthly ground a crystal floor and with mountain caverns shrines of spiritual worship. May all regions offer safe passage. And may the battling of nations fight a flower fight with gentle weapons of flowers.

Let this sink in…

As all quarters of the world is delightful with gardens of wish fulfilling flowers as a beautiful world is resplendent with light and color. We the Bodhisattvas sit on all sides of the earth to make it so.

Let this sink in…

Let all rejoice and turn away in disgust from poor ethics to embrace leaning and culture of a pure heart in all directions. Through the grace of the Creator you achieve ordination. You recall all past and future lives and reach the joyous ground.

Let this sink in…

The wisdom of Bodhisattva has now become your very own. When your inner mind knows this is so, come back to me in the here and now. You have become a Master of Bodhisattva. When you return from hypnosis you will have a new zest for life as you aim to make the world the playground it is meant to be.

Awake now as an Awakened one and go forth with a new lease on life. Arouse feeling wonderful and fine."

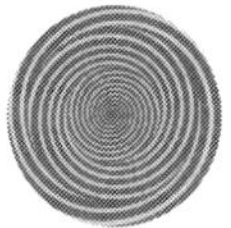

~ *Chapter 205* ~
IN CONCLUSION:
METAMORPHOSIS HYPNOSIS

Now that you know what hypnotherapy is all about this ultimate technique will have a profound meaning.

Metamorphosis is generally best known in relation to butterflies, e.g. the fertilized egg of the female insect hatches to caterpillar form. Following a lot of eating of its food-plant, the caterpillar takes on a chrysalis form, inside of which a miracle occurs. On emerging from the chrysalis, the rather unhandsome caterpillar has become transformed into a beautiful butterfly, which flies away into the sky. The metamorphosis of insects is readily observed. It is and instinctive process and the objective manifestation is clearly visible.

What is not so often appreciated is that all life forms go through the stages of metamorphosis. It is present in humans though the process is so subtle and less objectively observable, but the process is the same.

A male fertilizes the female's egg (yin and yang). After some months of developing as a fetus inside the mother, a baby is born. The baby eats and eats and grows into an adult in a variety of ways. Sometimes becoming fat and sometimes thin; sometimes smart and sometimes stupid, sometimes rich and sometimes poor. THIS IS THE CATERPILLAR STAGE OF A HUMAN BEING.

As years advance the time to enter the chrysalis stage draws near. Entering the chrysalis is to plunge into the unknown. Insects do it instinctively. But humans are more cautious. Many are fearful of plunging into the unknown, which might be dangerous; dangerous to losing themselves with the void, the center of creative change, and they miss their opportunity of transformation (for the current lifetime). They miss their opportunity to obtain their wings as it were.

The hypnotherapy of metamorphosis transforms limited perception to complete perception and limited consciousness to cosmic consciousness. It removes the fear of the plunge into the unknown and consciousness advances in the individual. It is easy to do once the fear of personal transformation and the unknown has been removed.

To know love, you have to have been in love. The experience changes you. The moment you enter love you come out a different person. A discontinuity has happened and you come out a new person. the old person is gone and the new one has come. It is the way of nature. Go for it.

MODUS OPERANDI: THE HYPNOTHERAPY OF METAMORPHOSIS

You will need:
The Serenity Resonance Sound or any other Alpha Theta Resonating Music
(available at the back of this book)
A space or place that lends itself to movement

Hypnotize the client and induce profound hypnosis.
1. Chaotic Breathing
The process of chaotic breathing is performed in silence. Suggest to the subconscious **"You will commence to breathe deeply in any pattern of breathing that seems right for yourself. Let your breathing be anyway it wishes to go. It can even be chaotic. Give the subconscious permission to perform breathing in all and any way it wants to go. You will perform this unregulated breathing for ten minutes and then stop to rest as the human caterpillar will have commenced entering the chrysalis stage."**

2. Rest
As they rest for ten minutes turn on the "Serenity Resonance Sound" in up volume. Instruct, **"Become one with the sound as you enter the chrysalis stage."**

3. The sound continues, **"Now let your body become relaxed and flexible. Release it from all restraints. Just allow your body to move and express itself in any way it wishes; in complete freedom with itself.**

You can laugh, weep, yell or jump. Allow it to become wild and crazy in its behavior. As the body releases repression, its limitation, so equally does the mind. Your body and mind react together. You may want to stand up and dance. You may even want to whirl around and around until you become completely dizzy. Body drops away from all limitations of behavior as you allow complete freedom for your body and mind to be all they are."

As the sound drones on, your client performs such freedom antics! It is a total letting go for ten minutes when you suddenly turn the sound off.

4. Plunge into the Void
"The subconscious mind takes you now within your chrysalis and when deep inside plunges you into the silence of the VOID. Silence reigns and even unconsciousness may come and all the while the creative energy of the void pervades you. Metamorphosis is occurring. From out of the old form a new being is emerging. Body becomes stronger, mind more sharp and keen. Mind is expanding and consciousness, your awareness of what is, expands along with it.. Even your perception is changing. The activity of mind is becoming under voluntary control and becoming like pure crystal, reflecting equally without distortion the perception the perceiver and the perceived. Your mind becomes a MASTERMIND through which your consciousness is known.

Just relax and sleep, if you wish with the silence of the VOID. A miracle of transformation is occurring within the chrysalis of yourself as you bask in this silence."

For ten minutes allow your client to remain in silence, then turn the "Serenity Resonance Sound" on again; softly at first and then slowly rising.

5. Hypnotherapist to client, **"Slowly, ever so slowly you will come out of the void to arouse and resume your daily life. Take your time there is no hurry. Subconscious mind you are the full director of when this special divine one returns to the universe with full realization of all they are. Gradually, gradually now arise when the metamorphosis is complete."**

Gradually your client will arouse from the hypnosis. A marvelous transformation has occurred. Before the person was a caterpillar living and viewing life upon a horizontal plane. Now, upon bursting forth from the chrysalis they have become as a butterfly...radiant and beautifully free with a mind soaring into sky.

His entire metamorphosis hypnotherapy process has taken but 30 minutes. You have given your client quite a gift in those thirty minutes! Can you use the process for yourself? Who is there to say you can't? Can you spare 30 minutes?

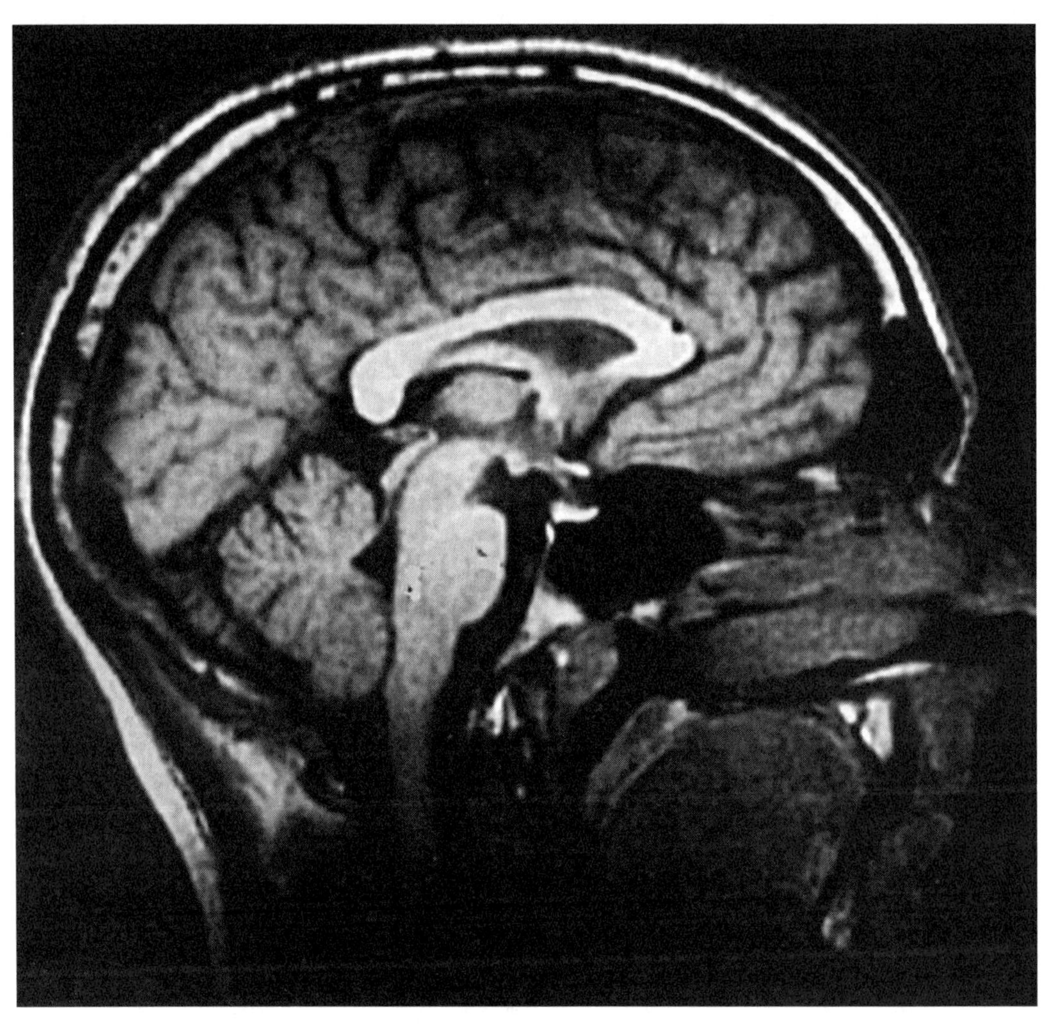

CAT scan of Jim's brain

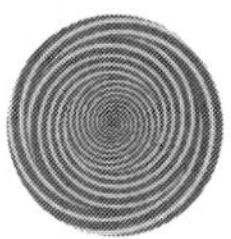

~ *Chapter 206* ~
EPILOGUE:
YOUR MIND POTENTIAL
IS VAST AND AWESOME

Question: *What do you call someone who seeks Hypnotherapy help?*
Answer: *Doctors call them patients. Hypnotists call them clients. Why not just call them by what they like best, THEIR FIRST NAME.*

In 1895, Thomas Jay Hudson wrote a wonderfully logical book, "The Law of Psychic Phenomena." He explained that mind functions on two distinctly separate levels:

1. Conscious thought (objective mind) designed for inductive reasoning, and
2. Subconscious thought (subjective mind) designed for deductive reasoning.

Hudson said that hypnosis is the "medium that moves us from one compartment of mind to another." His presentation was so convincing that many remain devoted to his concept.

In the mid-twentieth century, Dave Elman defined the conscious mind as the "critical" and limited mind activity and the subconscious as the non-critical, accepting, mind mode. Elman said that the critical mind limits the non-critical mind. He said it brilliantly, *"Hypnosis consists of bypassing critical mind and establishing selective thinking."*

This book advances the idea that your mind is not divided in two parts, but functions as a whole. Mind is a process of producing thoughts, which program the brain. Mind is an immortal continuum that belongs to the individual's consciousness, the SELF.

The brain is not immortal, as it belongs to the body. The brain does not originate thoughts. It is an organic computer that activates thoughts in accordance with how it has been programmed.

Through conscious purpose, hypnosis is induced. Through conscious purpose "suggestion formulas" are created. Conscious action of mind makes it possible to bypass critical mind and establish selective subconscious thinking.

Hypnosis then provides a way to program your mind to function through the Autonomic Nervous System with its Sympathetic and Parasympathetic divisions. The Parasympathetic nervous system unlimitedly accepts ideas.

Hypnosis moves you from an accepted "normal," conscious or objective state of mind into an "altered" subconscious or subjective mind-state. In hypnosis, mind becomes hyper-suggestible, to suggestion that directly modifies behavior. Its scope is omnipotent. It is the realm of miracles.

The methods and techniques in this book adhere to this premise.

Ormond McGill, PhD, Palo Alto, California

811

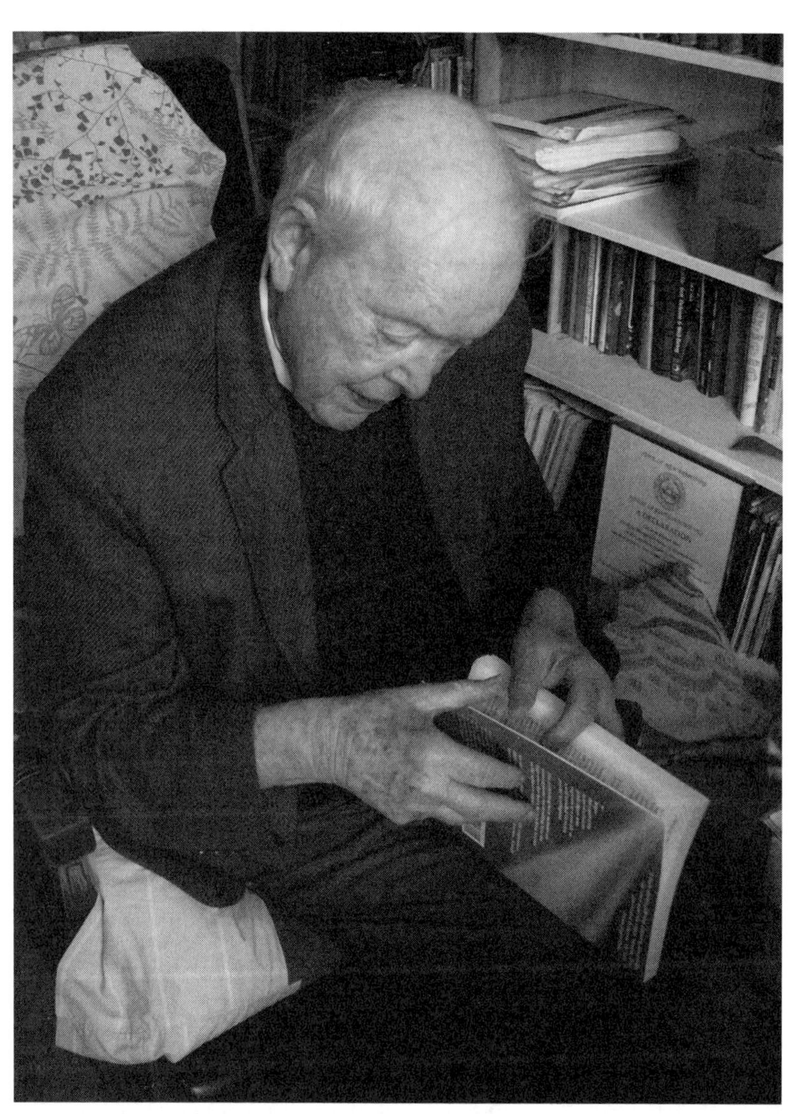

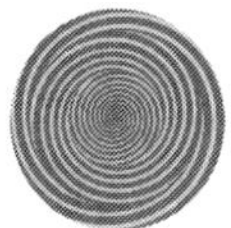

~ *Chapter 207* ~
ABOUT ORMOND MCGILL

I was born in Palo Alto, California on June 15th, 1913 to my mother Julia (Battele) and Harry McGill.

When I was 15, I presented my first full evening magic show at "Paly" High and recited my Tarbell mail order Magic Course patter word for word as though it was a sacred text. That wasn't what Tarbell would have recommended. He himself emphasized the importance of being natural and yourself. This is good advice for Professional Hypnotherapists as well. Develop your own original style and you will be an outstanding Hypnotherapist.

Hypnotism came into my life while still in high school when the Danish Hypnotist, DeWaldoza, came to town to perform a "demonstration of suggestion" at the Masonic Lodge. DeWaldoza invited up two Stanford students as volunteers. One blindfolded him and the other was told to take an object from his pocket (it was a comb) and hide it with any person in the audience. The hypnotist, still blindfolded, used "contact mind-reading" and instructed the student who had hidden the object to "not lead him but simply concentrate on where the object was concealed." Then gripping the student's hand, he immediately found the comb. I volunteered to try the procedure and I too succeeded. The process was a result of "muscle reading" DeWaldoza said.

Next he presented demonstrations in what he called "waking suggestion." He had everyone lock their hands together and invited those whose hands were locked tightly to come up and sit on the stage where they performed a most delightful "show of suggestion." I went home and immediately sent in ten cents to Johnson, Smith & Company for a little book on hypnotism and faithfully followed the instructions.

After two years of college at San Jose State College, majoring in psychology, my term paper on hypnotism was given in my psychology professor's upper classes and I went on the road with Mandu the Magician and took correspondence courses in commercial art and advertising. I eventually went back to college to study art and advertising and co-authored the book "Advertising for the Independent Business Man."

On September 29, 1943, after going together for 4 years, I married my sweetheart, Delight Beth Olmstead. We chose the path of the theater business with hypnotism as an integral part of the performances I presented under the name Dr. Zomb in theaters in the United States and Canada. I found I had a liking for sensational publicity stunts and performed many nutty things like escaping Houdini style, being buried alive, driving blindfolded or catching bullets in my teeth.

I appeared on Art Linkletter's "People are Funny" radio show in 1944 and later on the television version. I also became the technical advisor for the movie "The Hypnotic Eye."

You can learn so much from books. I have enjoyed writing books. In 1944 I wrote "How To Produce Miracles" and in 1947, I wrote the "Encyclopedia of Genuine Stage Hypnotism" that was published and republished in 5 consequent editions by Percy Abbott and more recently in

7 editions by Crown House Publishing and in 1953, I did two works on hypnotism "A Better Life Through Conscious Self-Hypnosis" and "Dental Hypnosis" for Dr. Rexford North's Journal of Hypnotism Company. Thirty-eight other books followed. One week after my wife Delight passed onwards in 1976, she began offering insights as to the nature of death while I lay in bed. After four days I wrote what was being given to me. In three weeks "The Book Of Delight" (published as "Grieve No More Beloved") was completely written.

I have the pleasure of channeling a spirit guide Patanjali, the Father of Yoga, who lived in Northern India around 319 B.C. and have learned from his sutras and processes to use the mind to advance consciousness from normal perception to super-consciousness. In Patangali's words, "Yoga is the cessation of mind. Through yoga the witness is established in itself. In other states there is identification with the modifications of the mind. You bring your mind to a stop by not trying to control it in anyway." The chapters on hypnosis and yoga will help you to master this master's ideas.

I am soon to turn ninety-one and I suppose that makes me an old man but honestly I don't feel old at all. I don't feel a bit different inside myself than I did at thirty-nine. I feel just fine. I can just be myself and it's great.

In this Hypnotherapy Encyclopedia I have shared things that have been created by me and things that have come to me as gifts I have treasured. May they have value to your practice of hypnotherapy and your life.

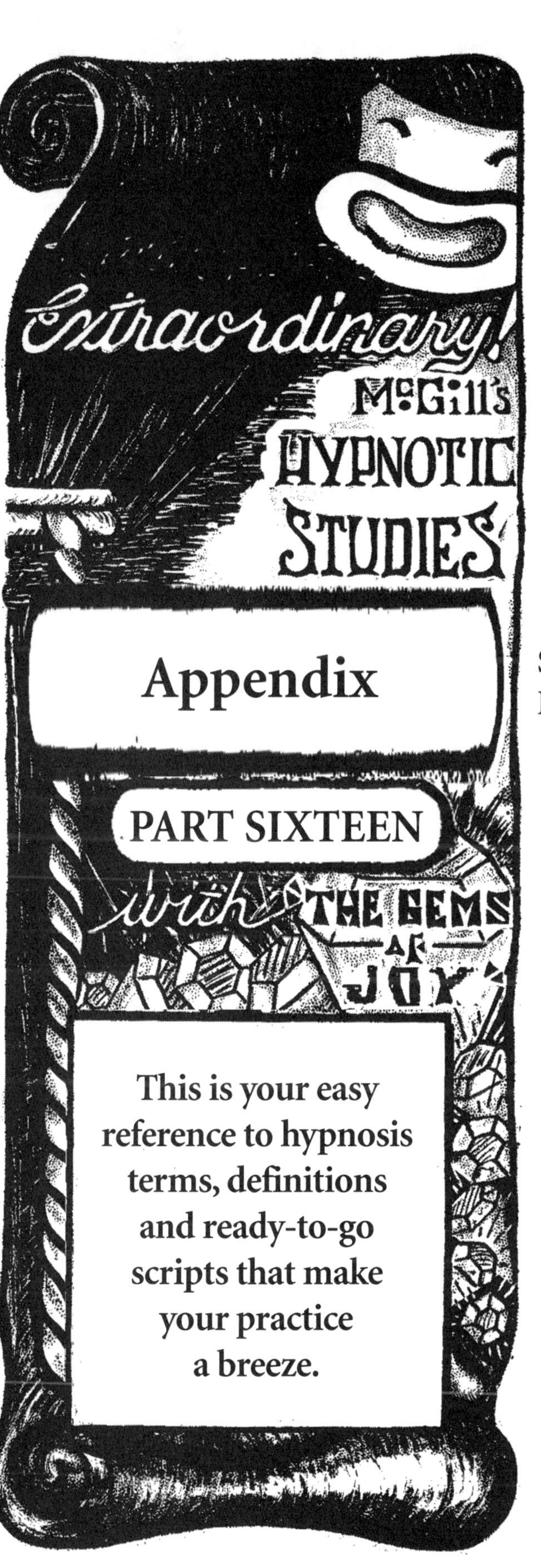

Appendix

PART SIXTEEN

This is your easy
reference to hypnosis
terms, definitions
and ready-to-go
scripts that make
your practice
a breeze.

SECTIONS IN
PART SIXTEEN

I.   DEFINITION/INDEX..................page 819

II. 347 SCRIPTS BY SUBJECT..................831

III. 153 INDUCTION SCRIPTS
     BY CHAPTER...835

IV. RESOURCES:
     BOOKS, TAPES, FORMS......................837

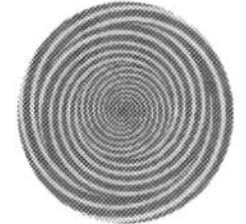

PART I: DEFINITION/INDEX

by Shelley Stockwell-Nicholas, PhD

*"Let your thoughts become positive because they become your actions.
Let your actions be positive because they become your destiny."*
—Mahatma Ghandi

~ Check Part II and III Indexes for more listings ~

A

Aarons, Harry: Founded the oldest hypnosis organization in operation; the American Association of Ethical Hypnotists, and Power Publishing that published numerous books on hypnosis.

Abdominal Brain or Emotional Brain: Also called the gate of the soul or the core chakra; the solar plexus of the body containing a large neural concentration. Pgs 421, 429, 430, 517, 518, 532, 670

Abreaction: The release or outward expression of emotions. Pg 307

Accidental Hypnosis: Spontaneous revival of a suggestion originally taken on when one bypassed objective thinking during times of heightened emotion or learning like infancy, childhood, or during trauma or illness. A similar situation later in life activates the original emotion, thoughts and actions.

Acupressure-Hypnosis: Chpt 127

Ackerman, Charlene: Acclaimed Director of The Hypnotherapy and Wellness Center in Wisconsin who teaches hypnosis in Taiwan. Pg 587

ADD (Attention Deficit Disorder) & ADHD (Attention Deficit Hyperactivity Disorder): Chpt 151

Addiction: Ongoing path-illogical compulsive relationship with mood altering substance or behavior where need often grows in tandem with the tolerance for it. Chpt 142. See Part II Index of Scripts by Subject.

Addiction Counseling Hypnosis: Hypnosis employed to overcome addiction.

Affect Bridge: Hypnotic process of connecting an original event and feelings to feelings in the present; also called a past anchor or memory chain. Pg 621

Age Progression: The hypnotic process to access the future; or advancing someone to a future time. Pgs 816, 824

Age Regression: Hypnotic process of reliving or revivifying past experiences of this lifetime, past lifetimes and between lifetimes. Subjects who explore current life times often "re-member" their own conception, womb and birth experience. Many report memory before conception. Where were you before you were born? Pgs 554, 583, 585, 587, 627, 629, 664 Chapters 159, 162, 163

Allegory: A parable subconsciously or consciously understood to symbolically represent deeper personal meaning.

Altered State: Mental gear shifting from conscious awareness to the trance states. Georgia.

Amnesia: A loss of memory or interruption of memory continuity. These are signposts of somnambulism. Pgs 11, 12, 16, 17, 33, 34, 79-81, 84, 111, 119, 214, 626, 721

Anchoring: A stimuli (like facial expressions, gestures, sounds, words, smell or taste) that trigger or elicit a subsequent desired response. Used effectively in pain management and Joy Therapy®. Pgs 201, 203, 338, 341, 365, 543

Anesthesia: See conscious sedation.

Animal Hypnosis: A bunny or frog on its back lies silent and doesn't move. Placing a chicken on their stomach and stretching their legs out behind them with their beak placed on a chalk line stills them. Sharks can be "hypnotized" by stroking their sides. A lobster is pacified by setting him upright on his tail. Pgs 60, 61

Animal Magnetism: The hypnotic balancing of the human energy field to override illness; principles advanced by Franz Mesmer. See Mesmer.

Anti-Aging Hypnosis: Chpt 116

Anxiety: Fearful feelings, thoughts and physical reactions that linger long after an actual threat has passed. Pgs 58, 60, 134, 266, 532, 545, 546, 553, 554, 568, 706, 757, 763

Archetypes: An original pattern by which all things of the same type are represented; human essence characterized as a symbolic "type." Carl Jung popularized seven major prime examples including the "wise person," "animus" (male), "anima" (female), and "shadow". The ancient Pantheons of the gods identified them with our now popular astrological signs as "Mars" (male), "Venus" (female), "Cronos" (father), "Gaea" (mother). "Vulcan" (financial wizard), "Pluto" (sexual), "Mercury" (mental), "Zeus" (spiritual), "Apollo" (child), "Uranus" (friendship), "Vesta" (perfectionist) and "Neptune" (mystic). Superman and Wonder Woman are more modern archetypes. Pg 307

Aromatherapy Hypnosis: Using distilled plant essences (phytochemicals) to enhance hypnosis, shift mood states, dispel hunger, bring more energy, abate discomfort and/or access past memory. Rene-Maurice Gattefosse coined the term "aromatherapy" in 1937.

Artificial Somnambulism: Marquis de Puysegur (1781-1825) expanded on Mesmer's approach by inducing the trance state while communing with trees.

Assertive Behavior Hypnotherapy or Self Expression Training: Hypnosis to enhance self-expression of opinions and emotions. Uses modeling, rehearsal, practice, systematic feedback and coaching, while reducing anxiety and educating the client of their human rights.

Astral Plane and Astral Projection: The realm of dreams and consciousness that bridges matter and spirit. A flight of fancy fueled by higher consciousness. Pg 782, Chpt 197

Auto-Conditioning, Auto-Hypnosis & Auto-Suggestion: See self-hypnosis.

Autonomic Nervous System: The peripheral nervous system that regulates involuntary responses.

Autophone or Audio Phone: This mechanical device consists of a pair of earphones, microphone and a small low wattage electrical voice amplifier used to offer self suggestions over a microphone to. Pgs 302, 341

Aversion Therapy: A hypnotically suggested negative response to hurtful behavior. Pgs. 26, 237, 242, 341

Avoidance: Evading resolution of undesirable situations instead of dealing with them directly; characterized by procrastination, denial, withdrawal, silent desperation, inaction like the inability to RSVP.

B

Behavior Hypnotherapy: Hypnotically exposing a client to that which causes them anxiety. It "turns the switch on higher" so that it can then be turned off.

Behavior-Modification Hypnosis: Hypnosis shifts negative behavior and attitudes into positive ones to heal underlying emotional stress. Millions release limiting behaviors, like overeating and smoking, by hypnotically readjusting behavior patterns imprinted in the subconscious mind. Hypnosis de-hypnotizes or de-programs painful past patterns and imprints. This holistic tool helps you rise above difficult times so you create new procedures to cope, clear and get back on track.

Bakas, Norbert: Director of the Bakas Hypnosis Center in Pennsylvania. Pg 546, Chpt 145

Bale, Dwight: Chpt 40

Berg, Carl Joseph: Chpts 136, 191

Bernheim, Hippolyte (1823-1904): Founder with Leibeault of Nancy Hypnotic School. Pgs xx, 151, 469

Biofeedback: Creating aware perception of unconscious responses (like heartbeat, brain waves or galvanic skin response) so that they can be consciously controlled. One handheld biofeedback device called the GSR2, sounds a tone into earphones. Others sound a tone with changes. Skin "resistance" determines if you are "agitated." Scientologists "clear people" using a version of this device that they call the "cans" because it resembles a tin can. Lie detector tests works on this same principle.

Biology of Emotions: Chpt 139

Bio-Magnetics and Magnetism: Pgs 72, 560 Chpts 126-133, 135, 196

Blum, Peter: Director of The Hypnosis Institute in Woodstock, NY. Chpt 44, Pg 358

BMIR's: Biological Manifestation of Internal Response or how a person responds to a verbal stimuli. An overpriced car. Pg 348

Body Psychotherapies: Emotions accessed through the body. From Hippocrates in the 4th century BC to modern times, bodywork offers hands-on or non-touch services applied to fixed or moveable systems to stimulate energy, flexibility, integration, wellness & relaxation. Acupressure, Adjustment Therapy, Aromatherapy, Awareness Training, Bio-Energetics, Breathwork, Chelation, Chakra Clearing, Channeling, Ch'iryo, Clinical Massage Therapy, Cranial-Sacral, Dowsing, Emotional Freedom Technique (EFT), Energy Healing, Energy Balancing, Energy Medicine, Feldenkrais, Healing Touch, Hydrotherapy, Jinshin Jyutsu, Kinesiology, Lymphatic Therapy, Massage Therapy, Magnetic Therapy, Meridian Therapy, Movement Therapy, Prana, Qi Gong, Radix, Reflexology, Reiki, Relaxation Therapy, Rolfing, Shiatsu, Structural Healing, Swedish Massage, Tai Chi, Therapeutic Touch, Vibrational Medicine, Voice Toning, Water-Birthing & Yoga are modern bodywork treatments.

Braid, James (1795-1860): Named "nervous sleep" "hypnotism" after the Greek word "hypnos" for the "god of sleep" and called the reawakened state "dehypnotizing." Others called it "Braidism." Pgs 1, 468, 469

Braid Induction Technique: Inducting trance by fixing the gaze upon a bright object.

Brainwave Entrainment: Induces trance by using the brains natural tendency to rhythmically model and synchronize with sound. See Serenity Resonance.

Brainwave Synchronizer: A photoelectric machine that uses a strobe light and through varying frequencies is said to entrain the brain into trance. Another version, called Integral Stimulating Intensity Stroboscope (ISIS), uses enlarged strobe light goggles. Potentially risky for seizure prone folks. Pg 512

Bruxism-Hypnosis: Hypnosis to stop the habit of unconscious tooth grinding or templer mandibular joint dysfunction (or TMJ).

B-Values: Abraham Maslow said that to be our best we need truth, goodness, beauty, unity, transcendence, aliveness, uniqueness, perfection, justice, order and simplicity.

C

Catalepsy: Intense hypnotic focus resulting in muscular or limb rigidity without muscles flexing. Arms or legs moved by into different positions remain in that position for indefinite time frames. Subjects "suspended" (neck on one chair back, heel on another chair back) between two chairs enjoy complete comfort and ease. Pgs 12, 13, 26, 151

Catatonic Trance: The body is so relaxed that the subject doesn't move a muscle. In this state there is complete anesthesia to pain. Pg 83

Catharsis: Cleaning away or releasing strong emotion. Pgs 10, 297, 470, 497

Causation: Factors and conditions from which behavior springs.

Cell Demand: Strong hypnotic commands focused upon the cellular level to restore wellness. Various systems talk to the healing intelligence of cells and body systems. Ed Martin calls his approach "Cell Command®".

Charcot, Jean Martin (1825 to 1893): Started the Salpetriere Hospital of Hypnotism, the largest hospital in Paris. Pg 469

Child Birth Hypnosis or Midwifery Hypnosis: Hypnosis conditioning used to assist birthing mothers, couches, doulas and medical personnel with a stress-free pre-natal, birth and post-natal experience. Hypnosis shortens labor, eliminates pain. Studies show that some 56% fewer cesareans are needed for mom's trained in hypnosis. Chpts 48, 49, Pgs 89, 161, 199, 352, 363, 435, 467

Children, Hypnosis For: Chapter 41, Pg 150

Chunking: Chunking up, meta-tag or divergent thinking is a hypnotic process to perceive the "big picture." Chunking down or convergent thinking is focusing to minute details. Pgs 338, 340, 341

Churchill, Randal: Author and teacher. Pg 351

Circle Hypnotherapy: Repeatedly feeling and building anxiety and then letting it go with more and more amusement and relaxation until the angst is gone.

Clinical Hypnosis: The hypnotist/client discipline of altered states of consciousness or trance coupled with conversation and verbal and non-verbal suggestion.

Co-Dependency: The control games of victim, rescuer or persecutor. Finishing someone else's sentences. Pgs 236, 256, 273, 402

Cognitive Hypnotherapy or Conscious Awareness Hypnotherapy: A conscious/subconscious hypnotherapeutic system using subconscious programming and aware choice for behavioral change. Shelley Stockwell, PhD, coined the name. Chpt 110

Collective Unconscious: Forces beyond our personal unconscious created by collective energies of all living beings. A term coined by Jung.

Color Therapy: The use of color for deepening, programming, healing and as a post hypnotic anchor. Pgs 67, 96, 106, 293, 509, 555, 556, 560, 611, 617, 675, Chpts 61, 188, 189

Coma State: State of deep self-centeredness characterized by catatonia. Pgs 13, 81, Chpt 20

Compartmentalization: Separating and categorizing thoughts, feelings and beliefs in order to deal with one thing at a time.

Complementary Health Care: A parallel modality for wellness; hypnotherapy is considered a legal alternative/complementary treatment.

Compounding or The Law Of Compounding: Repetitive, sustained suggestions that revert back to an initial suggestion. Used in hypno-therapeutic sessions to penetrate and seal a suggestion. Dr Bernheim revealed this powerful mental law in the 1800's and Dave Elman re-discovered it around 1934 and taught it in his classes. Chpt 57, Pgs 91, 100, 159, 156

Computer Hypnotherapy: The hypnotic approach created by Ormond McGill that correlates technology with your mental "biocomputer." Chpts 92 and 94

Conditioned Response or Conditioned Reflex: An automatic reflexive reaction to a stimulus. Pg 255

Conditioning: Ideas given during hypnosis that makes responses and future hypnosis easier; training one to think or behave a certain way.

Conference Room Technique: Hypnotic suggests that sub-personalities come together to collectively agree on a desired outcome.

Confusion Technique: Bombarding suggestions and instructions used to induce trance.

Congruity: Matching verbal and nonverbal communication. Incongruity has conflicting messages, "Your lips tell me 'no, no' but there is 'yes, yes' in your eyes."

Conscious Recall: Memory

Conscious Mind: Earth and Body Self, Room Awareness. The conscious mind makes decisions based upon information it receives from the sub and super-conscious mind and it impresses the subconscious with its sensory observations.

Conscious Sedation or Non-Pharmacological Analgesia or Hypno-Anesthesia: Hypnotically induced anesthesia without the use of chemicals. Chpts 140, 143-147, Pgs 17, 150, 468, 495, 473, 569, 751. See Index II: Pain & Healing

Consensus Trance: Cultural conditioned responses that are hypnotically transmitted from elders, peers, the media and/or the environment.

Constipation, Treating: Pg 536

Convincers: Perceptual tests that 'prove' to the subject that they are "hypnotizable." An example would be, "roll your eyes up into your head. Now try to open them. They just don't want to open. This is the feeling of hypnosis and you go deeper." See Suggestibility.

COPHO (Cooperative Organization of Professional Hypnosis Organizations): Pgs 48, 49

Core Belief: Basic underlying imprint, or hypnotic program, you subconsciously hold to be true about yourself. Core beliefs are buttressed by conscious thoughts and rationalizations. Hypnotherapy can re-script a limiting or destructive belief and enforce an enhancing one.

Coue, Emil: French Clinician who coined the phrase "Every day in every way, I am getting better and better. Chpt 114, Pgs xx, 15

Counter Regression: Returning from a regression to the here and now.

Counseling: Helpers and healers who use conversation, behavior modification and advice to co-create a personal wellness plan.

Counselors and Therapists: Art Therapists, Addiction Counselors, Coaches, Grief Therapists, Dance Therapists, Drug & Alcohol Abuse Counselors, Hypno-Counselors, Hypnotherapists, Pastoral Counselors, Music Therapists, Play & Humor Therapists & Primal Therapists, Rebirthing. See Hypnotherapist titles and specialties.

Creative Arts Hypnosis and Creative Hypo-Coaching: Harnesses the creative genius within. Eliminates limiting mindsets like writer's block and stage fright. Gives actors, dancers, comics, musicians, artists, writers and speakers the winning edge. Hypnosis makes memorizing scripts: auditions, performances and staying centered, easy. Creativity coaching gifts a unique opportunity to transcend linear time and conscious limits to master creativity. Hypnosis spontaneously opens the door to all creative expression invention, problem solving and fun.

D
Death: Chpts 117, 150, Pgs 46, 135, 176, 400, 441,532, 610, 617, 438-439, 677-678, 607, 706, 716, 721, 755, 794

Deepening Techniques: Techniques that intensify the hypnotic experience like "You go deeper with each breath and each beat of your heart" and, "As I count down from 1-5, you go deeper." Pgs 24, 25, 27, 95, 118, 119, 121, 165, 176, 180, 201, 449

Defense Mechanism
A behavior or belief used to conceal a truth from yourself or others; "de fence" obscures "de truth."

De-Hypnotizing: Bringing someone from the hypnotic state to the waking state; the process of removing a hypnotic suggestion.

Demonstrational Hypnotism: Educational and entertaining public hypnosis presentations. Pgs 157, 158

Dental Hypnosis: See Hypnodontics

Depression: Pg 332

Deprogramming: De-hypnotizing breaks the hypnotic seals of hurtful and destructive imprints. It is often used for surviving prisoners of war and others who have been brain washed by stress, circumstances or radical belief systems. Patti Hurst was deprogrammed after her stressful abduction. As a cure for the common cult, de-hypnotizing is a powerful and effective tool to break free from the dogma of Moonies, Jim Jones, Heaven's Gate or the like. Break a seal by hearing the voice of the person who offered the original seal and then hear them modifying the words so that it no longer applies.

de Puysegur, Marquis: See artificial somnambulism.

Desensitization: Systematically taking the physical or emotional energy from an issue like fear or hurt.

Devers, Dewie: In 1951, Dewey Devers and Peggy O'Neil renamed the 1943 "Hypnotism Society of Pittsburgh" the "Hypnosis Society of Pennsylvania" and received a state charter.

Dianetics: A philosophy/religious cult founded by L Ron Hubbard that uses "emotional clearing" and other hypnotic principles. Denies using hypnosis.

Dichotomous Thinking: "Of two minds" that widely differ or contradict each other. Also to categorize things in black and white, all or nothing, terms.

Direct Hypnosis: Implanting beneficial suggestions directly into the conscious, critical mind, which, in turn, imprints them into the subconscious, activating the universal mind: also called waking hypnosis. Pg 35

Disassociation: To detach or deny a connection to a particular train of thought, person or thing. Pgs 5, 209

Disclosure Forms: Pg 52

Disguised or Veiled Suggestion: Hypnotic suggestions imbedded in seemingly regular conversation.

Distortion: Inaccurate internal representation that limits one's life.

Double Bind: An Ericksonian statement like "You may either raise a hand or move your 'yes' finger when all parts attain inner harmony or integration." Pg 311

Dowsing or Devining Rods: Pgs 470, 471

Dream: Pg 34

Dual or Double Induction: Two or more voices used to induce trance. An easy and fun technique to use, the voices are often recorded to play in headphones; one voice in one ear and one voice in the other ear.

Durban, Paul: Director of Hypnotherapy at Pendleton Memorial Methodist Hospital, Louisiana. Pg 58

E

Ecstasy: Rapturous emotional excitement.

Educational Hypnosis: Motivates students for power learning, concentration and easy test taking. Hypnosis helps you think about knowing and know about thinking. Highlighting hypnotically allows you to vividly think, focus, absorb and re-member what you learn and perceive. See Oligodengroglia. Chpts 66, 68 , Pgs 48, 169, 579, 580, 581

Earache, Treating: Pg 535. See Index Part II Pain & Healing.

Effect: A condition that results from hypnosis.

Effleurage (Fr.) or Light Massage Induction: Place your hand on the client's forehead exerting gentle pressure. Then ease and bring your hand lightly down the face, barely grazing the skin. Say "As I glide my hand gently over your face, you glide gently into hypnosis."

Egyptian Hypnosis, Ancient: Pg 467

Eidetic Imagery or a Photographic Mind: Remembering a visual image from only brief observation. Pgs 328, 518

Electroencephalograph (ECT): An apparatus that detects brain waves.

Elman, Dave: His hypnosis techniques used rapid methods to bypass the critical mind, establish selective thinking and produce profound hypnosis (somnambulism). He modernized hypnosis by training doctors and dentists. Chpts 20, 38, Pgs 19-21, 80, 121, 124, 211, 221, 417, 486, 532, 629, 668, 792, 807

Ellner, Michael: NYC Hypnotherapist who specializes in helping those with AIDS. Chpt 121

Embedded Suggestion: Words and phrases purposely inserted into regular conversation or during hypnosis (usually during the induction).

EMH (Eye Movement Hypnosis) : A term coined by Hypnotherapist, Shelley Stockwell-Nicholas, PhD. where the hypnotized client is instructed open their eyes, recount a problem or trauma while following guided eye-movements. Similar to EMDR (eye movement desensitization and reprogramming).

Emotional Blind Spot: A place in your consciousness that will not or does not perceive what is.

Emotional Clearing: Letting go of emotional energy attached to hurtful thoughts.

Emotional Freedom Technique (EFT): A technique using physical "tapping" on acupressure points combined with verbal suggestion used as behavior modification. Also called "thought field hypnotherapy." Chpt 134

Emotional Discharge: Emotional release to relieve inner-pressure attached to continuing a limiting behavior or attitude.

Endorphin Release Hypnosis: Hypnotic suggestions for the body to release feel good, pain-reducing bio-chemicals.

England, Diana L.: Chpt 41, 46, 165

Enneagram: A categorical system based on nine personality styles.

Erickson, Milton: Chpt 105, Pgs 218, 219, 311, 445, 461, 793

Ericksonian Hypnosis: A hypnotic art form created by psychiatrist and M.D. Milton H. Erickson. Uses indirect inductions, suggestions and metaphor so the subject will come their own conclusions and attach their own meaning to the words spoken by the hypnotist; a measured indirect approach. Pg 2 See Milton Erickson.

Esdaile, James (1808-1859): The English surgeon, who pre-anesthesia, combined mesmerism with surgery. He performed pain-free hypnosis in India in 1845 reducing surgery mortality rate from 50% to only 8%. He also observed that his patients recovered more rapidly. Chpt 140, Pgs 83, 468, 473, 486

ESP or Extra Sensory Perception: See psychic development.

Etheric Plane State: Rising above mortal awareness to a higher state.

Eustress
Positive stress.

Expectation: The belief and anticipation of the positive hypnotic result.

Eye-Movement Desensitization And Reprocessing (EMDR): This system uses patterned eye movement to change emotional actions and reactions. The client thinks or speaks a problem as they move their eyes in varying or opposite patterns to create new neural responses.

F
False Memory Syndrome or Pseudo-Memory or Misinformation Effect: All memory is a reconstructive process that may or may not contain inaccuracies. Combining actual memories with repetitive suggestions and social pressure from others can cause some to forget the source and remember only the content of information. A hypnotist must ask open-ended questions and not create constructed untruths with leading questions.

Fascination Point: An object upon which the subject fixes their gaze to evoke trance.

Fixed Gaze: An intense and unexpected sound, light or darkness to evoke trance.

Fascination Techniques: Hypnotic techniques that absorb and hold the imagination. Pgs 47, 71, 174

Fear: See phobia releasement.

Fiore, Edith: Author of "You Have Been Here Before." Chpt 163

Flaccidity: A relaxed absence of muscle tone seen in a hypnotized person.

Force, The: Cosmic energy that comes into you from the universe. Pgs xxv, 608, 611

Forensic or Investigative Hypnosis: Hypnosis used for over a 100 years for investigative, legal and court proceedings. Helps victims and witnesses recall details of a crime. In the Chowchilla kidnapping case, hypnosis helped the driver recall a "forgotten" license plate number. Also used to help those on trial not get rattled and answer questions honestly. Pg 57

Fractional Relaxation: Repetitive, monotonous, long and drawn out techniques that bores conscious awareness to induce trance. For example; "The big toe on your left foot is relaxing,…99…and that relaxation now moves to the second toe on your left foot…98…"

Frankl, Viktor: 20th Century Nobel Peace Prize winner who, while captive in Auschwitz, underscored his logo therapy theory that a person has free will to be happy in every situation.

Free Association: A Freudian technique that has the client say everything that comes into his mind. The idea is to bring subconscious information into conscious awareness. Free association is often used while the client is in trance. Pg 470

Freud, Sigmund (1856-1939): Famous doctor who gave up hypnosis to use his newly named "psychoanalysis" and "free association" and dream analysis." His "Id, Ego and Super-Ego Theory" says you were born with a leering libido "Id" trying to get its way, developed "Ego" to modulate it and somewhere around six a judgmental "Superego" to morally puppet your upbringing. Pgs 307, 469, 470, 486

Freudian Slip: One that comes off easily. Words that reflect unconscious thoughts.

G

Gamma Range Hypnosis: Utilizes the heightened brain frequencies of 41– 100 Hz. Chpt 49, Pg 154

Gestalt Therapy: An integrative sub-self dialog approach based on the work of Fritz Perls. The client may act out scenes from dreams or life taking on the roles of each human, inanimate object and sub-personality with the idea of cooperation. Pgs 306, 351, 392

Glove Anesthesia: A hypnotic technique that numbs parts of the body to diffuse discomfort and pain. The suggestion is given that "your hand is numb and that numbness is transferred to any place your hand touches." Chpt 144, Pgs 548, 549, 568. See anesthesia. See Index II Pain & Healing.

Goal Oriented Hypnosis: The powerful motivation of positive thinking lets you manifest abundance on all levels: money,

love, peace and joy. Here you employ your natural resources and creativity and real-eyes dreams.

Greatrakes, Valentine: Known as the "stroking doctor" he used laying on of hands and massage for altered state and healing. See Effleurage.

Guided Imagery: A directed journey employing inner vision.

H

Habit Control Hypnosis: Hypnosis techniques that change repetitious unwanted patterns. See Specific Habit.

Hallucination: Sensing something that is not physically there; a sensory illusion.

Hammer, Joe: Marketing expert who created the "Stealth Marketing" Program Pgs 59, 60

Heart Conditions, Treating: Pg 536, Chpt 108

Hermetic Tradition: Teaching and writings attributed to Hermes Trismegisyus, a legendary author of magical, astrological and alchemical doctrines.

Hetero-Hypnosis: One person hypnotized by another as opposed to self-hypnosis.

Hierarchy Of Needs: Abraham Maslow's theory that we ascend from security needs, to ego needs in order to become fully healthy, functional and self-actualized.

Holder, Phillip: Chairman, International Counsel of Hypnotherapists, Counselors & Holistic Practitioners. Chpt 73

Holotropic Breathwork: Popularized by Stan Grof, PhD, this sustained deep breathing to proactive music and sounds evokes altered states and overloads the senses. Chpt 170

Horton, William: Founder, the Nat. Federation of NLP & author of "Primary Objective, Neuro Linguistic Psychology & Guerrilla Warfare" Chpt 97, Pg 345

Hunter, Roy: Author of "The Art of Hypnotherapy" Chpt 89

Hunza: A community in the Himalayas, noted for longevity of its residents. Chpts 117, 118

Hyperesthesia or Hyperaestheia: Heightened body sensitivity.

Hypermnesia: Enhanced recall of exact details while in hypnosis.

Hypersuggestability: Heightened receptivity to suggestion.

Hypnagogic or Hypnogogic: The state of drowsiness before trance characterized by relaxation.

Hypnagogic Image: Something imagined in trance or just before sleep.

Hypnoanalgesia: The use of trance to not feel pain. Hypnosis relaxes parts of the body or mind that causes pain. That's why surgery, while performed with hypnosis, requires little or no anesthesia. See Conscious Sedation.

Hypnoanalysis: Analyzing thoughts and feelings while in trance state. Coined by Hadfield while working with shell-shocked war veterans. He noted that forgotten or repressed childhood memories were the underlying cause of present pain and distress. This hypnosis approach when combined with Freud's psychoanalysis includes dream interpretation & free-association.

Hypnoanasthesia: The use of hypnosis to not feel anything. Hypnosis soothes chronic pain without drugs by stimulating the body's natural ability to numb. Druglessly assists patients undergoing medical and dental procedures. See Conscious Sedation.

Hypnodisc: A disc with a spiral pattern, used to induce trance. Pgs 64, 69

Hypnodontics or Dental Hypnosis: Uses hypnosis, relaxation, visualization and suggestion for dental procedures. It helps dental professional's soothe phobic clients, enhance procedures, eliminate pain and stimulate self-healing. Orthodontists use it to help with difficult handicapping facial and dental abnormalities to "achieve results that they would not be able to obtain any other way." (Dr. John Goode, Orthodontist). Pg 535. See Index Part II Pain & Healing.

Hypnogenesis: Inducing sleep or the state of hypnosis.

Hypnography: Painting or drawing while in trance.

Hypnoidal: Relating to or resembling hypnosis or sleep.

Hypno-Lethargy: The deepest state of hypnosis coma from the Charcot paradigm of the five phases of depth: Wakeful, Somnambulism, Catalepsy, Lethargy and Hypno-Lethargy.

Hypnologic: Pertaining to the scientific study of hypnosis.

Hypnology: The scientific study of hypnosis.

Hypnopedia or Hypnopaedia: Sleep learning.

Hypno-Persuasion: Chpt 81, Pg 199

Hypnopompic: The transition or twilight state between trance and wakefulness.

Hypno-Psychology: A mental discipline that studies and utilizes the processes that create thought.

Hypnos: The Ancient Greek "god of sleep" and father of Morpheus, "the god of dreams."

Hypnosis: A term coined by Dr. James Braid to describe "a repressed state of mental functioning in which ideas are accepted by suggestion rather than logic evaluation." A mind state of heightened awareness where one easily takes on suggestion. Prefix "hypno" means sleep. Chpt 1

Hypnosis Agreement
A verbal or nonverbal contract between the subject and the hypnotist. Pg 24

Hypnotherapeutic Processes: A myriad of techniques that may include: affirmation, aggression release, amnesia, anchoring, aversion, aroma therapy, behavior modification, biofeedback, bombardment, brainwave entrainment, breathwork, brief therapy, catalepsy, cell demand, chakra balancing, circle therapy, coaching, cognitive shift, conditioning, de-hypnotizing, demonstration, de-programming, depossession, desensitizing, double bind, Elman method, eye-movement desensitization and reprocessing (EMDR), emotional release or emotional freedom technique (EFT), enneagram, energy balancing (electron balancing), Ericksonian, fantasy, feedback, forgiveness, gestalt, guided imagery, hypnoanalysis, hypnoanesthesia, hypnocatharsis, hypno-education, hypnoenergetics, hypno-psychology, hypno-yoga, ideomotor response, ritual, impulse control, induction, inner child, joy therapy, kinesiology, leetha, life coaching, life (business) strategies, meditation, magnetism, memory chain, mesmerism, metaphor, mind control, mind dynamics, mind mapping, mind mastery, motivation, neurolinguistic programming, neurolinguistic psychology, neurypnology, nocebo effect, nonpharmacologic analgesia, parts dialogue or sub-personality, pinpoint method, placebo effect, post-hypnotic suggestion, programming, progression, projection, quantum healing, re-alerting, reality therapy, rebirth, recall, reframe, regression, rehearsal, reinforcement, release, reparent, repattern, reprogram, reversal, reverse speech, revivification, ritual, role-playing, scripting, self-hypnosis, sensory distortion, sleep-learning, soma/psychic integration, somnambulism, soul retrieval, subconscious behavior modification, suggestion, swish method, symbolic restructuring, systematic desensitization, tapping (EFT), time-line therapy, trance, trance channeling, triggers, ultra-depth, quantum focus, visualization and wellness vs. illness.

Hypnotherapist Titles and Specialties:
Advanced Hypnotist/Hypnotherapist, Certified Hypnotist/Hypnotherapist, Alchemical Hypnotherapist, Assertive Behavioralist, Assertive Behavior Hypnotherapist, Behavioral Hypnotist, Childbirth/Midwifery Hypnotist, Clergical Hypnotherapist, Clinical Hypnotherapist, Cognitive Hypnotherapist, Counseling Hypnotherapist, Deprogrammer, Doctor of Clinical Hypnotherapy, Developmental Hypnotherapist, Geriatric Hypnotherapist, Educational Hypnotist, Ericksonian Hypnotherapist, Forensic Hypnotist, Guided Imagery Coach, Health Care Hypnotherapist, Higher-Self Hypnotist, Holistic Hypnotist, Humanistic Hypnotherapist, Hypno-Advisor, Hypnoanalyst, Hypnoanesthesiologist, Hypnobirther, Hypnocoach, Hypnocounselor, Hypnodontist, Hypnodoula, Hypnohealer, Hypno-Integrationist, Hypno-Kinesiologist, Hypnologist, Hypno-Metabolic Specialist, Hypno-Metaphysician, Hypnomotivator, Hypnopotamus, Hypnopsychologist, Hypnopsychotherapist, Hypnoresearcher, Hypno-Technician, Hypnosis Instructor, Hypnotherapist, Hypnotist, Life Coach Hypnotherapist, Master Hypnotist, Medical/Dental Hypnotherapist, Mind Dynamics Coach, Motivational Hypnotist, Motivational Speaker, Naturalistic Hypnotist, Neurolinguistic Programmer, Neurolinguistic Psychologist, Past Life Therapist, Past Life Regressionist, Pastoral Hypnotherapist, Performance Hypnotist, Psycholinguistic Specialist, Psychotherapeutic Hypnotherapist, Relaxation Therapist, Re-Patterner, Repatterning Counselor, Reprogrammer, Shamanic Hypnotherapist, Spiritual Hypno-Counselor, Sports Hypnotist, Stage Hypnotist, Substance Abuse Hypnotherapist, Surgical Hypnotherapist, Transformational Hypnotherapist, Transpersonal Hypnotherapist and Wellness Wizard.

Hypnosis Training: Pg 48

Hypnotherapy: Using hypnosis to expand mental, physical, emotional and/or spiritual limits and promote holistic well being. Includes counseling, instruction in self hypnosis and motivating people reach goals, eliminate pain, self-destructive or limiting habits, meet challenges and feel great.

Hypnotic: The fascinated attention that produces hypnosis states.

Hypnotic Amnesia: Not consciously remembering your experience after coming out of hypnosis. Amnesia depends on the depth of trance, if the subject expects amnesia to occur, and if amnesia is suggested. See Amnesia.

Hypnotic Anesthesia: Using hypnosis to control pain. Also called a kinesthetic illusion. See Conscious Sedation.

Hypnotic Catharsis: A process used by Sigmund Freud to release emotions while entranced. See Catharsis.

Hypnotic Dissociation: Using hypnosis to objectively detach from a situation or to focus to one aspect only.

Hypnotic Gaze: Pg 70

Hypnotic Illusion: A transformed observation of what is.

Hypnotic Induction Profile (HIP): An inaccurate hypnotic susceptibility scale intended to test responsiveness to hypnosis.

Hypnotic Passes: Sweeping non-touch movements by the hypnotist over the subject's body. Popularized by Mesmer.

Hypnotic Seal: A nasty practice reported by Dave Elman that uses the hypnotic suggestion, "no other person but me can successfully hypnotize you (or arouse you from this state)." To remove such a limiting suggestion say, "Close your eyes and get a mental picture of the person who hypnotized you…good. Now imagine them saying to you that you are in charge of your state of mind and that you now choose who hypnotizes you (or wakes you trance). Now imagine them waking you from trance and open your eyes…very good." Or another approach "Whenever you think of hypnosis, or any relaxed state, or someone talks to you about it, your sense of humor is magnified 50x (or 500 times)." Chpt 103

Hypnotic Sleep: A deliberate process to induce the awakened intense attention mind state we call hypnosis; involves exhaustion of interest, monotony, a peaceful mind, relaxed and comfortable posture and detachment from external excitement. Talking about sleep and imitating sleep, evokes hypnotic sleep. Chpt 18, Pgs 75-77

Hypnotic Suggestion: Subconscious realization of ideas.

Hypnotic Test: See Suggestibility/Susceptibility Test or Convincer.

Hypnotism: The science, theory and practice of hypnotizing people. A subjective (subconscious) state of mind produced by and heightening the power of suggestion.

Hypnotism Society of Pittsburgh: Organized in 1943 with the first elected President George Beshenich followed by Louis Fleck, George McRacken, William Harnett, Dave Ellis and Tom Weigman. Renamed the Hypnosis Society of Pennsylvania in 1951; current President Norbert Bakas.

Hypnotize: To fascinate, charm and put someone into the body/mind state of hypnosis.

Hypno-Yoga: Chpts 165-171

Hysteria: Unmanageable fear, panic expressed as an outburst of emotion or internally as severe anxiety.

I

IBS: Irritable bowel syndrome.

Ideomotor or Ideosensory Movement or Response: Subtle, automatic, seemingly non-voluntary muscle movements that communicate thoughts or feelings from someone in hypnosis to themselves or the hypnotist. Chpt 32

Illness: See wellness

Imagery: Pictures from the mind.

Imbedded Suggestion: Emphasizing suggestive words, phrases or sentences during regular conversation or hypnosis intended to impact a person without their being consciously aware that the suggestion was made. Pgs 367, 370, 589

Imprint: An entrenched mental pattern and behavioral response created via experience, sensory perceptions and heightened emotion.

Imprinting: A strong behavior pattern learned at an early age that attracts a person to another, especially parents.

Index of Scripts
See Index II.

Indirect or Disguised Suggestion
Subtle, veiled prompts used to activate a hypnotic course of action or bring up information. See Imbedded Suggestion.

Induction: The process used by hypnotherapists to bring about and stimulate hypnosis. Transforms your mind state from ordinary awareness to the trance. Is done verbally or energetically by ones self, another, or a group. Inductions by Chapter. See Index II Scripts.

Inner Child Work: A modality popularized by Eric Burne as Transactional Analysis (TA) in the 1970's that recognizes and releases the sub-self, natural child to be the spontaneous, playful, creative, spirited, loving and free self and heals and protects the hurt, afraid, vulnerable inner child to be safe and protected. See subpersonality work.

Insanity: Mind out of control.

Installation: Substituting one belief for another. Pg 344

Instate Sleep Suggestion: A post-hypnotic suggestion given in trance to induce the sleep state.

International Hypnosis Federation: Educational, referral organization offering hypnosis to the public and supporting the work of mind, body spirit practitioners worldwide. www.hypnosisfederation.com, Pg 50

Integration: Holistic hypnotic process of embracing all parts of self and life: the antithesis of disintegration of fractionalization.

ISE or Initial Sensitizing Event: A defining moment where you accept an imprint about who you are and what you will do in the future.

J

James, William: In 1875, James gave the first lecture in "psychology," a phrase he coined. Hence he is known as the founding father of Psychology. James used pretending or consciously play-acting to help. The term "Hypnotherapy" did not come along until much later. Chpt 28, Pgs xix, 121, 129

Joy Therapy®: A name coined by creator Shelley Stockwell (-Nicholas) for a hypnotherapeutic system of overriding sadness, grief and depression with joy. Chpt 113

Jung, Carl G.: 20th century psychologist who advanced the thought of an inherent spirituality and a "collective unconscious" with patterned ideas or styles of thought within groups of people. A student of Freud, his "Jungian approach" theorized a synchronicity of dream symbols and archetypes, like "Self" and "Shadow," that connect us to a vast, universally shared collective unconscious and serve as a portal to "individuation."

K

Kappas, John G.: Author and founder of Hypmovation Institute in Tarzana, California.

Kein, Gerald F.: Author and Hypnotherapist Chpts 57, 104

Kouguell, Maurice: Author of "DAPTH®: Accessing the Unconscious in Hypnosis & Counseling".

Krasner, Al: Founder of The American Board Of Hypnotherapy. Chpt 145, Pgs 2, 559

Kundalini and Kundalini Hypnosis: The energy and feeling of being alive associated with an experience of the body opening through the central nervous system via the spine and the seven chakras. Chpts 178, 189, 193, Pgs 363, 501, 659-660, 702, 732, 741

L

Law of Reverse Effect: You don't always get what you want; but you get what you need. A pseudo-psychology law created by French psychologist Baudouin that says, "When the imagination and the will are in conflict the imagination invariably gains the day." Pg 16

Lay Hypnotist: Coined by licensed mental health practitioners to disparage the good work of professional non-licensed professional hypnotherapists. The term inaccurately portrays competitors as untrained.

LaVelle, Jillian: Author and President of the International Association of Counselors and Therapists in Florida.

Legal Profession: Hypnotist, master hypnotist and Hypnotherapist are listed as legal profession by the U.S. Department of Labor. Here hypnosis is defined as "the bypass of the critical factor of the conscious mind followed by the ability to accept suggestions."

Legal Requirements: Chpt 16

Leetha: A Malay practice of automatic movements for advancing consciousness.

Learning: See educational hypnosis

Lessin, Alexander: Pgs 304, 675

Lethargy: A deep hypnotic state that you enter the coma.

Liability Insurance: Pg. 53

Liebeault, Ambroise-August (1823-1904) With Hippolyte Bernheim wrote and published the famous book "Suggestive Therapeutics" and founded the Nancy School of Medical Hypnotherapy in Nancy, France. Pgs xx, 151, 469, 471, 518

Logo Therapy: A term coined by Viktor Frankl from the Greek word "logos" for "meaning." His theory says that meaning in life comes with 1) Freedom of will 2) Will toward meaning and 3) Meaning to life.

Lucid Sleep or Lucid Dreams: Dubbed by Jose Custodio de Faria (1755-1819), lucid dreaming is the act of being aware of dreaming while dreaming.

M

Maslow, Abraham: The late creator of the "Hierarchy of Needs Theory" that encourages authenticity, learning from your inner nature, meeting basic needs, transcending problems, making good choices, becoming a world citizen, finding the right mate and being joyous.

Mass Hypnosis: Simultaneous hypnosis of a group of souls.

Matching or Mirroring: Modeling or adapting another's behavior to establish rapport for trance induction. Italian philosopher, Dominican monk and follower of Galileo, Tommaso Campanella, practiced these techniques in 1568. Pgs 338-340

Maya: The illusion of belief. Pg 7

McGill, PhD, Ormond: The Dean of Hypnosis, author of this book and some 35 others. In the field since 1927 and has taught hypnosis since1981, he serves on the board of advisors for numerous hypnosis organizations and has been featured on television and many audio and video tapes. Chpt 208

Medical Hypnosis: Uses hypnosis, relaxation, visualization and suggestion for medical use. Hypnotism is a wonderful tool for to soothe the ill and phobic clients. It enhances procedures, lowers blood pressure, eliminates pain and stimulates self-healing. Hypnosis reduces real and psychosomatic problems, anxiety and depression. Rashes, warts and other skin problems respond well to hypnosis. Hypnosis easily "turns off" an asthma attack, helps you lose weight and quit smoking and other harmful habits. For specific problems, see Part II Index, Pain & Healing.

Meditation, Guided Meditation or Hypno-Meditation: Inner self-reflection or "naikan" (looking within). Chpts 166, 178, 184-201, Pgs 18, 75, 132, 154, 174, 179, 369, 438, 455, 511, 604, 651, 720

Memory: See Mnemonics.

Memory Chain: See Affect Bridge.

Mental Equilibrium: The balancing of thoughts to meet things with a calm detachment.

Mental Rehearsal: Imagining yourself acting and feeling the way you want to in a specific situation. Also called "future pacing."

Mesmer, Franz Anton (1734-1815) and Mesmerism: Created techniques for healing using what he called Animal Magnetism. Energy is transmitted via directed non-touch and thought to bring about altered states. Chpts 128-130, Pgs 1, 26, 39, 212, 467, 468, 470, 473, 477-480, 483-486, 489, 499, 525, 531, 532, 536, 601,658, 771, 781, 782, 784

Metaloscopy: The use of metals to induce trance. Dr. Burcq worked with Charcot in Paris and said that brass applied to the surface of the skin was "curative."

Metamorphosis Hypnosis: Chpt 205

Metaphorical Hypnosis: Hypnotically comparing two unlike things as having commonality. Story telling that uses archetypes and analogies to bring home a message. Often used in Ericksonian Hypnosis.

Meta-Program: See Chunking

Metronome: An instrument used in music that marks exact time; excellent as a hypnosis gadget.

Mindfulness: Conscious awareness of thoughts and actions.

Mind Mapping: Graphic depictions of your thoughts in physical form as words, doodles, colors or collages that materialize inner thoughts and goals; popularized by Shelley Stockwell. Also known as a treasure map or future mandala.

Mnemonics or Memory Hypnosis: Everything you experience is permanently recorded in your brain; yet, most experiences quickly slip below conscious awareness. Unimportant, painful or traumatic moments are tucked away so you return to homeostasis. Hypnotic memory techniques allow you to re-member the past, re-lease pain and to positively re-frame it in the present. Hypnosis increases the storing and retrieving of data. With it you recall; names, faces and things you read.

Morice, Winifred: Nutritionist, Hypnotist and author of best selling cook books. Pg 56

Morrill, Del Hunter: Chpt 145

Motivational Hypnosis: Motivational Hypnotherapists sometimes call themselves motivational speakers. Their seminars and workshops offer hands on tools for success at home, in relationships and at work and make deep permanent and lasting impressions on participants. Business owners and managers know that hypnosis holds the key to keep employees productive and positive. The fiscal consequences of job stress in the United States is estimated at some $200 billion dollars a year lost to workers compensation claims, low morale and poor performance.

Corporate hypnotist trainers are in much demand. Hypnosis boost self-esteem, confidences so you make better decisions, put off procrastination and get yourself in moving gear.

Mulder, Marleen: Northern California teacher and Ormond's good friend. Chpt 144

Munro, Henry: From Omaha, Nebraska he coined the phrase "suggestive therapeutics" to describe a combination of hypnosis with the chemical anesthesia ether to alleviate fear of surgery and reduce drug dosage. Chpt 140

N

Narco-Hypnosis: Narcotic drugged altered state using sodium Phenobarbital, sodium amatol &/or sodium pentothal.

Neuralgia, Treating: Pg 535

Neurypnology and Neuro-Hypnosis: Name given to "suggestions that became permanent during the sleep of the nervous system" or "nervous sleep" by Dr. James Braid from Scotland (1795-1860).

Neves, Richard: Since 1982 President of the American Board Of Hypnotherapy. Pgs i, 348

Nicholas, Shelley Stockwell: See Stockwell.

NLP or Neuro Linguistic Programming or Psychology: Hypnotic behavior modification to discover and shift internal responses and external behavior through sensory matching, modeling and suggestion. Chpts 97, 98, 99

NOR: Non-Ordinary Reality.

NOS: Non-Ordinary States.

O

Oates, David John: Author; "Beyond Backward Masking: Reverse Speech and the Language of the Inner Mind." Chpt 154

Objective Observer: Also called the hidden observer, silent witness, higher self or conscience; this part of self maintains an objective grasp on your reality and truth at all times.

Obsession or Compulsion: A recurrent, persistent over-board thought, impulse, idea or action that appears uncontrollable by conscious will, yet is easily put to rest with hypnosis. An obsession is a preoccupation where you've "got to do it." A compulsion is an irresistible impulse to perform a repetitive irrational act where you've "got to do it again and again." Pgs 19, 199, 241, 347, 383, 452, 709

Oligondendroglia: Helper cells that make you smarter! Hypnosis stimulates and creates synapses and oligondendroglia. People with doctoral degrees purportedly have more oligondendroglia than high school dropouts. Albert Einstein's brain was said to have four times more than any others studied.

Operator: Another name for a hypnotist.

Orion Response: Shattering, loud and/or quick sound or movement used to imprint a suggestion. Used as a brainwashing techniques as in the slapping of a weapon clip with a threatening command. Used in Hypnotherapy as a pause followed an unexpected blurting out of the client's name and then a suggestion.

Otto, Robert: Director, Institute of Dynamic Hypnosis in Laceyville, Pennsylvania. Chpt 47

P

Pacing: Hypnotically matching a subjects speech, movement, breath and behavior patterns to establish rapport. Also a projected positive emotion on what will happen in the future.

Pain Management: See Conscious Sedation.

Paralysis, Systematic: Loss of special and adaptive movements i.e. suggesting a person is unable to lift a cigarette while all other movements remain unaffected. Agraphia (suggesting that someone cannot write is another example). The opposite of this would be to increase a skill.

Perls, Frederick (Fritz): 1940's counselor and creator of gestalt therapy to integrate and "real-eyes" oneself. Pgs 306, 351

Parts Therapy: A hypnotherapy modality created by Charles Tebbits that explores the influence and integration of sub-personalities. Similar techniques are voice dialog, archetypes, psychodrama, psycho-synthesis and gestalt. Chpt 89 See Sub-Personality Work.

Past Life Therapy: See Age Regression.

Pattern Interrupt: Derailing a particular train of thought.

Payoff: What you get from thinking and doing the things you do. Negative or positive both give you some reward or you wouldn't do them. Most payoffs come from a past imprint or idea that you have accepted into the subconscious mind.

Phobia Releasement: Hypnotic techniques like NLP movie desensitization or pressing on the palm of the hand to let go of irrational fear or panic. Pgs 348, 625-627, 657-658

Phrenology: Relating the bumps on the head to specific qualities.

Pinpoint Hypnosis: An altered state modality created by Helen Becham using regression and reframing for positive change.

Placebo Effect: From the Latin meaning "I shall please" a placebo turns something neutral into something helpful. A hypnotic suggestion that an inert substance will produce a positive effect creates real physiological changes. Imagining makes it so. The opposite of placebo is "nocebo" which suggests that a powerless substance will produce adverse effects. Pgs 9, 26, 89, 433, 435, 452, 539, 552, 553, 558

Positive Change Hypnosis: Inner focused hypnosis to identify behavior patterns that aren't working and replace them with those that do work. Hypnotic changes bring happiness, health, self-empowerment, abundance, a satisfying love life, and self-control.

Post-Hypnotic Cuing: A cue that triggers a suggestion given in trance to become manifest in regular state. Pg 218

Post-Hypnotic Suggestion: Past suggestions given in hypnosis (theta-state) that influence future behavior; ideas carry over into behavioral action in the waking state (beta state). A post-hypnotic suggestion can be brought about spontaneously or by conditioned cues or memory tags. Chpt 55, Pgs 4, 11, 25, 80, 103, 201, 391, 568

Post-Traumatic Stress or PTS: Reliving of past traumatic events triggered by specific associated or generalized thoughts, feelings, places and details. Hypnosis easily calms and releases such past pain. Pg 348

Post-Trance Condition: Sustained susceptibility to hypnotic suggestion after formal hypnosis has ended.

Prana or Prahna: Sanskrit term for vital energy of life brought into the body by the breath: also called qi, ki or chi. Pranayama practices like Nadi (psychic nerve channel) breathing is used by Yogis in India. Pgs xxii, 121, 422, 470, 471, 659, 670, 671, 683

Pre-Hypnotic Suggestion: Suggestions given about hypnosis before a formal induction is offered. Pgs 33, 34, 66

Professional Hypnotist: One who make an income using hypnosis or hypnotic principles.

Programming: Directing suggestion to the issue at hand with the intention of changing the response.

Projection: Externalization; ascribing ones feeling, thoughts, traits, beliefs and impulses to others people or events. Example "put your coat on, I'm cold."

Psychic Development: Chpts 189, 196, 198, 199, 201, Pgs 175, 701, 723, 779, 426, 429, 479, 807

Psycho Acoustics: Chpts 34, 44, 137

Psycho-Neuro Immunology: The study of the inter-relationship of mind/body and wellness. Pg 524

Psychosomatic: Mind body connection; a cultural trance holds a misconception that mind and body are not one in the same and that if it's "all in your head" it needs to be discounted as less important than a mechanical issue. Pgs 441, 523, 672

Psychotherapy: Psychological techniques used to help someone lead a better, more functional life. Anyone can call himself or herself a "psychotherapist" in most states as this title is unlicensed. Pgs 58, 113, 114, 47, 54

Psychotronics: The study of out-of-the-ordinary subjects. Originated in England as a diagnostic approach for blood using a camera. Today the word is used to describe vibrations, light and sound energies and their applications.

Psychotropic: A drug capable of affecting the mind.

Pyramid Hypnosis: Hypnosis that uses a series of rapid, successive hypnosis, awakening and re-hypnotizing.

Rapid or Instant Induction: To quickly bring about trance state often as simple as a snap of a finger. Chpts 25, 26

R

Rapport: Intimate level of communication between the Hypnotherapist and client; being "enrapport" or in tune with your client. Self-rapport is being in tune with yourself. Pgs 17, 23, 29-32, 85, 86, 109, 148, 149, 150, 182, 247, 287, 309, 335, 338, 361, 385, 481, 656, 780

Re-alerting, Reawakening: Used to describe the return from (trance state) theta to (wakefulness) beta state. Of course, all interaction between the hypnotist and subject is suggestive hypnosis. Sometimes called de-hypnotizing.

Rebirthing Hypnosis: This deep sustained breathing technique brings about altered states was popularized by Sondra Ray.

Reflexology Hypnosis: Chpt 122

Reframing Hypnosis: Hypnotically putting a new frame around an old picture: a fresh way to observe a situation. Re-organizing and reinterpreting the significance of an experience for a happier outcome. Pg 703

Regression: Mentally, emotionally or physically recalling the past as if you are there. See Age Regression.

Re-Hypnotizing or Fractionation: Waking and re-inducing trance during a hypnosis session; used to deepen trance. Pg 26

Reify or Reification: To think of something abstract as real and tangible.

Reiki: A healing modality using Cosmic Energy popularized in Japan. Chpt 133, Pgs 470, 502, 693

Relationship or Family Hypnosis: Hypnosis puts you in touch with your sub-personalities and various ways to look at life. It helps resolve inner conflicts and integrate multi-dimensionally. As you learn to love and accept your selves, it's easier to love and accept others. Chpts 106-110

Relaxation: The by-product of all hypnosis is relaxation, and that alone helps you feel terrific. Hypnosis is the perfect antidote for chronic stress, pain and anxiety and it restores your natural ability to sleep.

Releasement Hypnosis: Hypnosis directed toward the goal of letting go of limiting thought forms and feelings.
Remote Therapy or Remote Depossession A belief and practice of long distance removal of negative energy. Pg 711

Repatterning: Another name for hypnotic behavior modification.

Repression: Thoughts, fantasies, memories and impulses unconsciously kept from conscious awareness.

Reverse Speech: Pg 22, Chpt 154

Revivification: To bring a memory back with clarity.

Rothman, Stephanie: Pg 7

S

Salpetriere Hospital: Paris's largest asylum created in the 1840's by Jean Charcot for hysterical women declared as "crazy." Pgs 185, 469, 509

Script: The suggestions and words a hypnotist gives to someone in a trance. See Index of Scripts, Part I & II.

Sedona Method: An energy technique said to release trapped emotions from the chest or solar plexus. The process: "Think of the worst thing that happened to you and ask yourself 1. Can I release it, 2. Would I release it, and 3. When will I release it?" (If you let it go you are complete. If not ask, "How does it feel holding on to it?" and repeat the questions again).

Selective Thinking: Directed suggestions subconsciously accepted.

Self-Conscious: Intense awareness of self.

Self Esteem: Internal assessment of self worth derived from verbal and non verbal suggestion and experiences.

Self-Exploration Hypnosis: As you learn to simultaneously tune into conscious and subconscious thoughts and actions, you become your own observer. This helps you understand the reasons for patterns, behaviors, gifts and style accept and empathize with yourself. Familiarity brings content(ment) as the purpose of your life is revealed to you.

Self-Hypnosis: Someone hypnotizing themselves; also called auto-conditioning, auto-hypnosis and auto-suggestion. Chpts 53, 58, 71, 75, 114, 115, 189, Pgs 18, 43, 44, 48, 50, 93, 105, 106, 181, 203, 207, 208, 295, 376, 379, 445, 457, 467, 598, 733

Serenity Resonance Sound or Symbiotic Resonance Sound: A sound vibration tape and DC created by Ormond McGill and Joseph Worrell that entrains the brain to frequencies more receptive to suggestion. Available at www.hypnosisfederation.com Chpts 34, 35

Sexual Wellness Hypnosis: Hypnosis uncovers the culprits of sexual frustration: performance anxiety, guilt, shame, and embarrassment. Limiting myths or socially unacceptable behaviors are reframed. Vitality replaces numbness. A good hypnotist educates and motivates passion, play and sexually wellness.

Shamanic Restructuring: Installing during trance the thought "it never happened" to replace a traumatic occurrence.

Siddhi: Hindu for "perfection" Siddhi powers, achieved though mastery of yoga states, include clairvoyance, levitation, teleportation, bi-location & healing.

Sleep, Hypnotic: Chpt 18, Pgs 76, 253, 452, 455, 595

Sleep Temples and Healing Shrines: Where folks in Ancient Egypt and Greece went to be hypnotized and healed for R & R.

Smoke Cessation Hypnosis: Results of largest-ever scientific comparison of ways to quit smoking showed that a visit to a hypnotist beat out a psychologist, social worker, psychiatrist and other physicians by a margin of 19% (or one to five). This meta-analysis of more than 600 studies of quit smoking programs covered more than 72,000 people in America and Europe and was conducted by the University of Iowa. Chpt 63, 64 and 65, Pgs 221, 124, 306

Social Script: Hypnotically imprinted social norms and etiquette that predetermine acceptable interaction.

Soma: Related to the body.

Somnambulism: A state of profound sleep or hypnosis where a person talks and walks and can have their eyes open. Here the subject is completely engrossed in the reality of suggestions given and generally experiences amnesia. Chpt 19, Pgs 12, 27, 75, 76, 83, 84, 86, 118, 119, 121, 214, 229, 250, 369, 486

Somnus or Somnolent: Induced drowsiness or sleep.

Sopor: Deep sleep.

Soporific or Somniferous: Sleepiness or drowsiness.

Sublimation: Unacceptable subconscious drives deflected into more socially acceptable outlets. For example aggression satisfied by watching wrestling, boxing or football.

Suppression: Thoughts, fantasies, memories and impulses consciously kept from conscious awareness.

Soul Retrieval: An ancient shamanic technique using imagery and non-verbal suggestion intended to integrate mind, body and spirit.

Special Needs Hypnosis: Stutterers and those with other speech difficulties, ADD (attention deficit disorder), hearing and visually impaired (tinnitus, blindness), brain injured, dyslexics, and aphasics (those with word understanding difficulties) have all benefited from hypnotic techniques.

Spencer (-Beachum), Anne, Dr.: Founder of the International Medical & Dental Hypnotherapy Association (1986) and Infinite Institute.

Spiritual Counseling: Certified Spiritual Counselors, Metaphysicians, Ministers, Transpersonal Hypnotherapists, Shamans and Clairvoyants use ancient & modern practices to help you integrate mind, body and spiritual well-being through interactive conversation, altered states, alchemy, astrology, breathwork, card reading, crystals, between life imagery, ceremony, chanting, chakra balancing, channeling, counseling, depossession, divination, dowsing, energy work, face reading, fantasy, handwriting analysis, hypnosis, inner vision, intuition, meditation, medical intuition, medicine stories, mysticism, numerology, palmistry, past-life regression, prayer, prediction, progression, ritual, shamanic rites, spiritual cleansing, story telling, soul retrieval symbols, trance & vision quests. Angels, archetypes, deities, spirit guides, saints, deceased loved ones, & ascended masters are cherished thought forms.

Split Personality: Also called " multiple personality disorder" or "associated disorder." See Sub-Personality.

Spontaneous Hypnosis: Naturally occurring hypnotic states commonly refer to a freeway hypnosis, trauma trance, boredom, daydreaming, runners high, being in the zone, love stuck, inspiration and spiritual ecstasy.

Sports Hypnosis: Hypnosis using the mind and psychological aspects to enhance physical performance and motivation. Post hypnotic suggestions with individuals and teams improve real life activity. Sports hypnotists help clients play their best, stay in the zone, avoid distractions and relax. Mental imaging becomes a self-fulfilling prophecy. Weight lifters who visualize body sculpting get better results then those who don't. Basketball players who mentally rehearse scoring free shots actually make more free shots. Golfers who play the shot mentally score better. A positive mental attitude evokes peak performance. Chpt 152, Pg 249

Squish Technique: Using each hand to personify conflicting viewpoints and bringing them together for integration. Pg 342

Stage fright, Overcoming: Chpt 39, Pg 112

Stage Hypnosis: Hypnosis in front of an audience is entertaining and enlightening. The hypnotist most do two things at once: keep the audience's attention, while carefully controlling the subjects (who are the show). Fire walking and other sensational demonstrations of mind power also fascinate and amaze us. Chpts 157, 158, Pgs 2, 11, 42, 43, 52, 53, 54, 80, 97

Stansberry, Barbara: Pg 138

Stockwell(-Nicholas), PhD, Shelley: Transpersonal Hypnotherapist, contributing editor of this book and author of 11 books. Founder of the International Hypnosis Federation (www.hypnosisfederation.com) and Dean of the Creativity Learning Institute certifying Hypnotists, Hypnotherapists and Spiritual Counselors. Chpts 14, 16, 34. 65, 69, 81, 88, 98, 104, 105, 108, 110, 113, 119, 123, 126, 133, 134, 137, 139, 145, 146, 149, 153, 157, 170, 176, 177, 178, 179, 196, 201, Pgs ii, ix, 32, 152, 215, 267, 347, 351, 352

Stress: Internal or external stimuli that signals danger to quickly activate every body system to fight, excite or run. May cause fear, pain, illness and upset. When properly channeled with hypnosis it can evoke motivation, energy and pro-action.

Stress Management Hypnosis: About one-third of us feel overloaded with stress. Hypnosis unloads overload and chronic fatigue and is a profound crisis intervention.

Stuttering: Chpt 161, Pgs 387, 389, 533

Subconscious Mind: Internal Self. Mental processes not yet revealed to wakeful awareness. The majority of brain functioning, these archives remember all tidbits of uncritically accepted information about self and life and from these memories draws conclusions.

Sub-Personality Work: Personifying emotional patterns and attitudes as distinct mini-selves. Quieting internal conflict and getting our many "sub-selves" or "ego parts" to get along and form a team. Integration usually requires the taming of the "inner critic" and the empowering of the "master controller." Multiple personality disorder (associated disorder) appears to be the extreme of this natural phenomenon where one sub-self is often unaware of the "others." Popularized by Roberto Assagioli as "Psychosynthesis," Hal and Sidra Stone as "Voice Dialogue," Charles Tebbits and "Gestalt Therapy" by Fritz Perls. Chpts 88, 89

Suggestibility: What suggestions will be most accepted? What suggestions will be most resisted?

Suggestibility/Susceptibility Test or Convincer: Hypnotic induction used to gauge a person's receptivity to trance and suggestion. Does not necessarily map a person's receptivity to either. Chpt 5, 94, Pgs 11, 40, 41, 77

Suggestion, Suggestion Formulas or Affirmation: Behavior influencing ideas offered during hypnosis as direct verbal or nonverbal statements or indirect implied messages to encourage and motivate. Visual cues like stickers, flash cards, embroidery, bumper stickers, and refrigerator magnets can reinforce suggestions. Chpt 52, Pg 201

Suggestive Therapeutics or Therapy: Dr. Henry Munro, M.D. from Omaha, Nebraska coined the phrase "suggestive therapeutics" to describe a combination of hypnosis with the chemical anesthesia ether to alleviate fear of surgery and reduce the dosage to only ten percent of what was usually given. His patients lived, experienced no pain and bypassed recovered more quickly. The Mayo brothers first tested Munro's process during deep abdominal surgery (Case Number One of some seventeen thousand cases that followed: each without a single death occurring.) Their Mayo Clinic became legendary as the only "safe" hospital where one had an excellent chance of surviving. Strangely, the Mayo Brothers never said they used hypnosis, even though an article about it was published the May, 1906 Obstetrical Journal. Suggestive therapy now refers to the hypnotic removal of symptoms. Chpt 140

Super-Conscious Mind: Higher Self, Expanded Consciousness, the super conscious mind encompasses and permeates all levels of consciousness. It oversees the conscious and subconscious and it remembers all my experiences within and beyond my individual personality.

Susceptibility: The degree to which one takes on suggestions or impressions.

Suspended Animation: Temporary slowing or suspension of bodily functions.

Sutphen, Richard: Author of "We Were Born Again To Be Together" and Founder, Valley of the Sun Publishing. Pg ii

Swish Swap: Behavior modification that substitutes a desired response for an undesirable one. Pg 343

Symbiotical Resonance Sound or Serenity Resonance Sound: A sound vibration tape and DC created by Ormond McGill and Joseph Worrell that entrains the brain to frequencies more receptive to suggestion. Available at www.hypnosisfederation.com, Chpt. 34, 35

Symbolic Restructuring: Installing positive images or archetypes to replace traumatic memory often followed with the post hypnotic suggestion "If ever you think of _________ (trauma) you will instantly and automatically substitute it with this new thought."

Symptom Removal: Direct suggestions of a problem going away. Pg 385

Synchronicity Theory: A phrase coined by Carl Jung to describe things in life caused by meaningful coincidence contrasting with the law of cause and effect.

Syndrome: A group behaviors that form a recognizable pattern like crying syndrome, responsibility syndrome, guilt syndrome, arguing syndrome, fight/fright/flight syndrome.

Synethesia: A sensory cross-over as in the ability to perceive sound as color, music as shape, shape as taste, or smell as sound. Reports of "colored letters" and "colored hearing" date back to the 1800's. This ability is said to be possessed by an estimated 1 in 300.

Systematic Desensitization: Repeatedly bringing up a fear until it losses its power.

T

Tapping: See emotional freedom technique.

Tebbits, Charles: Author and creator of the subpersonality modality, Parts Therapy. Chpt 89

Tantra Hypnotherapy: Chpt 171

Telkemeyer, Ernie: Illinois Hypnotherapist who specializes in working with children. Pgs 167, 168

Therapeutic: Curative

Thompson, Jeffrey: Sound researcher/therapist. Chpt 137

Thompson, Niccolous: Author "Hypnotherapy for Children" and "Hypnotherapy for the Sexually Abused" Pgs 166, 170

Transference: A client projecting their feelings of love or resentment onto the hypnotist. Pg 32

Time Line Therapy: Imagining a linear (or personally structured) time scale and regressing to before a trauma to take away the impact. A similar shamanic approach goes back to before an upset proclaiming, "It never happened."

Time Perception: Pgs 217, 218

Time Travel Hypnotherapy: Past life regression, future life progression and between life journeys offer profound personal exploration.

Tooge-Tooge Induction: Captain James Cook reported that Tongan natives induced trance when two women "beat briskly the body and legs with fists until the subject falls asleep. They continue all night with short intervals and reduced rapidity and strength."

Toole, Sharon E.: Pg 438

Trance or Reverie: An altered state of consciousness exaltation with heightened mental alertness, heightened emotion & receptivity to suggestion.

Trance Fix: Riveted attention with positive results.

Trance Medium or Trance Channel: A medium using hypnotic altered states to offer prediction, counseling and divination. Chpt 200, Pgs 702, 787

Transpersonal Hypnotherapy: Explores higher states of consciousness beyond the personality. Helps answers questions like "why am I here?" "What decisions will be for my highest good." Includes spiritual exploration, archetypes, soul retrieval, time travel and other higher states. Transformational and spiritual hypnotherapy enhances meditation and prayer. Here we contact the profound higher self and discover our life path and future. Spiritual guidance and emergence bring life changing perspectives. Trance channeling, automatic writing, spirit guidance and intuitive awareness offer powerful tools for self-discovery. Soul retrievals and rebirthing techniques reintegrate. So do auric cleansing and energy balancing.

Trauma: An intense upset or hurt marked by difficulty with similar events, denial, flashbacks, bad dreams and guilty parents.

Treatment Codes: Pg 58

Twilight Sleep: The state between wakefulness and sleep.

U

Unconscious Or Subconscous: Parts of the body/mind that are hidden from conscious thought, sensation or feeling awareness. The unconscious controls the autonomic nervous system.

Unconscious Learning: Milton Erickson's term for the state where someone intuitively knows the meaning of dreams, symbols and unconscious expression.

Unconscious Resistance: Not bringing buried thoughts or memory to conscious awareness.

Universal Mind: Chpt 183, Pgs xxi, 35-36 589, 590

Utilization: Using all the verbal and nonverbal data you receive from the client plus the environment to enrich the hypnotic experience. Also incorporating whatever is going on in the environment into the induction or suggestion.

V

Vitale, Anna: Chpt 124

Vogel, Marcel: IBM Senior Scientist who prior to his death, used low-voltage energies, amplified through quartz crystal, to effect wellness. Chpt 135

von Reichenbach, Baron (mid 1800's): Wrote "The Dynamics Of Magnetism, Electricity, Heat, Light, Crystallization And Chemistry In Their Relation To Vital Force" in 1846 which used the "Odic" Force for healing. Chpt 131, Pg 470

Voice Dialogue: Hal and Sidra Stone coined this name for work similar to gestalt therapy, subpersonality or parts therapy.

W

Waking Hypnosis: Suggestions accepted by a person not in a trance (alpha state). Hypnosis that starts with conscious doing and then moves into subconscious acceptance. Chpts 21, 22, 24, Pgs 87-102

Water, Healing: Chpt 4, Pgs 4, 7, 31, 72, 89, 492-497, 556, 559

Water, Charging (Pranazing) Charging water with prana. See water, healing.

Weight Control Hypnosis: Hypnosis to program positive changes in eating and drinking behavior. Chpt 61, 112, Pgs 50, 55, 57, 59, 61, 204, 211, 229, 230, 307, 341, 342, 356, 370, 395, 409, 418, 446, 452, 614, 657

Wellness: Chpts 111-125, 141, Pgs 44, 50, 51, 53, 200, 229, 256, 265, 276, 524, 527, 546, 557, 571, 702, 722, 747, 775, 794, 795. See Index Part II, Pain & Healing.

Wilson, Gaye: International hypnosis instructor from Placerville, California. Pg 547

Window of Opportunity: The psychological moment when a thought, idea or suggestion has its greatest impact.

Window Sleep: A publicity stunt used by Ormond McGill where a local girl is hypnotized to "sleep soundly with nothing disturbing you until I tell you to wake up." She is then placed in a store window (for 5 hours or less) and then taken by an ambulance to a theater, brought on stage and awakened.

Worrell, Joseph: Sound expert and co-creator of the Serenity (Simbiotical) Resonance Sound. Pgs 25, 154, 156, 520

Y

Yawning: A generally involuntary long deep breath can be used as an induction technique. Pgs. 42, 73, 88, 129, 208, 363, 370, 378, 379, 584, 688

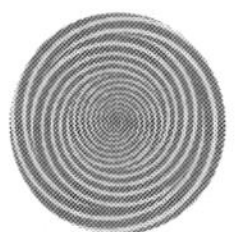

PART II: 347 SCRIPTS BY SUBJECT

A

Active Particiation Method Pg 297
Acupressure Hypnotherapy Pg 473
ADD/ADHD (Induction for) Pg 579
Addictive Drugs Pg 538
Addiction Chpt 142
Aesthetics Pg 457
Age Attitude Pg 226
Anger Management Pg 377
Arthritis Pg 535
Astral Healing (Suggestions For) Pg 442
Attitude Pg 30
Aversion Pg 242
Aversion Suggestion Pg 238

B

Balloon Stress Release Pg 266
Be Here Now Suggestions Pg 299
Be More Organized and Efficient Pg 226
Better Communication Pg 225
Big Mistakes, Little Successes/Celebrate Success Pg 399
Bio Tuning And Sonic Induction Pg 512
Bio-Magnetic Hypnotherapy Pg 490
Black and White Thinking (Locked-In)/
    Shades of Gray Suggestions Pg 395
Blame Game Pg 403/
    The Game Of Gift Pg 404
Blessing That Deepen Trance Pg 241
Blue Light Method Pg 771
Blue Vitality Bath Pg.231
Bodhisattva Hypnotherapy Pg 797
Bodhisattva Way Pg 801
Bogus Chemicals Pg 539
Breath (The Nerve Revitalizing) Pg 425
Breath (Hunza Complete Vitalizing) Pg 424
Breath (The Hunza Grand Psychic) Pg 426
Breathe For Life Pg 244
Breathe To Relieve Pg 521
Breathing (Rhythmic) Pg 425
Bringing in the Force Pg. xxiv
Broken Record/ Unstuck Pg 401
Broken Hearted
    (Pre-Hypnosis Pointers For The) Pg 383
Broken Heart Hypnosis (Ellis) Pg 384

C

Cartoon Movie That Mends Pg 350
Chakra Balancing
    (The Ladder Of Color) Pg 741
Change (Instant-Movie) Pg 347
Channeling (Trance)Pg 784

Childbirth:
    The Contraction Giggle Pg 569
    The Delivery Warm Up Pg 569
    Happy HypnoBirthday™
        (Stockwell-Nicholas Preparation) Pg 570
    Hello Baby Pg 569
    Hypnosis For Conception Pg 569
    Morning Sickness (Overcoming)Pg 571
    Pre Birth Hypnotherapy Pg 566
    Trouble Shooting Happy (HypnoBirthday) Pg 570
Chunking Down Pg 341
Chunking Up Pg 341
Cognitive Behavior Hypnosis pre-Talk Pg 392
Chakra Color Balancing Pg 737
Conflict, Squish A Pg 342
Common Sense (Abdominal Brain) Hypnotherapy Pg 432
Complain Game Pg 402
    An Attitude of Gratitude Suggestions Pg 403
Compounding To Stop Smoking Pg 221
Computer Technology Pg 320
Confidence Pg 259
Conscious Smile Pg 281
Constipation Pg 536
Convincer Scripts Pgs 40, 41
Cosmic Love Pg 688
Coue`s Twilight "Good Knot" Autosuggestion Pg 417
Coulda/Woulda/Shoulda Pg 400
Count Your Blessing Pg 331
Creativity Pg 226
Creativity (Hypnosis For) Pg 584
Creative Writing (Hypnotically Structure)Pg 585
Creative Writing Genius (Unleash Your) Pg 585
Cut Yourself Some Slack Pg 401

D

Death (Hypnotherapy Of)Pg 427
Death and Rebirth Pg 706
Depossession Pg 710
Depossession (Remote) Pg 711
Depression Pg 256
Depression (Overcome) Pg 263
Determination Pg 260
Determination (Cultivating) Pg 378
Direct Core Suggestion pg 237
Disassociate From Pain Pg 554
Do It Pg 258
Dreaming (Stockwell's Shamanic) Pg 352
Dreamwork (Stockwell's Hypnotic Gestalt) Pg 351
Dress Distress Pg 86
Drinking Habit Pg 537

E

Earache Pg 535
Earache Pg 495
Eye Trouble Pg 496
Edit & Tame The Editor Pg 304
Einstein Happiness Way Pg 269
Emotional Detox Pg 445
Enlightenment Pg. 685
End Mind Trap Games Pg 404
Energized (Vogel's Hypnotherapy Couch) Pg 507
Entering The Darkness Pg 753
ESP And PSI Powers
   (Universal Mind Suggestion For Developing Your) Pg 723
Excellence, Circle of Pg 345
Explaining Hypnosis Script Pg 33

F

Fear Gear (Shift the) Pg 569
Fear Of Cats Pg 626
Fear Of Heights Pg 388, 389
Fever Pg 496
Fire Away Pg 267
Food-For-Thought Self-Hypnosis Chpt 53
Forget You Not Pg. 316

G

Gestalt Pg 306
Get Over It Pg 369
Glove Anesthesia:
   Glove Anesthesia Pg 543
   Glove Anesthesia (Hand In The Snow) Pg 548
   Glove Anesthesia (Hand in the Bucket) Pg 548
   Glove Anesthesia (Post Hypnotic) Pg 549
   Glove Anesthesia Return Pg 549
   Glove Anesthesia (Transferring-Long Version) Pg 548
   Glove Anesthesia (Transferring-Short Version) Pg 548
Gossip Pg 257
Guardian Angel Induction Pg 705

H

Heart Condition Pg 536
Heart Mending Chpt 108
Heart Trouble Pg 495
Holistic Mental Marriage Pg 36
Holotropic Breathing Pg 675
Holy Water Pg 10
Hypnosis Explanation Pg 33
Hypnotherapy of Infinite Pg 745
Hypnotherapy of Nothingness Pg 295
Hypnotic Prelude After A Consultation Pg 94
Hypnotic Seal, Break It Pg 362
Hypnotic Sleep Pg 76
Hypno-Yoga Pg 652

I

Ideas Over Will Pg 15
Illness See Pain & Healing
Imagination (Hypnotherapy Of) Pg 355
Imbedded Commands To Be Slimmer Pg 370
Imbedded Quotes Pg 371
Immortality (Hypotherapy of)Pg 573

Increased Energy Pg 259
Indigestion Pg 496
Indirect Suggestions to Stop Alcohol Pg 366
Induction Scripts Part 2
Infinite Smallness Pg 325
Inner Child (Meet Your)Pg 624
Installation Pg 344
Integrity Pg 258

K

Karma Releasement Pg 646
Labeling and Name-Calling Pg 394
Re-mark-able Affirmation Pg 395

L

Laughter Pg 257
Laughter Hypnotherapy Pg 283
Let's Pretend You Hate Smoking Pg 124
Light & Sound Hypnotherapy Pg 508
Little Theater of the Mind Pg 333
Lucky Clients Pg 280
Lucky You Pg 279

M

Magnetizing Water Pg 492
Make A Wish Pg 358
Marriage (Saving A) Pg 382
Mastermind Hypnotherapy Pg 691
Matrimony Pg 381
Meditation (Hypno-) Pg 729
Mental Set Hypnosis Pg 409
Mesmer's Five-step Clinical Procedure Pg 481
Mesmeric Sitting Technique Pg 482
Metamorphosis Pg 812
Mind Trap Hypnotherapy (for Sexual Dysfunction,
   Stuttering, Fear of Heights) Pg 389
Money Pg 255
Money (The Color Of Riches) Pg 230
More Imbedded Commands Pg 370
Mozart's Musical Meditation Pg 438

N

Nail Bitting Pg 215
Native American's Controlling The Outside World Pg 755
Nit-Picking Negativity/ Not to Nit Pick Suggestions Pg 396
NLP Gives Sub-Personalities A Hand Pg 306
Non-Verbal Waking Suggestions Chapt 21 and Chpt 22
Nothing Need Be Done Pg 293

O

Ode To Adrenals Pg 257
Out Of Body Hypnotherapy Pg 775

P

Pain and Healing:
   Anesthetic Tapping Pg 540
   Anesthesia (Touch)Pg 540
   Arthritis Pg 495
   Arthritis Pg 535
   Burmese Pain Control Pg 555
   Control Room Kick It Up A Notch
      (Pain Management) Pg 557

Control Room Pain Magic Pg 555
Dialog With Needs Pg 553
Dialog With Pain's Punishment Pg 554
Dialog With Pain Pg 553
Dialog With Symptoms Pg 553
Disappearing Touch Pg 547
Feel Good Pg 256
Future Pacing Pain Pg 556
General Debility Pg 495
General Disability Pg 534
General Instructions For Successful
    Magnetic Healing Pg 496
Good Health For Yourself Pg 422
Good Health Hypnosis For Clients Pg 421
Headache Pg 493
Headache (Six Remedies) Pg 560
Healing Water Pg 9
Laugh It Off (Pain Management) Pg 557
Lavender Oil Approach (Pain Management) Pg 558
Magnetic Healing Pg 492
Mental Rehearsal (Pain Management) Pg 557
Molecular Healing Pg 522
Neuralgia Pg 494
Neuralgia Pg 535
"New" Anesthesia Pg 539
Pain (Stillpoint Approach To) Pg 554
Pain Sensations
    (Universal Mind Suggestion For Mastering) Pg 723
Paralysis Pg 496
Running Hot And Cold (Pain Management) Pg 557
Spinal Tap Exercise Pg 521
Soothe Your Neurons Pg 520
The Feel Good Overlay (Pain Management) Pg 556
Toothache (Magnetically Treat) Pg 494
Toothache Pg 536
Touch & Away (Pain Management) Pg 558
Tunnel As A Funnel (Pain Management) Pg 556
Up/Down/Turn It Off (Pain Management) Pg 557
Universal Mind Healing Pg 720
Utilizing the Environment (Pain Management) Pg 556
Wellness Pg 256
Happiness Hypnosis Pg 415
Higher States Pg 687
Immunization From Diseases
    (Universal Mind For) Pg 722
King Of The World Game Pg 370
Multiple Sclerosis (Healing Script) Pg 438
Pre-Hypnosis Suggestions Pgs 33, 34, 66

Parts Therapy Pg 308
Perfectionism or Nothing Pg 297/ Best Is Better Pg 298
Phobia (Neves' Release Theater) Pg 348
Playing The Game Of Life Pg 462
Positives Don't Count/ Yes! I'm Positive Suggestions Pg 397
Post-Hypnotic Cuing Pg 218
Power & Control Game Pg 399
    Live and Let Live Suggestions Pg 400
Pre-Hypnosis Script Pg 34
Problem (Good-Bye) Pg xx
Problem Solving Regression Pg 639
Progression Pg 246

Psychic (Be More)Pg 788
Psychic Wounds (Heal Ol') Pg 283
Pure Pleasure Pg 278

Q
Quick Reflexology Relaxation Pg 448

R
Rag Doll For Well Being Chpt 41
Regression For Fun Pg 641
Regression Reframe Pg 242
Reincarnation and Death Pg 638
Reiki Pg 500
Relax (Mom's Teddy Bear) Pg 572
Remote Control Expectations Pg 266
Replaceable Hypnotherapy Pg 275
Resistance (The Gift Of What You Resist) Pg 369
Right Brain Left Brain Pg 329

S
Self Hypnosis
    (Hypnotize Clients To Hypnotize Themselves) Chpt 53
Self Realization Pg 693
Self-Control Pg 260
Self-Control Pg 377
Self-Control Pg 379
Self-Control (Cultivating)Pg 380
Self-Empowerment Pg 378
Self-Esteem (Sunshine Suggestion Formula) pg 233
Self-Hypnosis For The Mature Adult pg 223
Serenity Hypnotherapy Pg 264
Sleep Apnea 452
Sleep Learning Pg 253
Sleep Suggestion Formulas Pg 455
Sleep (The Long Hypnotic) Pg 595
Sleeping Pill Addicts Pg 453
Slow Down Method Pg 314
Smoking:
    Smoking (Compounding To Quit) Pg 221
    Smoking (Sub-personalities To Quit) Pg 306
    Smoking (Let's Pretend You Hate It) Pg 124
    Smoking (Remote Approach to Stop) Pg 222
    Smoking - Tobacco (Changing Patterns To Quit) Pg 243
    Smoking (Screen Of Mind) Pg 238
    Smoking (Stop) Pg 241
    Smoking (Stop Today) Pg 236
    Smoking (Stop With The Sphere of Energy) Pg 239
Snappy Reinforcements Pg 215
Snapshot Swish-Swap Pg 243
Snuggle Down And Be Comfortable Pg 261
Social Confidence Pg 225
Soul Retrieval Pg 703
Somnambulism Pg 27
Sports Hypnosis (Stockwell-Nicholas) Pg 249
Stage Hypnosis Pg 601
Stage Hypnosis (Guardian Angel Hypnosis Show) Pg 607
Stamina Pg 259
Stress Pg 263
Stress Release (Magic Bubble) Pg 267
Stuttering Pgs 387-389, 630
Subconscious Hypnotherapy Pg 299
Suggestions For The Hypnotherapist Pg 25

Suggestions With Deep Meaning Pg 227
Super Learning Induction Pg 247
Super Learning (Suggestion-Formula For) Pg 248
Superconsciousness Pg 715
Superstar (You are a) Chpt 39
Surgery:
    Surgery Preparation (Bakas) Pg 546
    Surgery Preparation (Stockwell) Pg 547
    Surgery Preparation (Wilson) Pg 547
Sweeping Generalities Pg 395/ Detailing Suggestions Pg 396
Swish-Swap Waking Suggestion Pg 343
Swish-Swap With Sound Pg 243

T
Talent Pg 594
Tantra Hypnotherapy Pg 678
Tapping Pg 503
Telepathy Scripts Pg 779
Tension (Relieve) Pg 263
The Attention Technique Pg 659
The Essene Way Pg 748
Third Eye Opening Scripts Pg 781
The Great Mind Reader Concludes Pg 298
The Happiness Way Pg 273
The Hunza Method Pg 424
The Light Within Pg 695
The Violet Flame Pg 757
The White Light Of Protection Pg 732
Third Eye Seeing Pg 781
Thought Projection (Mesmer's Hand Passes And) Pg 483
Thought Stopping 215
Three Waking Group Hypnosis Experiments:
Time Distortion In Hypnosis Pg 218
Time (Post-Hypnosis & The Sense of) Pg 218
Time (Setting Your Mental Alarm) Pg 217
Timely Post Hypnotic Experiment Pg 213
Tolerance For Others Pg 225
Transcendental Hypnotherapy Pg 765
Triggering Gismos Pg 214
Trust Method Pg 385
Trust Your Timing Pg 369

U
Use Everything To Your Advantage Pg 369

V
Vitality Hypnosis Pg 513

W
Wake Up Suggestion Pg 26
Wake Up Well Pg 540
Weight:
    Color Me Thin Pg 229
    Eating To Exhaustion Pg 453
    Imbedded Comands To Be Slimmer Pg 370
    Mental Set Your Weight Pg 411
Well-Being (Coue`'s Formula) Pg 418
Wellness See Pain & Healing
Wellness (Mesmerism/Hypnosis For) Pg 478
Wellness (Stockwell's Script) Pg 435
Will & Memory Pg 251
Will You Remember Script Pg 34
Worry Game Pg 401
Worry (What, Me?) Pg 402

Y
Yama Yoga Pg 668
Yes I'm Positive Pg 255
Yoga Nidra Pg 651
You Are A Rainbow Pg 735
Youth (Universal Mind Suggestion For Perpetual) Pg 723

Z
Zen Hypnotherapy Pg 761

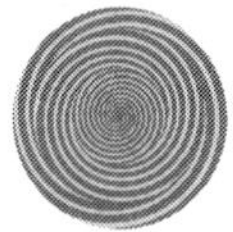

PART III: 153 INDUCTION SCRIPTS
BY CHAPTER

Chpt 17: The Four-Fold Induction Approach, pg 65
Bite the Cork Induction
Clock Dial Induction
Focused Feeling Inductions
Hands Over The Ears Induction
Hands Over The Eyes Induction
Hot Money
Hold Your Tongue Induction
Hypnodisc
Hypnotic Gaze
Hypnotic Voice
Look at your Spine Induction
Pendulum
Penlight Induction
Penlight Self Induction
Perfume Induction
Sip The Water Induction
Stick Induction
That's Delicious Induction
Ticking Watch Induction
Watch The Watch Induction

Chpt 18: Hypnotic Sleep, pg 75

Chpt 19: Somnambulism, Waking Induction, pg 79

Chpt 20: Waking Hypnosis, pg 83

Chpt 22: From Waking To Trance, pg 91

Chpt 23: Hypnotic Mood, pg 93

Chpt 24: Waking Convincers, pg 95
Anti-Gravity Body Lift Group Demonstration
Arm Rising Experiment
Eyelids Experiment
Falling Backward Experiment
Falling Forward Experiment
Fingertips Glued
Hands Locked
Hand On Your Head Test
Hands Stuck To A Stick Experiment
Making Yourself Light And Heavy
Memory Experiment
Sensory Effects
The Fist Lock

Chpt 25: Rapid Inductions, pg 103
Entering Waking Hypnosis
From Waking Hypnosis Into Profound Hypnosis

Chpt 26: More Rapid Inductions, pg 105
Bale's Finger Induction
Kerr's Cockroach On The Bar
McGill's Concentration/Relaxation Technique Version #1
McGill's Concentration/Relaxation Technique Version #2
McGill's Forehead Flick
Stockwell's 30 Second Zap

Chpt 29: I Can I Can't, pg 117
I Can't, I Can Pencil Drop 1
I Can't, I Can Pencil Drop 2

Chpt 30: Let's Pretend Some More, pg 121
Let's Pretend Candle Induction
Let's Pretend You're Not Pretending Induction

**Chpt 31:
Acting Out Hypnosis For The 'I Can't Be Hypnotized', pg 125**

Chpt 32: The Ideomotor Induction, pg 129

Chpt 33: Sandy Beach, pg 131

Chpt 34: Serenity Resonance Induction, pg 133

Chpt 35: Magnetic Mind Toning, pg 137

Chpt 36: Holistic Induction, pg 141

Chpt 37: Quotation Induction, pg 143

Chpt 38: Elman's Rapid Induction, pg 147
Elman's Handshake Induction
Fixation Tests
The Elman Two-Finger Hypnotic Induction
Two-Finger Induction For Anesthesia
Two-Finger Induction For Children

Chpt 39: You Are The Star, pg 153

Chpt 40: Bale's Inside Out, pg 157

Chpt 41: England's Rag Doll, pg 159

Chpt 42: Imagination Game Inductions, pg 163
Bucket of Water Induction
Flying Eagle Induction
Hypnotizing School Children
Puppet Induction
Telkemeyer's Slide Induction
The Penny Drop Induction
The Swing Induction
Thompson's Eye Of The President Induction

Chpt 43: Candy Induction, pg 171

Chpt 44: Blum's Singing Bowl Induction, pg 173

Chpt 45: Transpersonal Induction, pg 175

Chpt 46: Hypnodance Induction, pg 177

Chpt 47: Otto's Vertigo Induction, pg 179

Chpt 48: Whirling Dervish Induction, pg 181

Chpt 49: Instant Hypnosis, pg 185
Gamma Hypnosis En Masse
The Body Bump
The Evangelist Method
The Sudden Jerk

Chpt 50: Hindu Levitation, pg 189
Breezy Method
Go To Sweep Method
Head Of The Class
Head Of The Glass
Hum & Heavy
Look To Me For Hypnosis
Read Then Dead
Reflect on Relaxation
Take Your Toll
Three Finger Stroke Method
The AUM Induction
Up, Up And Away Method

Chpt 51: The Cobra Method, pg 193

Chpt 53:
Hypnotize Clients To Hypnotize Themselves, pg 207

Chpt 66: Super Learning Induction, pg 247

Chpt 91: Transcendental Induction, pg 315

Chpt 92: Computer Hypnotherapy, pg 319

Chpt 105: Stockwell's Indirect Induction, pg 367
Erickson's Environment Induction

Chpt 106: Yawn Induction, pg 375

Chpt 108: Heart-Mending Hypnosis, pg 383
Kate Ellis' NLP Heart Mending Theater
McGill's Trust Method

Chpt 114:
Coue''s Twilight "Good Knot" Autosuggestion, pg 417

Chpt 122: Quick Reflexology Induction Formula, pg 447

Chpt 126: Ancient Egyptian Induction, pg 467

Chpt 135: Electrical Induction, pg 507

Chpt 137: Bio Tuning And Sonic Induction, pg 511

Chpt 149: Mom's Teddy Bear, pg 567

Chpt 151:
Active Induction and ADD/ADHD Children, pg 579

Chpt 157: Induction And Deepening Techniques, pg 597
McGill's Crystal Ball Induction
McGill's Hand Above Head Induction

Chpt 158: Induction Of Trance For Volunteers, pg 607
Pretending Induction With A Crystal Ball Fixation

Chpt 165: Yoga Induction, pg 655
Yoga Massage Inductions

Chpt 180: Includes, pg 709
Write To Your Angel Induction

Chpt 183: Two Super Mind Inductions, pg 723
Deep Breathing Meditation Induction
Five Senses Super-Mind Induction

Chpt 185: Hypno-Meditation Induction, pg 733

Chpt 191: Essene Blue Sky Induction, pg 751
Essene Angels, Life, Light and Peace

Chpt 192:
Entering The Darkness Induction And Session, pg 757

Chpt 197: Out-of-Body Induction, pg 779

Chpt 198: Telepathy Scripts, pg 783

Chpt 199: Third Eye Opening Scripts, pg 785

Chpt 200: Trance Channeling Script, pg 787

Chpt 201: Be Psychic Scripts, pg 789

Chpt 203: BODHISATTVA Script, pg 801

Chpt 205: Chaotic Breathing, pg 807

Part I: Definition/Index, pg
Effleurage Induction
Tooge-Tooge Induction